OXFORD MEDICAL PUBLICATIONS

SOCIETY, STRESS, AND DISEASE

VOLUME 3

THE PRODUCTIVE AND REPRODUCTIVE AGE— MALE/FEMALE ROLES AND RELATIONSHIPS

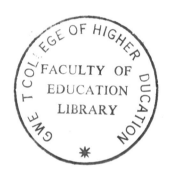

SOCIETY, STRESS,

The symposium on which this volume is based was sponsored jointly

by

THE UNIVERSITY OF UPPSALA

and

THE WORLD HEALTH ORGANIZATION

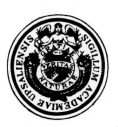 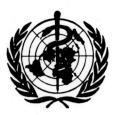

Oxford   OXFORD UNIVERSITY

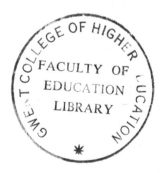

AND DISEASE

VOLUME 3

THE PRODUCTIVE AND REPRODUCTIVE AGE— MALE/FEMALE ROLES AND RELATIONSHIPS

Edited by LENNART LEVI, M.D.

*Director, Laboratory for Clinical Stress Research,
Karolinska Institute, Stockholm*

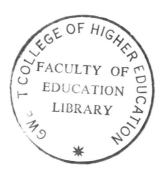
PRESS   *New York, Toronto 1978*

Oxford University Press, Walton Street, Oxford OX2 6DP

OXFORD LONDON GLASGOW NEW YORK
TORONTO MELBOURNE WELLINGTON CAPE TOWN
IBADAN NAIROBI DAR ES SALAAM LUSAKA ADDIS ABABA
KUALA LUMPUR SINGAPORE JAKARTA HONG KONG TOKYO
DELHI BOMBAY CALCUTTA MADRAS KARACHI

© *Oxford University Press 1978*

British Library Cataloguing in Publication Data

Society, stress and disease.
  Vol. 3: The productive and reproductive age.
  — (Oxford medical publications).
  1. Medicine, Psychosomatic — Congresses
  2. Stress (Physiology) — Congresses
  I. Levi, Lennart   II. Series
  616.08   RC49

  ISBN 0-19-261306-5

*The symposium on which this volume is based
was made possible through the generosity of
The Trygg-Hansa Insurance Group,
Stockholm*

*Printed in Great Britain
by William Clowes Ltd., London, Beccles, Colchester*

CONTENTS

SESSION 1

THE CONCEPT OF NORMALITY: MALE/FEMALE ROLES AND RELATIONSHIPS

SESSION 2

POTENTIALLY PATHOGENIC PSYCHOSOCIAL STIMULI ORIGINATING FROM MALE/FEMALE ROLES AND RELATIONSHIPS

SESSION 3

PSYCHIATRIC AND PSYCHOSOMATIC DISEASES POSSIBLY ASSOCIATED WITH MALE/FEMALE ROLES AND RELATIONSHIPS

SESSION 4

THE PREVENTION (PRIMARY AND SECONDARY) OF STRESS ORIGINATING FROM MALE/FEMALE RELATIONSHIPS

LIST OF CONTRIBUTORS

JOHN BANCROFT, M.D., M.R.C.P., D.P.M., M.R.C.Psych., First Assistant and Honorary Consultant, Unit of Reproductive Biology, 2 Forrest Rd, Edinburgh, Scotland.

BÖRJE CRONHOLM, M.D., Professor and Head, Department of Psychiatry, Karolinska Hospital, S-104 01 Stockholm 60, Sweden.

JOHAN CULLBERG, M.D., Associate Professor, Boo psykiatriska mottagning, Kommunalvägen 4. S-13200 Saltsjö-Boo, Sweden.

JOHN CULLEN, M.D., Director of Research, Department of Psychiatry, University College, Earlsfort Terrace, Dublin 2, Ireland.

LARS DAHLGREN, Ph.D., Managing Director, Trygg-Hansa Insurance Group, S-106 26 Stockholm, Sweden.

BENGT EDGREN, M.A., M.Sc., Senior Researcher, Laboratory for Clinical Stress Research (WHO Psychosocial Centre), Fack, S-104 01 Stockholm 60, Sweden.

ARNE ENGSTRÖM, M.D., Professor, Secretary, Swedish Science Advisory Council, Ministry of Education, Mynttorget 1, Stockholm, Sweden.

LARS ENGSTRÖM, M.D., Associate Professor, Department of Gynecology and Obstetrics, Löwenströmska Hospital, S-194 03 Upplands Väsby, Sweden.

WALTER D. FENZ, Ph.D., Professor, Department of Psychology, University of Waterloo, Ontario, Canada.

MARIANNE FRANKENHAEUSER, Ph.D., Professor and Head, Department of Psychology, University of Stockholm, Box 6706, S-113 85 Stockholm, Sweden.

JAN FRÖBERG, Ph.D., Ass. Director, Laboratory for Clinical Stress Research (WHO Psychosocial Centre), Fack, S-104 01 Stockholm 60, Sweden.

PAUL H. GEBHARD, B.S., M.A., Ph.D., Professor and Director, Institute for Sex Research, Indiana University, Morrison Hall 416, Bloomington, Indiana 47401, USA.

JAMES A. GOODMAN, B.A., MSW, Ph.D., Acting Director, Division of Special Mental Health Programs, National Institute of Mental Health, Room 12-105, Parklawn Building, 5600 Fishers Lane, Rockville, Maryland 20852, USA.

FERDINAND R. HASSLER, M.D., M.Sc., Associate Director for International Programs, National Institute of Mental Health, Parklawn Building, 5600 Fishers Lane, Rockville, Maryland 20852, USA.

JAMES P. HENRY, M.D., Professor, Department of Physiology, University of Southern California, 815 West 37th Street, Los Angeles, California 90007, USA.

PREBEN HERTOFT, M.D., Consultant Psychiatrist, University Clinic of Psychiatry (Rigshospitalet), Blegdamsvej 9, D-2100 Copenhagen, Denmark.

JOSEF HYNIE, M.D., D.Sc., Professor and Director, Sexuological Institute of Charles University, Karlovo nám. 32, Prague 2, Czechoslovakia.

AUBREY R. KAGAN, F.R.C.P., F.F.C.M., D.P.H., Professor, Laboratory for Clinical Stress Research (WHO Psychosocial Centre), Fack, S-104 01 Stockholm, Sweden.

CLAES-GÖRAN KARLSSON, M.Sc., Chief, Division of Biotechnology, Laboratory for Clinical Stress Research (WHO Psychosocial Centre), Fack, S-104 01 Stockholm 60, Sweden.

RICHARD S. LAZARUS, Ph.D., Professor, Department of Psychology, Tolman Hall, University of California, Berkeley, California 94720, USA.

LENNART LEVI, M.D., Director, Laboratory for Clinical Stress Research (WHO Psychosocial Centre), Fack, S-104 01 Stockholm 60, Sweden.

LARS LIDBERG, M.D., M.A., Professor and Head, Department of Forensic Psychiatry, Fack, S-10270 Stockholm, Sweden.

RITA LILJESTRÖM, Ph.D., Department of Sociology, University of Gothenburg, Karl Johansgatan 27 A-B, S-414 59 Gothenburg, Sweden.

BIRGITTA LINNÉR, LL.B., Svartmunkegränd 2A, SF-20100 Åbo, Finland.

MARGARET MEAD, B.A., M.A., Ph.D., Curator Emeritus of Ethnology, The American Museum of Natural History, 15 West 77th Street, New York, N.Y. 100 24, USA.

RICHARD P. MICHAEL, M.D., D.Sc., Ph.D., Department of Psychiatry, Emory University School of Medicine, Atlanta, Georgia 303 22, USA.

JOHN MONEY, Ph.D., Professor, Phipps 400, Johns Hopkins Hospital, Baltimore, Maryland 212 05, USA.

CAMILLA ODHNOFF, D.Sc., Associate Professor, formerly Cabinet Minister; Governor, Länsstyrelsen i Blekinge län, Box 59, S-371 01 Karlskrona, Sweden.

GORAN OLHAGEN, Ph.D., Chief, Division of Sociology, Laboratory for Clinical Stress Research (WHO Psychosocial Centre), Fack, S-104 01 Stockholm 60, Sweden.

HAROLD PERSKY, B.S., Ph.D., Professor, Department of Psychiatry, University of Pennsylvania, 465 Stouffer Building, Philadelphia, General Hospital, 34th and Civic Center Boulevard, Philadelphia, Pennsylvania 191 04, USA.

RICHARD H. RAHE, M.D., Director, Navy Medical Neuropsych. Research Unit, San Diego, California 92152, USA.

BROR REXED, M.D., Professor, Director-General of the Swedish National Board of Health and Welfare, S-106 30 Stockholm, Sweden.

NORMAN SARTORIUS, M.D., Director, Division of Mental Health, WHO, CH 1211 Geneva 27, Switzerland.

TORGNY SEGERSTEDT, Ph.D., Professor of Sociology, Rector Magnificus of Uppsala University, Box 256, S-751 05 Uppsala, Sweden.

MALCOLM TOTTIE, M.D., Senior Medical Officer, The Swedish Board of Health and Welfare, S-106 30 Stockholm, Sweden.

JAN TROST, Ph.D., Associate Professor, Department of Sociology, University of Uppsala, Drottninggatan 1, S-752 20 Uppsala, Sweden.

MARGARET VESTIN, B.A., Graduate from the Stockholm School of Social Studies, Head of Division at the Swedish Board of Education, Karlavägen 108, S-106 42 Stockholm, Sweden.

ALBERT ZAHRA, M.D., D.P.H., D.T.M. & H., Director, Family Health Division, WHO, CH-1211 Geneva 27, Switzerland.

PREFACE

In developing and developed countries rapid, fundamental social changes are taking place (e.g. in mating; breeding and rearing children; work relations and environment; and care of the old and sick). These changes are influenced by, and influence, phenomena such as population growth; urbanization; industrialization; environmental pollution; uneven distribution of resources; and the shortage of food, water, work, and housing for hundreds of millions of people. At the same time, increased communication is accompanied by increase in expectation. All this has strongly accentuated the effects — both beneficial and harmful — of psychosocial factors on health.

This has become increasingly recognized by the international medical community. In his report to the 29th World Health Assembly, the Director-General of the World Health Organization (WHO 1975) defined psychosocial factors as 'factors influencing health, health services and community wellbeing stemming from the psychology of the individual and the structure and function of social groups. They include social characteristics such as patterns of interaction within kinship or occupation groups; cultural characteristics such as traditional ways of solving conflict; and psychological characteristics such as attitudes, beliefs and personality factors.' He further points out that 'these factors are interdependent, and the way in which they affect the healthy development and functioning of individuals cannot be understood without considering the more global aspects of society — the organization and division of work, the institutions and structures forming the sociopolitical systems, the values, norms and codes regulating the behaviour of individuals and groups, and the cultural heritage'.

Closely related considerations constituted the background for a series of five international, interdisciplinary symposia on 'Society, Stress, and Disease'. The series started in 1970 and ended in 1976, covering the entire human life span, from birth to old age. It was jointly sponsored by the World Health Organization and the University of Uppsala, organized by the Laboratory for Clinical Stress Research (WHO Psychosocial Center) of the Karolinska Institute in Stockholm, and made possible through the generosity of the Trygg-Hansa Insurance Group.

The first symposium in this series aimed at a bird's-eye view of the entire area of man's psychosocial environment and his morbidity and mortality in psychosomatic diseases (Levi 1971). The second symposium focused on problems specific to the most formative years, namely childhood and adolescence (Levi 1975). The third symposium concerned itself with problems due to change in male/female roles and relationships, and the proceedings of this third symposium are now presented in an expanded and updated form.

The organizers have aimed to bring together researchers, practitioners, and decision-makers from many disciplines and parts of the world to discuss many aspects of male/female roles and relationships as psychosocial human stressors, and their possible influences on health and wellbeing. The participants were chosen to represent many different fields of knowledge and many different methods of scientific and practical approach. No attempts were made to reach any consensus of opinion. It is hoped, however, that this volume does present not only a selection, but also a meaningful *pattern*, of facts, theories, hypotheses, speculations, and value judgements concerning the various components of the 'psychosocial factors–stress–disease' system and their interrelationship, with particular reference to problems specific to male/female roles and relationships.

According to a Persian proverb 'one pound of learning requires ten pounds of common sense to apply it'. Although problems of application were extensively discussed and a number of proposals put forward, it will be up to the reader to provide the 'ten pounds' and to consider, in each specific case, the possibilities for application.

This book is intended to furnish a *'smörgåsbord'* of ideas and information. It is hoped that a wide variety of readers will be able to chose from it in accordance with their specific background and needs.

I would like to express my deep gratitude to the two sponsors of the symposia series and particularly to its President, Professor Torgny Segerstedt. I am further indebted to the publishers of the proceedings of the entire series, the Oxford University Press, for their helpfulness and cooperation.

The English in some of the chapters has been revised by Mr. Patrick Hort, M.A., whose help is gratefully acknowledged. Last but not least, I would like to express deep indebtedness to Dr. Aubrey R. Kagan and Mrs. Gun Nerje for their personal involvement and invaluable work in the organization of this symposium and in the compilation of the proceedings.

Laboratory for Clinical Stress Research,   LENNART LEVI
Fack,
S-10401 Stockholm, Sweden.

September 1977

REFERENCES

LEVI, L. (ed.) (1971). *Society, stress, and disease, Vol. 1: The psychosocial environment and psychosomatic diseases*. London.
LEVI, L. (ed.) (1975). *Society, stress, and disease, Vol. 2: Childhood and adolescence*. London.
WHO (1975). *Psychosocial factors and health*. Report of the Director-General, EB57/22.

ACKNOWLEDGEMENTS

John Money, who wrote Chapter 2, was supported in research by Grant No. 5-RDI-HD00325, USPHS, and by a grant from the Grant Foundation, Inc.

Grateful acknowledgement is made to the Foundations' Fund for Research in Psychiatry, the Grant Foundation, the National Institute of Mental Health (MH 19506), and the Georgia Department of Human Resources for providing support for the original work described in Chapter 4.

The study described in Chapter 6 was supported in part by grant number MH 21044 from the National Institute of Mental Health, U.S. Public Health Service. Dr. Persky is a recipient of Research Scientist Award number MH 18374 from the National Institute of Mental Health, U.S. Public Health Service.

Birgitta Linnér presented an earlier version of Chapter 19 at the 1971 annual meeting of the American Orthopsychiatric Association, Washington DC, and this was published in the *American Journal of Orthopsychiatry* (**41**).

Marianne Frankenhaeuser gratefully acknowledges financial support from the Swedish Medical Research Council (Project No. 997) and the Swedish Council for Social Science Research for the work described in Chapter 20.

The writing of Chapter 25 was facilitated by a grant from The Canada Council, and was prepared at the Laboratory for Clinical Stress Research, Karolinska Institute, Stockholm, Sweden. Barry R. Fogle contributed in the preparation of this manuscript as research assistant to Walter D. Fenz.

Chapter 26 first appeared as Report No. 72-34, and was supported by the Research and Development Command, Bureau of Medicine and Surgery, Department of the Navy, under Research Work Unit MF51.524.002-5011DD5G. Opinions expressed are those of the author and are not to be construed as reflecting the official view or having the endorsement of the Department of the Navy. Dr. Rahe expresses his gratitude to William M. Pugh, M.A., for his statistical assistance in the preparation of the chapter.

The research described in Chapter 27 was supported in part by NASA Grant NGL 05-018-003 and NIH Grant MH 19441.

Chapter 28 has also been published in *Acta psychiatrica et neurologica Scandinavica*.

John Cullen would like to thank sincerely his staff in the Department of Psychiatry and especially Dr. Austin Darragh, who is Director of the Psycho-Endocrine Unit, for their help with the case-material described in Chapter 29.

INTRODUCTION: INAUGURAL SPEECHES

A. ZAHRA

Madam Minister, Mr. Chairman, Ladies and Gentlemen: It gives me great pleasure, on behalf of Dr. Candau, the Director-General of the World Health Organization, to address this symposium and to wish the participants fruitful discussions.

Dr. Lambo, our Assistant Director-General, sends his apologies for not being able to inaugurate the proceedings today, owing to other engagements in Geneva.

The excellence of Swedish work in the field of psychosocial factors and disease is well-known, and this is manifested by the many distinguished participants in all or part of this conference, and, in particular, by the presence of Dr. Odhnoff, Minister for Family and Youth, Ministry of Social Affairs, at this session.

I wish to thank you, Professor Segerstedt, and you, Dr. Levi, and your colleagues, for the magnificent organization of this symposium, and to thank Trygg-Hansa, in the person of Mr. Dahlgren, for their generous support.

This series of symposia coincide with a crucial stage in the development of long-term health programmes in many countries in the world. In recent years the need for rational planning and evaluation of health services has gained in importance and has led to an increasing awareness of disease in its natural context, that of society as a whole. The focus of activities in the field of health is becoming broader, and disease control is no longer the one and only target of health efforts. In this ecological concept, disease is only one of the factors which must be studied, although an important one; others include social and economic conditions in countries, including national development plans, available manpower, and other resources. In this series of five symposia on society, stress, and disease this is the third, focusing on male/female relations and roles in the productive age.

The first of the series — on psychosomatic disease — was published by Oxford University Press in 1971. It justified many of the organizers' expectations; thus some of the notions discussed in it were found to be of value in structuring the second symposium — on childhood and adolescence — and will probably be of use in this and subsequent symposia. The first two symposia also demonstrated areas of similarity between workers in various disciplines that were previously hidden by differences in terminology. So we may say they have also served to break down barriers in communication.

These symposia have stimulated many ideas, much discussion, and concrete proposals for further research. Thus, some participants have been moved to write post-conference papers. Many have had ideas for new research, and some have already commenced joint research studies that were inspired during previous meetings. We in WHO have been stimulated and guided by them in our thinking on WHO's role in the studies of psychosocial factors in prevention of disease and promotion of health.

WHO activities in this field have included important collaboration with countries in the development of their plans for health, especially in the area of family health with emphasis on maternal and child health and mental health aspects. We are also working closely with other UN agencies in collaborative programmes: for example with UNESCO, on the changing role of women in society; with the United Nations Development Programme, in overall development of country resources; with the United Nations Fund for Population Activities in programmes relating to population; and with the United Nations Social Defence Research Institute in such areas as mental health aspects of crime and juvenile delinquency; we are also participating actively in preparations for the United Nations Conference on the Human Environment in Stockholm which will discuss both the physical and psychosocial environment.

This symposium comes at a time when dramatic, rapid change is taking place in developed and developing countries in fundamental social relationships in sexual relations, reproduction, child-rearing and male and female roles at home and at work. Already, there is evidence that while some of these changes may be necessary and some are beneficial, they have also harmful aspects.

I hope that, by reviewing existing knowledge and exchanging ideas, you will be able to suggest areas for health action and areas for research to support action designed to optimize the benefits of change and minimize the harm. In this way the Conference may help to develop a strategy for dealing more efficiently with disease in all its aspects, particularly the crucial one of the interrelationship between disease and the society in which it occurs.

The rich resources in participants, the balance of disciplines represented here, the quality of the pre-conference papers and the ability of the organizers, all give the assurance that contacts between experts in health and experts in other disciplines will be strengthened by this meeting. I am sure, too, that you will find these deliberations interesting and rewarding, and wish you all success.

CAMILLA ODHNOFF

Ladies and gentlemen: On behalf of the Swedish Government I have the pleasure to wish all of you welcome to this country.

In your series of international symposia on society, stress, and disease, you are now to discuss the productive and reproductive age — male and female roles and relationships. Already the title as I understand it reflects a radical attitude promising a constructive outcome of your discussions. It is clear that we all have productive as well as reproductive ages, men and women, and that we have to plan our private lives as well as our society to fit into a way of living where family and parenthood are natural and essential features as well as studies, work, and participation in public life.

Equal roles and equal responsibilities has been the generally accepted sex role ideology in the constructive and progressive debate in Sweden during the last 10 years. This ideology was also expressed in the Swedish government report to the United Nations in 1968 on the status of women. There it was stated, among other things: 'A decisive and ultimately durable improvement in the status of women cannot be attained by special measures aimed at women alone; it is equally necessary to abolish the conditions which tend to assign certain privileges, obligations, or rights to men. No decisive change in the distribution of functions and status as between the sexes can be achieved if the duties of the male in society are assumed *a priori* to be unaltered.'

The division of functions as between the sexes must be changed in such a way that both the man and the woman in a family are afforded the same practical opportunities of participating in both active parenthood and gainful employment. This aim can be realized only if the man is also educated and encouraged to take an active part in parenthood and is given the same rights and duties as the woman in his parental capacity.

In Sweden we have a fairly open approach to sex questions, a relatively unprejudiced attitude towards unmarried mothers, and a comparative rarity of the so-called 'double standard' may have created an impression that equality exists. It is true that women and men have largely the same legal rights and that all education, except military, is open to both sexes. Therefore it seems that we have achieved equality between the sexes, and consequently, we should have very little psychosocial dysfunction arising from sex roles or the relationships connected therewith. However, if we define equality between men and women in terms of equal influence and power, an equal position on the labour market, equal responsibility for home and children, equal pay, we must admit that in Sweden we have a long way to go and we do not compare very well even with many other industrialized countries: and that, with our various social policy measures, we have made only a relatively small advance towards a real freedom for both men and women to combine their roles at work, in the family and in society.

Many suburbs of the big cities are as little prepared for equal roles as the family itself may be. They seem to be planned from the economical aspect of two incomes per family, but function only if one of the parents stays at home.

At least a superficial equality characterizes the life of boys and girls up through school and vocational training. At marriage both are usually employed or studying. But it is when these 'equal' youngsters marry that their differences show up. Odds are high that they embody fundamentally different expectations. The one has right from the cradle been expected to be self-reliant, career-minded, to attain a status in society, the other to be soft and dependant, with only her husband's career in mind and the attainment of the status of the good mother of a flourishing family. The overwhelming evidence of television, films, magazines, and daily life is simple and clear. The unequal distribution of duties in the household will be a shock for the girl, especially one who up till then has had the same education, same job, and same pay. Another shock may be the gap between dream and reality as regards the role of the housewife. On the surface she is praised as the good wife, the source of family happiness, but within themselves many housewives feel that, in fact, they function more as the family door mat and dustbin. I saw a German investigation on matrimony as seen from the male and female angle. The great majority of men considered marriage, kitchen, and nursery to be the highlights of happiness for the women and a great satisfaction to themselves. While 92 per cent of the men claimed that their marriage was happy, only 19 per cent of the women joined this song of praise — the rest of them complained bitterly.

The question of sex roles is merely a part of the apparently confused pattern of modern society. The pattern is a mixture of will, reality, need, and resources. A gap between old and new is found in all areas. Therefore, we must find the least common denominator in order to push the pace of development and eliminate the obstacles that rise in our way. To neutralize the negative consequences of, for instance, sex-role prejudices is one such denominator.

René Dubos, microbiologist at the Rockefeller University in New York, says in his book *So human an animal*:

History confirms present-day observations in demonstrating that man can become adjusted, socially and biologically, to ways of life and environments that have hardly anything in common with those in which civilization emerged and evolved. He can survive, multiply, and create material wealth in an over-crowded, monotonous, and completely polluted environment, provided he surrenders his individual rights, accepts certain forms of physical degradation, and does not mind emotional atrophy.

What we strive for is a society of variation and integration. In social planning we must go out with an active strategy to create a society in which people can function on a basis of co-operation and mutual help, in which every individual is given the chance for personal development in contact and companionship with his fellow human beings, men and women, young and old.

In this connection I am naturally looking towards the younger generation. They are going to build the new society and we must clear the way for them. Children and their living environment must therefore be given priority. For their benefit we must take prophylactic measures and at the same time try to repair the damage done to the older generation. Public planning must also take both men and women into account. If people are to function well the planning of work-places, dwellings, and service facilities must be co-ordinated.

You are all of you distinguished experts. Mass media will listen to you with respect and consideration. You will be quoted as unprejudiced speakers of the truth. You know best yourselves that the truth looks different depending upon from which angle you regard it. Your expert resolutions are conditioned by the goals you set.

Technical obstacles and economical strain are hard to overcome. To solve such difficulties may become a goal in itself. But when you look deeper into these questions you will find that human needs are essential, and no solution on human problems, however elegant, will be successful if man is not its objective. Most societies may be good for the strong ones; and only a strong society may be good also for the weak ones, the old people, the handicapped, the children. To attain this, society needs the active participation of both men and women.

TORGNY SEGERSTEDT

Ladies and gentlemen: This is the third time I have had the honour of extending a hearty welcome to members of our stress symposia. I should especially like to thank you, Mrs. Minister, for the great personal interest that you have shown these symposia. We know that at this time of the year you are extremely busy, and we do really appreciate that you are taking such an active part in this gathering.

This time too it has been possible to bring together an outstanding group of experts. Some of them are old friends of these symposia: they are, if I may use the expression, 'regular customers', and that will guarantee a necessary continuity in our approach.

We are fully aware that the symposia would never have been possible without the support and authority of WHO, and I would for that reason like to thank the representatives of that important world organization for all the help they have given the organizers of this meeting.

I believe that one reason that these symposia attract so much interest is the fact that the subjects chosen are on the borderline of many different academic fields of research. I suppose the concept of 'stress' makes it necessary to treat stress problems in an interdisciplinary way. There must be a dialogue between scholars from different biological fields, as well as social scientists.

As we are mainly treating the problem of change, the development must be analysed in a historic perspective. I do not know whether our generation has experienced change as more painful than have earlier generations. In any case it is evident that the rapid change is creating a feeling of uncertainty and unrest. We do not quite know our social roles, particularly with regard to our female and male roles and relationships and our roles as parents. It is quite evident that such a subject can be treated only by experts from various fields in co-operation.

I think the honour of having brought all these people together is Dr. Lennart Levi's. He is well worth our admiration for his enthusiasm and his effective way in which he has been handling all the administrative problems of this conference. I should like to thank him very much for all he has done.

Once more, I should like to thank you for coming here and to express my hope that this symposium will be as successful as the two others. *Hjärtligt välkommen!* And so I declare this symposium open.

LARS DAHLGREN

Madam Cabinet Minister, Representatives of the World Health Organization, Mr. President, ladies and gentlemen scientists representing many disciplines and many parts of the world: On behalf of the Trygg-Hansa Insurance Group I wish to express a warm and hearty welcome to Stockholm and this week of symposium work and 'friendly co-existence', a welcome to number three of a series of five international symposia dealing with questions fundamental to the continued existence of civilization and social life, and maybe even to the survival of our species. It is a pleasure to meet again several friends from the first two symposia and to get an opportunity to make new friends.

Our enterprise, the Trygg-Hansa Insurance Group, has a strong and traditional interest in socially oriented activities with a natural connection to the insurance field — that is to say activities aiming at the prevention of damages to man or property or the repair and rehabilitation after damages. In that state of mind we support — financially or by organization — basic research and practical activities considering traffic security and traffic medicine, physical training and physiology, life-saving, ethics, and questions of human environment like stress. Our function should not be restricted to mere bookkeeping of premium income and various damage costs, but naturally comprises a responsibility for a broader field of human welfare.

Our group administers 27 per cent of the Swedish insurance market — more than 3 million of insurance policies, about equally divided among insurance for man's life and man's property. Our role in the market makes it possible and natural for us to engage in research activities related to damage prevention or rehabilitation for man and property, where relatively limited 'pilot contributions' at strategic points sometimes can prove to be of a great value.

The pattern of life has a deep impact on man's harmony and happiness, and thereby upon society. Destructive impacts are frequent in the societies of today: malnutrition; pollution; defective adaptation to quick changes in technical or social conditions; urbanization; and the overcrowding, anonymity, and criminality of big cities. We in the insurance sector of society are, in our daily work, made only all too well aware of the rapidly growing economic effects of these factors.

Finally — based upon our good experiences from the first two symposia in this series — I will express from us in the Trygg-Hansa group wishes for an interesting and productive symposium week — a week of international and interdisciplinary cross-fertilization and thereby of contributions to science and, indirectly, to the practical politics of our societies!

SESSION 1

The concept of normality: male/female roles and relationships

1. BACKGROUND, OBJECTIVES, DEFINITIONS, AND PROBLEMS

AUBREY KAGAN

THE THEME OF THE SYMPOSIA

The underlying premises of the series of symposia on 'Society, stress, and disease', from which this series of books originated, are that:

(1) stimuli arising from changing psychosocial situations may promote health or cause disease;

(2) if such situations are adapted to the organism's needs or the organism can adapt to the situation, health ensues; if not, disease results;

(3) when changes are slow, e.g. over periods of 100 000 years or so, natural selection and survival of the fittest is nature's method of adaptation;

(4) our innate characteristics must still carry the lessons of our formative aeons up to a few thousand years ago;

(5) when changes in the organism are faster (over periods of two or three generations), the process of adaptation depends much on man-made efforts. The time-honoured method of dealing with this is to see trouble coming — or, more usually, after it has come — and to make corrections. This has sometimes been described as 'planning from crisis to crisis'.

(6) changes are so fast and so extensive that ill-effects might occur on too large a scale with too little warning to be able to make a rational correction in time. (This is the prospect of people in developing and developed countries today. Environmental change — physical and psychical — is frequent, extensive, often incomplete, and, when planned, its significance is, at best, only partly known.);

(7) the rate of change is probably still increasing;

(8) since these changes are man-made, we can, in theory, reduce risk by: trying to slow the tempo; obtaining a better understanding of the effects; and introducing rational control of environmental change.

The purpose of this series of books is thus to consider how psychosocial stimuli cause or prevent disease, what health actions can be recommended on the basis of present knowledge, and to decide on priorities for increasing our knowledge.

The purpose of this Volume is to consider all this in relation to psychosocial stimuli arising from relations between men and women.

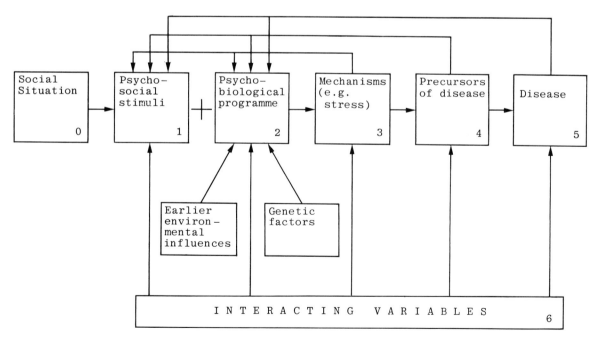

FIG. 1.1.   The relationship of stimuli arising from psychosocial factors (from Kagan and Levi 1974).

3

DEFINITIONS
(see Kagan and Levi 1974)

Figure 1.1 shows diagrammatically our concept of the relation of stimuli arising from psychosocial factors (first box on the left) to disease (last box on the right).

Psychosocial stimuli
'These are stimuli, suspected of being able to cause disease, which originate in social relationships or arrangements (i.e. in the environment) and affect the organism through the medium of higher nervous processes.'

Psychobiological programme
'A propensity to react in accordance with a certain pattern, e.g. when solving a problem, or adapting to an environment. Determinants of this programme in an organism are genetic factors, and earlier environmental influences.'

Mechanisms
'These are physiological reactions in the organism, induced by psychosocial stimuli, which, under some conditions of intensity, frequency or duration, and in the presence or absence of certain, interacting variables, will lead to disease.'

Precursors of disease
'These are malfunctions in mental or physical systems which have not resulted in disability but, if continued, will do so.'

Disease
'Disease is disability, caused by mental or somatic malfunction. Disability is failure in performance of a task. This must always include tasks considered essential, might include tasks considered normal, and, when more is known, will include tasks that are considered optimal. In applying this, it is necessary to state the level of the biological hierarchy to which it refers. Disease, as defined, is different at the cell, organ, organism, family, community level.' In this book, we will be concerned mostly with the individual, family, and community.

Interacting variables
'These are intrinsic or extrinsic factors, mental or physical, which alter the action of causative factors at the mechanism, precursor or disease stage. By "alter" I mean they promote or prevent processes that might lead to disease.'

The concept of the relationship between factors defined above, as shown in Fig. 1.1, is that stimuli arising from social situations, acting through the higher nervous processes in individuals or groups with a particular type of psychobiological programme, cause physiological changes which produce or prevent precursors of disease, or disease. Interacting variables, by modifying the stimuli or mechanisms, may enhance or reduce the precursor or disease-forming tendency.

Interacting variables may act on the precursors to prevent or enhance disease and may act on the disease processes to reduce or enhance it.

This concept is general. Below, I will try to specify characteristics in the various boxes in Fig. 1.1, to adapt it to the subject of this book.

CONCEPTS APPLIED TO MALE/FEMALE ROLES AND RELATIONSHIPS

This book is concerned with psychosocial stimuli arising from male/female encounters thought to affect health. This does not mean that we are concerned exclusively with mating, copulating, and pre- or post-copulatory activities. These are undoubtedly an important source of psychosocial stimuli from male/female relationships, but there are others of importance, e.g., in work, in play, and in the family. The book is not concerned with stimuli arising from similar male/male or female/female encounters, e.g., masturbation, homosexuality, lesbianism, and bestiality, except where these subjects are regarded as diseases arising from psychosocial stimuli which are the result of male/female encounters.

The psychobiological programme
This differs in each person, and within each person changes with environmental change. Nevertheless, it would be reasonable to suppose that a large part of the innate programme, being inherited from common ancestors or ancestors adapting to similar environmental hazards, is likely to be common to the whole of mankind. This is particularly likely to be true for sex roles and relationships because they are likely to have played an important part in survival. By identifying the common heritage, we may be able to draw speculative but useful conclusions about the social conditions to which man is adapted and from this hypothesize the conditions under which he is likely to be adapted.

'Sexuality' and 'pair bonding'. Anatomically, the human species is well designed for sexual activity. Distinctive features are:

(1) the extensive erogenous zones in male and female, e.g., everted lips, sensitive nose and ear lobes, relatively hairless skin;
(2) sensitive buttocks in the male and female and breasts in the female;
(3) relatively large penis and clitoris;
(4) anatomical propensity to face-to-face copulation.

The distinguishing physiological features are that:

(1) intercourse is relatively prolonged and frequent;
(2) the female often has an orgasm;
(3) there is virtually no closed season to copulation;
(4) face-to-face copulation is common.

4

A distinctive social pattern is not so clear-cut. This may be because it is more difficult to study and also because it is affected by culture. Nevertheless, it does seem likely that there is a prevailing, but by no means unique form of behaviour, characterized by:

(1) a tendency to a prolonged trial period with one or more successive persons to form a pair bond;
(2) a tendency to a prolonged pre-copulatory phase;
(3) a tendency to form a long-standing pair bond for mutual care and child-raising.

Celibacy, polyandry and polygamy, and communal intercourse and child-rearing occur, but are relatively uncommon.

The result of man's unique anatomical, physiological. and social factors could be to strengthen the pair bond by intense sexuality. Thus, even in the more 'permissive' or 'polygamous' societies, there is a tendency to form pair bonds for mutual care and child-rearing. Nevertheless, such is the intensity of sexuality that even in the least permissive societies there is a tendency for sexual intercourse to pass the bounds of the pair bond.

These strong tendencies could have been of survival value in the hunter/food-gathering tribe era. High sexuality contributes to reproduction and strong pair bonding, which itself, makes possible prolonged child-rearing, so necessary for the human young. But prolonged child-rearing could also have been provided by communal care. An argument sometimes used in favour of pair bonding is that it would support co-operation amongst the males whilst hunting. The latter was undoubtedly a *sine qua non* for survival, but I would have thought that it would have been supported as much by communal mating. However, for the latter to be effective, it would have had to be complete. Loss of a junior hunter's rights to mate in favour of a senior member would be likely to cause trouble. Pair bonding can to some extent tolerate promiscuity and *'les droits de Seigneur'*.

'Pair bonding' and susceptibility to disease. This is particularly important because there is some suspicion that, in modern societies, those that are pair bonded have an advantage over the non-pair bonded with regard to health. The alternative interpretations of this kind of data — that unhealthy people find it difficult to achieve or maintain a pair bond — is equally of interest if, as is often the case, this affects family-raising and genetic survival.

Susceptibility to disease and early distribution of labour. It is very likely that some roles within the hunter tribe were sex-related at an early stage, and remained so throughout the long era.

The hunter had to range afar and this must have been essentially a man's role. The women would, most of the time, be unable to take part in the hunt because of pregnancy, or the need to look after small children. Their role would therefore be the care of the young children, maintenance of the cave, and food-gathering from nearby.

The male role as the main provider probably did not change till the advent of farming, probably as little as 20 000 years ago. From then until present times, women have shared the function of providing for the family, although their ability to do so has been limited to a considerable extent by their productive and child-care functions. It is only in very recent times that this limitation has been substantially reduced.

One of the important consequences of the 'stay-at-home' role of women is the female role in caring for the sick and injured. Sickness in the male adult in the hunter tribe was probably largely due to trauma, with a smaller contribution from parasites and infections. In the women, susceptibility to disease would have been increased by frequent pregnancy and child-bearing and prolonged breast-feeding. Apart from trauma, the men would probably have had less sickness than women. It may be that, as a result of this, survival depended upon the development of a more disease-resistant woman, and it does seem that in general females are now more resistant than males to death, from the embryo stage onwards (see Chapter 21, pp. 143-8).

Male dominance and status. In today's society, however egalitarian, there is a tendency for the male to be dominant and to be given higher status than the female. In so far as this depends upon aggression, the male has a natural advantage in that his endocrine secretions encourage aggressiveness from an early age (in historical times, it has been shown that castrated males made very good subordinate servants).

Male dominance and status is seen in present-day arboreal primates. Whether it existed in prehistoric hunter tribes is unknown. It is very likely that the leader of the tribe was the wisest hunter, and therefore a male. The male role as the provider, and the female role of giving care may have strengthened the tendency for the female to be regarded as subservient to the male.

Limitations of this approach. The above approach to identifying a part of the psychobiological programme common to the majority of mankind is naïve and speculative, and has many weaknesses. Although the anatomical data are strong, the physiological data have some weaknesses, and the socio-behavioural data are unsupported by studies of representative samples. The best studies on sexuality are of quite unrepresentative samples of North Americans. A relation between the factors identified and survival is entirely speculative. Even if they are related to survival, and have become part of our innate make-up, it does not follow that all interference would always be harmful. And if interference is harmful, it does not follow that it will be equally harmful in all communities and all individuals in all communities. Group and individual variation has to be taken into account.

Conclusion. My conclusion is that factors such as
  (1) high sexuality,
  (2) pair bonding, and
  (3) male dominance
might be an important part of the present-day psycho-biological programme in man. Further evidence should be sought if social change is likely to affect these factors on a large scale. In particular, evidence should be sought to determine whether such changes are likely to result in benefit or harm. In doing so, it will be necessary to take into account communal and individual variation of the psychobiological programme.

Social situations and psychological stimuli that may arise

Some *social situations* that may interact with 'high sexuality', 'pair bonding', and 'male dominance' are attitudes towards and facilities for:

  (1) male/female sexual intercourse;
  (2) child-rearing;
  (3) mutual care;
  (4) male/female home roles;
  (5) male/female community roles (e.g. at work).

In theory, a situation is likely to be harmful if it cannot be adapted to, or if it calls too frequently for adaptation. This is irrespective of whether the emotions it arouses are pleasant or unpleasant.

Psychological stimuli that may arise include deprivation, excess, or threat to:

physiological needs or safety of the individual, family, or community;
sense of belonging;
self-esteem and status;
sense of purpose and self-realization.

Threat must be perceived, but need not be real. Degree of psychological stimulus would be expected to depend to a large extent on the difference between expectation and the situation as perceived.

The stimulus is likely to be enhanced or prolonged when there are no guidelines or rules to decision or correct action. This is particularly likely to occur when the situation is new, when the rules are changing, when they appear irrational, or when there is no accepted leadership.

Mechanisms

A number of processes are suspected of being mechanisms whereby psychosocial stimuli cause disease, e.g. mental, endocrine, immuno-reactive, and social. Relatively little is known about them. Most is known about hypothalamo-adrenomedullary and hypophyseal/adrenocortical reactions. They are characterized by increased catecholamine and 17-OH-corticosteroid secretion respectively, and are often assessed by measurement of these substances in the urine. These reactions, which involve other endocrine secretions and other systems, are often referred to as 'Selye stress' and occur with most, perhaps all forms of stimulation, whether they are physical or psychical, pleasant or

unpleasant. Their relation to a wide variety of precursors of disease, e.g. anxiety, raised blood-pressure platelet aggregation, attenuated immune response, has been demonstrated in man and animals.

These secretion reactions parallel 'arousal', are a useful preparation for adaptation to the needs of fight or flight, and are phylogenetically ancient. Whether psychosocial stimuli cause disease by such mechanisms is not known. Possibilities are:

  (1) that they are the common pathway by which stimuli cause disease;
  (2) that disease occurs only if the reaction is prolonged or frequent;
  (3) that disease occurs only if the normal response to the reaction — fight or flight — is not allowed to follow;
  (4) that the reaction is not a disease mechanism at all, but is an index of response to stimulus.

It is clear that conclusive evidence is needed.

Change and concern for the future

Is there reason for concern? Precursors, diseases, and interacting variables that may result from social changes in the five social situations acting on important aspects of the psychobiological programme are considered in Chapter 21. Here we may make some speculative associations.

Attitudes towards and arrangements for all the social situations are in a state of flux. For example, permissiveness towards premarital and extramarital sexual intercourse has developed very rapidly (*pari passu* with permissiveness to many other kinds of social arrangements) in the Western world. This may have advantages for some people in some ways, but it is not clear what these advantages are. Furthermore, we have seen severe disadvantages already in the form of venereal disease, unwanted pregnancy and its associated problems, and interpersonal conflict. There are probably preventable, but either because we are not yet permissive enough, or for other reasons, we have not yet found a practical approach. Further, there may well be other unsuspected risks of advantages that permissiveness encourages.

Attitudes to and arrangements for child-rearing are also undergoing change in developed and developing countries. But we know little of the benefits and risks of different forms of child-rearing. What kind of care gives an infant the best chance of development, hopefully better than the traditional form, and is compatible with further emancipation of women and of human well-being in general? The same can be said for changes in social situations relating to mutual care, other domestic roles of men and women, and their roles at work. In short, for each one of these social situations undergoing change, sometimes haphazard and sometimes deliberate, we are unable to say what is beneficial and what is harmful, and for whom.

But each of the social situations are interrelated. It is very likely that change in child-rearing arrangements will make desirable, make possible, or bring about changes in mutual care, other domestic roles, and work roles, and so on for other combinations of social situations. It is possible that change in male/ female roles will bring about changes in expectation from sexual arrangements. It would not be surprising if complete permissiveness in sexual relations, freed from risk of ill-health and freed from obligations relating to child-rearing, would bring about voluntary restrictions and different expectations.

Great changes are taking place in all these areas and will continue to do so as far as we can see. They may have most important effects, for good or evil, on our health and well-being. Yet our understanding of what is going on is very nearly nil.

Future action
We must cut through the cloudy wrappings of emotion in which our speculations are wrapped, identify hypotheses worthy of test, and find ways of testing them.

I think that this book will bring together a number of hypotheses and suggestions for health action. I hope we do not prevaricate by suggesting ways of looking for further *supporting* evidence for hypotheses, nor evangelically clamour for health action of *unproven* value.

If we are to progress as rapidly as possible, we should set up ways of *testing* our hypotheses and *evaluating* proposed health actions. Some ways in which this may be done are mentioned in Chapter 30.

SUMMARY

Rapid social change is a characteristic of life today in developed and developing countries. This calls for adaptation, and when demand is too frequent, too intense, meets with the wrong response, or cannot be met, disease is likely to occur. On the other hand, many social changes are beneficial.

When such changes took place slowly, nature's slow but cruel method of natural selection was adequate. But in the last 200 years or so change has been quicker in industrialized communities, and adaptation has been through rational social measures, usually taken after disaster had signalled the need — planning from crisis to crisis.

In the last 30 years, in developed and developing countries, change has taken place even faster, and our fear is that it will be too fast and too extensive to allow rational preventive measures to be determined. Our problem is to understand effects of social change so as to optimize benefits and decrease risks of harm.

A model is discussed, and the parts defined, of the concept (Fig. 1.1) of how social situations can give rise to psychological stimuli which, according to the individual or group's psychobiological programme may give rise to physiological changes (mechanisms) that may lead to precursors of disease or disease.

I postulate — by relating anatomical, physiological, and cultural characteristics of man of today, in general, to possible survival value during the aeons when their genetic characteristics were being formed — that important aspects of their psychobiological programme are:

(1) high sexuality;
(2) strong tendency to pair bonding; and
(3) male dominance.

REFERENCES

KAGAN, A. R. and LEVI, L. (1974). Health and environment — psychosocial stimuli: a review. *Soc. Sci. Med.,* **8**, 225–41.

2. DETERMINANTS OF HUMAN SEXUAL BEHAVIOUR

JOHN MONEY

PRINCIPLE OF DIFFERENTIATION AND DEVELOPMENT

Sexual behaviour in man, like the sexual anatomy itself, is by reason of man's place in the phyletic scale, dimorphic. That is to say, its growth from its inception onward is simultaneously a process of differentiation as well as of development. This fact tends to have been overlooked historically in psychiatry and psychology, which have spoken mainly of psychosexual development. Sexual theory has been impoverished thereby.

Reduced to its barest essentials, traditional sexual theory in psychiatry and psychology is built on two constructs: libido and identification. Libido, the instinctual sexual force, has not been conceived of as sexually dimorphic *per se*, though possibly as bisexual. Manifest difference in behaviour between the sexes has been regarded conceptually as secondary to libido and mainly as the developmental product of identification: to somewhat over-simplify, little girls identify with their mothers, little boys with their fathers. It is possible, though by no means justified, to account for identification exclusively in terms of stimulus/response and reward/reinforcement theory. Thus, there has grown up a strong current tradition of explaining differences in behaviour between the sexes — or deviations therefrom — as social environment or cultural in origin.

A theory in which the totality of dimorphism in sexual behaviour is attributed exclusively to postnatal social and cultural determinants is, *a priori*, open to the charge of being too narrow and simple. Moreover, notwithstanding the cogent evidence of the power of postnatal events in shaping gender identity and gender role† in human beings, one would be hard-pressed to defend an exclusively cultural theory against the newly accumulating evidence of animal sexology on the foetal influence of hormones on the governance of sexual behaviour by way of the central nervous system.

2. PRINCIPLES OF SEQUENTIAL DIFFERENTIATION

The antecedents of sexual dimorphism in human development are typically sequential (Fig. 2.1), beginning with the genetic dimorphism of the sex chromosomes, XY for the male and XX for the female. Then follows the differentiation of the gonads and their differentiated foetal hormonal functioning, differentiation of the internal reproductive anatomy, differentiation of the external genital morphology, differentiation of hypothalamic and associated brain regulatory pathways, differential sex assignment at birth, differential rearing as a boy or girl, differentiation of a gender role and

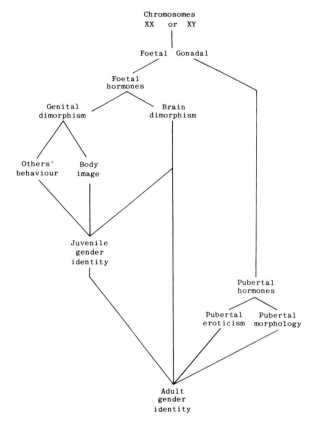

FIG. 2.1. Schematic and sequential relationship of the components of dimorphism in gender identity differentiation.

identity, differentiation of hormonal puberty, and differential response of falling in love, courtship, mating, and parenthood.

CRITICAL-PERIOD PRINCIPLE

Differentiation of the embryonic gonads is normally governed by the sex chromosomes, but only if the genetic code written into the chromosomes is permitted to express itself normally (the genetic norm of reaction)

†*Gender role* is defined as everything that a person says and does to indicate to others or to the self the degree that one is male or female or ambivalent; it includes but is not restricted to sexual arousal and response. Gender role is the public expression of gender identity, and gender identity is the private experience of gender role.

Gender identity is defined as the sameness, unity, and persistence of one's individuality as male or female or ambivalent, in greater or lesser degree, especially as it is experienced in self-awareness and behaviour, gender identity is the private experience of gender role, and gender role is the public expression of gender identity.

8

without interference or disruption at a critical period from an environment liable to produce distortions. The most dramatic distortion of the genetic code of the sex chromosomes is one in which their role as sex determinants is completely reversed. Yamamoto (1962) was able to bring about such a complete reversal in the killifish, *Orizeas latipes*, by exposing larvae to sex hormone. Exposed to oestrogen, the female sex hormone, an XY larva destined to have differentiated into a male, thereupon differentiated into a female. Amazingly enough, this XY female was able to breed with a normal XY male and produce young. Twenty-five per cent of the second generation larvae were then chromosomally XX (female), 50 per cent XY (male), and 25 per cent YY, which, if left untreated, would differentiate as males, but if treated with oestrogen, would become YY females. In the succeeding generation, it was then possible to breed YY females with YY males, the resultant progeny all being YY and differentiating as males, if left unexposed to experimental hormonal treatment. Yamamoto was also able to produce XX males by treating XX eggs with male sex hormone. The strongly and competitively masculine mating behaviour of YY males has been studied by Hamilton *et al*. (1969).

Yamamoto's experiment is not the first in which the germ cells have been reversed to produce ova instead of sperms, or vice versa, while still retaining their reproductive fertility. Many years ago, Witschi demonstrated that over-ripe toad eggs all developed as morphologic males. Not only the genetic males, but also the genetic females had the appearance of males and produced sperms, but without the male sex chromosome present in any of the sperms from the genetic females (Witschi 1956, 1965). Witschi and his co-workers (Chang and Witschi 1955, 1956; Mikamo and Witschi 1963) also succeeded in producing a similar reversal of genetic sex in toads by implanting sex hormones into the developing larvae. In 1964, Turner and Asakawa made a first step toward achieving the same result in a mammal by transplanting the gonads of foetal mice into a host animal, so that the foetal testis turned the foetal ovary into an ovotestis in which spermatogenesis progressed to the point of secondary spermatocytes. Burns (1961) had in 1956 used oestradiol in the foetal opossum to convert a would-be testis into an ovotestis producing ovocytes.

It has not yet been reported experimentally possible to reverse the sex differentiation completely from that of the genetic sex of the fertilized egg in mammals. Nonetheless the fish and amphibian experiments demonstrate how profound can be the reversal of everything pertaining to genetic sex: morphology, behaviour, and fertility. These experiments require that one keep an open mind with regard to possible partial reversals of the expression of genetic sex in human beings, perhaps of direct relevance to sexual psychopathology, from causes as yet unknown.

The fish and amphibian experiments also point out a profoundly important principle in the theory of heredity versus environment (perhaps more approriately designated as genetics versus environmentics). It is a principle that transcends the old dichotomy between nature and nurture by introducing the concept of the critical period. There is only a limited period during which a fertilized egg may be tampered with and forced to reserve the program for which it is genetically coded. After this limited, or critical period, the die is cast and the programe cannot be changed or, having been changed, cannot revert.

The die is cast regarding the differentiation of the gonads in the human species at around the sixth week after conception. In the XY embryo, the core of the undifferentiated gonad proliferates to form into a testis, and the rind becomes vestigal; whereas in the XX embryo at around the twelfth week the rind proliferates, while the core becomes vestigal, to form an ovary.

PRINCIPLES OF DIFFERENTIATION: VESTIGIATION V. HOMOLOGUES

The principle of commencing with the anlagen for both sexes, then allowing one to proliferate while the other vestigiates, is one which nature extends from the differentiation of the internal reproductive structures from the Müllerian and Wolffian ducts, both of which are initially laid down in parallel. Here another principle first becomes evident, namely this: for the differentiation of a male, something extra must occur — something must be added. In the total absence of gonads, whether by experimental castration of the foetus *in utero*, or by reason of a cytogenetic defect as in Turner's syndrome (typically 44 + XO = 45 chromosomes), the foetus will develop as a female. There is no doubt that nature's first disposition is to make a female. Morphologically, for a female to be differentiated it is not necessary to have foetal gonads able to release hormonal substances; whereas for the differentiation of a male, it is absolutely necessary to have them, and they must be testes. These foetal testes must release the so-called Müllerian-inhibiting substance which causes the homolateral Müllerian duct to regress, thus preventing the formation of the uterus and Fallopian tube on that side. The foetal testes must also release an androgenic or male-hormonal substance which prevents regression of the Wolffian ducts, thus ensuring the differentiation of the male internal sexual structures. When the Müllerian-inhibiting substance fails, it is possible to have a male born with fully differentiated uterus and tubes. So far as is known, this rather extraordinary anomaly does not have any subsequent primary influence on sexual behaviour. In the case of unilateral failure of the Müllerian-inhibiting substance, only a half uterus and one Fallopian tube is formed; subsequent external sexual development is liable to be hermaphroditic, with attendant risks of anomalously affecting sexual behaviour.

Differentiation of the external sexual organs comes after that of the internal organs and proceeds on the basis of an entirely different principal — the principal of homologues. Here nature begins with the same anlagen and uses them for sexually different purposes: the genital tubercle becomes either the clitoris or the penis; the genital folds become either the hood of the clitoris and the labia minora, or the foreskin and the wrap-around of the penis which forms the penile urethra; and the genital swellings become either the labia majora or the scrotal sac joined by the same median raphé that fuses the penile urethra. It is between the second and third month of foetal life in the human species that external-organ differentiation takes place.

MASCULINE DIFFERENTIATION: ADDITIVE PRINCIPLE

The differentiating principle at the embryonic stage of external-organ development is once again: add something to obtain a male. The something added is androgen. In the absence of androgen, a foetus will differentiate externally as a female, regardless of chromosomal sex; and in the partial absence of androgen, differentiation will be as an unfinished male, that is with incomplete fusion of the penile and scrotal skin, the penis being diminished in size and the testes possibly being undescended. Conversely, in the presence of a sufficient quantity of androgen even an XX foetus will differentiate externally as a male.

Brain differentiation
At around the same time as the external genitalia differentiate, foetal androgens also exert an influence on the developing central nervous system. In the lower, oestrous species, androgen administered to the foetus at the appropriate critical developmental period counteracts its primary disposition to develop, subsequently, the cyclic oestrous function of the female. The findings of different investigators using different techniques (reviewed by Harris 1964; Money 1965; Money and Ehrhardt 1972) converge on the hypothalamus as the responsible area of the brain. Nuclei in the hypothalamus govern, by way of their neural releaser-hormones, the pituitary gland's activity. The pituitary, in turn, cyclically or non-cyclically releasing its gonad-stimulating hormones, the gonadotropins, regulates the production of sex hormones from the ovaries or testicles.

The overall principle emerging from the foregoing neurohormonal (or neurohumoral) research is once again the familiar one: add something, androgen, to obtain a male. Whether the differentiation regulated by androgen follows the homologous pattern of the external genitals, or the vestigiation pattern of the gonads and internal organs, remains to be ascertained. One piece of evidence in favour of the vestigiation hypothesis is that of Fisher (1956, 1966) who was able to elicit simultaneous female (maternal or parental) and male (mating) behaviour in a male rat by injecting minute amounts of testosterone directly into the pre-optic area of the hypothalamus. The threshold for the release of parental behaviour is, under ordinary circumstances, more resistant in the male as compared with the female.

Masculinized female monkeys
Prenatal androgenizing experiments that have so far been performed on primates have not shown so direct an effect on hormonal cyclicity of menstruation as the corresponding experiments have done on hormonal cyclicity of oestrus in rodents. However, prenatally androgenized female rhesus monkeys tend to be about a year late in beginning to menstruate, and it is possible that the program of menstrual cycling over a lifetime may be changed. There is some evidence also to indicate a foetal effect on the central nervous system that will eventually influence sexual behaviour. For example, investigators at the Regional Primate Research Center, Beaverton, Oregon (Young *et al.* 1965; Phoenix 1966; Goy 1970) have produced genetic female rhesus monkeys so effectively virilized *in utero* by androgen injections of the mother that they were born with a normal male-appearing penis and empty scrotum instead of a clitoris and vaginal orifice. In the juvenile years, these animals gained behaviour scores for initiating play, engaging in rough-and-tumble play, chasing, making threatening gestures, and adopting the mounting position in sexual play that approximated to the scores of normal control males and were higher than those of normal control females. As they approached puberty and adolescence, these anatomically masculinized females tended to lose the masculine trend in their behavioural scores, but the complete story has not yet been ascertained, and the complete repertory of appropriate tests remains to be performed.

Masculinized human females
In human beings, there are two clinical syndromes that are the counterpart of foetal monkey androgenization. One is the syndrome of progestin-induced hermaphroditism in females. The other is the female adrenogenital syndrome of hermaphroditism, specifically in cases where masculinization is restricted to foetal life, its continuance after birth being prevented by treatment with cortisone. It is superfluous to the needs of this chapter to digress into a full clinical description of these two syndromes and their differential aetiology, prognosis, and therapy; see instead Wilkins (1965) and Money (1968). It is sufficient for present purposes to note that, regardless of aetiology, one has here examples of females subjected to masculinization in foetal life sufficient to enlarge the clitoris and partially fuse the labia, so as to create the appearance of hypospadias in the male. This anatomical abnormality is surgically corrected soon after birth, so that the appearance looks correctly female, in agreement with the sex of assignment and rearing. Hormonal function, either spontaneously or by regulation, is female, and puberty is normal in onset. What then of behaviour?

The evidence to date (Ehrhardt and Money 1967; Ehrhardt *et al.* 1968; Money and Ehrhardt 1972) is that foetal androgenization in the above two syndromes does indeed influence the subsequent development of behaviour, though only to a limited extent. It does not induce a complete reversal of gender role and gender identity in the sense that a girl feels she ought to be a boy or would like to change her sex, even though she might feel she would have opted to be a boy had she been able to choose. Nor does it automatically steer her in the direction of lesbianism. But it does tend to make of her a tomboy, as judged by self-declaration and confirmed by parents and friends. Her tomboyism is defined, perhaps above all else, by vigorous, muscular energy expenditure and an intense interest in athletic sports and outdoor activities in competition with boys. This competitiveness is not especially associated with aggression and fighting. It is compatible with rivalry for dominance in the dominance hierarchy of boyhood, as evident in those few prenatally androgenized genetic female individuals who are assigned and reared as boys, though such dominance rivalry tends to be subdued in those who are reared as girls. The girls who are the tomboys typically scorn fussy and frilly feminine clothes and hairdos in favour of utility styles. Tomboyism is incompatible with a strong interest in maternalism or parentalism as revealed in the rehearsals of childhood doll play or in future ambitions for the care of tiny babies. It does not exclude the anticipation of romance, marriage, and pregnancy, but these are regarded in a somewhat perfunctory way as secondary to a non-domestic career. Career ambitions are consistent with high academic achievement and with high IQ, which tends to be a characteristic of girls with foetal androgenization (Money 1971).

Anti-androgenism: rats
The experimental opposite of foetal androgenization of the female is non-androgenization or anti-androgenization of the male. The former can be achieved by means of foetal castration, a technically difficult operation even in a species like the rat in which the young are delivered foetally immature. Neonatal castration of the male rat does indeed preserve cyclic functioning of the pituitary, as is normal in the female (Harris 1964). The use of anti-androgen is even more dramatic in its effect. When such a hormone is injected, with the proper timing, into the pregnant mother, then the foetal testes of the genetic males become dormant and fail to supply androgen to the anlagen of the external genitalia. In consequence, the animal, to be specific a rat (Neumann and Elger 1965), is born with normal-appearing female genitals. By castrating the animal to eliminate all further influence of its own testes and giving replacement doses of female hormones at puberty, it is possible to obtain normal female mating behaviour from these genetic males (Neumann and Elger 1966). The stud males of the colony do not distinguish them from normal females. The sex-behaviour reversal is complete.

Foetal de-androgenization: human
In human beings, two clinical syndromes† are close counterparts of experimental anti-androgenism in animals, namely Turner's syndrome and the testicular-feminizing or androgen-insensitivity syndrome (Wilkins 1965; Money 1968). In both instances, foetal androgenization of the external genitals fails so that the baby is born with normal-appearing female external genitalia. In Turner's syndrome, there are neither ovaries nor testes as a result of the chomosomal error responsible for the syndrome, so that foetal androgenization is an impossibility. In the androgen-insensitivity syndrome, the testes are present and the chromosomal sex is 46,XY = male. The testes produce male sex hormone in an amount normal for a male; and at puberty, they produce also female sex hormone in an amount normal for a male. It is not the testes that are at fault in this condition, but all the cells of the body, which manifest a genetic inability to respond to male sex hormone. The body therefore responds to the testes' output of female hormone; it develops a normal female appearance, including breasts, at puberty. There is no uterus, however, since the testes produced their Müllerian-inhibiting substance early in embryonic life, thus causing its vestigiation.

The behaviour of girls and women with either Turner's syndrome (Money and Mittenthal 1969) or the androgen-insensitivity syndrome (Money, Ehrhardt, and Masica 1868; Masica, Money, Ehrhardt, and Lewis 1969) is indisputably feminine. They are not tomboys. In childhood their interest is in traditionally feminine play and activities. They show strong maternalistic interests in doll play from an early age, generally like to take care of children as they grow through childhood, and rehearse fantasies of romance, marriage, and motherhood as their primary ambition for the future. They are bitterly disappointed when their case is diagnosed and they learn the prognosis of sterility and motherhood by adoption. When eventually they do adopt children, they make good mothers. Their sex-lives in marriage are the same as for anatomically normal wives selected at random, and are subject to the same vicissitudes — except for the probability of needing long-term hormonal therapy and, in some cases of androgen insensitivity, surgical lengthening of the vagina for ease in sexual intercourse.

CORE GENDER IDENTITY: PRINCIPLE OF DISSOCIATION

Babies who will in future be diagnosed as having the androgen-insensitivity syndrome are almost never diagnosed at birth or in early childhood, for the obvious

†The syndromes of 17α-hydroxylase deficiency and gonadotropin deficiency also qualify when they are so complete that the baby is born with female external genitalia. They are of sparse occurrence and too few individuals have been followed psychologically to warrant inclusion here, though preliminary findings are not discordant with those herewith presented. The 3β-hydroxysteroiddehydrogenase deficiency also produces a genetic male with female external genitals, but such a baby is not viable unless the deficiency is partial only, which is very seldom.

reason that they look normally female, unless the testes should happen to be descended into the groin or the labia. The same is true for Turner's syndrome, except that various of the possible congenital defects of this syndrome, unrelated to the missing gonads, may bring the child to earlier medical attention. It therefore happens that the differentiation of gender identity in these female-appearing people cannot be studied except under the reinforcement of a rearing that is female, like their appearance. The real test of the influence of sex of assignment and rearing on psychosexual differentiation is better studied in cases of sexual anomaly where the visible appearance is hermaphroditically ambiguous so that two people of the same diagnosis can be found, one having been assigned, reared, and surgically and hormonally treated as a boy, the other as a girl.

This condition, though rare, is met often enough to demonstrate the extraordinary power of postnatal events on the differentiation of gender role and identity. The typical finding is that gender role and identity differentiate in conformity with the sex of assignment and rearing. This conformity can withstand various partial contradictions which include: (1) even such extreme contradictory hormonal puberty that a person raised as a girl virilizes like a boy or, being raised as a boy begins to grow breasts and pass menstrual blood through the urethra; (2) tomboyism of energy expenditure in a person raised as a girl; (3) imperfect pubertal virilization with a non-erectile stub of a penis in a person raised as a boy; and (4) a masculine type of threshold, in a person living as a woman, for erotic arousal in response to visual and narrative erotic representations as contrasted with the more feminine threshold of dependence on tactile stimulation and romantic symbolism.

There are exceptions, nonetheless, when gender identity does not differentiate in conformity with sex of assignment. Disparity between the two is most likely to arise when the assignment itself is ambivalent. The parents may be given no medical conviction about their infant's sexual diagnosis, or even may be told to half expect that a sex change might be necessary later. Parental ambivalence can be further reinforced if the genitalia are left surgically uncorrected during childhood so that they not only are a reproach to the child, when he or she looks at them, but also may be the source of teasing from siblings, cousins, or friends. Under such circumstances the child, sensing and then knowing full well that something is wrong, does not tolerate the cognitive dissonance of his ambiguity. It is very rarely that an hermaphrodite settles for an ambiguous or hermaphroditic gender identity. A resolution of ambiguity is achieved instead by the simple binary arithmetical expedient of repudiating the attributed status, so obviously wrong and unsatisfactory, in favour of its opposite — which at least has the virtue of not having yet been proved wrong and unsatisfactory.

This process of resolving dissonance by means of a formula for reassignment may be inchoate or articulate,

when it occurs. It usually takes place early during an hermaphrodite's childhood, for the resolution of an ambiguous gender identity cannot feasibly be postponed. To achieve formal recognition of the change then becomes something of a *cause célèbre* and a strong driving force in life.

The question of whether or not the influence of foetal hormones on sex differentiation of nuclei of the hypothalamus may have any bearing on an hermaphrodite's conviction of the need for sex reassignment cannot at present be answered. One can simply note (Money 1969) that the decision seems to be arrived at more frequently by male than female hermaphrodites, and is more likely to require a female-to-male change of status than vice versa — which may have more to do with ambiguity of anatomy and of diagnosis in male hermaphroditism than with assigned sexual status *per se*. Moreover, a genetically male hermaphrodite with highly feminized genitalia who was originally assigned as a female and later requests reassignment to live as a male is less likely to meet with opposition from conservatives in the medical profession than is a genetically female hermaphrodite of similar appearance who makes the same request. Few hermaphrodites who do not consolidate their gender identity from infancy onward, but reach a point of self-reassignment, contrast strongly with those whose gender identity is consolidated, and for whom a sex reassignment by edict would be a disaster.

In the sex assignment of hermaphrodites, it is still relatively common for an on-the-spot decision to be made in the delivery room or at home at the time of birth, and then to have to be changed later, after completion of a full diagnostic work-up. As a result, a reannouncement of the baby's sex has to be made. Provided the parents are correctly guided through this dilemma, reannouncement need have no long-term adverse effect, then or subsequently, on the differentiation of the child's gender identity.

It is somewhere between the ages of 12 and 18 months, dependent on a baby's facility in the understanding and use of language, that a sex reannouncement becomes more than an adjustment problem for the parents alone, and one for the child as well. By the time he has command of names, nouns, pronouns, and clothing differentiating the sexes, a boy has a clear concept of himself as a boy, and a girl of herself as a girl. There is now no such simple thing as a sex reannouncement: it will be a sex reassignment involving the child as a person. Psychologically, it is very serious business, for the child already has a self-identity as a boy or girl. The core gender identity, to use a term increasingly in vogue, is already on the way to being firmly established. This is an aspect of psychosexual differentiation not accounted for in the traditional Freudian scheme of the oral, anal, and genital stages of psychosexual development.

The differentiation of a core gender identity would appear to follow the same priciple as the differentiation of the gonads and the internal reproductive organs. In other words, two systems are present to begin with. Only one of them becomes finally functional. In the case of gender identity, however, the non-functional system does not become vestigial in the true sense, but is dissociated — coded as negative and not manifested by oneself. Thus, a boy grows up to know how to do all the boy things, because he also knows how not to do all the girl things, or vice versa for a girl. It must be much the same type of coding as happens in the brain in bilingualism. Under special circumstances in the boy, the negatively coded girl pattern may be brought to the fore — as when, for example, a child reaches a decision of sex reassignment. The same may occur under circumstances of severe personality disorganization associated with adolescent psychosis. A behavioural sex change may emerge still later in life, in certain rare cases of temporal lobe epilepsy, or as a consequence of senile brain deterioration, and may be manifest in the form of personality changes, among others, toward transvestitism or homosexuality. When the temporal lobe is involved and the epileptic focus can be removed surgically, then both the seizures and the psychosexual anomaly may be relieved.

PRINCIPLE OF IDENTIFICATION AND COMPLEMENTATION IN GENDER IDENTITY DIFFERENTIATION

The system coded as negative for oneself but positive for members of the other sex is also the system that represents to oneself the complement or reciprocal of one's own positively coded system. It is, so to speak, a template in one's brain for monitoring actions and reactions of the other sex which complement or reciprocate one's own, and with which one must interact.

Postnatal gender-identity differentiation is a product of experience assimilated or learned by way of the twin principles of identification and complementation. Identification learning is manifested as behaviour which imitates or impersonates that of a model or models of the same sex. Complementation learning is manifested as behaviour which reciprocates that of a model or models of the opposite sex. Typically the chief models are a child's own parents or parent substitutes. Other people in the domestic environment, including other siblings, or even television figures may function as secondary models. When identification and complementation behaviour are appropriately manifested, they may be contingently reinforced by any observer of either sex who happens to approve of them, and likewise for the reverse, namely, negative reinforcement of inappropriate behaviour. It is not imperative that both an identification or a complementation model always be present, since a person of either sex can be the agent of appropriate positive and negative contingency reinforcement. Thus, theoretically a mother can reinforce the behaviour of her young son when, even though separated from his father or other male identification model,

he exhibits behaviour toward her that is appropriately complemental of her own. Usually, of course, the boy will not be permanently separated or secluded from all male models, and ideally he should not be — likewise, conversely, for a girl.

As the development of gender identity by way of identification and complementation is also a process of differentiation, it is facilitated if the two alternatives, masculine and feminine, are experienced by a developing infant and young child as having, in some degree, non-overlapping boundaries in the precepts and behaviour of those whom he encounters. To cite an extreme negative example: if the father who sired a child is a transexual who subsequently undergoes complete sex reassignment then, in his new role as a female, he cannot function any more as a masculine model. His role overlaps too completely that of the child's mother and other normal females — so much so that the reassigned male-to-female transexual can serve as a feminine model for a young child as, say, an adoptive mother, foster mother or stepmother. Likewise, in reverse, for a female-to-male transexual.

The boundaries of masculine and feminine may become confused and overlapping if the parents or other important people in a child's life are in some way ambivalent about masculine and feminine. Thus, it is difficult for a boy to differentiate an unambiguous gender identity should he have a mother who is ambivalent about her son's maleness because she is phobic of the male penis, his father's and his own included. It is similarly difficult if the boy has a father who is ambivalent about masculine eroticism in so far as he is phobic of the female's vagina, even though, being a father, he has sometimes managed to copulate. Likewise, it is difficult for a girl whose mother is an ambivalent martyr to menstruation, intercourse, and childbirth; or whose father reacts ambivalently to the femininity of all females, his wife and daughter included, because he sees them as martyrs to be exploited, as though they were males lacking something.

Apart from ethical and political considerations, it does not much matter, so far as the process of gender-identity differentiation is concerned, what is defined or stereotyped as masculine and what feminine, in any given epoch or culture. It is more important that there be consensus among important individuals in the child's life, and lack of ambiguity and contradiction in the gender-learning signals transmitted to him or her from all sources of identification and complementation.

On the basis of historical and ethnopsychologic data, it is well established that there are many viable definitions or stereotypes of a masculine and a feminine gender role. The common denominator of them all is that women menstruate, gestate, and lactate, and men do not. Until this basic dictate of mammalian phylogeny can be reversed, there will always be an authentic basis to the differentiation of gender role and, by implication, of gender identity, in the two sexes. Even in the most radical human sexual reversal therapeutically achieved to date, that of hormonal and surgical sex reassignment of the transexual individual, reversal of fertility is technically quite impossible. Parenthetically, transexuals show that planned reversal of gender identity is also technically impossible. A transexual is a person who has spontaneously differentiated a gender identity discordant with morphologic sex, as a result of which he or she requests and may receive sex reassignment.

As already indicated, it is not imperative for effective gender-identity differentiation that a child have as father a genetic and gonadal male, or as mother a genetic and gonadal female. The annals of hermaphroditism and of transexualism show that paradoxes on the basis of the genetic and gonadal criteria are irrelevant to effective parentalism. It is more important that the parent have the appropriate secondary sexual appearance — which can be hormonally induced and/or augmented by means of plastic surgery, as needed. It is even more important that the parent behave in the culturally appropriate sexually dimorphic way toward the child as a mother or father.

In a child's developmental differentiation of gender identity, there are two universal disparities between identification and complementation that may cause developmental trouble, namely, disparities with respect to dominance and to genital incest. The parent inevitably has a status of dominance over the infant and juvenile child. Should a young child's identification with the parents be total and complete, then he or she would become dominant over the parents. Dominance-struggles between child and parent — or sibling and sibling — may become evident early in infancy. They may become acute in prepuberty and sometimes disastrous in the crises of adolescence, the phyletically decreed age of establishing autonomy.

Gender-identity differentiation in the early juvenile years logically should be expected to include identification with the romantic and sexual behaviour of the older model. Thus, at the appropriate developmental age, the small child should be expected to include romantic, coquettish, seductive, or protosexual behaviour in his or her repertoire of behaviour toward members of the other sex. Such behaviour is readily recognizable in the pre-school years in our society, but far less so than if it were under a more lenient cultural taboo.

In our society, the developing child is subject to an injunction to impose a constraint on assertion of dominance over older people of the parental generation. A similar constraint applies to sexual eroticism. In so far as it applies to relationships of the child to members of the parental generation, this constraint on literal genito-erotic identification with the parent of the same sex constitutes what is conventionally subsumed under the term Oedipus complex. In our own society it is an even more extensive conventional constraint, since it applies also to imitating the same-parent coital role in relationships with one's age mates of the opposite sex. In some ethnic groups, such age-mate relationships are not prohibited, and they are part of the behaviour of primates lower than man.

PRINCIPLE OF MASCULINE VULNERABILITY

It is widely acknowledged that, disregarding impotence and frigidity, the incidence of psychosexual disorders is higher in males than females. The variety of psychosexual disorders is also greater in males than females; some of the more bizarre and exotic anomalies simply are not recorded in the female. It is quite likely that one has here a by-product of yet one more manifestation of the principle of sexual differentiation, namely that something must be added to differentiate a male. The something added that makes the difference between female and male in psychosexual erotic functioning might well, once again, be androgen. Its site of action, or absence thereof, would undoubtedly be the brain. Its mechanism of action would most likely pertain to threshold sensitivity for erotic arousal from a visual stimulus or, perhaps, its evocation in imagery from a marrative stimulus. After puberty, it is males who are girl-watchers, more than females who are boy-watchers. Teenage boys use nude pictures as masturbation stimuli, but girls do not. At puberty, the boy is self-presented with realistic erotic images in dreams accompanied by orgasm; the girl is not. The very sexual performance of the boy is categorically different from that of the girl, in that his penis must be aroused to erection before he can begin; and it must ejaculate in orgasm if reproduction is to be effected. In the girl, by contrast, it is possible for conception to occur without either arousal or orgasm. It is possible for the male to be erotically aroused by touch alone, a fact to which many husbands can attest. But it is typically the visual image that lends an element of excitement and, above all, incites the male to be the one who takes erotic initiative. This principle of male initiative is widespread in the animal kingdom, and in many species is dependent on visual stimulation, the closest competitor being smell.

If nature seems always to need to add something to make a male, then she seems also more likely to fail in her effort. The birth ratio, usually quoted at 106:100, in favour of males, allows for the more rapid wastage of the male, and the conception ratio, estimated at as high as 140:100, shows even more dramatically how easy it is for a male to fail. There are no definite figures available, but the vulnerability of the male is again demonstrated at puberty, when, in the clinic, partial or complete failure of hormonal puberty is more common than in the female (excluding the postpubertal problems of ovulatory and menstrual irregularity). In the matter of psychosexual arousal, nature's difficulty in differentiating a male again manifests itself in the greater number of males than females who are 'turned on' by an atypical, bizarre, or erotic stimulus, that is, one that has positive arousal value when it should be either neutral, negative, or partial. All the paraphiliac anomalies in a textbook of sexual psychopathology can be interpreted

14

in terms of being aroused by an atypical stimulus. Sometimes it is almost possible to glimpse how atypical connections between behavioural components can be established, by reason of their proximity of representation in the nervous system, as MacLean (1965) pointed out with respect to oral/anal representations in the limbic system.

Vulnerability to errors of psychosexual functioning has no single source of origin. In a few cases genetics can definitely be implicated, as in some cases of the XXY (Klinefelter's) syndrome or the XYY syndrome. Men with either of these cytogenetic anomalies are vulnerable to some or other peculiarity of sexual behaviour. XXY men are also weak in libido, as well as sterile.

Whether events in intrauterine life may predispose human beings to psychosexual errors later in life is uncertain. In animal experiments it has been found that attempted experimental androgenization of the female foetus can be blocked by barbiturates and by the antibiotics puromycin and actinoymycin-D (Gorski 1971). One wonders what effect, if any, sleeping pills or other pharmacological products taken by a pregnant mother may have on the unborn foetus. The intrauterine effects of maternal stress, presumably hormone-mediated, may also affect the unborn foetus, according to the data of Ward (1972). Pregnant rats stressed by being constrained under glaring light produced sons with lessened testicular weight and penis length. As adults they were deficient in male mating behaviour when tested with receptive females. They also had a lowered threshold for display of the crouching (lordosis) response of the female when experimentally tested with stud males. Another intrauterine effect, also presumably hormone-mediated, was found by Clemens (1974) in female rats from litters with large numbers of brothers: the larger the number of brothers, the greater the likelihood that the sisters would display masculine mounting behaviour when hormonally primed with androgen in adulthood.

The bulk of today's evidence points unquestionably to events in early postnatal life and infancy as of prime importance in relation to eventual psychosexual normalcy. Harlow's (1965) work with rhesus monkeys raised on dummy mothers and in isolation from playmates is too well known to need retelling here. It points to the hitherto unsuspected importance of clinging and the sense of touch in primate development. It points also to the need to be able to play at the appropriate critical period — sexual play included — if normal reproductive behaviour and parenthood is subsequently to be achieved. A report from the chimpanzee colony in New Mexico (Kollar, Beckwith, and Edgerton 1968) shows that, like the rhesus monkey, these primates also are vulnerable to errors of psychosexual function when captured from their normal jungle troop and imprisoned in captivity. In fact, their sex-behaviour problems are uncannily human.

As for human beings themselves, there is no highly systematic body of knowledge concerning the contin-gencies between rearing and subsequent sexual behaviour, though there is a store of clinical knowledge and hypotheses, too vast to be reviewed here. It is perhaps a safe generalization to say that almost any major disruption of a child's developmental experience, regardless of its origin or type, is a potential source of disturbance in subsequent psychosexual development — the more so the younger the child. The vulnerability of the psychosexual system to disturbance may simply reflect the fact that its differentiation is actively in progress during early childhood. It may also be a reflection of the fact that, in many societies, our own included, psychosexual development is subject to an excess of taboos, such as the taboo on sexual play in childhood. If one judges from the evidence of the other primates, then childhood sexual play is a necessary and normal rehearsal in preparation for adolescence and adulthood. Perhaps we would do well to re-examine our policies on childhood sexual play as a determinant of adult sexual behaviour.

PRINCIPLE OF LOVE AS AN IMPRINT

After the advent of hormonal puberty, a new milestone in psychosexual development is reached, namely the capacity to experience falling in love. Children in kindergarten have play romances, and children in the so-called latency period (not so very latent, either!) may play at copulation games, but they do not fall in love, unless precocious falling in love may itself be a specific sign of psychosexual maldevelopment. The capacity to be aroused and possessed by the stimulus of the love object is not simultaneous with puberty. It does not occur, for instance, in children with precocious puberty of infantile onset until they become older — twelve is probably about the youngest. By contrast, in children, most notably boys, with long-delayed puberty, it is possible though not routine to observe the experience of falling in love at some time from middle to late teenage, even when complete hormonal infantilism still persists (Money and Alexander 1967). One suspects, therefore, that whereas one neurohumoral mechanism (or biological clock) in the hypothalamus turns on puberty by way of activating the pituitary, another mechanism, site unknown, activates the capacity to fall in love.

Falling in love resembles imprinting, in that a releaser mechanism from within must encounter a stimulus from without before the event happens. Then that event has remarkable longevity, sometimes for a lifetime. The kind of stimulus that, whether it be acceptable or pathological, will be the effective one for a given individual will have been written, so to speak, into his psychosexual program, in the years prior to puberty and dating back to infancy. Especially in the case of psychopathology, a boy or girl may be shocked and guilty to be 'turned on' by an abnormal stimulus, while at the same time secretly fascinated and obsessed with it because of the sexual feeling it releases. The effective

15

erotic stimulus may not initially be revealed in full, so that there is some element of discovery and expansion in erotic experience with the passage of time. By and large, however, human beings stay remarkably stable in their erotic preferences. Thus, it is not possible to teach a man or even a teenager to be, say, a masochist or a peeping-Tom; and a few teenage exposures to homosexuality do not create an appetite for more. The appetite has to be there in the first place. Earlier in childhood, the power of exposure and experience is probably far more impressive and lasting. However, a great deal more work needs to be done on the after-effects of childhood sexual experiences.

There seem to be distinct personality types so far as falling in love is concerned, and they may correspond to the augmenters and diminishers of sensation as described by Petrie (1967). At one extreme are people of psychopathic or sociopathic personality disposition, the Don Juan and nymphomaniac types who are the experts at one-night stands. These are perhaps diminisher-people whose experiences fade quickly and stand in need of constant repetition and novelty.

By contrast, at the other extreme are the augmenter-people who cannot let an experience go. It reverberates and enlarges in their memories, and haunts them. The love affairs of many schizoid and schizophrenic people have this quality. They may have an anguished love affair without ever declaring themselves to the partner; or even possibly conduct the whole love affair with an imaginary partner by way of a photograph.

The majority of mankind, of course, falls somewhere between these two extremes. Each tends to judge the other from within the solipsism of his own 'egg shell' as being like himself. But the fact is that we are quite differently determined so far as sexual behaviour goes.

ANDROGEN/LIBIDO PRINCIPLE

When a teenager who has a syndrome of sexual infantilism nonetheless has a falling in love experience, it is not as intense and full-bodied as it will be once he is given effective hormone replacement therapy. The sex hormones do not in any way govern the cognitional content of eroticism — they do not cause homosexuality, for example — but they do affect the intensity and frequency of its expression, though without exercising total responsibility in this respect. Androgen is probably the libido hormone for both sexes (Money 1961; Herbert 1966; Trimble and Herbert 1968) though some women, notably those with androgen insensitivity, seem to be able to function adequately without it. Female-to-male transexuals report heightened intensity of orgasm and erotic feeling in the clitoris (which is preserved in reconstructive surgery) after they are hormonally reassigned and receive testosterone replacement therapy. They retain the typical female capacity for multiple orgasm.

Normal women tend to report a more receptive attitude of wanting to be possessed at around the time of ovulation, which is when the oestrogenic phase of the menstrual cycle is in the ascendant. A correlate of the ovulatory phase in the rhesus monkey is the secretion of a vaginal pheromone, biochemically constituted of short-chain aliphatic acids (Michael, Keverne, and Bonsall 1971). This odoriferous substance is a sex attractant for the male, stimulating him to copulate.

Oestrogen tends to be an inhibitor of androgen. At the menstrual phase, when progesterone levels are higher and androgen may be less inhibited, women are more likely to take an initiating role of inducing the male. The birth-control pill may change this cycle, but in a way that seems to depend on the formulae of the different brand names (Grant and Pryse-Davies 1968).

Anti-androgens (Money 1970; Money *et al.* 1975) may prove to be very beneficial in enabling certain sex criminals to gain a measure of control over their otherwise ungovernable sexual behaviour. The effect is reversible when the medication is stopped, without adverse side-effects. The same medication promises also to be helpful in the regulation of violent rage outbursts in some temporal lobe epileptics (D. Blumer, personal communication).

The hormonal changes of pregnancy have no routinely systematic effect on a woman's sex life. The mechanics of carrying a baby affect different women differently, as does the psychological effect of the meaning of pregnancy and parenthood. Being a parent affects husband and wife equally and may have a profound effect, it goes without saying, on their opportunities for sexual behaviour.

As with the hormonal changes of pregnancy, those of the menopause have no systematic effect on a woman's sex life, except in so far as the vaginal mucosa may become atrophic and too dry, with an adverse effect on sexual intercourse. This effect can be reversed by the judicious prescription of oestrogen (which also will serve as a protection against osteoporosis). The direct effect of the hormonal changes of the menopause on mood and temperament varies widely, as does the effect of the psychological meaning of having reached the end of child-bearing; consequently, both of these effects themselves bear no systematic relationship to post-menopausal sexual behaviour. It is important for many couples to know that the menopause does not mark the end of a woman's sexual desire and ability. Her sexual life may continue, and even be improved, far into old age.

The male's sex life also may continue far into old age, unmarked by any such dramatic hormonal event as the menopause of the female. The refractory interval between erections and between orgasm lengthens as age increases, but with great individual variation. Failing potency can generally be improved in older men whose own androgen levels have declined by the judicious prescription of testosterone. Impotence not associated with a falling-off in androgen production is not improved by treatment with hormones, and the same holds true for so-called frigidity in women.

16

Apart from the ageing effect, deficit or impairment of sexual behaviour and its frequency has many different aetiologies, requiring considerable astuteness to establish diagnosis. The symptom of deficient or impaired sexual activity may be a sequel to: a genetic defect; an error of metabolism; an endocrine error; a mechanical, neurological, or circulatory defect; a traumatic injury; an adverse psychological reaction to illness (for example, after a heart attack); a primary psychiatric disorder (especially depression); a disturbance of personality and the interpersonal relationship of sex; or a lack of sufficient timing, variety, or novelty of stimulation.

An excess of sexual activity is more often regarded boastfully as an asset rather than as a symptom. Yet it may be a symptom, especially when it represents a change from a former lesser level, together with a change in the type of behaviour. The most likely diagnostic considerations then are: an endocrine error; a neurological error (particularly a trauma, tumor, or senile atrophy of the brain); a primary psychiatric disorder (especially mania or hypomania); or a disturbance of personality and the interpersonal relationship of sex.

PRINCIPLE OF GENITO-PELVIC SENSATION

It seems obvious that one of the determinants of sexual behaviour is the integrity of the sexual organs with which coitus is performed. Yet large amounts of sexual tissue can be removed without destroying the capacity for erotic response (Money 1961). Following amputation of the penis, whether by accident or because of malignancy, orgasm is retained. Sexual desire remains as before, creating a serious problem of morale in being unable to satisfy the partner.

A more complete loss of penile tissue is entailed in sex-reassignment surgery for male transexualism, for the corpora are extirpated and only the skin retained as a lining for the new vagina (Jones, Schirmer, and Hoopes 1968). Post-operatively and living as females, transexuals claim they experience erotic satisfaction in the female sexual role, and some report a climactic feeling of orgasm which, if different than they formerly experienced as males, satisfies them more because they are able to be in the female role.

Penile tissue is not lost as a sequel to priapism, but the corpora are, in many cases, functionally destroyed. Erection is impossible. Here again orgasm and desire for intercourse are retained, and the morale seriously injured.

The morale problem is, by contrast, quite different in cases of paraplegia (Money 1960) where the loss is not of genital tissue, but of all spinal cord connection with the brain. The genitalia are able to respond reflexly to local tactile stimulation, but the patient has no feeling and awareness of what has happened. A paraplegic male has no erection in response to erotic thoughts and imagery. The nearest he gets to an orgasm is by dreaming one, and even sexual dreams disappear as the years pass after the paraplegic injury occurred. The paraplegic knows that he has lost his sex life and would elect, if he could, to have it returned, but there is none of the quality of urgency and frustration found in men whose genitals can perform only a part of their sexual function without completing it. Signals from the genitals are obviously a principal component or determinant of sexual behaviour.

In women as in men, ablation of genital tissue is compatible with the retention of erotic sensation and orgasm. The evidence comes from women who undergo radical resection of the vulva for epidermoid cancer, and from hermaphroditic females whose hypertrophied clitoris is resected or extirpated. According to the evidence of genital ablation, an orgasm is an orgasm regardless of the stimulation that triggers it — which is precisely the verdict of the Masters and Johnson (1966) research into the human sexual response. These authors effectively put to rest the ghost of the old controversy of the clitoral versus the vaginal orgasm as a determinant of mature sexual behaviour in the female.

PRINCIPLE OF DIMORPHIC SIGNALS

Over and beyond the specifics of genito-pelvic sexual behaviour, there is a vast amount of human behaviour that is sexual in the sense that it is dimorphic in relation to gender: what men do one way, women do another. This kind of gender-related behaviour ranges from fashions of dress to conventions of work and earning a living, and legal status; from rules of etiquette and ceremony to recreation and labour-sharing in the home. Though these various stereotypes of what is masculine and what is feminine may ultimately derive from such fundamental sex differences as urinary posture, menstruation, child-bearing, lactation, stature, weight, and muscular power, the conventions themselves are defined by custom and may be arbitrary and subject to sudden changes of fashion or slow changes in the cultural pattern. It does not matter that they change. It is the fact that they exist in any given time and place that counts, for we human beings are sensitively dependent on our cognition of the signals and cues emanating from others — they are determinants of our own sexual behaviour, just as are plumage differences in birds. We differ from birds in being able to adapt and change the signals historically, but we cannot obliterate them altogether. There is no more convincing evidence in support of this principle than the fact that the average man or woman tends to accept the impersonation put forth by a transvestite or a transexual — provided of course, that it is a perfect or near-perfect impersonation. It is then possible to accept the impersonation, even after the truth is known, as being more genuine than the sex of the sex organs. It is even possible for a psychosexually normal person to fall in love with a transexual impersonator. Resolution of the incongruity between impersonation and the sex organs is then achieved by responding to the impersonator as someone beset by misfortune who is deserving or needing medical or surgical help. There is no more cogent illustration of how compelling is the influence of the senses over that of judgement in determining human sexual behaviour!

PRINCIPLE OF CULTURAL DETERMINANTS

Cultural tradition determines not only the criteria of sexually dimorphic behaviour, but also various criteria of sexual interaction. The variety of possibilities is extensive but not limitless, although the limits have not yet been catalogued. Variability can be classified as pertaining to the following characteristics of partnerships:

(1) age: same or disparate;
(2) physique: juvenile, adolescent, or adult;
(3) sex: same or opposite;
(4) kinship: related or not related by blood, clan, or race;
(5) caste or class: same or different;
(6) number: unity or plurality of partnerships;
(7) overlap: sequential or contemporaneous partnerships, or one partnership only;
(8) span: transient or constant partnerships;
(9) privacy: public or concealed;
(10) accessories: plain or modified by material artifacts, e.g. personal adornment, contraceptive device, etc.

To illustrate: the people of the Lake Toba region of northern Sumatra live in a cultural tradition that permits an age difference in a sexual partnership, ranging over the spectrum of physique from puberty to young manhood, but only in homosexual and not heterosexual partnerships. In late childhood, it is not decent for children to stay sleeping in their parents' single-roomed house. A girl takes her sleeping mat to the home of a widow or old woman who accommodates about half a dozen girls who range in age from puberty to late adolescence. A boy joins a group of a dozen to fifteen males, his own age or older, who sleep in a boy's house specially constructed for them.

Among males, information about the sexuality of unmarried females is conjectural, as talk about sexual activities, except between husband and wife, is taboo between the sexes. There is, however, among males overt information about their own sexual activities. When a boy goes to sleep in the boys' and young men's house, he learns from adolescents and young unmarried men how to participate in paired homosexual play with them or other boys; primarily mutual masturbation of penis held against penis, maybe anal coitus, but never fellatio. Each member of the group may become partner to the others, in rotation. Relationships are not necessarily unobserved, but they are always in pairs, not in larger groups. Partnerships among group members do not involve falling in love, but they are constant up to the point where a young man opts to leave the group by marrying. No man is permitted to remain a bachelor.

When he is ready to marry, a young man asks a close friend to join him in a prescribed etiquette of approaching the chosen girl and his own family, to see if they have the wealth to pay the bride price and put on a wedding festival.

The young man in search of a wife narrates the procedure of his courtship to his companions in the boys' house. Once married, he discloses details about sexual intercourse. In this way information is transmitted down the generations, and a young adolescent is prepared to anticipate his graduation from the era of homosexual experience to heterosexual falling in love and marriage.

The homosexual era in adolescence, by sequestering the sexes, ensures that young women will be virgins until married. The sanctions against premarital sex are stringent, so that a pair who are discovered in transgression probably commit suicide. Once a marriage is effected, the parties discontinue homosexuality, though men away on working parties in the jungle may temporarily resume them.

By contrast with the allowable age disparities in homosexual partnerships, the heterosexual partnership is formed between people of like age in young adulthood, or else the girl may be younger, in her teens, than the man, in his twenties. The relationship between the pair may be as close as cousins, but there is no special kinship obligation in the choice of a partner. There is a preference for partnerships within the racial/linguistic group. Marriage is the first and only heterosexual partnership. Neither party is permitted additional heterosexual partnerships, except for remarriage after the early death of one of the spouses. A marriage cannot otherwise be broken. Being married is, of course, publicly announced. The coital relationship of marriage is, by convention, private and unobserved, except that young children may awaken when the parents are copulating. They must then not disclose their observation, but ignore it. According to the formalities of the culture, they learn about sex not at home, but from their adolescent and young adult friends.

The cultural traditions of a lakeside village in Sumatra have been able to survive intact for an unspecified number of generations, but now, under the impact of cultural contact through education and broadcasting, these traditions are yielding to change. Change is a hallmark of the cultural traditions of our own society in the present age of instantaneous broadcast communication, nuclear-space technology and, in matters sexual, effective contraception. Whereas to some the change in sexual traditions is anathema, to others it is Utopia, but to none is it very clear, what, exactly, is happening. In terms of the ten schematic categories listed above, one may suggest the following as applicable in the United States. There has been no change of tradition

18

with respect to a preference for pairing couples of similar age, except for continuing toleration of a few cases of disparity within the adult years. There is still a rigid rule against juvenile sexual play, though the age of 'sex education' is subject to radical downward revision, amidst sometimes acrimonious social controversy. There is no issue more heated than that of the rights of adolescents and young adults to have sexual and love affairs premaritally, with or without contraception and the intention to marry and/or have children. The trend is toward greater freedom. Sanctions against homo-sexuality are being examined and eased, though ambivalently, in favour of consensual agreements between adults. Problems of kinship in mating continue to be singularly unimportant, so long as the incest taboo is respected. The issue of miscegenation is so explosive that it can scarcely be mentioned in public and political discussion, perhaps because it is a foregone conclusion that black/white intermarriage will become routine. Class and caste preference and distinctions in sexual pairing remain otherwise about the same as ever.

The leading pressure-point of change in our society's sexual traditions would seem to be toward a greater plurality of sexual relationships, for females as well as males, on a basis of mutual reciprocity. This change is registered in sequential more often than contem-poraneous plurality of relationships, before or after marriage. Even contemporaneous relationships are constant, over a period of time, rather than transient. Availability of effective contraception is undoubtedly the material artifact that underlies this cultural change, though in the case of serial marriage and divorce, with children to be supported, the economic and legal eman-cipation of women is also a major factor. Despite the plurality of partnerships, the preference is still for episodic monogamy or fidelity, rather than running more than one affair, contemporaneously. However, a new institution, its future still uncertain, is the 'swinging scene' of partner exchanging and group sex, coexistent and compatible with contractual marriage and long-term loyalty and emotional allegiance to one partner.

Participation in any sexual relationship outside of marriage is still subject to at least a partial need for concealment, though increasing freedom is accorded to young adults to be frank and open about their non-marital sexual liaisons, and living together. Coitus itself is still subject to the rule of privacy, though some group sex participants are indifferent to being observed or to engaging in activities with more than one partner simultaneously.

Whether or not these changes in sexual tradition con-stitute a sexual revolution or are simply variations of basic primate behaviour has become a subject for rhetoric and politics as well as for science and medicine. The reader must formulate his own conclusions.

The juxtaposition of nature versus nurture has long been a favourite topic of argument pertaining to the behaviour of human beings. Fascination with the topic stems ultimately from the issue of free will versus deter-minism. Nature is cast in the deterministic role of imperatively governing an inevitable and inexorable destiny variously named as biological, hereditary, con-stitutional, instinctual, and innate or inborn. Nurture by contrast is cast in the probabalistic role of optionally governing a modifiable and reversible fate, variously named as social, environmental, acquired, learned, and developmental.

Irrespective of terminology, the conceptual problem lurking in the nature/nurture dichotomy is that the two interact. They are not independent variables. Table 2.1 presents a different conceptualization of how to dif-ferentiate the inevitable from the optional in a $2 \times 2 \times 2$ scheme which simultaneously differentiates the phylo-graphic from the idiographic, and the nativistic from the

TABLE 2.1

Nativism and culturalism as determinants of gender identity/role, classified simultaneously with phylographic versus idiographic, and imperative versus optional determinants (with permission, from Money (1975)).

		Nativistic	Culturistic
Phylographic (species shared)	Imperative	Menstruation, gestation, lactation (women) vs. impreg-nation (men)	Social models for identification and complementation in gender-identity differentiation
	Optional	Population size, fertility rate and sex ratio	Population birth/death ratio. Diminishing age of puberty
Idiographic (individually unique)	Imperative	Chromosome anomalies, e.g., 45,X; 47,XXY; 47,XYY. Vestigal penis. Vestigal uterus. Vaginal atresia.	Sex announcement and rearing as male, female, or ambiguous.
	Optional	Getting pregnant. Breast feeding. Anorexic amenorrhea. Castration.	Gender-divergent work, play, and status. Gender-divergent cosmetics and grooming. Gender-divergent child care.

culturistic. That which is phylographic is species shared, whereas the idiographic is personally unique. Both may be either nativistic or cultural in origin, and, either way, may exist as imperatives or options.

The cells of Table 2.1 may be filled in for a variable other than that of gender identity role, the variable which is here appropriate.

SUMMARY

Chromosomal sex programs the differentiation of the foetal gonads which program the presence or absence of foetal testicular secretions, which program whether sexual morphology will be male or, in their absence female; and whether hypothalamic regulatory pathways will be masculinized or remain feminine. External genital morphology programs dimorphism of social response to a baby and developing child, and also the child's own body image, during the early period of life when gender identity differentiates. Psychosexual errors have their genesis at this early time. Pubertal hormones program adult secondary sexual dimorphism and lower the threshold for falling in love. Androgen in both sexes lowers the threshold for erotic response and participation. Adult hormones do not determine the content of erotic imagery nor the application of atypical imagery to sexual practice.

REFERENCES

BURNS, R. K. (1961). Role of hormones in the differentiation of sex. In *Sex and internal secretions* (ed. W. C. Young). Baltimore.

CHANG, C. Y. and WITSCHI, E. (1955). Breeding of sex-reversed males of *Xenopus laevis* Daudin. *Proc. Soc. expl Biol. Med.*, **89**, 150–2.

—— and WITSCHI, E. (1956). Genetic control and hormonal reversal of sex differentiation in *Xenopus*. *Proc. Soc. expl Biol. Med.*, **93**, 140–4.

CLEMENS, L. G. (1974). Neurohormonal control of male sexual behaviour. In *Reproductive behaviour* (ed. W. Montagna and W. A. Sadler). New York.

EHRHARDT, A. A. and MONEY, J. (1967). Progestin-induced hermaphroditism: IQ and psychosexual identity in a study of ten girls. *J. Sex Res.*, **3**, 83–100.

——, EPSTEIN, R., and MONEY, J. (1968). Foetal androgens and female gender identity in the early-treated adrenogenital syndrome. *Johns Hopk. med. J.*, **122**, 160–7.

FISHER, A. E. (1956). Maternal and sexual behavior induced by intracranial chemical stimulation. *Science* (*N.Y.*), **124**, 228–9.

—— (1966). Chemical and electrical stimulation of the brain in the male rat. In *The brain and gonadal function*, Vol. III of *Brain and behavior* (ed. P. A. Gorski and R. E. Whalen). Berkeley, California.

GORSKI, R. A. (1971). Gonadal hormones and the perinatal development of neuroendocrine function. In *Frontiers in neuroendocrinology 1971* (ed. L. Martini and W. F. Ganong). New York.

GOY, R. W. (1970). Experimental control of psychosexuality. In 'A discussion on the determination of sex' (ed. G. W. Harris and R. G. Edwards). *Phil. Trans. roy. Soc.*, B, **259**, 149–62.

GRANT E. C. G. and PRYSE-DAVIES, J. (1968). Effect of oral contraceptives on depressive mood changes and on endometrial monoamine oxidase and phosphatases. *Brit. med. J.*, iii, 777–80.

GREEN, R. and MONEY, J. (ed.) (1969). *Transsexualism and sex reassignment*. Baltimore.

HAMILTON, J. B., WALTER, R. O., and DANIEL, R. M. (1969). Competition for mating between ordinary and supermale Japanese medaka fish. *Anim. Behav.*, **17**, 168–76.

HARLOW, H. F. and HARLOW, M. K. (1965). The effect of rearing conditions on behavior. In *Sex research, new developments* (ed. J. Money). New York.

HARRIS, G. W. (1964). Sex hormones, brain development and brain function. *Endocrinology*, **75**: 627–48.

HERBERT, J. (1966). The social modification of sexual and other behaviour in the rhesus monkey. Progress in Primatology. *Cong. int. primatol. Soc.*, **1**, 222–46.

JONES, H. W., SCHIRMER, H. K. A., and HOOPES, J. E. (1968). A sex conversion operation for males with transsexualism. *Amer. J. Obstet. Gynaec.*, **100**, 101–9.

KOLLAR, E. J., BECKWITH, W. C., and EDGERTON, R. B. (1968). Sexual behavior of the ARL colony chimpanzees. *J. nerv. ment. Dis.*, **147**, 444–59.

MACLEAN, P. D. (1965). New findings relevant to the evolution of psychosexual functions of the brain. In *Sex research, new developments* (ed. J. Money). New York.

MASICA, D. N., MONEY, J., EHRHARDT, A. A., and LEWIS, V. G. (1969). IQ, fetal sex hormones and cognitive patterns: Studies in the testicular feminizing syndrome of androgen insensitivity. *Johns Hopk. med. J.*, **124**, 34–43.

MASTERS, W. H. and JOHNSON, V. E. (1966). *Human sexual response*. Boston.

MICHAEL, R. P., KEVERNE, E. B., and BONSALL, R. W. (1971). Phermones: Isolation of male sex attractants from a female primate. *Science* (*N.Y.*), **172**, 964–66.

MIKAMO, K. and WITSCHI, E. (1963). Functional sex-reversal in genetic females of *Xenopus laevis*, induced by implanted testes. *Genetics*, **48**, 1411–21.

MONEY, J. (1960). Phantom orgasm in the dreams of paraplegic men and women. *Arch. gen. Psychiat.*, **3**, 373–82.

—— (1961). Components of eroticism in man. I: The hormones in relation to sexual morphology and sexual desire. *J. nerv. ment. Dis.*, **132**, 239–48.

—— (1961). Components of eroticism in man. II: The orgasm and genital somesthesia. *J. nerv. ment. Dis.*, **132**, 289–97.

—— (1965). Influence of hormones on sexual behavior. In *Ann. Rev. Med.*, **16**, 67–82.

—— (1970). Use of an androgen-depleting hormone in the treatment of male sex offenders. *J. Sex Res.*, **6**, 165–72.

—— (1969). Sex reassignment as related to hermaphroditism and transsexualism. In *Transsexualism and sex reassignment* (ed. R. Green and J. Money). Baltimore.

—— (1971). Pre-natal hormones and intelligence: a possible relationship. *Impact Sci. Soc.*, **21**, 285–90.

—— (1975). Hermaphroditism and pseudohermaphroditism. In *Gynecologic endocrinology* (ed. J. J. Gold) (2nd edn). New York.

—— and ALEXANDER, D. (1967). Eroticism and sexual function in developmental anorchia and hyporchia with pubertal failure. *J. Sex Res.*, **3**, 31–47.

20

MONEY, J. and EHRHARDT, A. A. (1972). *Man and woman boy and girl: The differentiation and dimorphism of gender identity from conception to maturity*. Baltimore. (In press)

—— and MITTENTHAL, S. (1970). Lack of personality pathology in Turner's syndrome: Relation to cytogenetics, hormones and physique. *Behav. Genet.*, **1**, 43–56.

——, EHRHARDT, A. A., and MASICA, D. N. (1968). Fetal feminization induced by androgen insensitivity in the testicular feminizing syndrome: Effect on marriage and maternalism. *Johns Hopk. med. J.*, **123**, 105–14.

——, WIEDEKING, S., WALKER, P., MIGEON, C., MEYER, W., and BORGAONKAR, D. (1974). 47,XXY and 46,XY males with antisocial and/or sex-offending behavior: antiandrogen therapy plus counseling. *Psychoneuroendocrinology*, **1**.

NEUMANN, F. and ELGER, W. (1965). Proof of the activity of androgenic agents on the differentiation of the external genitalia, the mammary gland and the hypothalamic-pituitary system in rats. *Androgens in normal and pathological conditions*, pp. 169–85. International Congress Series No. 101. Amsterdam.

—— and —— (1966). Permanent changes in gonadal function and sexual behavior as a result of early feminization of male rats by treatment with an antiandrogenic steroid. *Endokrinologie*, **50**, 209–25.

PETRIE, A. (1967). *Individuality in pain and suffering*. Chicago.

PHOENIX, C. (1966). Psychosexual organization in nonhuman primates. *Conference on Endocrine and Neural Control of Sex and Related Behavior*. Puerto Rico.

TRIMBLE, M. R. and HERBERT, J. (1968). The effect of testosterone or oestradiol upon the sexual and associated behaviour of the adult female rhesus monkey. *J. Endocrinol.*, **42**, 171–85.

WARD, I. L. (1972). Prenatal stress feminizes and demasculinizes the behavior of males. *Science (N.Y.)*, **175**, 82–4.

WILKINS, L. (1965). *The diagnosis and treatment of endocrine disorders in childhood and adolescence* (third edition). Springfield, Illinois.

WITSCHI, E. (1956). Etiology of gonadal agenesis and sex reversal. In *Gestation, Transactions of the Third Conference* (ed. C. A. Villee). Princeton.

—— (1965). Hormones and embryonic induction. *Arch. Anat. micro. Morph. exp.*, **54**, 601–11.

YAMAMOTO, T. (1962). Hormonic factors affecting gonadal differentiation in fish. *Gen. comp. Endocrinology.*, Suppl. 1, 311–45.

YOUNG, W. C., GOY, R. W., and PHOENIX, C. H. (1965). Hormones and sexual behavior. In *Sex research, new developments* (ed. J. Money). New York.

3. SOCIAL DETERMINANTS OF MALE AND FEMALE ROLES AND RELATIONSHIPS

MARGARET MEAD

WEIGHT GIVEN TO CHILD-BEARING AND CHILD-REARING

The major determinant of sex roles in human societies has been the degree of weight given to the child-bearing and child-rearing functions in the social arrangements through which men and women co-operate with each other. For example, all social arrangements may hinge upon women's child-bearing functions: the way in which a dwelling is constructed, a canoe built, or a garden planned may be strictly related to the fact that women bear children. On the other hand, women's child-bearing functions may be seen completely to define her role but this role may be viewed as unimportant or dangerous or disqualifying for the activities that are valued most. In still a third type of society, especially where emphasis is placed upon valuable contributions that can be made by youth and by those past middle age, child-bearing and its attendant requirements may be overshadowed by other expected contributions.

Other variations on this central theme may be found in the extent to which food-getting, shelter-building, social control, and the other normal social activities are compatible with the specific characteristics of women as pregnant, lactating, menstruating, or menopausal. For example, in a nomadic society where the nomadism may be precariously related to a change of season or to intervals in which food is very scarce, it may frequently be necessary for the group to press on. In such a society, delivery of a child becomes an episode dangerous to the group and less likely to have a successful outcome if a newly delivered woman must immediately resume the march.

In general it may be said that where there is more diversification of roles and occupation, more complex division of labour and greater social stratification, there is less likelihood that the difference between men and women will be structured into the social expectations for each sex. Where the major division of labour is sexual, reproductivity will loom much larger and failure to bear a child will be more conspicuous and more likely to be compensated for by adoption and continuation of the child-bearing role, although in rare cases childlessness may become an advantage for specialized ritualistic activities.

ROLE CONFLICTS AND STRESS

Stress is introduced when the expected character and roles of men and women are less compatible with the requirements of parenthood. For example, if women are expected to be hardy and capable of very strenuous work, this may result in conflict between the requirements of maternity and her other economic or social activities. If men are expected to play a nurturing role towards young children, this may interfere in their carrying out such activities as aggressive defence of the group, dangerous raiding parties, long-distance trading, and similar pursuits. Whenever there is an incompatibility between social and parental expectations, as for example in the role expectations of a reigning queen or head of household, or the role of a subsidiary husband under a polyandrous structure, the result may either be heavy stress, or very elaborate social arrangements to overcome the discrepancies in the expected role performance. Examples of the latter are the chastity belts crusaders put on their wives as they left them for many years to be their administrative representatives; castration of males who are to be in close protective contact with women; or the introduction of women police and women warders with the growth of female criminality.

All societies display cultural expectations which are in many ways contrary to the observed actualities, especially when a trait to which cultural expectations are attached has wide variation or occurs discontinuously in a population. Stress on the individual occurs whenever he or she has traits falling outside of the expected range of deviation. This is illustrated for the trait of height in cases of dwarfism or gigantism. In most of the physical traits which differentiate men and women, there is great overlap: although males are on the average taller than females, many females are taller than males. But since the role expectations for men and for women often do not overlap, the stress accompanying such deviations will be felt differently: the male dwarf will suffer more than the female dwarf, the over-tall female more than the over-tall male. Where physical defects such as deafness or mutism are concerned, they may be seen contrastingly. For example, a deaf man who is a good provider of food may be able to obtain a wife, but a deaf woman who cannot hear her husband's voice may be unacceptable as a mate.

As the skills required of human beings become more complex, they may be assigned to one sex or the other in such a way that differential ability will be crippling to one sex. Thus, where only males of a selected social class are expected to learn to read, males of other classes and all females may suffer no stigma from the particular optical or cerebral defects which make reading difficult. In the rare cases where it is customary to give girls a greater degree of formal education than boys, the situation may be reversed and the girl who fails to learn to read may be more stigmatized than such a boy.

Where marriages are arranged on grounds which largely ignore the physical and mental qualities of the two partners, as occurs when there is child betrothal, kinship-regulated marital choice, or use of a go-between where considerations of wealth and social standing are paramount, married couples will manifest and deviate from the various expected contrasts between males and females in a wide variety of ways. The wife may be taller, the husband more garrulous, the wife more muscular, the husband better with fine work with his hands, to mention only a few combinations.

Where free mate selection and a large number of possible mate choices coincide, new factors enter. Although the individual who displays those qualities believed to be most desirable in members of his or her sex will apparently have the best chance to marry, many obscure compensations may enter in as one partner attempts to compensate for defects in the self, such as height or beauty, in the choice of the other. Marriages contracted on grounds of formal suitability — in height ratio, for example — may be found to differ markedly in other respects where sex roles are expected to be systematically differentiated. Thus, a tiny woman may prove to be able to dominate her large slow husband; a small weak-kneed man to be extremely prolific as a progenitor.

ATTRIBUTED BEHAVIOURAL TRAITS

Traits which may be arbitrarily assigned as either male or female far outnumber and outweigh any traits which have so far been found to be correlated with primary sex characters. For this reason, the more that a society emphasizes the importance of attributed rather than innate sex-related physical behavioural traits, the more likely it will be that stress will be introduced in individuals, as they will more frequently fail to conform to the cultural expectations. The more variety there is in the upbringing of girls and boys, the greater the opportunity for each to develop types of behaviour deemed appropriate only for the other sex. Schooling boys and girls together inevitably aggravates this situation, no matter how great an attempt may be made not to allow the appearance of abilities considered inappropriate for the sex of the pupils. Rebellion against the restrictions of culturally defined sex roles may be expected to correlate positively with such factors as an increase in schooling — for both sexes — in availability of occupational choice, and in the removal of restrictions on free movements. When one or more of these conditions, or similar ones, are present, more feminine rebellion demanding greater freedom and more male rebellion demanding exemption from the expected parental role may be expected.

CULTURAL STRESS

Within each sex, the emphasis placed upon the concomitants of primary sexual difference will also be instrumental in the amount of stress. Where the distinctively female physical crises of menarche, menstruation, defloration, conception, gestation, delivery, lactation, weaning, and menopause are heavily burdened by expectations of physical stress or by heavy social ceremonial emphasis, the cultural stress will be greater upon the individual whose physical make-up varies from the expected form. In societies which do not recognize menstrual pain, the occasional girl who experiences violent menstrual contractions will be anomalous and consequently under stress; in societies in which all women are expected to display morning sickness during first pregnancy, the woman who fails to do so may be treated as unfeminine. However, deviance in the form that physical events take is not the only important contributor to stress. The very ways in which such events are conceived by the culture will contribute to stress, and in some cases may also provide a solution for stress. In females, if first menstruation is accompanied by a tremendous amount of fuss and ceremonial, costuming and gift-giving, where the girl is the centre of attention, it may be the size and importance of the ceremonial itself that becomes the point of stress; girls without economic means who will go without ceremony may suffer less stress.

In none of these cases can arbitrary statements be made such as that defloration is or is not more stressful if institutionalized in virginity tests and public display. Rather it must be recognized that the way in which each sexually correlated but physiologically varying event is placed in the total social context is crucial. However, the more a society stresses those aspects of behaviour which have a recognized physical base, the sharper the contrast between men and women, even where the physical capacity in question — e.g. procreation — may be shared between the two sexes. Although modern research methods can often allocate responsibility for infertility to one partner or the other, the difference in the mechanisms involved still accentuates the primary difference between the sexes. Thus the identification of infertility may have very different effects on men and women, releasing in woman the capacities which are more usually expressed after the menopause, but crippling the creative capacities of men and in turn the creative capacities of their potentially fertile wives.

DIFFERENT CAREER LINES

A peculiar kind of stress is introduced by the different career-lines of men and women. In all societies to date, public achievement has been demanded of men, and child-bearing and child-rearing have been the principal demands made upon women. In the instances where male achievement levels off in middle age, as happens when purely physical skills are demanded, as in fishing or hunting, athletics or warfare, or where there are highly graduated career lines where the failure to ascend another step on the ladder is sharply accentuated, males experience a sense of defeat and depression which may require some outside stimulus — like a new wife — to dispell. Females, on the other hand, experience at menopause a renewed sense of energy and zest whether or not their reproductive role has been fulfilled. They are now free to pursue other tasks, often other roles. Indeed, in many societies, the postmenopausal woman, whether as queen mother, mother-in-law, or village elder freed from disabling taboos and restrictions, takes on new authority and new satisfactions.

Where both men and women live into late middle age, these differences in response to completed periods of a career-line may occasion a sharp break in monogamous marriages, as the husband finds his wife independently zestful, or the wife finds the husband seeking for new external stimuli to restore his confidence in his own powers. Such differences in response become particularly stressful in those societies where women are also permitted some degree of competitiveness in public life, and where the attribution of success and failure to men is much more definite and specific. A differential survival rate may result, as is the case between men and women in the United States, and the expectation on the part of males that their wives will outlive them and gather the fruits of their labours may in turn add to the stress for young married men. The difference in the sex-related incidence of ulcers — a predominantly female disease 70 years ago; a predominantly male disease in the 1940s — is an example of one way in which such contrasts in career lines may be expressed. Stress for married women is greater when the expectation of death in childbirth is greater; such expectations have been enormously reduced for women, while the expectation of death from degenerative disease for men who live to late middle age, under modern conditions, has increased.

INNATE PHYSICAL STATE
AND ATTRIBUTED TRAITS

It may be said that stress will result whenever social expectations link any mental or physical trait to some innate physical state that cannot be altered or can be altered only by most violent and exceptional means, when the innate physical state is not actually related to the attributed trait. This is true of skin colour, of secondary sex characters — such as size of breasts or size of genitals — or specific lineage, such as whether one is of a princely line. It should be possible to construct a multi-dimensional matrix within which an individual's actual and measurable traits can be arranged so as to show the extent to which actual capacities are correlated with expected capacities on the basis of cultural expectations. Such measurable traits would include height, IQ (as measuring relative expectation of success within a given educational system), skin

sensitivity, musical capacity, mathematical ability, eye/hand co-ordination, and many other attributes normally associated with some other innate condition like sex or skin colour.

Yet, in constructing such a matrix for an individual, it would be necessary to recognize that there are both primary and more subtle sources of stress. Primary stress may be introduced during adolescence and later, to the extent to which an individual deviates from expectation in a negative direction. Thus stress occurs for the overly short male, the overly tall female, the weak first-born in a society where primogeniture is important, the female first-born where the first-born should be a male, the aggressive young male Negro in the United States where docile caste behaviour is demanded by superordinate whites. Nevertheless, additional elements of stress may also be introduced. The male or female who seems to possess all of the expected characteristics may also be overly weighted with expected success, with guilt, and with far heavier demands than those made on individuals who conform less to the cultural expectations. Such differences may be compounded in various ways and often explain reversals between generations; where women are first emancipated, the least 'feminine' women may have the easier time, as an expectation of deviance may actually promote their success in a new, hitherto male role. However, a style of successful deviance may then be set, which will handicap those who follow: the 'masculine' woman may be forced into a role she does not wish to fill; the 'feminine' woman may be debarred from a role that was originally stylized merely as deviant.

RESEARCH AND SOCIAL POLICY

There is an urgent need for more research on the extent to which the exercise of procreative functions in women is positively correlated with health and with performance of other social roles. On the results of such research it would be possible for society to project a future in which sex roles become progressively less significant, or a future within which women's reproductivity — as individuals — must be safeguarded. There is no doubt, as comparative cultural and historical studies show, that almost any trait can be attributed and so produced into either sex and denied the other. We are less much less certain about the consequences. We do not even know whether the kind of creative result which can sometimes be attained by celibacy or abstinence, in which all of an individual's energies are channelled into activities other than sex and reproduction, can in fact be attained in women as well as men. We do know that the cessation of any expectation of maternity can release women's energies, but we do not know at what price. We do know that all of a man's capacity for individual achievement can be muted in the interests of his wife and children, and that this indeed has happened for almost all men since the dawn of history. We do not know what a release from parental responsibility would do for a man's motivation toward achievement and ability to contribute as an individual.

Considerations of stressfulness in the various arrangements for educating males and females and for division of labour inside and outside the home, need to be accompanied by an assessment of the social and individual costs and benefits of such stress. Too little stress may, like too little anxiety, so lower creativity as not to be worth working for.

REFERENCES†

ABRAHAM, K. (1922). Manifestations of the female castration complex. *Int. J. Psychoanal.*, 3, 1–29.

ABU LUGBOD, J. (1961). Egyptian marriage advertisements: Microcosm of a changing society. *Marr. Fam. Liv.*, 23, 127–36.

AGRIST, S. S. (1969). The study of sex roles. *J. soc. Issues*, 25, 215–32.

AINSWORTH, M.D. (1962). *Deprivation of maternal care*. Public Health Papers 14. Geneva.

APPEL, F. W. and APPEL, E. M. (1960). Intracranial variation in the weight of the human brain. In *Handbook of aging and the individual — psychological and biological aspects* (ed. Birren, J. E.), pp. 137 *et seq.* Chicago.

ARIWOOLA, O. (1965). *The African wife*. London.

ASWAD, B. C. (1967). Key and peripheral roles of nobel women in a Middle Eastern Plains village. *Anthrop. Quart.*, 40, 139–52.

BABCHUK, N. and BATES, A. P. (1962). Professor or producer: The two faces of academic man, *Soc. Forces*, 40, 341–8.

BALINT, M. (1937). A contribution to the psychology of menstruation. *Psychoanal. Quart.*, 6, 346–52.

BANKS, J. A. (1954). *Prosperity and parenthood: a study of family planning among the Victorian middle classes*. London.

BARRY, H. III, BACON, M. K., and CHILD, I. L. (1957). A cross-cultural survey of some sex differences in socialization. *J. abnorm. soc. Psychol.*, 55, 327–32.

BASTOCK, M. (1967). *Courtship: an ethological study*. Chicago.

BATESON, G. (1947). Sex and culture. *Ann. N.Y. Acad. Sci.*, 47, 603–64.

BEARD, M (1947). *Woman as force in history*. Toronto.

BEAUVOIR, S. (1953). *The second sex*. New York.

——— (1959). *Memoirs of a dutiful daughter*. Cleveland, Ohio.

BEIGEL, H. G. (1954). Body height in male selection. *J. soc. Psychol.*, 39, 257–68.

BEIGEL, H. G. (1963). *Advances in sex research*. New York.

BELL, D. (ed.) (1968). *Toward the year 2000: work in progress*. Boston.

BENEDEK, T. (1952). *Psychosexual function in women*. New York.

——— (1960). The organization of the reproductive drive. *Int. J. Psychoanal.*, 41, 1–15.

——— and RUBENSTEIN, B. (1939). Correlations between ovarian activity and psychodynamic processes: I. The ovulative phase; II. The menstrual phase. *Psychosom. Med.*, 1, 245 *et seq.*, 461 *et seq.*

BENEDICT, R. (1938). Continuities and discontinuities in cultural conditioning, *Psychiatry*, 1, 161–7.

——— (1946). *The chrysanthemum and the sword*. Boston.

BETTELHEIM, B. (1962). *Symbolic wounds: puberty rites and the envious male*. New York.

BIBRING, G. L., DWYER, T. F., HUNTINGTON, D. S., and VALENSTEIN, A. F. (1961). A study of the psychological processes in pregnancy and of the earliest mother–child relationship. *Psychoanal. Stud. Child.*, 16, 9–72.

BIRD, C. (1970). *Born female: the high cost of keeping women down*. New York.

BIRREN, J. E. (ed.) (1960). *Handbook of aging and the individual—psychological and biological aspects*. Chicago, Illinois.

———, BICK, M. W., and FOX, C. (1969). Age changes in the light threshold of the dark adapted eye. In *Handbook of aging and the individual — psychological and biological aspects* (ed. J. E. Birren), p. 513. Chicago, Illinois.

BLOOD, R. O., Jr and WOLFE, D. M. (1960). *Husbands and wives: the dynamics of married living*. Chicago, Illinois.

BOHANN, P. (ed.) (1970). *Divorce and after*. New York.

BOOTH, G. C. (1946). Variety in personality and its relation to health, *Rev. Religion*, 385–412.

BOWLBY, J. (1951). *Maternal care and mental health*. Monograph Series No. 2. Geneva, Switzerland.

BRECKINRIDGE, M. (1952). *Wide neighborhoods: a story of the frontier nursing service*. New York.

BRENTON, M. (1966). *The American male: a penetrating look at the masculinity crisis*. New York.

BRIFFAULT, R. S. (1927). *The mothers: a study of the origins of sentiments and institutions* (3 vols). London.

——— and MALINOWSKI, B. (1956). *Marriage: past and present*. Boston, Massachusetts.

BROFENBRENNER, M. and BUTTRICK, A. (1969). Population control in Japan: An economic theory and its application. *Law Contemp. Prob.*, 25, 536–57.

BROWN, F. (1961). Depression and childhood bereavement. *J. ment. Sci.*, 107, 754–77.

BROWN, J. K. (1963). A cross-cultural study of female initiation rites. *Amer. Anthrop.*, 65, 837–53.

——— (1970). Sex division of labor among the San Blas Cuna, *Anthrop. Quart.*, 43, 57–63.

BULLOUGH, V. L. (1964). *The History of prostitution*. New York.

BUXTON, J. (1963). Girls' courting huts in Western Mandari. *Man*, 63, 49–51.

CALHOUN, A. (1945). *A social history of the American family from Colonial times to the present*. New York.

CASSARA, B. B. (1962). *American women: the changing image*. Boston, Massachusetts.

CENTRAL STATISTICAL BOARD OF THE COUNCIL OF MINISTERS OF THE U.S.S.R. (1960). *Women in the U.S.S.R.*, Moscow.

CHAPMAN, J. D. (1968). *The feminine mind and body*. New York.

CHRISTENSEN, H. T. (1968). Children in the family: relationship of number and spacing to marital success, *J. Marr. Fam.*, 30, 283–9.

CITIZENS' ADVISORY COUNCIL ON THE STATUS OF WOMEN (1968). *American women 1968*. Washington, D.C.

CLARE, J. E. and KISER, C. V. (1951). Social and psychological factors affecting fertility: XIV. Preference for children of given sex in relation to fertility. *Milbank Mem. Fund Quart.*, 29, 440–92.

†There are a great many references to the status of women, and almost none to man, because the literature is so organized that the only time male roles are considered as one of two roles, with possible consequences, is when the role of women is being discussed.

CLARK, M. and ANDERSON, B. G. (1967). *Culture and aging: anthropological study of older Americans*. Springfield, Illinois.

CLARKSON, F. E., VOGEL, S. R., BROVERMAN, I. K., BROVERMAN, D. M., and ROSENCRANTZ, P. S. (1970). Family size and sex-role stereotypes. *Science (N.Y.)*, **167**, 390–2.

CLIGNET, R. (1970). *Many wives, Many powers: authority and power in polygynous families*. Evanston, Illinois.

COHEN, Y. A. (1964). *The transition from childhood to adolescence: cross-cultural studies of initiation ceremonies, legal systems, and incest taboos*. Chicago.

COMMISSION FOR INTERNATIONAL RELATIONS OF THE FEDERATION OF WOMEN'S ASSOCIATIONS OF YUGOSLAVIA (1961). *Women's rights in Yugoslavia*. Belgrade, Yugoslavia.

COSER, R. L. (1964). *The family: its structure and functions*. New York.

—— (ed.) (1969). *Life cycle and achievement in America*. New York.

COUNCIL OF MEDICAL WOMEN'S FEDERATION COMMITTEE REPORT (1957). An investigation of the menopause in one thousand women. In *Psychological development through the life span* (ed. S. L. Pressey and R. G. Kuhlen). New York.

COUNT, E. W. (1958). The biological basis of human sociality. *Amer. Anthrop.*, **60**, 1049–85.

CRAWLEY, A. E. (1931). Man and woman. In *The family* (ed. E. B. Reuter and J. R. Runner). New York.

CRESSY, E. H. (1955). *Daughters of changing Japan*. London.

CROOKE, W. (1922). The land and island of women. *Man India*, **2**, 216–19.

DAEDALUS (1964). The woman in America. *Daedalus*, Spring, 579–801.

DAHLSTROM, E. (ed.) (1971). *The changing roles of men and women*. Boston, Massachusetts.

DALY, M. (1968). *The church and the second sex*. New York.

D'ANDRADE, R. G. (1966). Sex differences and cultural institutions. In *The development of sex differences* (ed. E. Maccoby). Stanford, California.

DAVID, D. S. (1969). *Career patterns and values: a study of men and women in scientific, professional, and technical occupations*. New York.

DAVIS, K. (1965). The population impact on children in the world's agrarian countries. *Pop. Rev.*, **9**.

DEMARTINO, M. F. (ed.) (1963). *Sexual behavior and personality characteristics*. New York.

DEPREE, S. (1962). The influence of parental achievement expectations and role definitions on achievement motive development in girls. Unpublished honors thesis, University of Michigan, Ann Arbor.

DEUTCH, H. (1944–45). *The psychology of women* (2 vols). New York.

DEVEREUX, G. (1937). Institutionalized homosexuality of the Mohave Indians. *Hum. Biol.*, **9**, 498–527.

—— (1955). *A study of abortion in primitive societies*. New York.

DINGWALL, E. J. (1957). *The American woman*. New York.

DINITZ, S., DYNES, R. R., and CLARKE, A. C. (1954). Preferences for male or female children: traditional or affectional? *Marr. Fam. Liv.*, **16**, 128–30.

DIXON, M. (1949). The secondary social status of women: Class and caste applied to women's position. *Phylon X*.

DODGE, N. (1966). *Women in the Soviet economy: their role in economic, scientific, and technical development*. Baltimore, Maryland.

DRIVER, H. E. (1941). Girls' puberty rites in western North America. *Anthrop. Rec. Univ. California*, **6**, 21–90.

DURKHEIM, E. (1963). *Incest: the nature and origin of the taboo*. New York. (First published in French (1898) in Vol. 1 of *L'annee sociologique*.)

DYSON-HUDSON, R. (1960). Men, women and work in a pastoral society. *Nat. Hist.*, **69**, 42–57.

EARTHY, E. D. (1968). *Valenge women: the social and economic life of the valenge women of Portugese East Africa*. New York.

EISENSTEIN, V. W. (ed.) (1956). *Neurotic interaction in marriage*. New York.

ELLIS, H. (1927). *Man and woman* (6th ed.). New York.

ENGELS, F. (1941). *Origin of the family, private property and the state*. New York.

EQUAL EMPLOYMENT OPPORTUNITY COMMISSION (1967). *Guidelines on discrimination because of sex*. Washington, D.C.

ERIKSON, E. H. (1964a). *Childhood and society* (second edition). New York.

—— (1964b). Inner and outer space: reflections on womanhood. *Daedalus* Spring, 582–606.

—— (1968). *Identity, youth, and crisis*, New York.

ETZIONI, A. (1968). Sex control, science, and society, *Science (N.Y.)*, **161**, 1107–12.

EVANS-PRITCHARD, E. E. (1963). *Essays in social anthropology*. New York.

FAGLEY, R. M. (1960). *The population explosion and Christian responsibility*. New York.

FARBER, S. and WILSON, R. H. L. (1963). *The potential of woman*. New York.

FELDMAN, H. (1965). *Development of the husband and wife relationship: a research report*. New York.

FLEISCHMAN, D. E. (ed.) (1929). *An outline of careers for women: a practical guide to achievement*. New York.

FLÜGEL, J. C. (1947). *Men and their motives: psycho-analytical studies*. New York.

FORD, C. and BEACH, F. A. (1951). *Patterns of sexual behavior*. New York.

FORTUNE SURVEY (1946). Women in America. Part I. New York.

FOX, R. (1967). *Kinship and marriage: an anthropological perspective*. Baltimore, Maryland.

FRANK, L. K. (1954). The psychocultural approach in sex research. *Soc. Prob.*, **1**, 133–9.

FREEDMAN, R. (1963). *The sociology of human fertility: a trend report and bibliography*. Oxford, England.

FREEMAN, L. (1971). The changing role of women; a selected bibliography. *Bibliographic Series*, no. 9. III Title. Sacramento State College Library.

FREUD, S. (1918). *Totem and taboo*. New York.

GAGE, J. (1963). *Matronalia, essai sur les deviations et les organisations culturelles des femmes dans l'ancienne Rome*. Brussels, Belgium.

GEBHARD, P. H. (1958). *Pregnancy, birth, and abortion*. New York.

GEIGER, H. K. (1968). *The family in Soviet Russia*. Cambridge, Massachusetts.

GIFFEN, N. (1930). *The roles of men and women in Eskimo culture*. Chicago, Illinois.

GINZBERG, E. (1966). *Educated American women: self portraits*. New York and Londond.

—— and RAZAMOV, I. M. (1966). *Life styles of educated women*. New York.

GOODE, W. J. (1963). *World revolution and family patterns*. New York.

GOODY, J. R. (1956). A comparative approach to incest and adultery. *Brit. J. Sociol.*, **7**, 286–305.

GORDON, D. C. (1968). *Women of Algeria: an essay on change.* Cambridge, Massachusetts.

GORDON, R. E., GORDON, K. A., and GUNTHER, M. (1961). *The split-level trap.* New York and Toronto.

GORER, G. (1971). *Sex and marriage in England today.* London.

GOSHEN-GOTTSTEIN, E. R. (1966). *Marriage and first pregnancy; cultural influences on attitudes of Israeli women.* London and Philadelphia.

GREAT BRITAIN COMMITTEE ON HOMOSEXUAL OFFENCES AND PROSTITUTION (1963). *The Wolfenden Report: Report of the Committee on Homosexual Offenses and Prostitution.* New York.

HAAS, M. R. (1964). Men's and women's speech in Kosati. *Language*, **20**, 142–9.

HALL, E. T. (1966). *The hidden dimension.* New York.

HAMAMSY, L. S. (1957). The role of women in a changing Navaho society. *Amer. Anthrop.*, **59**, 101–11.

HARRINGTON, C. (1958). Sexual differentiation in socialization and some male genital mutilations. *Amer. Anthrop.*, **70**, 951–6.

HEATH, D. B. (1958). Sexual division of labor and cross-cultural research. *Soc. Forces*, **37**, 77–9.

HELLER, C. S. (ed.) (1969). *Structural social inequality: a reader in comparative social stratification.* New York.

HENRY, J. (1963). *Culture against man.* New York.

HILLIARD, M. (1960). *Women and fatigue.* New York.

HOBHOUSE, L. T. (1951). *Morals in evolution: a study in comparative ethics* (7th ed). London.

HOLLINGSHEAD, A. B. (1957). Cultural factors in mate selection. In *Psychological development through the life span* (ed. S. L. Pressey and R. G. Kuhlen). New York.

HOUGHTON, R. C. (1877). *Women of the Orient.* Cincinnatti and New York.

HUTCHINSON, G. E. (1959). A speculative consideration of certain possible forms of sexual selection in man. *Amer. Natur.*, **93**, 81–91.

ILIFF, F. G. (1954). *People of the Blue Water: my adventures among the Walapai and Havasupai Indians.* New York.

JACOBS, S. (1968). Berdache: a brief review of the literature. *Colorado Anthrop.*, **1**.

JACOBY, S. (1970). Women in Russia. *New Repub.*, **162**, 16–18.

JAFFE, F. S. (1964). Family planning and poverty, *J. Marr. Fam.*, **26**, 467–70.

JAHODA, M. and HAVEL, J. (1955). Psychological problems of women in different social roles — a case study of problem formulation in research. *Educ. Rec.*, **36**, 325–35.

JAMES, W. (1890). *The principles of psychology.* New York.

JOYCE, T. A. and THOMAS, N. W. (ed.) (1908). *Women of all nations.* New York.

KABERRY, P. M. (1952). *Women of the grassfields.* London.

KALISH, R. A., MALONEY, M., and ARKOFF, A. (1966). Cross-cultural comparisons of college student marital role preferences. *J. soc. Psychol.*, **68**, 41–7.

KEIFFER, M. G. and WARREN, P. A. (1970). Resource bibliography. In The impact of fertility limitation on women's life-career and personality. *Ann. N.Y. Acad. Sci.*, **175**, 781–1.1065.

KELMAN, H. (ed.) (1967). *Karen Horney: feminine psychology.* New York.

KESTENBERG, J. S. (1956). Vicissitudes of female sexuality. *J. Amer. Psychoanal. Ass.*, **4**, 453–76.

KHURI, F. I. (1970). Parallel cousin marriage reconsidered: a Middle Eastern practice that nullifies the effects of marriage on the intensity of family relationships, *Man*, **5**, 597–618.

KINSEY, A. C., POMEROY, W. B., and MARTIN, C. E. (1948). *Sexual behavior in the human male.* Philadelphia.

—— and THE STAFF OF THE INSTITUTE OF SEX RESEARCH, INDIANA UNIVERSITY (1953). *Sexual behavior in the human female.* Philadelphia and London.

KIRKPATRICK, C. (1938). *Nazi Germany: its women and family life.* Indianapolis, Indiana.

KLAUSNER, S. Z. (1968). Social aspects of sexual behavior. In *International encyclopedia of the social sciences*, (ed. D. L. Sills), Vol. XIV, pp. 201–8. New York.

KLEIN, V. (1948). *The feminine character: history of an ideology.* New York.

KOMAROVSKY, M. (1964). *Blue-collar marriage.* New York.

LANDES, R. (1940). A cult matriarchate and male homosexuality. *J. abnorm. soc. Psychol.*, **35**, 386–97.

LANDES, R. and ZBOROWSKI, M. (1950). Hypotheses concerning the Eastern European Jewish family. *Psychiatry*, **13**, 447–64.

LÉVI-STRAUSS, C. (1949). *Les structures élémentaires de la parenté.* Paris.

—— (1969). *The elementary structures of kinship.* Boston.

LEWIS, O. (1949). Husbands and wives in a Mexican village: a study of role conflict. *Amer. Anthrop.*, **51**, 602–10.

LOWIE, R. H. (1931). Woman and religion. In *The making of men* (ed. V. F. Calverton), pp. 744–57. New York.

LYNN, D. B. and SAWREY, W. L. (1959). The effects of father absence on Norwegian boys and girls. *J. abnorm. soc. Psych.*, **59**, 258–62.

MACCOBY, E. (ed.) (1966). *The development of sex differences.* Stanford, California.

MAKARENKO, A. S. (1967). *The collective family.* New York.

MALINOWSKI, B. (1953). *Sex and repression in savage society.* Londn and New York.

MALINOWSKI, B. (1962). *The sexual life of savages in North-Western Melanesia: an ethnographic account of courtship, marriage, and family life among the natives of the Trobrian Islands, British New Guinea.* New York.

MARRIOTT, A. (1948). *Maria: the potter of San Ildefonso.* Norman, Oklahoma.

MASON, O. T. (1894). *Woman's share in primitive culture.* New York.

MASTERS, W. H. and JOHNSON, V. E. (1966). *Human sexual response.* Boston, Massachusetts.

MATTHEWS, E. and TIEDEMAN, D. V. (1964). Attitudes toward career and marriage and the development of life style in young women. *J. Counsel. Psychol.*, **11**, 375–84.

MEAD, M. (1928). *Coming of Age in Samoa*, New York.

—— (1932). Contrasts and comparisons from primitive society. *Ann. Amer. Acad. polit. soc. Sci.*, **160**, 23–8.

—— (1935a). *Sex and temperament in three primitive societies.* New York.

—— (1935b). Woman: position in society: primitive. In *Encyclopedia of the social sciences* (ed. E. R. A. Seligman and A. Johnson), Vol. 15, pp. 439–42. New York.

—— (1936). On the institutionalized role of women and character formation. *Zeitschr. Sozialforsch.*, **5**, 69–75.

—— (1943). The family in the future. In *Beyond victory* (ed. R. N. Anshen), pp. 68–87. New York.

—— (1946a). Cultural aspects of women's vocational problems in post World War II. *J. Consult. Psychol.*, **10**, 23–8.

—— (1946b). What women want. *Fortune*, **34**, 172–5, 218.

—— (1947). The concept of culture and the psychosomatic approach. *Psychiatry*, **10**, 57–76.

—— (1949). *Male and female.* New York.

—— (1953). The impact of cultural changes on the family. In *The family in the urban community* (ed. D. Tyler), pp. 3–17, Detroit.

—— (1957a). American man in a woman's world. *N.Y. Times Mag.*, **11**, 20–3.

27

MEAD, M. (1957b). Changing patterns of parent-child relations in an urban culture. *Int. J. Psycho-Anal.*, **38**, 369–78.

—— (1957c). Review of *The American woman*, by J. Dingwall. *N.Y. Herald Tribune Book Review*, May 26, 10.

—— (1960). Problems of the late adolescent and young adult. In *Children and youth in the 1960's: survey papers prepared for the 1960 White House Conference on Children and Youth*. Washington, D.C.

—— (1961). Cultural determinants. *Amer. J. publ. Hlth.*, **51**, 1552–4.

—— (1962). A cultural anthropologist's approach to maternal deprivation. In *Deprivation of maternal care: a reassessment of its effects*. Public Health Papers No. 14, pp. 45–62. Geneva.

—— (1963a). Families and maternity care around the world. *Bull. Amer. College Nurse Midwifery*, **8**, 2–7.

—— (1963b). Some general considerations. In *Expression of the emotions in man* (ed. P. H. Knapp), pp. 318–27. New York.

—— (1963c). *Totem and taboo* reconsidered with respect. *Bull. Menninger Clin.*, **27**, 185–99.

—— (1965a). Introduction, and epilogue. In *American Women* (ed. M. Mead and F. B. Kaplan), pp. 3–6; 181–204. New York.

—— (1965b). Marriage isn't for every woman, *Chatelaine*, **38**, 74–77.

—— (1967a). Introduction. In *The peaceful revolution: birth control and the changing status of women*. New York.

—— (1967b). The life cycle and its variations: The division of roles. *Daedalus*, Summer, 871–5.

—— (1968a). Family life is changing. In *The new encyclopedia of child care and guidance* (ed. S. M. Gruenberg), pp. 675–82. New York.

—— (1968b). Incest. In *International encyclopedia of the social sciences* (ed. D. L. Sills), Vol. VII. New York.

—— (1969). The American woman today. In *The 1969 world book year book*, pp. 78–95. Chicago, Illinois.

—— (1970a). Anomalies in American post-divorce relationships. In *Divorce and after* (ed. P. Bohannan), pp. 97–112. New York.

—— (1970b). Working mothers and their children. *Manpower*, **2**, 3–6.

—— (1976). A comment on the role of women in Agriculture. In *Women and world development* (ed. I. Tinker and M. Bo Bramsen), pp. 9–11. Overseas Development Council (AAAS), Washington, D.C.

—— and KAPLAN, F. B. (1965). *American women*. New York.

—— and NEWTON, N. (1965). Conception, pregnancy, labor and the puerperium in cultural perspective. In *First International Congress of Psychosomatic Medicine and Childbirth*. pp. 51–4. Paris.

—— and —— (1967). Cultural patterning of perinatal behavior. In *Childbearing — its social and psychological aspects* (ed. S. A. Richardson and A. I. Guttmacher). Baltimore.

—— and —— (1969). Voluntary population control? Three experts debate possibility. *Planned Parent. News*, **1**, 3.

MEGGITT, M. J. (1964). Male–female relationships in the Highlands of Australian New Guinea. *Amer. Anthrop.* special publication, **66**, 204–24.

MENNINGER, K. A. (1943). Psychiatric aspects of contraception. *Bull. Menninger Clin.*, **7**, 36-40.

MIDDLETON, R. (1962). Brother–sister and father–daughter marriage in Ancient Egypt. *Amer. sociol. Rev.*, **27**, 603–11.

MOLL, A. (1921). *Handbuch der Sexualwissenschaften* (second edition). Leipzig.

MONEY, J. (ed.) (1965). *Sex research, new developments*. New York.

——, HAMPSON, J. G., and HAMPSON, J. L. (1957). Imprinting and the establishment of gender role, *Arch. Neurol. Psychiat.*, **77**, 333–6.

MUELLER, G. (1961). Legal regulation of sexual conduct. *Legal Almanac Ser.* No. 9. New York.

MUKHOPADHYAY, A. (1957). Sati as a social institution in Bengal. *Bengal Past Pres.*, **76**, 99–115.

MURDOCK, G. P. (1937a). Comparative data on the division of labor by sex. *Soc. Forces*, **15**, 551–3.

—— (1937b). Correlation of matrilineal and patrilineal institutions. In *Studies in the science of society* (ed. G. P. Murdock), pp. 445–70. New Haven, Connecticut.

—— (1949a). The social regulation of sexual behavior. In *Psycho-sexual development in health and disease* (ed. P. H. Hoch and J. Zubin). New York.

—— (1949b). *Social structure*. New York.

—— (1964). Cultural correlates of the regulation of premarital sex behavior. In *Process and pattern in culture: essays in honor of Julian H. Steward* (ed. R. Manners), pp. 399–410. Chicago.

MURPHY, R. F. (1959). Social structure and sex antagonism, *J. Southwest. Anthrop.*, **15**, 89–98.

MYRDAL, A. and KLEIN, V. (1956). *Women's two roles: at home and work*. London.

NELSON, C. (1968). Changing roles of men and women: illustrations from Egypt. *Anthrop. Quart.*, **41**, 57–77.

NEWTON, N. (1955). *Maternal emotions*. New York.

O'NEILL, W. L. (1967). *Divorce in the progressive era*. New Haven, Connecticut.

PARSONS, T. and BALES, R. F. (1955). *Family, socialization and interaction process*. Glencoe, Illinois.

PATAI, R. (ed.) (1967). *Women in the modern world*. New York.

PIERCE, R. I. (1970). *Single and pregnant*. Boston.

PLOSS, H. H., BARTELS, M., and BARTELS, P. (1935). *Woman: an historical gynaecological and anthropological compendium* (3 vols). London.

POLGAR, S. (1966). Sociocultural research in family planning in the United States: review and prospects. *Hum. Organ.*, **25**, 321–9.

POLLAK, O. and FRIEDMAN, A. S. (ed.) (1968). *Family dynamics and female sexual delinquency*. Palo Alto, California.

PRASAD, T. (1959). Fate of a barren woman in Hindu society, *Ind. Folklore*, **2**, 15–19.

PRINCE PETER OF GREECE AND DENMARK (1963). *A study of polyandry*. The Hague, Holland.

PUTNAM, E. J. (1910). *The lady*. New York.

RAINWATER, L. (1965). *Family design: marital sexuality, family size, and contraception*. Chicago, Illinois.

—— and YANCEY, W. L. (1967). *The Moynihan report and the politics of controversy*. Cambridge, Massachusetts.

RAPHAEL, D. (1973). *The tender gift: breastfeeding*. Englewood Cliffs, New Jersey. (In press)

REED, R. B. (1947). Social and psychological factors affecting fertility: VII. The interrelationship of marital adjustment, fertility control, and size of family, *Milbank Mem. Fund Quart.*, **25**, 383–425.

REITZENSTEIN, F. (1923). *Das Weib bei den Naturvolkern*. Berlin.

RICHARDS, A. I. (1961). *Chisungu: a girls' initiation ceremony among the Bamba of Northern Rhodesia*. New York.

ROBIN, F. (1967). *Kinship and marriage: an anthropological perspective*. Baltimore, Maryland.

RODGERS, D. A., ZIEGLER, F. J., ALTROCCHI, J., and LEVY, N. (1965). A longitudinal study of the psycho-social effects of vasectomy, *J. Marr. Fam.*, **27**, 1–222.

ROHEIM, G. (1932). Psychoanalysis of primitive cultural types. *Int. J. Psycho-Anal.*, **13**, 1–222.

ROSEN, L. (1969). Matriarchy and lower class Negro male delinquency, *Soc. Problems*, **17**, 175–88.

ROSENBLATT, P. C. (1966). A cross-cultural study of child rearing and romantic love. *J. Person. soc. Psychol.*, **4**, 336–8.

SANFORD, N. (1966). *Self and society: social change and individual development.* New York.

SCHEINFELD, A. (1944). *Women and men.* New York.

SEBBELOV, G. (1913). The social position of men and women among the natives of East Malekula: New Hebrides. *Amer. Anthrop.*, **15**, 273–94.

SEWARD, G. H. (1946). *Sex and the social order.* New York and London.

SHETTLES, L. B. (1961). Conception and birth sex ratios: a review. *Obstet. Gynecol.*, **18**, 122–30.

SILVERMAN, S. F. (1967). The life crisis as a clue to social functions. *Anthrop. Quart.*, **40**, 127–8.

SIMON, R. J., CLARK, S. M., and TIFFT, L. L. (1966). Of nepotism, marriage, and the pursuit of an academic career. *Sociol. Educ.*, **39**, 344–58.

SKARD, A. G. (1965). Maternal deprivation: the research and its implications. *J. Marr. Fam.*, **27**, 3.

SKULTANS, V. (1970). The symbolic significance of menstruation and the menopause. *Man*, **5**, 639–51.

SLATER, P. E. and SLATER, D. A. (1965). Maternal ambivalence and narcissism: a cross-cultural study. *Merrill Palmer-Quart.*, **11**, 241–59.

SODDY, K. (ed.) (1955–6). *Mental health and infant development* (2 vols). London and New York.

—— (ed.) (1961). *Identity: mental health and value systems.* London.

—— (1967). *Men in middle life.* London.

SOUTHALL, A. (ed.) (1961). *social change in modern Africa.* London.

SPARROW, G. (1970). *Women who murder.* New York.

SPINDLER, L. and SPINDLER, G. (1958). Male and female adaptations in culture change. *Amer. Anthrop.*, **60**, 217–33.

STEPHENS, W. N. (1963). *The family in cross-cultural perspective.* New York.

STERN, K. (1965). *The flight from woman.* New York.

STOLLENWERK, T. T. (1967). *Back to work ladies: a career guide for the mature woman.* New York.

STOLLER, R. (1968). *Sex and gender: on the development of masculinity and femininity.* New York.

STRACHEY, J. (ed.) (1965). *New introductory lectures in psychoanalysis.* New York.

STRATHERN, M. (1972). *Women in between.* Seminar Press, New York.

STROUSE, J. (ed.) (1974). *Women and analysis.* Grossman, New York.

STYCOS, J. M. (1967). Contraception and Catholicism in Latin America. *J. soc. Issues*, **23**, 115–34.

TANNER, J. M. and INHELDER, B. (ed.) (1956–60). *Discussions on child development* (4 vols). London and New York.

TAYLOR, G. R. (1953). *Sex in history.* London.

TERMAN, L. M. and MILES, C. M. (1936). *Sex and personality: studies in masculinity and femininity.* New York.

THOMAS, W. I. (1907). *Sex and society.* Chicago.

TIETZE, C. (1962). *Surgical sterilization of men and women: a selected bibliography.* New York.

TIETZE, C. (1965). History of contraceptive methods. *J. Sex Res.*, **1**, 69–85.

TIETZE, C. and LEHFELDT, H. (1961). Legal abortion in Eastern Europe. *J. Amer. med. Ass.*, **175**, 1149–54.

TIGER, L. (1969). *Men in groups.* New York.

TURNER, R. H. (1964). Some aspects of women's ambition. *Amer. J. Sociol.*, **70**, 271–85.

VAERTUNG, M. and VAERTUNG, M. (1932). *The dominant sex: a study in the sociology of sex differentiation.* London.

VAN DEN BERG, J. H. (1961). *The changing nature of man.* New York.

WESTERMARCK, E. A. (1921). The history of human marriage (5th ed) (3 vols). London.

WOLFENSTEIN, M. (1965). Changing patterns of adolescence. In *Transcultural psychiatry* (ed. A. V. S. de Reuck and R. Porter), pp. 195–215. London.

WOLFF, H. G. (1947). Protective reaction patterns and disease. *Ann. intern. Med.*, **27**, 944–69.

WORTIS, H. and RABINOWITZ, C. (ed.) (1972). *The women's movement: social and psychological perspective.* New York.

YOUNG, F. W. (1965). *Initiation ceremonies: a cross-cultural study of status dramatization.* Indianapolis, Indiana.

4. INTERRELATIONSHIPS BETWEEN AGGRESSION AND SEXUALITY IN RHESUS MONKEYS: RELEVANCE OF THE PRIMATE MODEL

D. ZUMPE and RICHARD P. MICHAEL

INTRODUCTION

Social organization and behaviour can be regarded as the resultants of a number of species characteristics (size, mobility, nutritional requirements, reproductive characteristics, etc.) that interact with various environmental factors (distribution of food, density of cover, presence of predators, etc.) in such a way as to produce life-support and reproductive strategies that are optimal for the survival of the individual and of the species (Crook *et al.* 1976). A given species in a particular habitat will be subjected to different selection pressures that sometimes operate in opposition to each other. For example, in a physically small species with restricted mobility, the distribution of food in the environment might promote territoriality that serves to space individuals over the available resources. In order to reproduce, however, a male and female must come together for mating, and frequently achieve this by advertising their sex and location by visual, auditory, or olfactory displays; this in turn exposes them to predation. On a broad level of analysis, knowledge of adaptive advantages enables predictions to be made about the social organization of a species. Thus, in a pelagic, marine environment, where conditions are stable and food supply is evenly distributed, a common form of social organization is the school that helps to protect its anonymous individual members from predation. In a more variable and unstable fresh-water environment, a greater proportion of territorial species exhibit temporary pair bonding: here, the adaptive advantage of parental care for larger eggs, permitting delayed hatching of more mature and less vulnerable young, is the overriding one.

Territoriality, either in the individual or in a social group of individuals, is intimately related to intraspecific aggression, an appetence for which can be demonstrated experimentally in a highly territorial species such as the damsel fish, *Microspathodon chrysurus* (Rasa 1971). The adaptive advantages of intraspecific aggression in the maintenance of closed social systems, and in reproductive selection, are also clearly apparent; however, there must be temporary or more permanent mechanisms for preventing injury or death when individuals have to come into close proximity for reproduction or for group cohesion. Studies on a number of species of fishes and birds have shown that there is a close relationship between reproductive activity and agonistic behaviour, and have provided evidence that many courtship displays originated from

the conflict between agonistic tendencies against, and sexual attraction for, the partner (Tinbergen 1959). The onset of the breeding season is often associated with increased aggressivity towards conspecifics, especially by males, which may lead to the establishment of breeding territories. Not surprisingly, when females first approach males in their territories, they are often attacked repeatedly, and even during early courtship, sexual displays may break down into overt aggression between the partners (robin, *Erythacus rubecula*: Lack (1943); chaffinch, *Fringilla coelebs*: Hinde (1953); ten-spined stickleback, *Pygosteus pungitius*: Morris (1958). However, such aggression may be redirected (Bastock, Morris, and Moynihan 1954) towards a third individual or towards inanimate objects as courtship proceeds (fishes of the family *Cichlidae*: Baerends and Baerends-Van Roon (1950); corn bunting, *Emberiza citrinella*: Andrew (1957); gulls and kittiwakes, *Larus argentatus, L. ridibundus*, and *Rissa tridactyla*: Moynihan (1955); Tinbergen (1959)). In some cases, threats directed just past or away from the partner have become ritualized into courtship displays (ducks, *Anatidae*: Lorenz (1941)).

All species of primates studied to date exhibit intraspecific aggression, but its frequency and intensity appear to vary widely between species (*Alouatta villosa*: Altmann (1959); *Macaca mulatta*: Altmann (1962); Southwick *et al.* (1965); *M. radiata*: Simonds (1965); *Papio ursinus* and *P. anubis*: Hall (1962); Hall and DeVore (1965); *P. hamadryas*: Kummer (1968); *Cercopithecus aethiops*: Struhsaker (1967); *Erythrocebus patas*: Hall (1965); *Cercocebus albigena*: Chalmers (1968); *Pan troglodytes*: Goodall (1965); Reynolds and Reynolds (1965); van Lawick-Goodall (1968); *Gorilla gorilla*: Schaller (1963), and between different groups of the same species (*M. mulatta*: Singh (1966); *P. anubis*: Paterson (1973)). Furthermore, within the group itself the frequency of agonistic interactions increases with social change (*M. mulatta*: Southwick (1967); Marsden (1968); Bernstein *et al.* (1974), and varies with the level of sexual activity, namely, increasing at the start of the breeding season and varying in relation to the female's reproductive cycle (*Lemur catta*: Jolly (1966); *Saimiri sciureus*: Latta *et al.* (1967); Baldwin (1968); *Cercocebus albigena*: Chalmers (1968); *M. mulatta*: Carpenter (1942); Altmann (1962); Rowell (1963), Vandenbergh and Vessey (1968); Vessey (1973); Gordon and Bernstein (1973); *M. fuscata*: Imanishi (1963); *P. anubis*: Bolwig (1959); *Pan troglodytes*: Köhler (1925); Yerkes (1939); Nowlis (1942)).

There is, therefore, overwhelming evidence that in a great many vertebrate species, and certainly in primates, intraspecific aggression is the rule rather than the exception, and that mechanisms exist which modify the level and intensity of the aggression exhibited towards conspecifics in different situations. It seems highly probable that the human is no exception, and that in man, too, mechanisms exist whereby agonistic tendencies are modified and utilized to ensure the formation and maintenance of social and sexual bonds. We have become particularly interested in the way in which bonds between prospective sexual partners are both established and fragmented by the normal interaction of sexual and agonistic tendencies (we exclude here highly pathological conditions), and by the causal factors underlying these mechanisms. In the human, such an analysis would be, of course, tremendously complex and very difficult to conduct even if the ethical and cultural problems could be overcome. Nevertheless, it now seems opportune, with the current state of knowledge, to study these matters on a comparative basis in a range of higher primates that exhibit both an aggressive potential and well-marked sexual bonding.

SOCIAL AND REPRODUCTIVE ORGANIZATION IN THE RHESUS MONKEY

Under free-ranging conditions, rhesus monkeys live in troops that may comprise as many as 100 or more males and females together with their young. Individual troops have well-defined home ranges which may overlap somewhat; however, troops tend to avoid each other in the areas of overlap. Males are generally dominant over females, and the adults of each sex, at least in captivity, exhibit hierarchical rank orders, with the male hierarchy being rather more linear and well-defined than the female hierarchy. Sexual activity is largely restricted to a 4-month period which, in the natural habitat in North India, lasts from October to February (Southwick *et al.* 1965; Lindburg 1971). During the mating season, females periodically begin to approach and mate with several different males and, after a few days, a female forms temporary consort (pair) bonds with a male and mates exclusively with him for from a few days up to 2 or more weeks. Thereafter, the female may again mate promiscuously but then becomes sexually inactive for a while before she again starts approaching males, approximately 1 month (28-day menstrual cycle) after the previous initiation of sexual activity. Copulation consists of a greatly variable number of mounts by the male on the female, each mount generally being associated with intromission and pelvic thrusting, and terminating in a mount with ejaculation. Mounts may be initiated either by the male or by the female; the female may refuse the male's mounting attempt or, conversely, initiate mounts by means of sexual invitations to the male (see below). Both between mounts and after the ejaculatory mount one partner typically grooms the other (Carpenter

1942; Altmann 1962; Koford 1965; Kaufmann 1965). Gestation lasts about 5·5 months, and in North India females give birth to a single infant during a period lasting from March till May (Southwick *et al.* 1961; Lindburg 1971). During the non-mating season, free-ranging males on Cayo Santiago undergo testicular regression (Conaway and Sade 1965).

EXPERIMENTS WITH RHESUS MONKEYS

As a first step in analysing the factors underlying sexual bonding in the rhesus monkey, we have used the adult, oppositely sexed pair in a cage situation as the basic unit of study. This eliminates several important variables such as spatial factors, effects of other conspecifics, dominance, and mother/infant relations (Southwick 1967; Harlow and Harlow 1962). In the studies reported below, behavioural observations were made on feral-raised adults that were imported directly from India. After a period of quarantine and acclimatization, observations on individual pairs were made in large observation cages from behind one-way vision mirrors. Tests were of 60-minute duration, and all social, sexual, and agonistic behaviours were recorded in sequence and timed to the nearest 30 seconds (Michael *et al.* 1966, 1967a; Michael *et al.* 1968). As a rule, males were tested on consecutive days with each of two female partners, and females with each of two male partners, in order to control for individual differences and partner preferences. Tests were conducted 5 or 6 days a week, and the timing and sequence of tests were kept constant to control for diurnal activity cycles. When not being tested, all animals were housed in individual cages to prevent unobserved behavioural interactions from influencing test scores. Despite the highly artificial testing conditions, social, sexual, and agonistic behaviours were remarkably similar to those seen under free-ranging conditions, except that their frequencies per hour were usually higher in the laboratory situation. Detailed accounts of the behaviour encountered in tests, and the behavioural indices derived from them, are given elsewhere (Michael and Welegalla 1968; Michael and Zumpe, 1970a, b; Zumpe and Michael 1970a, b).

Behaviour during the menstrual cycle
When males are paired with intact females whose oviducts have been ligated to prevent pregnancy, many behavioural changes occur in relation to the menstrual cycle that, at first glance, appear somewhat confusing. This is because the behavioural patterns vary from pair to pair and, within a given pair, from cycle to cycle. Changes in the total number of mounts per test were found to fall into four major patterns in relation to the stage of the female's menstrual cycle: (A) those with well-defined maxima near mid-cycle, sharp declines in the luteal phase, and a secondary rise just before menstruation; (B) those with sustained high levels during the follicular phase, again sharp declines early

31

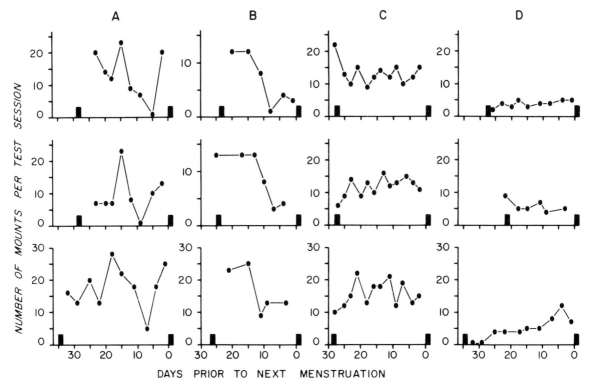

FIG. 4.1. Changes in the number of mounts per test by male rhesus monkeys in relation to the menstrual cycle of their female partners. Examples from 12 pairs of animals showing the four main types of mounting pattern, two with rhythmicity (types A and B) and two without rhythmicity (types C and D). Solid rectangles indicate vaginal bleeding. (From Michael 1971.)

in the luteal phase, and with low levels persisting until the next menstruation; (C) cycles without evidence of any rhythmicity but with high levels of mounting activity throughout; and (D) cycles with low mounting activity throughout (Fig. 4.1) (Michael 1971).

As mentioned earlier, mounts may be initiated either by the male or by the female's sexual invitations, and the male's mounting attempt may be refused or accepted by the female. It was therefore of interest to examine how behavioural changes in the male, on the one hand, and in the female, on the other, interact to produce the different types of mounting rhythm. In approximately half of the cases with mounting rhythms (types A and B), females remained receptive (did not refuse and continued making invitations throughout the cycle), but seemed to vary in their stimulus value to the male, so that the mounting rhythm resulted primarily from a decline in the number of male mounting attempts in the luteal phase. In addition, there was a decline in the number of female sexual invitations that were accepted by the male. In the other half of the cases, the stimulus value of the female remained relatively unchanged throughout the cycle, since males almost invariably accepted female invitations and attempted mounting. However, the females' receptivity appeared to fluctuate so that the mounting rhythm resulted from

an increase in the number of female refusals and a decline in the number of female sexual invitations during the luteal phase of the cycle. Fig. 4.2 shows two examples of the latter type of case and illustrates how

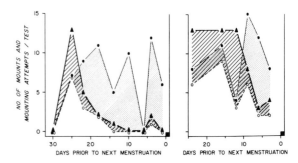

FIG. 4.2. Illustrating in two cycles how mounting rhythms (type A on left, type B on right) result from male mounting attempts, female refusals, and female sexual invitations. The female contributes positively, by initiating mounts, during the first parts of the cycles (hatched area), and negatively during the second parts of the cycles by actively refusing (stippled area). Where hatched and stippled areas overlap, the female is inviting and refusing in the same test. Triangles: mounts per test; filled circles: male mounting attempts; open circles: successful mounting attempts. (From Michael and Welegalla 1968.)

32

the behaviour of the male and female interacted to produce a type A and a type B mounting cycle (Michael and Welegalla 1968).

Under natural conditions it is hardly likely, of course, that an unreceptive female would remain in the close vicinity of a male with sexual ambitions towards her. Conversely, a male would not tolerate the sexual approaches of a female for which he has no sexual interest. Even under laboratory conditions, where a male and female are confined within a testing cage, changes in the female's sexual receptivity and sexual attractiveness (Michael *et al.* 1967*b*) interact to increase the chance of fertilization. This is achieved by maximizing the frequency of ejaculation near the time of ovulation (Fig. 4.3). The upper part of the figure compares our rhesus monkey data with some human data (Udry and Morris 1968); the lower part shows the rhesus monkey data smoothed by plotting 2-day means. The mean number of ejaculations occurring from the first to the twelfth reverse cycle days was significantly

lower than that from the thirteenth to the twenty-fourth reverse cycle days (*t* test, *P* < 0·001). The similarity between the timing of the behavioural changes in rhesus monkey and man points to the existence of a neuro-endocrine mechanism that is common to both species.

Hormonal factors influencing sexual interactions
The observations described above confirmed and amplified those made in the field and firmly related the behavioural changes to the stages of the menstrual cycle. Since ovariectomy abolishes all behavioural rhythms and, in many cases, greatly reduced sexual activity (Michael, Herbert, and Welegalla 1966, 1967), it seemed highly probable that ovarian hormones are playing a key role in determining the interactions of the pair. As in the human, plasma oestradiol levels in the female rhesus monkey rise sharply to a maximum 24–48 hours before ovulation but then decline to low levels in the luteal phase. Plasma progesterone levels are low during the follicular phase, start to increase just before the oestradiol peak, and reach high levels in the luteal phase of the cycle. Plasma testosterone levels are fairly low throughout but reach a maximum on the same day as the oestradiol peak (Bosu *et al.* 1972; Krey *et al.* 1973; Hess and Resko 1973). The effects of ovarian hormones on female sexual receptivity and attractiveness were therefore investigated by pairing males with ovariectomized females receiving hormone replacement treatments.

1. Female receptivity. Receptivity can be measured by (1) the number of male mounting attempts, and (2) the number of sexual invitations. The female can actively initiate mounting by the male by means of specific gestures and postures. The sexual presentation, whereby the female adopts the receptive stance with her hindquarters directed towards the male, is shared by many Old World primates (*Cercocebus albigena*: Chalmers (1968); *Macaca mulatta*: Carpenter (1942); Altmann (1962); *Papio ursinus*: Bolwig (1959); Hall (1962); *P. hamadryas*: Zuckerman (1932); Kummer (1968); *Theropithecus gelada*: Spivak (1968); *Hylobates lar*: Carpenter (1940); *Pan troglodytes*: Yerkes (1939); Goodall (1965); *Gorilla gorilla*: Hess (1973)). Rhesus monkeys also initiate mounting by means of three other gestures: the 'hand-reach' (a slap on the ground with one hand), the 'head-duck' (a quick lowering of the head relative to the shoulders), and the 'head-bob' (a rapid upward jerk of the head) (Michael and Zumpe 1970*a*). Although these three gestures are less effective than the presentation in stimulating male mounts, they are made with greater frequency and are responsible for initiating just as many mounts as the presentation posture. Using these measures as criteria, female receptivity was decreased by ovariectomy, and there were increased numbers of refusals and decreased numbers of sexual invitations (especially hand-reaches, head-ducks, and head-bobs). Fig. 4.4 shows changes in female sexual invitations and refusals, and changes in

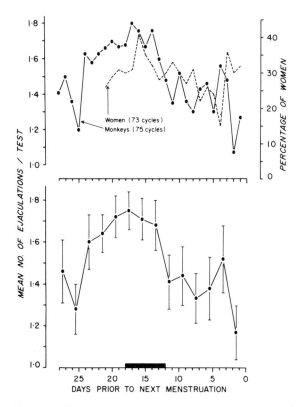

FIG. 4.3. *Upper part*: comparison of the copulatory activity of rhesus monkey and man in relation to the menstrual cycle. Filled circles: mean number of ejaculations per test (32 pairs of rhesus monkeys); dashed line: percentage of women reporting sexual intercourse (40 women) (Udry and Morris, 1968). *Lower part*: rhesus monkey data smoothed by plotting means of 2 consecutive days. Vertical bars give standard errors of means. Horizontal bar gives expected time of ovulation (Hartman 1932). (From Michael and Zumpe 1970*c*.)

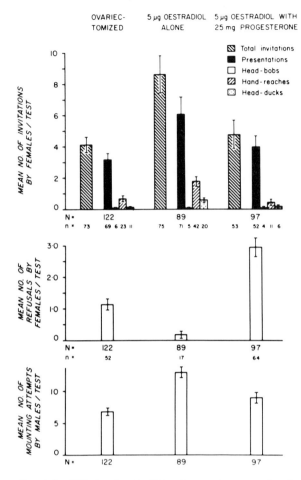

OVARIEC-TOMIZED   5 µg OESTRADIOL ALONE   5 µg OESTRADIOL WITH 25 mg PROGESTERONE

FIG. 4.4. Effects of oestradiol and progesterone on female receptivity (invitations and refusals) and attractiveness (male mounting attempts). Oestrogen enhances both the females' receptivity and their attractiveness to males while progesterone reverses these effects. Vertical bars give standard errors of means; N = numbers of tests; n = numbers of tests in which behaviours occurred (8 pairs). (From Zumpe and Michael 1970a, by courtesy of the Association for the Study of Animal Behaviour.)

male mounting attempts, when ovariectomized females were first treated with oestradiol alone and subsequently with progesterone in addition (Zumpe and Michael 1970a). Clearly, oestrogen enhances the receptivity of females and, although an increase in male mounting attempts occurred, the number of refusals declined and the number of female sexual invitations increased. When progesterone was given, these effects were reversed. Thus, oestrogen increases receptivity while progesterone suppresses it, and this action of progesterone contributes to the decline in the male's ejaculations during the luteal phase of the cycle.

2. *Female attractiveness.* Female attractiveness can be measured by several behavioural indices including (1) the number of male mountings attempts and (2) the

latency from the start of the test to the first male mounting attempt. As assessed by these indices, oestrogen increases female attractiveness and progesterone decreases it (Fig. 4.4, bottom histograms). It is now known that female attractiveness is mediated in part by olfactory cues, and that substances appear in the vaginal secretions of oestrogen-treated females that stimulate the sexual activity of males (Michael and Keverne 1970; Keverne and Michael 1971). These substances are volatile and, if males are made anosmic, the substances are without any behavioural effects (Michael and Keverne 1968). We take the view that they can be regarded as acting in a manner analogous to that of a pheromone in lower mammals. Gas chromatographic studies and mass spectrometry have characterized these chemicals as a series of short-chain fatty acids. Their production in vaginal secretions is stimulated by oestrogen and suppressed by progesterone but they are, in fact, products of bacterial action (Curtis *et al.* 1971; Bonsall and Michael 1971; Michael *et al.* 1971; Michael *et al.* 1975a). The role of hormones appears to be that of modulating the level of substrate available for microbial activity. It is of interest that these same substances are present in the vaginal secretions of women with normal menstrual cycles, and that concentrations are at maximum near the expected time of ovulation. However, in women using oral contraceptives (who do not ovulate), the midcycle increase is abolished (Michael *et al.* 1974, 1975b). We do not, however, know whether these volatile acids are used as olfactory signals in the human (Michael *et al.* 1976).

Effects of the behaviour of the partner on sexual interactions.

Olfactory signals are not the only factors that contribute to stimulating interest in the partner; numerous others do so too. Rhesus monkeys exhibit marked individual differences and partner preferences, and it is difficult to predict a male's level of performance with one female from his behaviour with another. This is reminiscent of the human situation. The factors responsible for these individual differences and preferences remain largely unknown but would include anatomical, hormonal, and behavioural characteristics, particularly the agonistic and grooming interactions. Unfortunately, many of the behavioural indices used to assess sexual motivation (the readiness to copulate) are not independent of each other. To give an extreme example: a female cannot express her lack of receptivity by refusing the male's mounting attempts if he fails to make any. Similar considerations apply in less extreme cases. For example, if an intact female makes fewer sexual invitations at midcycle than at other times (Michael and Welegalla 1968), it cannot be inferred that she is therefore less receptive, because the male is also mounting and frequently at midcycle and the female has less need and opportunity to invite.

A knowledge of the effects of ovarian hormones on behaviour enables us to use them rather specifically to

34

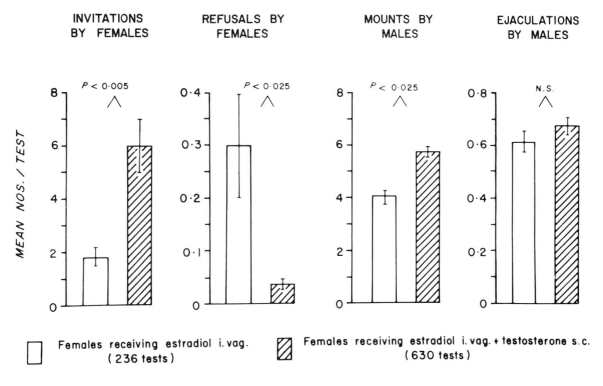

INVITATIONS BY FEMALES — REFUSALS BY FEMALES — MOUNTS BY MALES — EJACULATIONS BY MALES

MEAN NOS. / TEST

☐ Females receiving estradiol i. vag. (236 tests)

▨ Females receiving estradiol i. vag. + testosterone s.c. (630 tests)

FIG. 4.5. Administering testosterone to ovariectomized, oestrogen-treated females significantly increases their invitations and decreases refusals without any corresponding changes in ejaculations by their male partners. Vertical bars give standard errors of means. Wilcoxon matched-pairs signed-ranks test (12 pairs). (From Michael and Zumpe 1978.)

answer certain questions. Thus, testosterone increases the receptivity of ovariectomized females without much increasing their attractiveness to males (Michael *et al.* 1972). In the experiments described below, it is used to manipulate the female's receptivity. The intravaginal administration of small amounts of oestrogen, on the other hand, increases female attractiveness without much affecting her receptivity (Michael and Saayman 1968), and this treatment is used here to manipulate the sexual activity of her male partners. In the first experiment, oestrogen-treated females receive testosterone to examine its effects on female sexual invitations in a situation where males are mounting and ejaculating regularly. Fig. 4.5 shows that there is a significant increase in invitations and decrease in refusals although ejaculatory activity remains unchanged. When testosterone is withdrawn, invitations declined in the absence of any changes in male sexual activity (Fig. 4.6). This demonstrates that testosterone enhances female sexual motivation even when one controls for the rewarding effect of the male's copulation (Michael and Zumpe 1978).

In the second experiment, the effect of the male partner's ejaculatory activity on female sexual motivation is examined by relating the numbers of invitations made by testosterone-treated females to whether or not

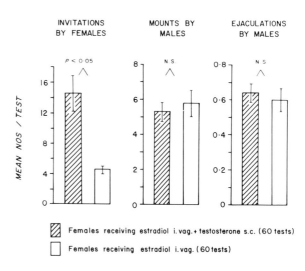

INVITATIONS BY FEMALES — MOUNTS BY MALES — EJACULATIONS BY MALES

MEAN NOS / TEST

▨ Females receiving estradiol i. vag. + testosterone s.c. (60 tests)

☐ Females receiving estradiol i. vag. (60 tests)

FIG. 4.6. Withdrawing testosterone from ovariectomized, oestrogen-treated females significantly decreases their invitations without any corresponding changes in the sexual behaviour of their male partners. Vertical bars give standard errors of means. Sign test (6 pairs). (From Michael and Zumpe 1978.)

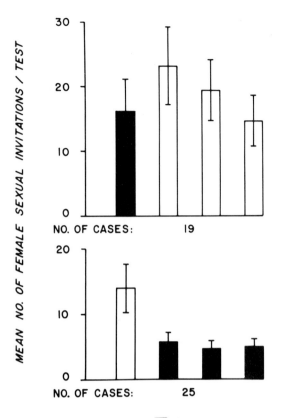

FIG. 4.7. The effects of ejaculation on female sexual invitations in sequences of 4 successive tests (5 pairs). *Upper part*: after invitations increase during the first and second non-ejaculatory tests (two-way analysis of variance, $P < 0.025$), they decline again in the third non-ejaculatory test ($P < 0.05$) to levels in the initial ejaculatory tests. *Lower part*: after a decrease in invitations during the first ejaculatory test ($P < 0.005$), there are no further changes. Vertical bars give standard errors of means. (From Zumpe and Michael 1977.)

the male ejaculates during a test. Fig. 4.7 shows that there is a significant increase in sexual invitations during the first and second non-ejaculatory tests following a test with ejaculation, and a subsequent decline to initial levels (upper part). In contrast, a decline in invitations during ejaculatory tests following a test without ejaculation is not followed by any further changes (lower part) (Zumpe and Michael 1977). These data demonstrate that the occurrence of ejaculation has a marked, if short-term, effect on the invitational behaviour of sexually excited female rhesus monkeys.

Factors affecting agonistic interactions

Changes in the rhesus female's endocrine status during the menstrual cycle can result in a lack of synchrony

between the motivational states of the partners. For instance, early in the luteal phase the sexual motivation of the female may decline rapidly while that of the male remains relatively high (Fig. 4.2). This can lead to a conflict of interests and a revival of agonistic tendencies between the partners. It is a matter of great interest to try to understand how the aggressive tendencies within the consort pair are used adaptively and resolved.

1. Direct aggression within the pair. Under our testing conditions, levels of agonistic interactions between intact males and females are generally quite low in the

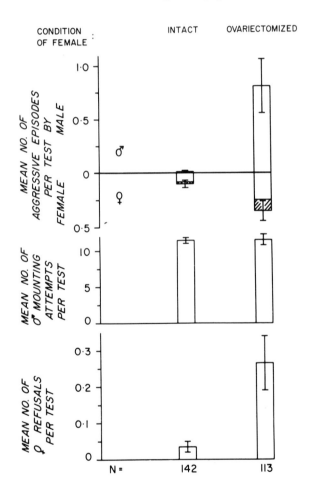

FIG. 4.8. Ovariectomy markedly increases the aggressive interactions between partners (4 pairs). Aggression by females is both in response to that initiated by males and also in response to male mounting attempts (hatched area) as receptivity declines. Vertical bars give standard errors of means; N = numbers of tests. (From Michael 1969.)

majority of pairs, so that it is desirable to administer hormones to ovariectomized females in order to accentuate the behavioural events. Even so, many pairs do not show aggression sufficiently often for quantitative analysis, so that some caution should be exercised in generalizing from the data presented below. Fig. 4.8 shows the effects of ovariectomy on direct aggression (number of episodes during which an animal threatened, hit, or bit the partner) where the male sexual interest, as measured by the number of male mounting attempts, did not decline significantly (lower part). Ovariectomy, which results in a decline in female receptivity, is associated with a marked increase in agonistic interactions within the pair, particularly with increased male aggression. Female aggression also increases, but a third of this increase is in response to male mounting attempts — 'unreceptive' aggression (hatched area). Fig. 4.9 shows the effects of oestrogen and progesterone on aggressive interactions where male sexual interest in females does not change very much. As female receptivity increases with oestrogen treatment, male aggression disappears. However, the overall level of agression by females remains unchanged, but that com-ponent associated with male mounting attempts (hatched area) is abolished. It would seem, then, that 'spontaneous' aggression by the female increases with oestrogen treatment. Progesterone administration, which decreases female receptivity, is associated with a very marked increase in female aggression, but this increase is entirely due to aggressive responses to male mounting attempts. Comparison with the untreated condition shows that there is about three times as much 'spontaneous' and about three times as much 'unreceptive' aggression by females that are treated with oestrogen and progesterone in combination. The males remain remarkably tolerant of the increased aggressivity of their partners.

These data indicate (1) that aggression arises between the pair when one but not the other partner is ready to copulate, and (2) that, contrary to expectations, oestrogen enhances the female's aggressivity while apparently affording her some protection from aggression by the male (Michael and Zumpe 1970b). This interpretation would be consistent with the observations made in the field (Carpenter 1942). Under free-ranging conditions, females spontaneously begin to approach males when they first become receptive although initially prone to being attacked. After establishment of consort bonds, however, females are shown a considerable degree of tolerance by their male partners. This raises the question of how the agonistic tendencies between the sexually interacting partners are prevented from expressing themselves in such a way as to disrupt sexual bonding and copulation.

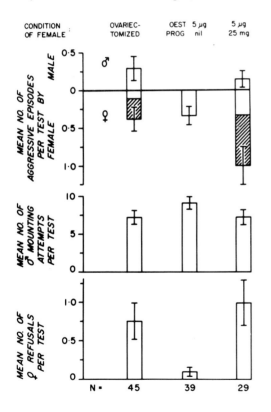

FIG. 4.9. Administration of oestradiol to ovariectomized females does not change their level of aggression although they become receptive (fewer refusals) and male aggression ceases. Progesterone increases female refusals and aggression, but only that component of the latter associated with male mounting attempts (hatched area) (3 pairs). Vertical bars give standard errors of means; N = numbers of tests. (From Michael and Zumpe 1970b, by courtesy of the Association for the Study of Animal Behaviour.)

2. *Aggression directed away from the sexual partner.* Under our testing conditions, about half the males and females exhibit aggressive gestures and movements that are characterized by being directed *away from*, rather than towards, the partner. Although our one-way vision mirrors are angled in such a way that animals can see neither their own reflections nor those of their partners, animals will suddenly begin to stare fixedly at some spot in front of or above the cage, as though they were catching sight of something, and will start making threats in that direction (threatening-away). The significance of this somewhat strange cage behaviour was not immediately apparent to us, but it gradually became clear that it was a 'vacuum activity'. Often the animal threatening-away glances over its shoulder at the partner as though enlisting its cooperation. Not infrequently, the partner will join in so that both animals are threatening together in the same general direction. The central feature of threatening-away behaviour is that it is never directed towards the partner. This behaviour pattern generally begins just before the start of a mounting series, continues between mounts, and invariably stops after ejaculation has occurred (Zumpe and Michael 1970b). Individuals vary greatly in the frequency with which they exhibit this behaviour, and for a given pair either the male or the female may be the main initiator.

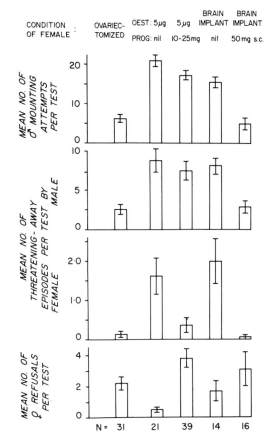

CONDITION OF FEMALE :	OVARIEC-TOMIZED	OEST: 5μg PROG: nil	5μg 10-25mg	BRAIN IMPLANT nil	BRAIN IMPLANT 50mg s.c.

FIG. 4.10. The upper two sets of histograms show a well-marked positive correlation between male mounting attempts and male threatening-away episodes. Male and female threatening-away episodes are positively correlated *only* when the female is receptive. When females receive progesterone, refusals increase, receptivity declines, and they no longer join in with the male's threatening-away behaviour (2 pairs). Vertical bars give standard errors of means; N = numbers of tests. (From Zumpe and Michael 1970*b*, by courtesy of the Association for the Study of Animal Behaviour.)

Fig. 4.10 shows changes in the frequency of threatening-away by males and females when their sexual interest in each other was changed by treating the females with ovarian hormones. Threatening-away by the male is closely associated with his sexual interest in the female; increasing when mounting attempts increase and decreasing when they decline. However, the female joins in with his behaviour only when receptive. Female threatening-away increases with oestrogen treatment, but declines with progesterone-induced unreceptivity. Threats by sexually interacting animals towards (1) other conspecifics,(2) mirror reflections, and (3) nothing in particular have been described previously (*Macaca mulatta*: Ball and Hartman (1935); Hinde and Rowell (1962); Altmann (1962); *Erythrocebus patas*: Hall (1967)). Joint threatening-away by sexual partners is obviously a useful mechanism for

directing onto the environment the aggression existing between the pair. In a social species under free-ranging conditions, of course, such threats will almost invariably be directed towards other conspecifics in the vicinity. This helps to isolate the sexually interacting pair from interference by other group members and will consolidate consort bonds. Threatening-away from the partner is high when direct threats towards the partner are low, and this lends further support to the view that it may be regarded as redirected aggression.

The findings outlined above demonstrate the extraordinarily closely knit interrelationships that exist between aggressive and sexual tendencies in a higher primate. This becomes apparent not only during the behavioural interactions of the animals themselves, but can also be demonstrated in phylogenetic terms. Thus, as in many fishes and birds, aggression directed away from the prospective sexual partner both discharges in a harmless way the aggression aroused by the partner and also serves to consolidate sexual bonds. Further, there is evidence that individual components of redirected aggression in the rhesus monkey have become ritualized into specifically female invitational gestures, namely, the hand-reach, head-duck, and head-bob (Zumpe and Michael 1970*a*). A similar derivation of courtship displays from agonistic behaviour has been elucidated in lower vertebrates, for example, 'inciting' in ducks (Lorenz 1941). In several social primate species, enlisting the aid of another individual in threatening at a third is not solely characteristic of the sexually bonded pair ('protected threat', *Papio hamadryas*: Kummer (1968). Of course, in the human family and in human societies, instances of the utilization of, at least, analogous mechanisms abound: the 'scapegoat', the 'straw man', 'identification with the aggressor', the use of 'an external threat' by national leaders, etc.

Effects of novel stimuli

Thus far, we have mainly considered the effect on agonistic interactions of changing the sexual behaviour of the pair, and this is fairly easily done by using hormone treatments. It is obviously of considerable interest to look at the reverse situation, and to see whether there are any effects on sexual activity when the agonistic interactions of the pair are changed; this is best achieved by altering environmental stimuli. This was done by introducing novel stimuli in the form of (1) unfamiliar female partners and (2) a large mirror in which both partners can see themselves (this mimics the presence of conspecifics). Four castrated, testosterone-treated males were paired for many months with the same four ovariectomized, oestrogen-treated females ('old' females); during this period, ejaculatory activity declined gradually. Fig. 4.11 (*left*) shows the effects on ejaculation and on redirected aggression when the 'old' female partners are abruptly replaced by four similarly treated unfamiliar females ('new' females). A marked increase in male and female

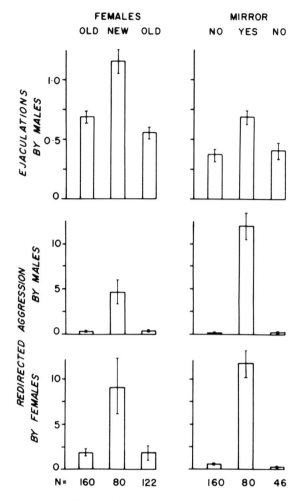

FEMALES
OLD NEW OLD

MIRROR
NO YES NO

EJACULATIONS BY MALES

REDIRECTED AGGRESSION BY MALES

BY FEMALES

N = 160   80   122   160   80   46

FIG. 4.11. Effects of changing environmental stimuli on the sexual potency of castrated, testosterone-treated male rhesus monkeys (16 pairs). Left-hand sets of histograms: replacing females that had been tested with males for many months by new, unfamiliar females results in an abrupt increase in ejaculations and in redirected aggression. Right-hand sets of histograms: exposure to mirrors, to give the illusion of other monkeys, produces similar effects. Vertical bars give standard errors of means; N = numbers of tests. (Michael and Zumpe, unpublished observations.)

redirected aggression is associated with almost twice as much ejaculatory activity (two-way analysis of variance, $P < 0.001$ in all males). Reintroducing the 'old' females immediately reverses the behavioural changes. After a year of regular testing, during which redirected aggression and ejaculatory activity again declined, large mirrors were placed outside the testing cages. Fig. 4.11 (*right*) shows that the presence of mirrors (conspecifics) changes levels of both redirected aggression and ejaculatory activity in the same direction as the presence of unfamiliar females (Michael and Zumpe, unpublished observations). These results are rather difficult to

understand, but may best be conceptualized in the following way. If the stimulating properties of the partner are held constant for excessively long periods of time, there is a decline in the level of arousal which adversely affects both agonistic and sexual activity. However, conditions that will stimulate either behaviour will also immediately and rapidly restore the other.

CONCLUSIONS

The rhesus monkey appears to be a very appropriate model for studying those aspects of the sexual and agonistic interactions that are relatively inaccessible to experimentation in the human for ethical reasons. This is not simply because the rhesus monkey has a 28-day menstrual cycle, a highly developed neocortex, and a complex social organization. More significantly, the rhesus monkey has a complicated system of communication (visual, auditory, tactile, and olfactory) which is partly genetically determined but which is also susceptible to modification by experiential factors. The resulting behavioural plasticity is expressed by the wide variation in the behaviour patterns of individual animals and, therefore, in the behaviour of a given animal with different partners. This is exemplified by the various types of mounting patterns shown by males during the menstrual cycles of their partners. This feature of primate behaviour is naturally something of a headache for the experimentalist because it makes for a certain lack of neatness in one's results. But it is this variation and plasticity, in contrast to the inflexibility and stereotypy of rat or cat reproductive behaviour, that makes the primate model germane to the human condition.

It is a complex task to develop the experimental tools needed to analyse primate communication systems, and it may take years rather than months for the experimental data to fall into place. Although we have not dealt here with factors operating principally in the male, it is now abundantly clear that sexual attraction in rhesus monkeys results in part from hormonally induced changes both in the female's sexual interest in the male and in his sexual interest in her. The changes in female receptivity and attractiveness are very closely interrelated with changes in aggressive tendencies, and consort bonds appear to become established when the sexual attraction between partners is associated with a redirection onto the environment of the aggression existing within the pair. Copulatory success seems to be greatest when agonistic tensions have declined, namely, after the establishment of consort bonds. However, in a situation where aggression has reached very low levels, male potency can be increased dramatically by reintroducing agonistic tension into the sexual situation, and this occurs entirely as a result of manipulating environmental factors in castrated, testosterone-treated males where there can be no activation of the gonads. The non-hormonal determinants of male potency clearly merit further study.

39

REFERENCES

ALTMANN, S. A. (1959). Field observations on a howling monkey society. *J. Mammal.*, **40**, 317–30.

—— (1962). A field study of the sociobiology of rhesus monkeys (*Macaca mulatta*). *Ann. N.Y. Acad. Sci.*, **102**, 338–435.

ANDREW, R. J. (1957). The aggressive and courtship behaviour of certain *Emberizinae*. *Behaviour*, **10**, 225–308.

BAERENDS, G. P. and BAERENDS-VAN ROON, J. M. (1950). An introduction to the study of the ethology of cichlid fishes. *Behaviour*, Suppl. 1, 1–242.

BALDWIN, J. D. (1968). The social behavior of adult male squirrel monkeys (*Saimiri sciureus*) in a semi-natural environment. *Folia primatol*, **11**, 35–79.

BALL, J. and HARTMAN, C. G. (1935). Sexual excitability as related to the menstrual cycle in the monkey. *Am. J. Obstet. Gynec.*, **29**, 117–19.

BASTOCK, M., MORRIS, D., and MOYNIHAN, M. (1954). Some comments on conflict and thwarting in animals. *Behaviour*, **6**, 66–84.

BERNSTEIN, I. S., GORDON, T. P., and ROSE, R. M. (1974). Aggression and social controls in rhesus monkey (*Macaca mulatta*) groups revealed in group formation studies. *Folia primatol.*, **21**, 81–107.

BOLWIG, N. (1959). A study of the behaviour of the chacma baboon, *Papio ursinus*. *Behaviour*, **14**, 136–63.

BONSALL, R. W. and MICHAEL, R. P. (1971). Volatile constituents of primate vaginal secretions. *J. Reprod. Fert.*, **27**, 478–9.

BOSU, W. T. K., HOLMDAHL, T. H., JOHANSSON, E. D. B., and GEMZELL, C. (1972). Peripheral plasma levels of oestrogens, progesterone, and 17α-hydroxy-progesterone during the menstrual cycle of the rhesus monkey. *Acta Endocrinologica*, **71**, 755–64.

CARPENTER, C. R. (1940). A field study in Siam of the behavior and social relations of the gibbon (*Hylobates lar*). *Comp. Psychol. Monogr.*, **16**, 1–212.

—— (1942). Sexual behavior of free-ranging rhesus monkeys (*Macaca mulatta*). *J. comp. Psychol.*, **33**, 113–62.

CHALMERS, N. R. (1968). The social behaviour of free living mangabeys in Uganda. *Folia primatol.*, **8**, 263–81.

CONAWAY, C. H. and SADE, D. S. (1965). The seasonal spermatogenic cycle in a free-ranging band of rhesus monkeys. *Folia primatol.*, **3**, 1–12.

CROOK, J. H., ELLIS, J. E., and GOSS-CUSTARD, J. D. (1976). Mammalian social systems: structure and function. *Anim. Behav.*, **24**, 261–74.

CURTIS, R. F., BALLANTINE, J. A., KEVERNE, E. B., BONSALL, R. W., and MICHAEL, R. P. (1971). Identification of primate sexual pheromones and the properties of synthetic attractants. *Nature (Lond.)*, **232**, 396–8.

GOODALL, J. (1965). Chimpanzees of the Gombe Stream Reserve. In *Primate behavior* (ed. I. DeVore), pp. 425–73. New York.

GORDON, T. P. and BERNSTEIN, I. S. (1973). Seasonal variation in sexual behavior of all-male rhesus troops. *Am. J. phys. Anthrop.*, **38**, 221–6.

HALL, K. R. L. (1962). The sexual, agonistic, and derived social behaviour patterns of the wild chacma baboon, *Papio ursinus*. *Proc. zool. Soc. Lond.*, **139**, 283–327.

—— (1965). Behaviour and ecology of the wild patas monkey, *Erythrocebus patas*, in Uganda. *J. Zool., Lond.*, **148**, 15–37.

—— (1967). Social interactions of the adult male and adult females of a patas monkey group. In *Social communication among primates* (ed. S. A. Altmann), pp. 261–80. Chicago.

—— and DEVORE, I. (1965). Baboon social behavior. In *Primate behavior* (ed. I. DeVore), pp. 53–110. New York.

HARLOW, H. F. and HARLOW, M. K. (1962). Social deprivation in monkeys. *Scient. Amer.*, **207**, 136–46.

HARTMAN, C. G. (1932). Studies in the reproduction of the monkey *Macacus (Pithecus) rhesus*, with special reference to menstruation and pregnancy. *Contr. Embryol.*, **23**, 1–161.

HESS, D. L. and RESKO, J. A. (1973). The effects of progesterone on the patterns of testosterone and estradiol concentrations in the systemic plasma of the female rhesus monkey during the intermenstrual period. *Endocrinology*, **92**, 446–53.

HESS, J. P. (1973). Some observations on the sexual behaviour of captive lowland gorillas, *Gorilla g. gorilla* (Savage and Wyman). In *Comparative ecology and behaviour of primates* (ed. R. P. Michael and J. H. Crook), p. 507–519. London.

HINDE, R. A. (1953). The conflict between drives in the courtship and copulation of the chaffinch. *Behaviour*, **5**, 1–31.

—— and ROWELL, T. E. (1962). Communication by postures and facial expressions in the rhesus monkey (*Macaca mulatta*). *Proc. zool. Soc. Lond.*, **138**, 1–21.

IMANISHI, K. (1963). Social behavior in Japanese monkeys, *Macaca fuscata*. In *Primate social behavior* (ed. C. H. Southwick), pp. 68–81. London.

JOLLY, A. (1966). *Lemur behavior. A Madagascar field study*. Chicago.

KAUFMANN, J. H. (1965). A three-year study of mating behavior in a free-ranging band of rhesus monkeys. *Ecology*, **46**, 500–12.

KEVERNE, E. B. and MICHAEL, R. P. (1971). Sex-attractant properties of ether extracts of vaginal secretions from rhesus monkeys. *J. Endocr.*, **51**, 313–22.

KOFORD, C. B. (1965). Population dynamics of rhesus monkeys on Cayo Santiago. In *Primate behavior* (ed. I. DeVore), pp. 160–174. New York.

KÖHLER, W. (1925). *The mentality of apes*. London.

KREY, L. C., BUTLER, W. R., WEISS, G., WEICK, R. F., DIERSCHKE, D. J., and KNOBIL, E. (1973). Influences of endogenous and exogenous gonadal steroids on the actions of synthetic LRF in the rhesus monkey. In *Hypothalamic hypophysiotropic hormones* (ed. C. Gual and E. Rosemberg), pp. 39–47. International Congress Series No. 263, Amsterdam.

KUMMER, H. (1968). *Social organization of Hamadryas baboons*. Chicago.

LACK, D. (1943). *The life of the Robin*. London.

LATTA, J., HOPF, S., and PLOOG, D. (1967). Observation on mating behavior and sexual play in the squirrel monkey, *Saimiri sciureus*. *Primates*, **8**, 229–46.

LINDBURG, D. G. (1971). The rhesus monkey in North India: an ecological and behavioural study. In *Primate behavior: developments in field and laboratory research* (ed. L. A. Rosenblum), Vol. 2, pp. 1–106. New York.

LORENZ, K. (1941). Vergleichende Bewegungsstudien an Anatinen. *J. Orn.*, Suppl. 3, 194-294.

MARSDEN, H. M. (1968). Agonistic behaviour of young rhesus monkeys after changes induced in social rank of their mothers. *Anim. Behav.*, **16**, 38–44.

MICHAEL, R. P. (1969). Effects of gonadal hormones on displaced and direct aggression on pairs of rhesus monkeys. In *The biology of aggressive behaviour* (ed. S. Garattini and E. B. Sigg), pp. 172–178. Amsterdam.

—— (1971). Neuroendocrine factors regulating primate behavior. In *Frontiers in neuroendocrinology* (ed. L. Martini and W. F. Ganong), pp. 359–398. London.

—— and KEVERNE, E. B. (1968). Pheromones in the communication of sexual status in primates. *Nature (Lond.)*, 218, 746–9.

—— and —— (1969). A male sex-attractant pheromone in rhesus monkey vaginal secretions. *J. Endocr.*, 46, xx–xxi (Abstract).

—— and —— (1970). Primate sexual pheromones of vaginal origin. *Nature (Lond.)*, 225, 84–5.

—— and SAAYMAN, G. S. (1968). Differential effects on behaviour of the subcutaneous and intravaginal administration of oestrogen in the rhesus monkey (*Macaca mulatta*). *J. Endocr.*, 41, 231–46.

—— and WELEGALLA, J. (1968). Ovarian hormones and the sexual behaviour of the female rhesus monkey (*Macaca mulatta*) under laboratory conditions. *J. Endocr.*, 41, 407–20.

—— and ZUMPE, D. (1970a). Sexual initiating behaviour by female rhesus monkeys (*Macaca mulatta*) under laboratory conditions. *Behaviour*, 36, 168–86.

—— and —— (1970b). Aggression and gonadal hormones in captive rhesus monkeys (*Macaca mulatta*). *Anim. Behav.*, 18, 1–10.

—— and —— (1970c). Rhythmic changes in the copulatory frequency of rhesus monkeys (*Macaca mulatta*) in relation to the menstrual cycle and a comparison with the human cycle. *J. Reprod. Fert.*, 21, 199–201.

—— and —— (1978). Effects of androgen administration on sexual invitations by female rhesus monkeys (*Macaca mulatta*), *Anim. Behav.* (In press).

——, BONSALL, R. W., and KUTNER, M. (1975a). Volatile fatty acids, 'copulins', in human vaginal secretions. *Psychoneuroendocrinology*, 1, 153–63.

——, ——, and WARNER, P. (1974). Human vaginal secretions: volatile fatty acid content. *Science (N.Y.)*, 186, 1217–19.

——, ——, and —— (1975b). Primate sexual pheromones. In *Olfaction and taste* (ed. D. A. Denton and J. P. Coghlan), Vol. v, pp. 417–24. New York.

——, ——, and ZUMPE, D. (1976). Evidence for chemical communication in primates. *Vitam. Horm.*, 34, 137–86.

——, HERBERT, J., and WELEGALLA, J. (1966). Ovarian hormones and grooming behaviour in the rhesus monkey (*Macaca mulatta*) under laboratory conditions. *J. Endocr.*, 36, 263–79.

——, ——, and —— (1967a). Ovarian hormones and the sexual behaviour of the male rhesus monkey (*Macaca mulatta*) under laboratory conditions. *J. Endocr.*, 39, 81–98.

——, KEVERNE, E. B., and BONSALL, R. W. (1971). Pheromones: isolation of male sex attractants from a female primate. *Science (N.Y.)*, 172, 964–6.

——, SAAYMAN, G. S., and ZUMPE, D. (1967b). Sexual attractiveness and receptivity in rhesus monkeys. *Nature (Lond.)*, 215, 554–6.

——, ——, and —— (1968). The suppression of mounting behaviour and ejaculation in male rhesus monkeys (*Macaca mulatta*) by administration of progesterone to their female partners. *J. Endocr.*, 41, 421–31.

——, ZUMPE, D., KEVERNE, E. B., and BONSALL, R. W.

—— (1972). Neuroendocrine factors in the control of primate behavior. *Recent Progr. Hormone Res.*, 28, 665–705.

MORRIS, D. (1958). The reproductive behaviour of the ten-spined stickleback (*Pygosteus pungitius L.*). *Behaviour*, Suppl. 6, 1–154.

MOYNIHAN, M. (1955). Some aspects of reproductive behaviour in the black headed gull (*Larus ridibundus ridibundus L.*) and related species. *Behaviour*, Suppl. 4, 1–201.

NOWLIS, V. (1942). Sexual status and degree of hunger in chimpanzee competitive interaction. *J. comp. Psychol.*, 34, 185–94.

PATERSON, J. D. (1973). Ecologically differentiated patterns of aggressive and sexual behavior in two troops of Ugandan baboons, *Papio anubis. Amer. J. phys. Anthrop.*, 38, 641–8.

RASA, O. A. E. (1971). Appetence for aggression in juvenile damsel fish. *Z. f. Tierpsychol.*, Suppl. 7, 7–68.

REYNOLDS, V. and REYNOLDS, F. (1965). Chimpanzees of the Budengo Forest. In *Primate behavior* (ed. I. DeVore), pp. 368–424. New York.

ROWELL, T. E. (1963). Behaviour and female reproductive cycles of rhesus macaques. *J. Reprod. Fert.*, 6, 192–203.

SCHALLER, G. B. (1963). *The mountain gorilla.* Chicago.

SIMONDS, P. E. (1965). The bonnet macaque in South India. In *Primate behavior* (ed. I. DeVore), pp. 175–196. New York.

SINGH, S. D. (1966). The effects of human environment on the social behavior in rhesus monkeys. *Primates*, 7, 33–40.

SOUTHWICK, C. H. (1967). An experimental study of intragroup agonistic behavior in rhesus monkeys (*Macaca mulatta*). *Behaviour*, 28, 182–209.

——, BEG, M. A., and SIDDIQI, M. R. (1961). A population survey of rhesus monkeys in Northern India: II. Transportation routes and forest areas. *Ecology*, 42, 698–710.

——, ——, and —— (1965). Rhesus monkeys in North India. In *Primate behavior* (ed. I. DeVore), pp. 111–59. New York.

SPIVAK, H. (1968). *Ausdrucksformen und soziale Beziehungen in einer DscheladaGruppe (Theropithecus gelada) im Zoo Zurich.*

STRUHSAKER, T. T. (1967). Social structure among vervet monkeys (*Cercopithecus aethiops*). *Behaviour*, 29, 83–121.

TINBERGEN, N. (1959). Comparative studies of the behaviour of gulls (*Laridae*): a progress report. *Behaviour*, 15, 1–70.

UDRY, J. R. and MORRIS, N. M. (1968). Distribution of coitus in the menstrual cycle. *Nature (Lond.)*, 220, 593–6.

VAN LAWICK-GOODALL, J. (1968). The behaviour of free-living chimpanzees in the Gombe Stream Reserve. *Anim. Behav. Monogr.*, 1, 161–311.

VANDENBERGH, J. G. and VESSEY, S. (1968). Seasonal breeding of free-ranging rhesus monkeys and related ecological factors. *J. Reprod. Fert.*, 15, 71–9.

VESSEY, S. H. (1973). Night observations of free-ranging rhesus monkeys. *Amer. J. phys. Anthrop.*, 38, 613–20.

YERKES, R. M. (1939). Social dominance and sexual status in the chimpanzee. *Quart. Rev. Biol.*, 14, 115–36.

ZUCKERMAN, S. (1932). *The social life of monkeys and apes.* London.

ZUMPE, D. and MICHAEL, R. P. (1970a). Ovarian hormones and female sexual invitations in captive rhesus monkeys (*Macaca mulatta*). *Anim. Behav.*, 18, 293–301.

—— and —— (1970b). Redirected aggression and gonadal hormones in captive rhesus monkeys (*Macaca mulatta*). *Anim. Behav.*, 18, 11–19.

—— and —— (1977). Effects of ejaculations by males on the sexual invitations of female rhesus monkeys (*Macaca mulatta*). *Behaviour*. (In press)

5. SOCIAL PSYCHOPHYSIOLOGICAL STUDIES OF THE SEXUAL DIFFERENTIATION OF BEHAVIOUR IN A MAMMALIAN SOCIETY

J. P. HENRY, D. L. ELY, and P. M. STEPHENS

For the past 10 years our laboratory has been studying the social interactions of one of the smallest of rodents — the common mouse — in the hope of gaining insights into the relations between society, stress, and disease. One objective of this chapter is to emphasize that although mice have very little neocortex or 'socio-cultural' brain, the neurophysiological basis of their instinctive behaviour and emotions is based on a complex array of brain structures known as the limbic system, which is very similar to the limbic system in man, the cultural animal. In our experiments, the effects of complex habitats, 'population cages' composed of standard caging connected by narrow tubing, are studied by tagging animals magnetically and following their activities. We are studying in particular the differentiation of the behaviour of murine societies into male and female behaviour patterns whose nervous and hormonal determination appear to be the same as in man.

INTRODUCTION

Colonies of mice can be used as an economic, rapidly maturing models for the demonstration of the sexual differences in behaviour patterns in a community of mammals. The term 'social psychophysiological' in the title of this chapter emphasizes that the work is not only directed upwards, towards the activities of the social brain, i.e. to long-range goals involving complex linguistic and mechanical manipulation, but also downwards, towards the hormonal and other physiological accompaniments of the primitive dichotomy into male and female behaviour.

PHYSIOLOGICAL DETERMINANTS OF SEXUAL DIFFERENTIATION

In the course of a discussion on comparative social behaviour in man and beast, Fox (1968) contributed a valuable essay on man, the cultural animal. He comments that man is dependent upon his environmentally stable inherited patterns of behaviour to a far greater degree than has been believed by many social scientists. One of the points he makes is that we must clearly identify the root stock of biological universals upon which the elaborate cultural patterns of human societies are grafted. Evidence is steadily accumulating on this score from a number of different disciplines.

In *The human animal*, ethologists Hass and Eibl-Eibesfeldt (Hass 1970) describe their use of a prismatic lens mounted on a motion picture camera. By shooting at right angles to the direction in which the camera was pointing, they could take 'candid camera' shots of the spontaneous behaviour of peoples all over the world. Their work supports the view that man has a considerable birthright of patterns which are held in common by all races and cultures. For example with regard to behaviour between the sexes, Haas and Eibl-Eiblesfeldt describe a universal smile of friendliness and also the flirtatious averted glance.

In his summary chapter in a recent collection of worldwide anthropological studies of human sexual behaviour, Gebhard gives a distillate of sexual practices common to all human groups with regard to such aspects as foreplay and coitus within and outside marriage (Gebhard 1971). His presentation supports Hass and Fox's conclusion that many of the patterns of human sexual behaviour appear to have an inherited basis and are not of purely cultural origin. As Gebhard puts it: 'There seems to be a basic similarity in physiological response to sexual stimuli and in psychological reactions. All men (and women) are one in sharing much the same interests, lusts, frustrations, loves, sorrows, and joys that are part of human sexuality.'

Ewer's work describing the ethology of mammals carries this point of common heritage one step further. She demonstrates that all species exhibit related patterns of courtship and mating. They all demonstrate elaborate maternal and often paternal patterns of attachment, i.e. of care and nurturance for the young, including nesting, feeding, and protection (Ewer 1968).

Carrying the analysis one stage further, psycho-endocrinological studies show that these behaviour patterns are dependent upon the right hormone combinations *in utero* and during maturation as well as after sexual maturity. Harlow *et al.* (1971) and Beach (1970) review the evidence derived by Young *et al.* (1964) that typical male and female behaviour cannot be explained in terms of learned variables. The aggressive role of the male and the response of the female to the male are respectively determined by a lifetime of exposure of the developing and mature brain to testosterone or by current oestrogen levels. Recent illuminating work along these lines shows that the dominant members of a group of Rhesus monkeys have a higher level of testosterone than the subordinate (Rose *et al.* 1971). Even in culture-bound man, it has been shown

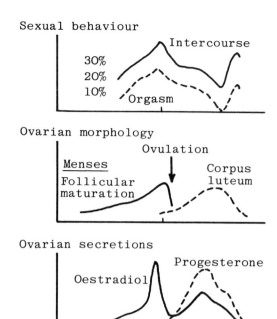

Sexual behaviour

30%
20%
10%

Intercourse

Orgasm

Ovarian morphology

Ovulation

Menses
Follicular
maturation

Corpus
luteum

Ovarian secretions

Oestradiol

Progesterone

Gonadotropin secretions

LH

FSH

−16 −12 −8 −4 0 +4 +8 +12 +16
Days from LH peak

FIG. 5.1. Schematic diagram representing the temporal inter-relationships of sexual behaviour, ovulation, and plasma oestradiol, progesterone, luteinizing hormone (LH), and follicle stimulating hormone (FSH) during the menstrual cycle. Note that the highest incidence of coitus and orgasm in a group of spontaneously reacting women coincides with the peak of oestrogen release. Slightly modified from Luttge (1971).

that the incidence of intercourse is hormonally determined and manyfold increased in the unconstrained female during ovulation when the oestrogen level peaks to its maximum (Luttge 1971) (Fig. 5.1).

Washburn and Hamburg (1968) have made the point that in man the brain is physically dominated by a new social brain which corresponds to his enormous and recently evolved neocortex. These huge association areas, several times larger than those of the chimpanzee, are concerned with the ability to work mathematical and linguistic abstractions, to remember, to plan, and to inhibit socially inappropriate action. But below this mushroom cap there remains the brain's 'stem' and the limbic system — an elaborate, primitive system already present in the reptilian brain. A generation of work by Papez and MacLean and others has

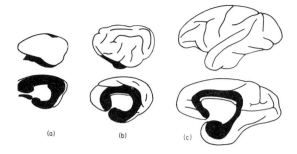

FIG. 5.2. Showing the relative sizes of the limbic lobe of (a) rodent, (b) carnivore, and (c) primate relative to the rest of the brain. Upper drawing is the lateral, and the lower, the medial view. The white enveloping neocortex mushrooms late in phylogeny. Modified from MacLean (1954). *J. Neurosurg.* **11**, 29. Reproduced with permission of the *Journal of Neurosurgery*.

shown that the action of this part of the brain is related to instinct and the emotions (Ganong 1971; MacLean 1970). It consists of rims of cortical tissue around the roots of the cerebral hemispheres and a group of associated structures, the amygdala, hippocampus, and septal nuclei (Fig. 5.2).

The combined evidence from ethology and from neurophysiological studies indicates that this region is responsible for certain basic patterns of environmentally stable function, such as social organization and territory formation, courtship and mating, and parent-child attachment behaviour (MacLean 1970). This limbic system and the structures below it in the brainstem, such as the hypothalamus and midbrain, are together responsible for the basic forms of emotional responses and are involved in motivation. As noted above, they have the same design characteristics in minute rodents, such as the mouse, as in man.

THE ROLES OF THE NEOCORTICAL SOCIOCULTURAL BRAIN AND THE LIMBIC SYSTEM AND BRAINSTEM

To summarize the argument of the preceding section: man's enormous sociocultural brain is responsible for the bewilderingly complex elaboration of acquired characteristics that our various cultures exhibit, but no new sets of principles have been elaborated. And although it is true that the human organism can supress these ancient patterns of behaviour, it is not without risk of physiological and behavioural disturbance.

All mammals, from the mouse with its relatively small neocortex to man with his overwhelming development of the same region, have the same mechanisms for forming social groupings. Basically, the primordial brain appears to be 'female', only differentiating into that of the male under the influence of the androgenic hormones. There are special periods of sensitivity in the brains of both sexes, to the learning of certain patterns which later become environmentally stable. All have some mechanisms for expression and communication, social organization and territory, for finding food and for its storage, for courtship and mating, and for parental or attachment behaviour (Ewer 1968). The weight of evidence points to the limbic system and regions below it as the critical mediators of these activities (MacLean 1970; Ganong 1971).

Two major pathways exist by which the organism makes physiological adjustments to any challenge to these drives which manages to get past the coping processes and to disturb the internal equilibrium. The defence response involves arousal of the sympathetic system and the adrenal medulla, and the alarm response of Selye involves hypothalamo-hypophyseal influence upon the adrenal cortex (Maso 1968). Chronic arousal of these mechanisms leads to disturbances of the various male and female behaviour patterns that are described by the ethologists, and carries the threat of physiological breakdown and disease. We are presently concerned with behaviour patterns that are associated

with sexual differentiation in the mouse. A later discussion will centre on coping processes and the pathology that ensues when they fail.

COMPLEX INTERCOMMUNICATING BOX SYSTEMS: POPULATION CAGES

Our study of the behaviour of mice uses complex cage systems in which six to a dozen standard boxes are connected by lucite tubing just sufficiently large to permit them to squeeze past each other. Each 300 mm × 150 mm × 150 mm box is to an average 25-g, 102-mm body length mouse about what an average room in a house would be to a human, i.e. 6 m × 3 m × 3 m (Fig. 5.3). In human architecture the function of regions is differentiated. Indeed even in quite primitive sites there will be male and female role areas, i.e. regions for nursery, latrine, sexual and sleeping activities, and for feeding and drinking. Further we enrich the environment by furniture which we arrange and rearrange in

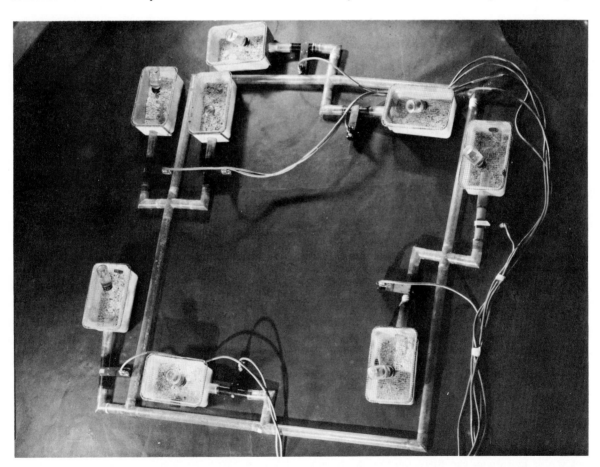

FIG. 5.3. This system of independent boxes, each with its own food and water supply, permits the animals to establish territory. The single entrance with a right-angle bend is easily protected. Hall-effect detector units at the portal of each box permit detection of mgnetically tagged animals and quantitative determination of behavioural patterns, such as dominance and subordination.

44

various patterns at will. The complex population cages used for the mouse have the rudiments of the same possibilities of structuring, i.e. fluffy wood shavings are provided by a 5-cm layer. Those boxes that are chosen for nesting are kept scrupulously clean by the females (Fig. 5.4(a)). On the other hand, in the latrine boxes the mice allow large accumulations of faeces and urine (Fig. 5.4(b)). Food and water are made available in various areas according to the design.

A MAGNETIC DETECTION SYSTEM

We study social behaviour by using an automatic counting device triggered by magnet implants in the back or belly of the mice. Two magnets are placed in all of the members of a standard colony of 5 males and 10 females. The animals can then be tagged two at a time by magnetizing and demagnetizing them with a simple solenoid. Magnetic detectors at the portal of each box will then make it possible to recognize box entry-exits, time spent in boxes, and events such as the isolation of an intruder or parturient female, nest building, and patrols in which a number of boxes are visited by the dominant and other high-status animals in rapid succession. Thus from the ensuing activity records we can identify the patterns typical of males and females. The

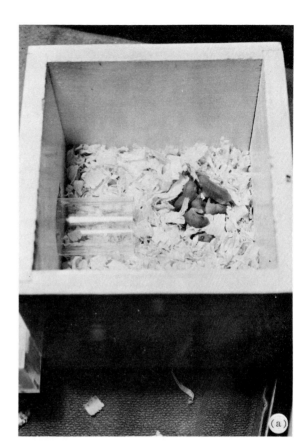

FIG. 5.4. (a) There is a sharp contrast between the clean nesting box from which most faeces are removed and the latrine box (b), where the scarred subordinates stay, only venturing out briefly for food and water.

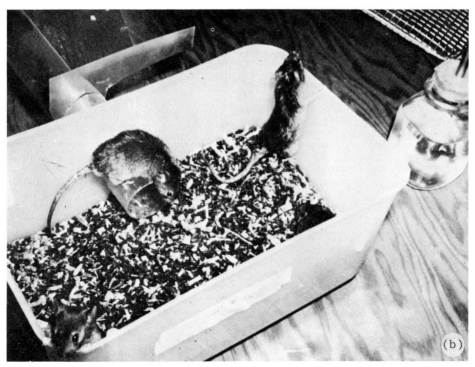

45

animal playing the dominant role enjoys a very general freedom of movement throughout the whole system. Rivals have less mobility, whereas confinement to the latrine area is the typical fate of the subordinate or of an intruder male (Fig. 5.5). Females are found in

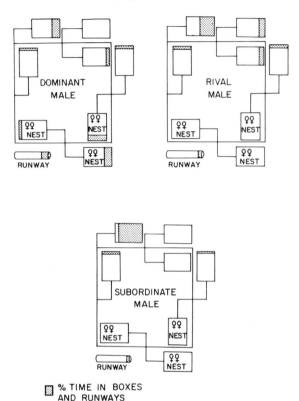

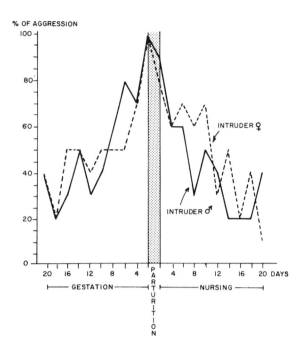

Fig. 5.6. Aggressivity of females during periods of gestation and nursing. Defence against intrusion by pregnant females increases progressively as they approach term and thereafter progressively declines. Modified from Beniest-Noirot (1956). *Un. int. Sci. biol.*

Fig. 5.5. Male territories, showing the differentiation of the males in the colony shown in Fig. 5.3. The nesting boxes will be clean in comparison with that occupied by the subordinates. The dominants have frequent access to all boxes and patrols them by making visits to four or more boxes in a period of less than 8 minutes.

nesting boxes, and, depending on population density and stability, many or few will be pregnant or lactating, i.e. the social situation determines the percentage of colony effort expended in the care of the young as opposed to other types of social interaction. In general the females are distinguished by displaying less aggressive activity and by their freedom from nicks and bites. However, a female will defend a nesting box from an intruding male or female and block it off with shavings (Fig. 5.6). In the socially healthy colony she remains unbitten and is not involved in fighting. Indeed the level of fighting even among the males in a socially adjusted colony is low; a state that can be achieved by raising them all together from birth so that they are in effect siblings.

HORMONES AND BEHAVIOUR IN A MURINE COLONY

Mice show a clear differentiation of that male versus female role behaviour which Hamburg (1968) and Harlow (1971) have so eloquently described in the wild primate as well as the caged Rhesus Macaque. There is increasing evidence that these behavioural differences are associated both with neonatal and later adult levels of the androgenic hormone, testosterone, and of the female sex hormones, oestrogen and progesterone.

The colonies in which food and water and shavings are freely available permit the differentiation of the typical female role activity of nest building. She will make many hundred passages from one box to another in a few hours carrying shavings in her mouth; and when agitated, she moves her infants in the same way (Fig. 5.7). The female confines herself to the nest boxes with her young for many hours in the day (Fig. 5.8); she displays nest-building activity and scrupulously cleans up the box in which she is located (Fig. 5.4(a)). The subordinate male is confined to a single box (Fig. 5.5). The alpha or dominant male gets access to all boxes, and the rival visits all except the nesting boxes (Fig. 5.5). To the most energetic and competent go the social resources, the breeding privileges. But a group of

46

castrated males will live peaceably with each other and with the females in a colony until their androgen level is raised by the administration of testosterone.

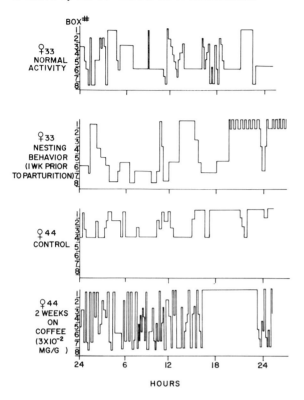

Fig. 5.7. Female behaviour profiles: record contrasting the activity of two females. Female 33 shows patrols and much movement between boxes until one week prior to parturition. She then shows less general activity, but engages in nest building during the period of 20–26 hours. Female 44 is a less dominant animal and moves less until put on coffee, when she engages in intense activity interrupted by an exceptionally long rest period from 16 hours to 23 hours in Box #1.

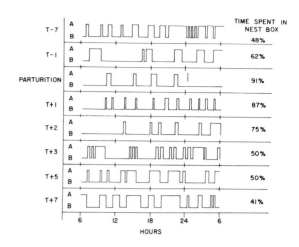

Fig. 5.8. Maternal behaviour: two-box system. As a pregnant female approaches parturition the percentage of time spent in the nest-box portion of a two-box system increases and then falls off again during the week following. A = Food and water area; B = nursery.

SOCIAL DEPRIVATION AND THE ENSUING SOCIAL DISORDER

The above clearly defined behavioural characteristics break down in animals that do not receive adequate socialization during their infancy and maturation. Aggressive competition is sustained as they fail to develop a strict ranking order, and no consistent avoidance behaviour patterns develop to separate out a group of subordinates. As Crook (1970) puts it, the assertive freely expressed utilization of available physical (food, water, nesting) and social (mating, social interaction) commodities by high-status animals constrains the behaviour of rivals and subordinates. If there is inadequate socialization during maturation, these constraints fail, each continues to challenge the

TABLE 5.1

Although the activity of females that have been raised in isolation is as high as that of a normal social group, their blood-pressure is elevated, their relative adrenal weight much greater, and the percentage of pregnancies per unit time is lower

	Entry/exits per hour	Patrols per 24 hours	Blood-pressure (mmHg)	Relative adrenal weight (mg per 100g)	Percentage of pregnancies per 2 months
Interacting socialized females	19	6·8	123	16·9	80
Interacting isolated females	20	5·8	147	22·9	30

other and social disorder prevails. There is evidence of strong psychosocial stimulation as the confrontations persist and the fighting is sustained. The females no longer build communal nests and raise litters together, and their level of such activity is low compared with the females in a normally socialized group, while that of the males rises above the norm (Table 5.1). The few pregnancies that do go to term and are successfully delivered are followed by failure to maintain an inviolate nesting region. Other females grab the young and move them at random, so too does the parent, and within a few hours they die of neglect and maltreatment.

This failure of male and female role differentiation is a sign of a breakdown of the murine social order. Powerful mutual stimulation ensues as the animals compete on an individual basis. This social breakdown and failure of the normal mutual role-associated teamwork processes of coping with the environment is connected with an arousal of the defence and of the alarm responses to varying degrees. The ensuing sustained responses either of the sympathetic system with activation of the adrenal medulla or of the anterior hypophysis with release of the hormone ACTH which controls adrenal cortical activity or of both systems can lead to pathophysiological disturbances. With a sufficiently prolonged and intense arousal, sexual activity ceases; then with further stress disease processes follow, whos precise nature is in part determined by the sex of the victim and on his or her role in the social grouping in which these events are occurring.

REFERENCES

BEACH, F. A. (1970). Some effects of gonadal hormones on sexual behavior. In *The hypothalamus* (ed. L. Martini, M. Motta, and F. Raschini), pp. 617–40. New York.

BOWLBY, J. (1970). *Attachment and loss*. London.

CROOK, J. H. (1970). Social organization and the environment: aspects of contemporary social ethology. *Anim. Behav.*, **18**, 197–209.

EWER, R. F. (1968). *Ethology of mammals*. New York.

FOX, R. (1968). The cultural animal. In *Man and beast: comparative social behavior* (ed. J. F. Eisenberg and W. S. Dillon), pp. 273–96. Washington, D.C.

GANONG, W. F. (1971). Neurophysiologic basis of instinctual behavior and emotions. In *Review of medical physiology* (ed. W. F. Ganong), pp. 173–85. Los Altos, California.

GEBHARD, P. H. (1971). Human sexual behavior: a summary statement. In *Human sexual behavior* (ed. D. S. Marshall and R. C. Suggs), pp. 201–17. New York.

HAMBURG, D. A. (1969). Observations of mother-infant interaction in primate field studies. In *Determinants of infant behavior* (ed. B. Foss), Vol. IV, pp. 271–95. London.

HARLOW, H. F., McGAUGH, J. L., and THOMPSON, R. F. (1971). *Psychology*. San Francisco.

HASS, H. (1970). *The human animal*. London.

LUTTGE, W. G. (1971). The role of gonadal hormones in the sexual behavior of the Rhesus monkey and human. *Arch. sex. Behav.*, **1**, 61–88.

MacLEAN, P. D. (1970). The limbic brain in relation to the psychoses. In *Physiological correlates of emotion* (ed. P. Black), pp. 130–44. New York.

MASON, J. W. (1968). 'Overall' hormonal balance as a key to endocrine organization. *Psychosom. Med.*, **30**, 791–808.

MINTURN, L. and LAMBERT, W. W. (1964). *Mothers of six cultures: antecedents of child rearing*. New York.

ROSE, R. M., HOLADAY, J. W., and BERNSTEIN, I. S. (1971). Plasma testosterone, dominance rank and aggressive behavior in male Rhesus monkeys. *Nature (Lond.)*, **231**, 336–8.

WASHBURN, S. L. and HAMBURG, D. A. (1968). Aggressive behavior in old world monkeys and apes. In *Primates: studies in adaptation and variability* (ed. P. Jay), pp. 458–68. New York.

YOUNG, W. C., GOY, R. W., and PHOENIX, C. H. (1964). Hormones and sexual behavior. *Science (N.Y.)*, **143**, 212–18.

6. NEURO-ENDOCRINE DETERMINANTS OF DIFFERENCES IN HOSTILITY AND AGGRESSION BETWEEN MALES AND FEMALES

HAROLD PERSKY

INTRODUCTION

The general problem of affect/endocrine relationship

Although psycho-endocrinology is a fairly recent word, the underlying concept of a relationship between physiological (i.e. 'bodily') processes and psychological (e.g. emotion, defence, and cognition) processes is not new. The Milesian physicians of Asia Minor, possibly subsequent to Babylonian contacts, attempted to associate one aspect of hepatic secretion with mood state.

The psycho-endocrine studies of the twentieth century were pioneered by Walter B. Cannon and Hans Selye on the role of neurohumours and hormones in various types of life stresses, and by Sigmund Freud, who demonstrated the centrality of affect, particularly anxiety, in human behaviour. Although many other investigators have contributed significantly to various aspects of the body of work collected together under the term 'psychosomatic', these three investigators provided the broad premises that have led to present-day studies.

Starting with specific hormonal or neurohumoral assessment in various 'stress' diseases, or describing the fluctuation in levels of experienced anxiety during the course of such illnesses, has resulted in the realization that frequently ordered relationships occur between two levels of biological organization: one best described in physiological and/or biochemical terms, the other in symbolic and/or sociological language. The transducer mechanisms connecting these disparate modes of description may soon be elucidated.

Our present knowledge of affect/endocrine relationships is not only based on static studies; experimental manipulation using neurophysiological, pharmacological, and sociological techniques has provided much information substantiating the static studies.

What kind of documentation has been offered in demonstration of affect/endocrine relationships? Emotions were, of course, recognized, identified, and even quantified way back in history. The poets, those most perceptive of scholars, have been concerned with emotions throughout the ages. Nevertheless, it remained the duty of the more prosaic scientist to bring the affects into the more conventional domain of scholarship. Books describe the unique characteristics of anxiety (Levitt 1967; Cattell and Scheier 1961; Basowitz *et al.* 1965), depression (Beck 1967; Grinker *et al.* 1961; Bellak 1952), and hostility (Buss 1961; Saul

1956; Scott 1958) to mention but a few of the mood states. It may well reflect a characteristic of our times that considerably more effort has been expended on these so-called 'negative' emotions than on the more felicitous ones of elation, joy, and love.

Considerable effort has been expended in attempts at quantification of moods. A wide variety of devices have been used, ranging from open-ended clinical rating scales culled from structured interviews to more covert instruments like the Rorschach inkblot test. In between lie checklists, questionnaires, etc. A major difficulty, reflected in the plethora of test instruments, occurs as a consequence of the fact that these psychological devices do not always agree with one another. Either the instrument does not truly measure the mood that it purports to assess, or the two instruments being compared tap different aspects of the same mood. For example, Zuckerman *et al.* (1967) have compared anxiety, depression, and hostility scores simultaneously obtained from five different devices intended to measure all three effects. They found considerable variation in the degree of correlation among the respective scales intended to assess the same mood. Objective devices (ratings, checklists, questionnaires) tended to yield significant correlations with one another but correlated poorly with projective test scales (inkblot, thematic apperception test).

In addition to this difficulty, Zuckerman *et al.* found that the individual scales derived from the same test instrument did not specifically assess the indicated mood as shown by significant correlation between the respective scales. Hamburg *et al.* (1958) have noted that anxiety, depression, and hostility ratings obtained from a clinical interview correlated significantly with one another. Zuckerman also noted a similar problem with checklist scores. Despite this apparent overlap, specific scales responded in appropriate fashion to imposed stresses calculated to increase the experience of the emotion under question. Thus, Levitt *et al.* (1960) found that direct suggestion of the experience of anxiety to normal individuals under hypnotic trance resulted in an elevation in checklist items for anxiety which clearly distinguished hospitalized, anxious patients from matched, normal control subjects.

What kinds of endocrine measures have been used in psycho-endocrine studies? In the past investigators have resorted to secondary indices of glandular activity since direct measurement of hormone levels was not feasible. As a result of the explosive development of

49

endocrine chemistry over the past two decades more direct estimates of endocrine function have become available. Even with such estimates, we do not know which index constitutes the 'best' measure of a particular gland's function. Until recently, the circulating level of a hormone was regarded as an adequate index; subsequently, it was recognized that only the tiny fraction of the circulating hormone not bound to the transport protein was the functionally active hormone. Investigators have used such diverse indices as circulating hormone level, metabolite excretion, and production rate and all of these indices have provided useful information for psycho-endocrine studies. That no single index is always the 'best' one is demonstrated by the finding of O'Brien et al. (1976) that although production rates of cortisol R_C and testosterone R_T correlate highly with trait measures of anxiety and aggression respectively, the plasma levels of these hormones correlate highly with the state measures of these same affects.

Anxiety/adrenocortical relationships
I would like to illustrate what is meant by affect/endocrine relationships by citing some examples concerned with anxiety/adrenocortical relationships. This psycho-endocrine relationship has received the most attention to date. One of the earliest reports is that of Bliss et al. (1956); using a then new technique for the measurement of the plasma concentration P_C of cortisol and a crude rating scale for anxiety, these investigators obtained a highly significant correlation between these two variables in a group of disturbed, schizophrenic patients. Persky et al. (1956) obtained significant differences between hospitalized, anxious patients and matched controls for both P_C and urinary hydroxycorticoid excretion (17-OHCS), an important metabolite of cortisol, with the higher values occurring in the patients. Using a more elegant clinical rating, the latter investigators were also able to show a progressive increase in association between P_C and anxiety rating following a disturbing interview which increased in intensity (Persky et al. 1958). Most recently, Sachar et al. (1970) demonstrated that a highly significant relationship occurs between R_C and a selected group of anxiety scores culled from a clinical interview with depressed patients. The interview was assessed for a variety of other moods, none of which bore any ordered relationship to R_C.

Many other studies of a valuable nature have been reported concerning the anxiety/adrenocortical relationship but it is not possible to give details here. One other study in this area is worth mentioning because of its connection to the central theme of this book. Persky et al. (1959a) attempted to raise P_C experimentally in a group of healthy volunteers by directly suggesting the experience of anxiety to them while under hypnotic trance. Only the female subjects responded with a significant elevation in P_C as compared to their basal hypnotic values. At first glance this finding would seem to suggest an unequivocal difference in sex response to stressful stimulation. However, the complexity of sex-difference research may be nicely illustrated by this example. The female subjects were similar in age and occupation (students) to the male subjects. They differed from the men with respect to their career choice (nurse v. doctor), their residential arrangements (nursing residence v. private quarters), and from each other in the fact that they were at different stages of their menstrual cycles, and possibly in other respects as well. In addition, the hypnotist was a man. It was never established whether any or all of these factors contributed to the sex-difference to the stressful stimulus. The possibility that they might have led us to change our subsequent experimental designs.

Depression/endocrine relationships
Since adrenocortical activation occurred in response to anxiety and since some investigators at the time felt that it probably occurred following any type of emotional arousal, a number of studies were undertaken to establish the facts of the matter. Board et al. (1956) first noted an elevated P_C in depressed patients with retarded patients yielding higher values than agitated ones. Bunney et al. (1965) demonstrated the fluctuation in urinary 17-OHCS which paralleled the psychological changes during the course of treatment of a group of depressed patients. Persky et al. (1976) demonstrated that experimentally induced depressive states yield higher P_C and 17-OHCS than similarly induced calm states in the same group of normal volunteers. These latter findings suggest a discrepancy with respect to the previously mentioned work of Sachar et al. (1970). Both Board and Fox et al. (1961) have attempted to relate the elevated adrenocortical response to the meaning of the experienced mood to the subject, rather than to the intensity of the experienced affect per se. Obviously, further studies are in order.

Other affect/endocrine relationships
Other affect/endocrine studies are far less numerous than those involving the relationship of the adrenal cortex to anxiety and depression. Corticotropin (ACTH) (Persky et al. 1959b), somatotropin (STH) (Greene et al. 1970; American Psychosomatic Society 1972), luteinizing hormone (LH) and follicle-stimulating hormone (FSH) (Persky 1964), thyroxine (Johansson 1970), oestrogens (Murawski et al. 1968; Nesbitt 1968) and androgens (Rose et al. 1969; Brooksbank and Pryse-Phillips 1964) have all been related to one or another mood state. Recently there has been an increase in interest in the relation of adrenomedullary hormones and their metabolites to various moods (Levi 1967; Frankenhaeuser and Patkai 1965; Hathaway et al. 1969; Maas et al. 1968).

Other psychological (non-affect) relationships
Of all psychological processes, emotions are the most readily visible (and audible) and consequently consti-

tuted the first of the psychological parameters to be examined for endocrine relationships. Longitudinal studies of the type described by Bunney et al. (1965) and Sachar et al. (1963) have shown that disruption of defence and eruption of emotion bear a close relationship to endocrine fluctuation. The possibility remains that breakdown of defence which precedes appearance of emotion may actually be the triggering mechanism for hormone response. The problem is still far from solved. As indicated above, Board et al. (1956) and Fox et al. (1961) consider that the cognition of the emotional state, regardless of its intensity objectively, may also trigger endocrine response. Here again, much work remains to be done.

THE RELATIONSHIPS OF TESTICULAR FUNCTION TO AGGRESSION

Historical background

Up to this point no mention has been made of the relationship of moods to testicular or ovarian function. The latter is beyond the scope of this book; the former has only yielded a few papers involving man until very recently. However, a considerable literature on the relationship between testicular function and aggression has existed for some time for infrahuman species and the data provide useful and interesting guidelines for the emerging human studies. To a large degree, the lack of human studies, until very recently, reflected the lack of adequate endocrine methodology. As a consequence the animal studies of the past resorted to secondary indices of testicular function, almost all of which could not be employed for man.

The early studies utilized overt behaviour to assess aggression; fighting and winning constituting successful aggression and losing constituting poor aggression. A good many of the early studies on aggression were carried out with mice. It was readily shown that intact mice consistently defeated castrates (Scott 1966); furthermore, exogenous administration of testosterone to castrates restored their fighting ability (Sigg 1969). Goy (1968) has shown that female monkeys androgenized in utero were considerably more aggressive than their non-androgenized female playmates.

Symbolic behaviour is an important aspect of aggression in monkeys, as it may well be in lower species. Consequently, Rose et al. (1972) were able to relate position in the dominance hierarchy to P_T. In another study, Kreuz and Rose (1971) were unable to relate extent of fighting behaviour alone to P_T for a group of prisoners, possibly because no attempt was made to assess other aspects of aggression.

Using an objective test measure of hostility and aggression, the Buss-Durkee hostility inventory (Buss and Durkee 1957), Persky et al. (1971) were able to show that both P_T and R_T were significantly related to that test measure. Since the Buss-Durkee inventory contains two factors, one measuring hostile feelings (hostility in), the other aggressive feelings (hostility out), it was possible in the latter study to demonstrate that R_T was highly correlated with the aggression factor score but only modestly and negatively correlated with the hostile feelings factor score.

Persky et al. (1972) attempted to validate this relationship experimentally by raising and lowering hostile feelings by suggestion to subjects under hypnotic trance and subsequently measuring P_T and R_C. Although appropriate affect response was elicited by the suggestions, the endocrine findings were equivocal. High P_T values were obtained on the calm suggestion while lower R_T values were obtained on the hostile suggestion. These results may reflect an inadequate suggestion as well as an effect of hypnosis itself on metabolic clearance rate.

Methodological aspects

Studies on aggression in man are complicated by a lack of adequate indices of aggression. Mere fighting behaviour was not associated with P_T although a psychological test measure of aggression was. For man aggression may include behavioural manifestations of fighting, symbolic representations, and cognitive awareness in a very complex mixture. Considerable improvement in assessment is essential for future studies.

To date manifest hostility and aggression have been assessed by a checklist device such as Zuckerman's MAACL hostility scale (Zuckerman and Lubin 1965), and trait hostility and aggression have been measured by the Buss-Durkee inventory. The latter instrument has been shown to be highly predictive of obtained scores in experimental aggression studies (Persky et al. 1972). The importance of the cognitive component of aggression has been nicely documented in the case of the young Quaker wrestler in the film entitled The friendly persuasion.

Assessment of testicular function has undergone a rapid revolution over the past decade. The crude index of urinary 17-ketosteroids has been discarded in favour of a variety of techniques for the direct measurement of plasma testosterone, including competitive protein binding (Horton et al. 1967) and radioimmunoassay (Ismail et al. 1972). By these methods as little as 10^{-12} g testosterone may readily be detected. The production rate of testosterone has likewise provided a useful criterion of testicular activity with highly sensitive techniques, which are also used in female subjects, for the determination of several micrograms per day. One cautionary word concerning testosterone assessment is in order. The availability of highly sensitive measurement techniques requiring small amounts of plasma and the utilization of in-dwelling catheters have enabled investigators to measure plasma levels almost continuously. Sachar et al. (1972) have recently demonstrated the rapid liability of P_T over very short periods of time. The finding raises serious question as to the mode of comparison of hormonal and psychological data.

TESTOSTERONE/AGGRESSION RELATIONSHIPS IN MALES AND FEMALES

At this point I would like to present some studies undertaken in my laboratory concerning testosterone/aggression relationships in men and women. Women, like men, produce testosterone, albeit in much smaller amounts. Essentially, all of the testosterone produced by women is derived from the liver rather than the testes (Horton and Tait 1967). Some investigators have attributed an important function, libidinal drive, to this small amount, although they do not have direct proof (Swyer 1968). (Nineteenth century novelists frequently subscribed to this hypothesis: their passionate heroines frequently possessed a light down upon their upper lips.)

Plasma testosterone levels, MAACL-hostility scores, and Buss-Durkee hostility scores are given in Table 6.1

TABLE 6.1

Plasma testosterone levels, MAACL-hostility scores and Buss-Durkee hostility scores of four groups of subjects

Group	N	P_T (ng per 100 ml)	MAACL	Buss-Durkee
Young men (1)	18	686	3·2	22·3
Older men (2)	15	404	3·7	21·5
Young women (3)	5	27	7·2	21·2
Older women (4)	5	27	6·2	19·0

for four groups of subjects: (1) a group of healthy young men ranging in age from 17 to 27 years (mean ± S.E.: 22·0 ± 0·8 years); (2) a group of healthy, older men ranging in age from 30 to 66 years (45·1 ± 2·7 years); (3) a group of healthy, young women ranging in age from 20 to 27 years; and (4) a group of older women ranging in age from 53 to 60 years. All of the young women were not using any contraceptive steroids and had normal menstrual cycles (26–34 days duration for the group). All of the older women were menopausal for at least one year as judged by absence of menses and elevated urinary gonadotropins. The young men and women were students in a local university; the older men and women were professionals.

Plasma testosterone levels were determined in the men by competitive protein-binding; in the women by radioimmunoassay. Good agreement was obtained between the two methods on identical samples. The P_T levels of Group 1 subjects were considerably higher than those of Group 2 (686 ± 46 ng per 100 ml v. 404 ± 39 ng per 100 ml). Groups 3 and 4 were identical with respect to P_T: 26·6 ng per 100 ml v. 26·7 ng per 100 ml. The young men had 25 times more testosterone in their plasma than the young women while the older men had 15 times more. Unfortunately, no estimate of the quantity of non-protein-bound testosterone ('free' testosterone) was available for any group.

The MAACL-hostility scores of the young men were almost identical with those of the older men (3·2 v. 3·7), both mean values being considerably lower than reported values in other normal studies. This finding may reflect the care used in selecting the subjects of this study. Female values were slightly higher: 7·2 and 6·2 for the young and older women respectively. Buss-Durkee hostility scores were almost identical for all four groups. However, the young men scored considerably higher on at least two of the subscales contributing to the aggression factor than the young women. Both the older men and women scored about the same on the aggression subscales; these values were considerably lower than those obtained in the younger subjects (see Table 6.2).

TABLE 6.2

Buss-Durkee aggression subscale scores of four groups of subjects

Group	Indirect	Verbal	Assault
Young men (1)	3·6	7·0	3·9
Older men (2)	2·9	6·3	4·1
Young women (3)	3·8	6·2	1·8
Older women (4)	2·4	4·6	2·0

Elsewhere (Persky *et al.* 1971) we have reported that a significant correlation r was obtained between P_T and the sum of the Buss-Durkee hostility scores for the younger men, but not the older ones. The aggression factor score correlated even more highly with P_T in the young men and only trivially in the older men; the negative hostility factor scores did not yield significant correlations with either group of men. No significant relationship as judged by inspection appears to occur betwen Buss-Durkee scores and P_T for either group of women; however, the aggression factor scores appear to correlate with P_T for the young women but not the older ones. Extreme caution in interpreting this preliminary finding is necessary because of the small sample size of the female groups. A suggestion of a possible relationship also occurs between degree of sexual activity and P_T but here again caution in interpretation is indicated. Incidentally, all of the young male subjects were potent as evidenced by ability to deliver semen samples on demand and high normal semen counts with good motility.

DISCUSSION

The data described in this chapter represent to our knowledge the first effort to relate plasma testosterone levels to measures of aggression in women. In so doing, the relation observed in young men has tentatively been extended to young women. Despite a P_T far lower than that obtained in young men, the data from the young women suggest that a similar relationship between aggression score and testosterone level occurs. While much speculation about this finding is possible, the most reasonable attitude to assume is a cautious one until additional data is obtained suitable for more powerful analysis.

The lack of relationship between P_T and aggression scores in older men and women is less dramatic but equally interesting. In our earlier report on male subjects we speculated that older men had developed some mastery over the aggressive feelings and that possibly as a consequence this mood state did not contribute to

any great degree to the variance in P_T. We also suggested that the flooding of the circulation with the potent hormone, testosterone, in the younger men released large quantities of aggression for which suitable controls had not yet developed. Perhaps the same explanation is valid for the female case.

Our principal difference is with respect to age rather than to sex even though the differences in P_T levels between all men and all women are great. We might speculate that here again our notions about aggression/hormone relationships have been conditioned by a stereotype concerning the respective sexes rather than the actual facts. Although females of all species are generally less engaged in fighting behaviour than males, fighting, as pointed out earlier, does not constitute the totality of aggressive behaviour. More careful studies are definitely in order concerning aggressive behaviour in women: its nature, the ways in which it is manifested, and its relationship to phases of the menstrual cycle.

We have illustrated in this chapter that psychoendocrine relationships are also present in the area of aggression and testosterone metabolism. From a psychosomatic standpoint they would suggest that a considerable degree of specificity occurs between individual mood states and individual hormones. Further discussion of the problem of specificity is beyond the scope of this chapter.

REFERENCES

AMERICAN PSYCHOSOMATIC SOCIETY (1972). Psychosocial, hormonal, and arrhythmia precursors of the early prehospital phase of myocardial infarction. Abstracts of Presentations, American Psychosomatic Society Annual Meeting, p. 24.

BASOWITZ, H., PERSKY, H., KORCHIN, S. J., and GRINKER, R. R. (1955). Anxiety and stress. New York.

BECK, A. T. (1967). Depression. New York.

BELLAK, L. (1952). Manic-depressive psychosis. New York.

BLISS, E. L., MIGEON, C. J., BRANCH, C. H. H., and SAMUELS, L. T. (1956). Reaction of the adrenal cortex to emotional stress. Psychosom. Med., 18: 56, 1956.

BOARD, F. A., PERSKY, H., and HAMBURG, D. A. (1956). Psychological stress and endocrine functions: blood levels of adrenocortical and thyroid hormones in acutely disturbed patients. Psychosom. Med., 18, 324.

BROOKSBANK, B. W. L. and PRYSE-PHILLIPS, W. (1964). Urinary 16-androsten-3-ol, 17-oxosteroids and mental illness. Brit. med. J., (i), 1602.

BUNNEY, W. E. Jr, MASON, J. W., and HAMBURG, D. A. (1965). Correlations between behavioral variables and urinary 17-hydroxycorticosteroids in depressed patients. Psychosom. Med., 27, 229.

BUSS, A. H. (1961). The psychology of aggression. New York.

—— and DURKEE, A. (1957). An inventory for assessing different kinds of hostility. J. cons. Psychol., 21, 343.

CATTELL, R. B. and SCHEIER, I. H. (1961). The meaning and measurement of neuroticism and anxiety. New York.

FOX, H. M., MURAWSKI, B. J., BARTHOLOMAY, A. F., and GIFFORD, S. (1961). Adrenal steroid excretion patterns in eighteen healthy subjects. Tentative correlations with personality structure. Psychosom. Med., 23, 23.

FRANKENHAEUSER, M. and PATKAI, P. (1965). Interindividual differences in catecholamine excretion during stress. Scand. J. Psychol., 6, 117.

GOY, R. W. (1968). Organizing effects of androgen on the behavior of rhesus monkeys. In Endocrinology and human behaviour. London.

GREENE, W. A., CONRON, G., SCHALCH, D. S., and SCHREINER, B. F. (1970). Psychologic correlates of growth hormone and adrenal secretory responses of patients undergoing cardiac catheterization. Psychosom. Med., 32, 599.

GRINKER, R. R., MILLER, J., SABSHIN, M., NUNN, R., and NUNNALLY, J. C. (1961). The phenomena of depressions. New York.

HAMBURG, D. A., SABSHIN, M. A., BOARD, F. A., GRINKER, R. R., KORCHIN, S. J., BASOWITZ, H., HEATH, H., and PERSKY, H. (1958). Classification and rating of emotional experiences. Arch. Neurol. Psychiat. (Chic.), 79, 415.

HATHAWAY, P. W., BREHM, M. L., CLAPP, J. R., and BOGDONOFF, M. D. (1969). Urine flow, catecholamines, and blood pressure: The variability of response of normal human subjects in a relaxed laboratory setting. Psychosom. Med., 31, 20.

HORTON, R. and TAIT, J. F. (1967). In vivo conversion of dehydroisoandrosterone to plasma androstenedione and testosterone in man. J. clin. Endocrinol. Metab., 27, 79.

——, KATO, T., and SHERRINS, R. (1967). A rapid method for the estimation of testosterone in male plasma. Steroids, 10, 245.

ISMAIL, A. A. A., NISWENDER, G. D., and MIDGLEY, A. R., Jr (1972). Radioimmunoassay of testosterone without chromatography. J. clin. Endocrinol. Metab., 34, 177.

JOHANSSON, S., LEVI, L., and LINDSTEDT, S. (1970). Stress and the thyroid gland: a review of clinical and experimental studies, and a report of own data on experimentally induced PBI reactions in man. *Reports from the Laboratory for Clinical Stress Research*, No. 17.

KREUZ, L. E. and ROSE, R. M. (1971). Assessment of aggressive behavior and plasma testosterone in a young criminal population. Abstract of Presentations, American Psychosomatic Society Annual Meeting, p. 23.

LEVI, L. (1967). Stressors, personality traits, emotions, and performance as related to catecholamine excretion. In *Emotional stress* (ed. L. Levi). Stockholm.

LEVITT, E. E. (1967). *The psychology of anxiety*. Indianopolis.

———, DEN BREEIJEN, A., and PERSKY, H. (1960). The induction of clinical anxiety by means of a standardized hypnotic technique. *Amer. J. clin. Hypnosis*, **2**, 206.

MAAS, J. W., FAWCETT, J., and DEKIRMENJIAN, H. (1968). 3-Methoxy-4-hydroxy phenylglycol (MHPG) excretion indepressive states: a pilot study. *Arch. gen. Psychiat.*, **19**, 129.

MURAWSKI, B. J., SAPIR, P. E., SHULMAN, N., RYAN, G. M., Jr, and STURGIS, S. H. (1968). An investigation of mood states in women taking oral contraceptives. *Fertil. Steril.*, **19**, 50.

NESBITT, R. E. L., HOLLENDER, M., FISHER, S., and OSOFSKY, H. J. (1968). Psychologic correlates of the polycystic ovary syndrome and organic infertility. *Fertil. Steril.*, **19**, 778.

O'BRIEN, C. P., Jr, SMITH, K. D., BASU, G. K., and PERSKY, H. (1976). Testosterone metabolism and hostility in normal young men. *Biol. Psychiat.* (In press)

PERSKY, H. (1964). Excretion of luteinizing hormone (LH) by normal human subjects. *J. Albert Einstein Med. Ctr*, **12**, 29.

———, GRINKER, R. R., HAMBURG, D. A., SABSHIN, M. A., KORCHIN, S. J., BASOWITZ, H., and CHEVALIER, J. A. (1956). Adrenal cortical function in anxious human subjects: plasma level and urinary excretion of hydrocortisone. *Arch. Neurol. Psychiat. (Chic.)*, **76**, 549.

———, HAMBURG, D. A., BASOWITZ, H., GRINKER, R. R., SABSHIN, M., KORCHIN, S. J., HERZ, M., BOARD, F. A., and HEATH, H. A. (1958). Relation of emotional responses and changes in plasma hydrocortisone level after stressful interview. *Arch. Neurol. Psychiat. (Chic.)*, **79**, 434.

———, GROSZ, H. J., NORTON, J. A., and McMURTRY, M. (1959a). Effect of hypnotically-induced anxiety on the plasma hydrocortisone level of normal subjects. *J. clin. Endocrinol. Metab.*, **19**, 700.

———, MAROC, J., CONRAD, E., and DEN BREEIJEN, A. (1959b). Blood corticotropin and adrenal weight-maintenance factor levels of anxious patients and normal

subjects. *Psychosom. Med.*, **21**, 379.

———, SMITH, K. D., and BASU, G. K. (1971). Relation of psychologic measures of aggression and hostility to testosterone production in man. *Psychosom. Med.*, **33**, 265.

———, ———, ———, and O'BRIEN, C. P., Jr. (1972). Effect of a hostile suggestion on testosterone production rate. *Int. J. clin. exp. Hypnosis*, **20**.

———, ZUCKERMAN, M., and CURTIS, G. C. (1976). Affective, autonomic and endocrine resposes to four suggested emotions. *J. nerv. ment. Dis.* (In press)

ROSE, R. M., BOURNE, P. G., POE, R. O., MOUGEY, E. H., COLLINS, D. R., and MASON, J. W. (1969). Androgen responses to stress II. Excretion of testosterone, epitestosterone, androsterone and etiocholanolone during basic combat training and under threat of attack. *Psychosom. Med.*, **31**, 418.

———, GORDON, T. P., and BERNSTEIN, I. S. (1972). Sexual and social influences on testosterone secretion in the rhesus. Abstracts of Presentations, American Psychosomatic Society Annual Meeting, p. 22.

SACHAR, E. J., MASON, J. W., KOLMER, H. S., Jr, and ARTISS, K. L. (1963). Psychoendocrine aspects of acute schizophrenic reactions. *Psychosom. Med.*, **25**, 510.

———, HELLMAN, L., FUKUSHIMA, D. K., and GALLAGHER, T. F. (1970). Cortisol production in depressive illness. *Arch. gen. Psychiat.*, **23**, 289.

———, ROFFWANG, H. P., HELLMAN, L., and GALLAGHER, T. F. (1972). Recent studies of 24-hour patterns of hormone secretion: implications for psychoendocrine research. Abstract of Presentations, American Psychosomatic Society Annual Meeting, p. 26.

SAUL, L. J. (1956). *The hostile mind*. New York.

SCOTT, J. P. (1958). *Aggression*. Chicago.

——— (1966). Agonistic behavior of mice and rats: a review. *Amer. Zool.*, **6**, 683.

SIGG, E. B. (1969). Relationship of aggressive behavior to adrenal and gonadal function in male mice. In *Aggressive behavior* (ed. S. Garattini and E. B. Sigg). Amsterdam.

SWYER, G. I. M. (1968). Clinical effects of agents affecting fertility. In *Endocrinology and human behavior* (ed. R. P. Michael). London.

ZUCKERMAN, M. and LUBIN, B. (1965). *Manual for the multiple affect adjective check list*. San Diego.

ZUCKERMAN, M., PERSKY, H., ECKMAN, K. M., and HOPKINS, T. R. (1967). A multitrait multimethod measurement approach to the traits (or states) of anxiety, despression and hostility. *J. project. Tech.*, **31**, 39.

7. EXPECTATIONS CONCERNING FEMALE AND MALE SEX ROLES AND THEIR CHANGE WITH TIME

JAN TROST

INTRODUCTION

In this chapter we will discuss and analyse some data obtained from a panel study concerning sex role expectations. The aim of the study was to analyse the fields of mate-selection and marital satisfaction. Couples in Westtown, Sweden were interviewed in 1965 and 1970. In 1965 the couples were newly established. The oldest marriage was about 6 months old, and some of the couples were to get married soon after the interview.

In 1965 the main interest was on the problem of mate-selection, whereas in 1970 the interest was on marital satisfaction and what had happened during the 5-year period from 1965 to 1970.

The basic sample consisted of 409 couples. Due to refusals and the fact that some people were impossible to find etc., the final sample in the 1965 part of the study was about 65 per cent for the men and 70 per cent for the women. For the same kinds of reasons the final sample in the 1970 study was about 65 per cent of the basic sample for the men and almost 70 per cent for the women. Since the drop-outs were not exactly the same persons in 1965 and in 1970 the final sample *in the panel* was 50 per cent for men and 56 per cent for women, out of the basic sample of 409 men and 409 women. (For more information see Trost (1971).)

The fact that the drop-out from the panel is as high as almost 50 per cent of the basic sample means that the data must be treated with care and that it is not possible to generalize about the population of Westtown or about the Swedish population from these figures. However, the data are valuable for several reasons. In practice it is almost impossible to make perfect panel studies in this field. Very few studies of this kind have been made anywhere in the world, and an analysis of the data from the panel can be seen as examples or illustrations of theoretical lines of thought. Also the analysis may provide important ideas in developing theoretical lines of thought in this field.

We were interested in analysing changes in sex role expectations between 1965 and 1970. The questions that were asked concerned the subject of married women working outside the home, as well as sex. The actual questions were formulated (translated here) as follows:

1. Should married women without children work outside the home? (Both 1965 and 1970)
2. Should married women with children of school age work outside the home? (1965)
3. Should married women with children aged 7–12 work outside the home? (1970)
4. Can the woman as well as the man take the initiative to coitus? (Both 1965 and 1970)

5. Whose sexual satisfaction has the greatest importance for marital satisfaction — the man's, the woman's, or both? (Both 1965 and 1970.)

It should be noted that all questions except the last one lay stress on the position of being a woman; in two cases a specified one: the attribute of having children or not having any children at all.

We define 'role' (Trost 1967*a*) as the ego's perception of expectations that a person, a group, or an aggregate has on the ego in a given, ego-perceived position. It is evident that from the data available here we cannot directly analyse the sex roles, but we can analyse sex role expectations.

The questions concerned the attitudes of the individuals in the final sample. There could be a bridge between the attitudes in these cases, and the norms or expectations. We think there is such a bridge. The actual attitudes are a result of, among other things, a process of socialization. This process of socialization is by definition a normative process, which means that we learn or are socialized to perceive other people's norms and we internalize these norms in our minds in such a way that they are attitudes of our own. However, these attitudes from 1965 were influenced and possibly changed, by what happened during the 5 years between 1965 and 1970 and by the perception of the attitudes of the other spouse.

It is obvious from what is said above that, according to our paradigm, some of the attitudes of an individual are expectations upon other persons or, stated otherwise, our attitudes are sent as norms. In the same way some of the perceived attitudes of the other spouse will act as perceived norms and thus they will be obeyed as more obvious norms are. For a more detailed discussion of these problems see e.g. Aronsson (1971).

DATA

In the following we will present data for only those persons and couples from which we have answers. This means that the number of cases will be about 200 and sometimes less than 200. This limitation in the data would be a serious one if our intention was to give a description of the population. But since our intention is merely to give an analysis of changes in sex roles over time the limitation is not very serious.

Question 1: married women without children

About 70 per cent of both the males and the females in 1965 answered 'yes' to the question whether they

TABLE 7.1

Should a married woman without children work outside home?

(a) *Answers from men*

1965	1970		
	Yes	Indifferent and no	Sum
Yes	99 (92)	32 (39)	131
Indifferent and no	39 (46)	27 (20)	66
Sum	138	59	197

(b) *Answers from women*

1965	1970		
	Yes	Indifferent and no	Sum
Yes	129 (117)	34 (46)	163
Indifferent and no	32 (44)	29 (17)	61
Sum	161	63	224

thought that married women without children should work outside the home, and the rest, about 30 per cent, said 'no' or were indifferent. The results are about the same for 1970, which means that there were no net changes. The gross changes are shown in Table 7.1. Numbers in parentheses are numbers of persons in each cell expected under the assumption that the two variables are independent of each other, and calculated upon the actual marginal frequencies.

We find that among the men there are 32 individuals who have moved from a positive attitude towards married women without children working outside home to an indifferent or negative attitude, and 39 who have moved in the other direction. For simplicity we call the former ones 'traditionalists' and the other category 'modernists'. Among the women we have 34 individuals who have become traditionalist and 32 who have become modernist.

Only 10 (31 per cent) of the 32 men who have become traditionalist perceive that the wife thinks that married women without children should work outside the home. Ten of them perceive their wife as being for and 12 (38 per cent) perceive that she is against married women without children working outside the home. On the other hand, out of those 39 who have become modernists, 37 individuals (95 per cent) perceive the wife to have the idea that the married woman without children should work outside the home. Thus, we can assume

that there is an influence upon the men from their perception of the wife's thinking.

The average number of children differs between those men who have become traditionalists and those who have become modernists. Among the former group less than 50 per cent have two children or more but among those who have become modernists about 75 per cent have two or more children. It seems reasonable that the experience of having children should influence one's mind in relation to one's attitudes towards married women without children and their position of working outside the home or not doing so. For comparison it could be mentioned that in the whole sample just over 50 per cent have two children or more.

Among those who have grown traditionalist about 40 per cent are married to a woman who is working outside the home and among those who have grown modernist there are about 60 per cent in the same situation. We assume that the experience has influenced at least some of the respondents.

If we compare the perception of the spouses' view in 1965 with the perception in 1970 we find that all of the men who are traditionalists (except one) in 1965 perceived that their wives thought that the married woman without children should work outside the home, but in 1970 one-third of them had changed their perception in the direction of perceiving that the wife says no, and one-third in the direction of perceiving that she is ambivalent.

The same comparison for the modernists in 1970 shows that almost all of them perceived the wife as a yes-sayer, but in 1965 more than 50 per cent perceived the wives as yes-sayers, and only 25 per cent perceived the wife as a traditionalist. From this we can conclude that there is a tendency for those who have become traditionalists not to be influenced by their perception of the wife's view to the same extent as those who have become modernists.

The women who have become traditionalists are somewhat younger than those who have become modernists; little over 40 per cent of those who have become traditionalists and only 25 per cent among those who have become modernists are younger than 26 years.

All of the women who have become modernists (except one) perceived that their husbands thought that married women without children should work outside the home. Among those who have become traditionalists the picture is somewhat different. Half of them perceived their husbands as being indifferent in these matters; and one-third of them perceived their husbands as being in favour of married women without children working outside the home.

There is a tendency for women who have become traditionalists to have a larger number of children than those who have become modernists — the difference is, however, very small between these two categories.

There is a weak tendency to be more housewives among those who have become traditionalists than among those who have become modernists — 13 out of 34 of the traditionalists and 9 out of the 31 who have become modernists.

If we compare the women's perception of their husbands' views in 1965 with their perception in 1970 we find that 25 out of the 28 women who have grown traditionalists in 1965 perceived that their husbands thought that the married women without children should work outside the home, but in 1970 about 60 per cent (16 women) had changed their perception in the direction of perceiving that their husbands say no or are indifferent. The same comparison for the modernists yields that in 1970 all except one perceived the husband as a yes-sayer but even in 1965 half of them perceived him as yes-sayer, while the rest perceived the husband as no-sayer or indifferent.

Questions 2 and 3: married women with children of school age

The next question was limited to the married woman with a child or children of school age (1965) and with a child or children aged 7–12 years (1970). It should be noted that the question was not the same in 1970 as in 1965. However, we assume that the real content is about the same in spite of the fact that the semantic content differs. There is no problem with the lower age limit, i.e. 7 years, since children in Sweden do not go to school until they are 7 years old. But the upper limit in 1970 is lower than the upper limit in 1965. In 1965 some of the respondents probably considered children aged 7–15 or 16. The reason why we assume that the real content of the two questions is about the same is that the upper age limit for the obligatory schools now is about 16 years, but this is fairly new. Fifteen years ago the children finished their obligatory school at the age of 13–14 years. We assume that most of the people have considered the lower school ages for another reason; this reason is that the discussion in Sweden has dealt with the lower school ages and, as far as we know, very seldom with the upper school ages (teenagers).

If we here also dichotomize between those who answered 'yes' to the question and those who answered 'no' or were indifferent we find that the net change for men is about 10 per cent (44 per cent saying yes in 1965 and 34 per cent in 1970) and for the women the net change is about the same, but the relative number of yes-sayers is higher among them than among the men (57 per cent yes-sayers in 1965 and 48 per cent in 1970). These net changes might be an effect of the difference in wording of the two questions but, as mentioned above, we do not think that wording is very important. The net change might be an effect of other things, for instance the discussions in mass media, etc. They have been very intensive during the last years of the 1960s and most of these discussions have dealt with the situation for married women with children in the school years and younger. At the same time one should notice that there is a *decrease* in the relative number of persons being positive towards married women in this situation

TABLE 7.2

Do you think that married women with children aged 7–12 years should work outside home? (1970)

Do you think that married women with children at school ages should work outside home? (1965)

(a) *Answers from men*

1965	1970		
	Yes	Indifferent	Sum
Yes	39 (35)	52 (56)	91
Indifferent and no	38 (42)	69 (65)	107
Sum	77	121	198

(b) *Answers from women*

1965	1970		
	Yes	Indifferent and no	Sum
Yes	70 (61)	53 (62)	123
Indifferent and no	40 (49)	58 (49)	98
Sum	110	111	221

working outside the home whereas the discussions mostly have propagated for an increase in the number of married women who have children of school age and are working outside the home.

The gross changes are shown in Table 7.2. We find among men that there are 52 persons who have moved from a positive attitude toward married women with children in the school years to a negative or indifferent attitude; and 38 who have moved in the other direction. Among the women we have 53 persons who have moved from a positive to an indifferent or negative attitude in 1970; and 40 who have moved in the other direction.

For this variable the same tendency can be found for men as was found concerning the attitude toward the married woman without children, i.e. those who have become traditionalists perceive more often that the wife says that a woman with children of school age should work at home (33 out of the 51 actual, which is about 65 per cent, whereas only 10 per cent of those who have become modernists). Ten (20 per cent) of those who have become traditionalists perceive that their wife thinks that a woman with children of school age should work outside the home, but 29 (about 75 per cent) of those who have become modernists have

57

this perception. The traditionalists are married to women working at home to a greater extent than the modernists are.

There is a tendency for the women who have become traditionalists to be younger than those who have grown modernist. Among those who have become traditionalists 45 per cent were 26 years old or younger in 1970; among those who have grown modernist 25 per cent are 26 years or younger and in the whole material the corresponding figure is 38 per cent.

We found in both men and women a tendency to perceive their spouses as similar to themselves. Only about 15 per cent of those who have grown traditionalist perceive that the spouse thinks that a married woman with children in the school years should work outside the home, but about 85 per cent of those who have become modernists perceive so.

There is a tendency among the men for the traditionalists to perceive their wives as similar to themselves, both in 1965 and in 1970; i.e. many of the traditionalists answered 'yes' on the perception question in 1965 and 'no' on the same question concerning their wives' views in 1970. Only about 5 per cent of the traditionalists (out of 51 persons) have changed their perception in the opposite direction. The tendency is exactly the same for the modernists, i.e. most of them perceived in 1965 that their wives were negative towards married women with school-age children working outside the home but in 1970 they have changed their perception. The same holds true for the women, both those who have become traditionalists and those who have become modernists.

Question 4: initiative to coitus

Can the woman as well as the man take the initiative to coitus? The alternative answers were slightly different in 1965 from 1970: in 1965 the alternatives were: 'yes, absolutely', 'yes, undecided', 'no, undecided', 'no, absolutely not'. In 1970 the alternatives were: 'yes', 'no', and 'undecided'. Very few in 1965 as well as in 1970 said 'yes, undecided'; for this reason we have dichotomized the variables in 1965 between 'yes, absolutely' and 'yes, undecided', and in 1970 the alternatives 'no' and 'undecided' are put together.

These differences in the answering alternatives might be important in the marginal frequencies; if in the 1965 interview situation a respondent answered 'yes' with some uncertainty the respondent was classified in the category, 'yes, undecided', but in 1970 the same kind of answer might well have been classified as 'yes', which means that the two answers, which are the same in content, have been classified in different categories. This means that one could assume that the number of yes-sayers (as they are classified here) would be higher in 1970 than in 1965. The figures show a clear tendency in this direction: the net change was 6 per cent for men and 14 per cent for women (92 per cent male yes-sayers in 1965 and 98 in 1970, for females 83 and 97 per cent respectively). But at the same time it is reasonable to

TABLE 7.3

Can the woman as well as the man take an initiative to coitus?

(a) *Answers from men*

1965	1970		
	Yes	Indifferent and no	Sum
Yes, absolutely	177 (175)	3 (5)	180
Yes, indifferent	13 (15)	2 (0)	15
No, indifferent No, absolutely not			
Sum	190	5	195

(b) *Answers from women*

1965	1970		
	Yes	Indifferent and no	Sum
Yes, absolutely	182 (179)	2 (5)	184
Yes, indifferent No, indifferent No, absolutely not	33 (36)	3 (0)	36
Sum	215	5	220

assume for instance that the marital experience would give a result in the same direction.

In our opinion, though almost everyone in this sample says that the woman as well as the man can take the initiativ to coitus, we cannot draw the conclusion that there is an equality in these senses between the two sexes. The reason for this is that it evidently might be assumed that people do not mean the same things or the same behaviour or activities when talking about the initiative to coitus coming from a woman as from a man.

The gross changes from 1965 to 1970 are found in Table 7.3. Since only 3 of the men have changed their minds from saying that a woman as well as a man can take the initiative to coitus in 1965 to saying 'no' or being undecided in 1970, we shall not try to analyse them — they are too few for this. However, we have 13 men who have changed their minds from being undecided in 1965 to saying (in 1970) that the woman as well as the man can take the initiative to coitus. We will compare these 13 men's answers with the answers from all men in our sample.

Those men who have changed their minds from 1965 to 1970 discuss sexual matters with their spouses much more seldom than the men in the total sample. Only 1

58

person (8 per cent) out of the 13 who have changed their minds says that he often discusses sexual matters with his wife. One third of the men in the total sample say that they discuss sexual matters with their wives very often or often. There are no age differences between those men who have changed their minds and the total group. The changers do not believe that sexual satisfaction is important for marital satisfaction to the same extent as the men in the total sample do.

There is no tendency at all as regards the perception of the spouses' views in relation to the question whether the women as well as the man can take the initiative to coitus. This has to do with the fact that almost all men perceive that their wives feel that the woman as well as the man can take the initiative to coitus.

The situation is about the same with the women as with the men as regards the number of changers in the two principal categories. We have only 2 who have changed their views from being positive in 1965 to being indifferent or negative in 1970. However, we have 33 cases of change in the opposite direction, i.e. from being indifferent or no-sayers in 1965 to being yes-sayers in 1970. Let us compare these 33 changers with the total sample.

There is a tendency, not very strong, however, that the women who have changed their minds in the more 'liberal' direction discuss sexual matters with their husbands more seldom than the women in the total sample do. Evidently, this is the same tendency as for the men. There are no age differences between this category and the total group. For the women there are no differences between the changers and the total group as regards their beliefs in the importance of sexual satisfaction for marital satisfaction.

As regards the perception of the other spouse's opinion concerning this topic, the same is true as for the men, i.e. there are no tendencies since almost everyone perceives the other spouse to think that both the man and the woman can take the initiative to coitus.

Question 5: sexual satisfaction

Whose sexual satisfaction has the greatest importance for marital satisfaction? The net change between 1965 and 1970 for men is 9 per cent (71 per cent of the men said 'both' in 1965 and 80 per cent said so in 1970, the answer 'the woman' was given by 19 per cent in 1965 and by 12 per cent in 1970 and the answer 'the man' 10 and 8 per cent respectively). The net change for the women is much more evident, it is 26 per cent (58 per cent of the women said 'both' in 1965 and 84 per cent said so in 1970, the answer 'the woman' was given by 3 per cent in 1965 and 1 per cent in 1970, and the answer 'the man' was given by 39 and 15 per cent respectively).

We can see here that when the spouses were newly married the difference in opinion on this question between the man and the woman was fairly large, but it has decreased after 5 years of marriage. There is, however, a small tendency in 1970 for more women to say that the man's satisfaction is the most important

TABLE 7.4

Whose sexual satisfaction has the greatest importance for the marital satisfaction?

(a) *Answers from men*

1965	1970			
	The woman's	Both	The man's	Sum
The woman	10 (5)	24 (29)	3 (3)	37
Both	13 (17)	110 (102)	7 (11)	130
The man	1 (2)	10 (13)	6 (2)	17
Sum	24	144	16	184

(b) *Answers from women*

1965	1970			
	The woman's	Both	The man's	Sum
The woman	0 (0)	5 (4)	0 (1)	5
Both	1 (1)	110 (104)	12 (18)	123
The man	1 (1)	65 (72)	19 (12)	85
Sum	2	180	31	213

one, and almost none of the women say that the woman's sexual satisfaction is the most important one.

The gross changes are found in Table 7.4. We will here analyse four types of changers. Among the men there are 7 who have changed from saying 'both' to saying 'the woman', 24 persons from saying 'the woman' to saying 'both', and 10 persons from saying 'the man' in 1965 to saying 'both' in 1970. Among the women the figures are 12 changing from saying 'both' to saying 'the man', 1 person from saying 'both' to saying 'the woman', 5 persons from saying 'the woman' to saying 'both', and 65 persons who have changed from saying 'the man' in 1965 to saying 'both' in 1970. Since there are so few among the women (1 and 5 respectively) who have changed to or from saying 'the woman' we will not try to analyse them. This means that we in reality have only two categories in which we are interested (but in principle there are more categories). They are: those who have changed their minds from saying that the sexual satisfaction of both partners is of the greatest importance in marital satisfaction to saying (in 1970) that the sexual satisfaction of the man is of the greatest importance, and those saying in 1965 that the man's sexual satisfaction has the greatest importance for marital satisfaction and in 1970 saying that the man's and the woman's sexual satisfaction are of equal importance. The fact that both in 1965 and in 1970 there are so few women who have said that the woman's sexual satisfaction is the most important, and that a fair number have said in 1965 that the man's sexual satisfaction is the most important, can be seen as an indication of the notion of sex roles, as regards the women, remaining among women. If this conclusion is correct one must conclude that this kind of sex role expectation is more seldom found among the men.

If the idea presented earlier (that the perception of the opinion of the other spouse influences the actual opinion) is correct, we should find that those who have changed their minds should have done so in the direction of what they perceived their spouse to think. There is a tendency in this direction for men who have changed from saying (in 1965) that the woman's sexual satisfaction is the most important one in marital satisfaction to saying 'both' in 1970, and for those men who in 1965 have said that the man's satisfaction is the most important and in 1970 saying 'both'. However, we do not find any tendencies for those men who have changed from saying 'both' in 1965 to saying 'the man' or 'the woman' in 1970. As is said above there are too few cases in the material for the women, so we can analyse only two categories. The assumption is verified for those women who in 1965 said that the man's sexual satisfaction was the most important and have changed their minds to saying 'both' in 1970. In fact, this change is very remarkable, since 57 out of the 61 changers perceive that their husband says 'both' in 1970. For those women who in 1965 have said that the satisfaction of both spouses is the most important, there is a tendency in the assumed direction, but not as strong as the one mentioned above.

We have asked the respondents to do a self-rating of their own marital happiness in 1970 on a seven-point scale, going from 'very unhappy' to 'very happy'. It is possible to assume that men who have changed their mind from saying 'both' in 1965 to saying 'the man' in 1970 have grown more selfish or dominant, those men who said 'both' in 1965 and 'the woman' in 1970 are assumed to have grown more submissive, and those who have changed their minds from either saying 'the woman' or saying 'the man' in 1965 to saying 'both' in 1970 can be assumed to be more co-operative. The corresponding assumptions for women would be that those who have changed from saying 'both' to saying 'the man' have grown more submissive, those who have changed from saying 'both' in 1965 to saying 'the woman' in 1970 have grown more dominant, and for the remaining two categories the assumptions are the same as for the men. Since the societal norms today can be said to favour a more co-operative mind than a submissive or a dominant one, we can assume that the categories here classified as co-operative should have a higher marital satisfaction than the other two categories. Data show that there are no clear tendencies for men in the assumed direction, nor in any other direction. The data for women show a tendency to satisfy the assumption (n.b. only the two categories that are analysed here).

Another measurement of the marital satisfaction is provided by the question concerning whether the respondents get enough affection from the other spouse. If we use this criterion on marital satisfaction and the same classifications mentioned above we find that the data for men tend to classify them as either submissive or co-operative. In the dominant category there are only 7 individuals and all say that they get enough affection. According to this measurement, the figures for the women show that the women here classified as submissive show higher marital satisfaction than those called co-operative do. This is in contradiction to the assumption that the co-operative categories should have higher marital satisfaction than the other categories.

The two types of male changers here named dominant and submissive say that they discuss sexual matters with their spouses much more than the men here classified as co-operative do; the tendency is the same for the women.

We asked the respondents how great an importance their sexual life had in their marital satisfaction. For the men there is a tendency for the submissive men to say, to a greater extent than the dominant or the co-operative men, that their sexual life has a very great importance for their marital satisfaction; we cannot find the same tendency for the women, since the submissive category contains only 1 person. There is an important difference (n.b. the small number of cases) between the dominant and the co-operative women — many dominant women claim that their sexual life has a very great importance in their marital satisfaction, but very few of the co-operative women say so.

CONCLUSION

We have found that the net changes in our panel data are small, except in one case — the answers from the women concerning their opinions about the importance that their sexual satisfaction has upon their marital satisfaction. This net change can be seen as an indicator of greater egalitarianism as regards sex roles.

The gross changes are, in all cases analysed here, smaller than the expected gross changes (expected from the marginal frequencies and under the assumption that the variables are independent); the differences between the observed and the expected gross changes are, however, fairly small. This means that the gross changes in relation to the net changes are on the average fairly noticeable. The majority of the gross changes are in a direction that is consistent with the assumed changes in the societal norms toward greater and greater egalitarianism as regards sex roles.

There is a clear tendency for those who have changed their minds in these questions to have a perception of the other spouse's opinion that it is similar to one's own opinion. This holds true for men as well as for women. We assumed that the similarity of one's own opinion and the perception of the other spouse's opinion is due to an influence, conscious or unconscious, from the spouse. It is reasonable that the two spouses in a marital dyad should influence each other and that after 5 years of marriage this influence should be fairly noticeable. But at the same time a somewhat contradictory assumption is reasonable too — the assumption that one perceives the other spouse as similar to oneself, independent of the other spouse's opinion. A tendency in this direction was found by Trost (1967b) in analysing the mate-selection process with data from the first step in the panel.

There is a tendency too for the results mentioned in the last paragraph to be more pronounced for those who have become modernists than for those who have become traditionalists. The modernists have changed from being negative toward married women with or without children working outside the home to a positive attitude; and the traditionalists have changed in the other direction. This difference between the modernists and the traditionalists may have something to do with the fact that the modernists have changed their minds in the direction that is in accordance with the now official societal norms. Those who have grown traditionalist can be said to be in opposition to the societal norms and it seems reasonable that they should be more independent, not only in relation to societal norms, but also in relation to the opinions in the family group.

As a concluding remark we assume that the personal effect on the individual differs between those who change their mind in the direction of the societal norms and those who change in the opposite direction. In the former category one receives overt or covert rewards from the surrounding social environment and from one's own internal mind but in the latter category one receives overt or covert punishment from the surrounding social environment to a greater extent and one risks feeling dissonant, because of the change as such, and because of feeling like an outsider or perceiving the social norms to be unreasonable — a state of anomie.

SUMMARY

Data from a panel study, collected in Sweden in 1965 and in 1970, are analysed with respect to changes in expectations regarding sex roles. Both spouses in marriages that were formed in 1965 were interviewed at both times. The examples on sex roles that are analysed concern whether married women should work outside home, who should take initiative to coitus, and the relation between sexual satisfaction and marital satisfaction. The results show that the net changes are fairly remarkable, that there is a connection between the perception of the spouse's opinion and one's own, and that most of the changes go in the same direction as the societal norms but an important number go in the opposite direction.

REFERENCES

ARONSSON, Å. (1971). 'Grupp och grupptillhörighet' [Group and group belongingness]. Research Report from the Department of Sociology, Uppsala University. Special Series on Alcohol Research, AF 20. Uppsala.

TROST, J. (1967a). *Om sociala roller* [On social roles]. Sociologisk Forskning, p. 96–138.

—— (1967b). Some data on mate-selection: homogamy and perceived homogamy. *J. Marr. Fam.*, **29**, 739–55.

—— (1971). 'A marriage panel: methods and distribution of frequencies.' Research Report from the Department of Sociology, Uppsala University. Special Series on Family Research, FF 16. Uppsala.

8. GENDER IDENTITY AND SEXUAL DYSFUNCTION IN THE MALE

JOHN BANCROFT

Gender identity is one aspect of human sexuality which begins to develop early, well before sexual orientation is established. If sexual maladjustment is to be prevented we need to understand the part that disturbances of gender identity play in its causation. If they are important then preventative measures might be taken in childhood or early adolescence before sexual relationships are established.

The possible association between gender identity and sexual behaviour has been explored in an earlier paper (Bancroft 1972). In that paper a general theoretical model for such relationships was suggested and examined in the particular cases of homosexuality and transvestism. The purpose of this chapter is to extend this examination to include male sexual dysfunction.

The theoretical model was based on the assumption that sexual behaviour, whether normal, dysfunctional, or deviant, depends on the interaction of many factors. The two principal components of sexual behaviour, the choice of sexual partner, and the method of relating to that partner, not only effect each other in a reciprocal manner, but also interact with gender identity. Thus the choice of sexual partner determines to some extent the method of relating to that partner and vice versa. The choice of a homosexual partner, for example, or a passive method of relating, may undermine the masculine gender identity of a male, whilst a feminine gender identity will in turn effect the choice of partner and so on. The purpose of the theoretical model was to suggest a mechanism based on cognitive consistency theory, to account for these interrelationships.

It was suggested (Bancroft 1972) that most factors influencing sexual behaviour are relatively non-specific, their effects depending on how they interact with other factors present. Some are relatively specific although their effects are likely to produce repercussions in the sytem as a whole. An example of a specific factor is the physiological dysfunction of the sexually inadequate male, resulting from either innate deficiencies or faulty autonomic learning (Bancroft 1971).

Though the effects of such physiological factors on sexual performance are obvious, their effects on gender identity are hardly less striking. Few experiences are as undermining to a man's sense of masculinity than sexual failures. But to what extent may disturbed gender identity cause sexual failure in the first place or alternatively serve to perpetuate it once it has happened? These questions are relevant both to the prevention and treatment of sexual dysfunction.

AETIOLOGICAL FACTORS RELATED TO GENDER IDENTITY

Let us next consider some other views of the aetiology of sexual dysfunction which may have a bearing on these questions. The majority of such views have been in the psychoanalytic literature, and are based largely on anecdotal evidence. Very few systematic studies of possible aetiological factors have been reported (for review see Cooper 1969).

Most writers have stressed the importance of anxiety from various sources as a cause of sexual failure. Fear of castration is one of the most common in the psychoanalytic literature, though there is very little systematically collected data to support this hypothesis. Such a fear, however, could be interpreted as a threat to one's masculinity. 'Inferiority feelings' are often mentioned and in some cases no doubt involve feelings of inferiority about gender. It is difficult, however, to separate such feelings that may have preceeded the sexual failure from those that stemmed from it. Fenichel (1945) considered that 'feminine identification' was important in some cases of impotence, whereas other writers have in some way blamed adolescent homosexuality (e.g. Stafford Clark 1954).

Masters and Johnson (1970), in reporting the treatment of their vast series of sexually inadequate couples, briefly mention some factors of aetiological significance. Most of these have no obvious association with gender identity but the following are probably relevant.

Of their 32 cases of primary erectile impotence, 3 reported an absent father and an overt sexual relationship with the mother. Of the 213 cases of secondary erectile impotence, 13 reported markedly dominant mothers (dominating both husbands and sons), and 5 markedly dominant fathers. In a further 5 one parent was absent. These workers equated an absent parent with dominance by the other parent and concluded that the presence of a dominant mother would lead to insufficient masculinity for the child to identify with, whereas a very dominant father would present too much masculinity for the child to attempt to achieve. In either case the result, they suggested, could be a sensitivity to any suggestion of personal inadequacy. In neither premature ejaculation nor ejaculatory incompetence, however, were any aetiological factors suggested which clearly involved gender identity.

One aspect of gender which is measurable is physique, particularly as reflected in the androgyny scores. Johnson (1968) in investigating the part that 'constitutional factors' play in sexual dysfunction, compared the androgyny scores in a group of 55 impotent males and 55 normal controls. The result showed considerable differences between patients and controls, which were largely accounted for by those patients with neurotic personalities and an early onset to their sexual problems. Coppen (1959) has already shown the difficulties in interpreting such findings in his study of the androgyny scores of homosexual and heterosexual psychiatric patients. Johnson, however, concluded on the basis of his results that constitutional factors were probably important in his cases. He did not go any further in explaining what such constitutional factors might be or how they might operate.

The relationship between gender identity and physique has not been investigated, though it is usually presumed that awareness of a feminine physique may undermine one's sense of masculinity. The presence of a relatively gynaecoid physique does not necessarily mean that the subject is aware of it; nevertheless, physique may have a direct effect on gender identity in this way. Alternatively, some common factor may be responsible for both physique and gender identity. Furthermore, it is not inconceivable that psychological factors may have an effect on physique. The factors determining the androgyny score are dependent on testosterone levels at puberty (Tanner 1962). It is certainly possible that hormone levels and even the timing of the onset of puberty may be influenced by psychological processes (Donovan 1963). At the present time it is difficult to see how these varied causal relationships could be differentiated.

Let us confine ourselves therefore to factors which could have an understandable psychological effect on the development of gender identity and which can be identified as existing before the establishment of any sexually dysfunctional pattern. The following are proposed as important, though many others may be involved:

(1) relationship with the mother;
(2) relationship with the father;
(3) awareness in pre-puberty and early adolescence of physical factors or abnormalities of possible gender significance;
(4) transvestite or transsexual fantasies or behaviour.

Let us then look at each of these in more detail.

Parental relationships
Considerable attention has been given to the role of parental relationships in homosexuals, much less in the case of sexually inadequate males.

There is general agreement between most workers that there is a high incidence of disturbed parental relationships in the childhood and adolescence of homosexuals, with somewhat more importance being attached to the paternal relationship (West 1959; Bene 1965; Bieber *et al.* 1962).

Bieber went as far as to say that a constructive, supportive, warmly relating father precludes the possibility of a homosexual son. O'Connon (1964) also reported a high incidence of absent fathers in homosexuals but this finding was not supported in Bieber's study, or that of Moran and Abe (1969). More recent studies have shown that disturbed parental relationships are not more common in homosexuals than heterosexuals, when homosexuals low in neuroticism are considered. There may, however, be some association for male homosexuals low in masculinity (Seigelman 1974).

Most explanations of the effect of disturbed parental relationships are not relevant to the development of gender identity, except in the special case of childhood transsexualism (Stoller 1968; Green 1969). Clearly, however, mothers may interfere in the development of masculinity in their sons by directly encouraging feminine attributes, by being overprotective and instilling a feeling of physical vulnerability in the boy, by being over-dominating and controlling in relation to the father and the son.

The father may cause difficulty by being both excessively masculine and competitive in his relationships with his son, so that the son feels unable to compete, or by being weak and unmasculine himself depriving the son of a good male model with which to identify. An absent father will result in both a lack of such a model and the possibility (though not inevitability) of an over-controlling mother.

Physical factors
We have already discussed the possible roles of physique in determining gender identity. In addition, chronic physical handicap may lead to an impaired sense of masculinity, as may obesity, gynaecomastia of puberty, abnormalities of the genitalia such as undescended testicle, and enuresis. A physical characteristic of particular interest is the size of the penis. This has received special attention in the study of homosexuals (Bieber *et al.* 1962; Bancroft 1972). It has a special significance because it is a physical characteristic which may be very much influenced by psychological factors. The size of the non-erect or erect penis is by no means fixed and concern about its size might perpetuate a smaller penis than would otherwise be the case, due to the effect on resting vaso-motor tone.

Transvestite or transsexual tendencies
Such tendencies occurring in childhood or adolescence may effect gender identity in ways which have already been discussed in a previous paper (Bancroft 1972).

CLINICAL DATA

To investigate the possible importance of these factors further, some of the author's clinical material has been examined. In recent years I have taken systematic histories from most patients with sexual problems referred to me for behavioural treatment. These histories have included the areas listed above. The 25 most recent cases of male sexual dysfunction (19 cases of erectile impotence, 4 cases of premature ejaculation, and 2 cases of ejaculatory incompetence) have therefore been looked at and compared with 25 homosexuals selected randomly from my clinical material. (Mean age of sexually dysfunctional group, 31·4 years, range 19 to 53; mean age of homosexuals 28·9 years, range 18–45). In both groups the information was collected in exactly the same way. The findings are given below. The presence of a particular factor is recorded only when it is striking and unequivocal.

Retrospective data of this type is inevitably of uncertain validity and, particularly with small numbers such as these and the absence of a normal control group, it is not possible to draw firm conclusions. It is hoped, however, that this data will be of value at least in generating hypotheses.

The following operational definitions were used in recording the data.

Operational definitions

Maternal relationships. Dominating/controlling mothers are those who throughout childhood and adolescence are both clearly dominant in the marriage and closely control the son's life. Such a son feels markedly influenced by his mother's will. Domination of the husband alone would not be included here. *Detached mothers* show a lack of affection and little attention to their son during childhood. *Over-protective mothers* worry about their sons' physical health and safety to the extent that they inhibit or prevent masculine play activities.

Paternal relationships. Absence or death of father before the age of 10 is indicated. *Detached/hostile fathers* show a lack of affection for their sons and spend very little time in their company during childhood. The relationship may or may not be a hostile one. *Weak fathers* are dominated by their wives, and are unable to give a lead to their sons, who feel little respect for them and see their fathers as failures. *Unremarkable parental relationships* are those in which no obvious disturbance of any kind is reported.

Physical factors. The following areas were investigated routinely: chronic physical illness or handicap in childhood and adolescence leading to a restriction of physical activities, feminine physical characteristics, obesity, gynaecomastia, any abnormality of the genitalia, enuresis after the age of 10. The unequivocal presence of or concern about any of these conditions was rated as positive in this category. In several cases more than one factor was present.

Anxiety about size of penis was rated as a separate factor, provided that it was reported as occurring in early adolescence.

Transvestite and transsexual tendencies. Any evidence of pleasurable cross-dressing or thoughts of wanting to be a girl recalled after the age of 5 and not occurring as part of a group activity (e.g. dressing-up group games) was included here.

Results

The results are shown in Tables 8.1–8.5.

TABLE 8.1

Maternal relationship

Type of relationship	Sexually inadequate (n = 25)	Homosexual (n = 25)	Difference between groups
Dominating/controlling	2	2	N.S.
Detached	1	3	N.S.
Over-protective	3	6	N.S.
Unremarkable	18	10	$\chi^2 = 3.99$ $p \leq 0.05$

TABLE 8.2

Paternal relationship

Type of relationship	Sexually inadequate (n = 25)	Homosexual (n = 25)	Difference between groups
Absent/dead	6	1	N.S.
Detached/hostile	7	4	N.S.
Weak	2	8	N.S.
Unremarkable	10	12	N.S.

TABLE 8.3

Both parental relationships disturbed

Sexually inadequate (n = 25)	Homosexual (n = 25)	Difference between groups
1	9	$\chi^2 = 6.15$ $p \leq 0.02$

TABLE 8.4

Factor	Sexually inadequate (n = 25)	Homosexual (n = 25)	Difference between groups
Physical factors present	14	14	N.S.
Anxiety about size of penis	6	11	N.S.
Transvestite or transexual tendencies	4	10	N.S.

TABLE 8.5

Accumulated incidence of factors

Factor	Sexually inadequate (n = 25)	Homosexual (n = 25)	Difference between groups
No factors	1	2	
One factor present	7	4	$\chi^2_3 = 10$
Two factors present	16	7	$p \leq 0.02$
Three or more factors present	1	12	

Conclusions

Comparison of the two groups shows that, as far as these recorded factors are concerned, they occur commonly in both sexually dysfunctional and homosexual males. Only one of the first and two of the second group were free from all of them (Table 8.5). However, when each factor is taken in turn, no significant difference between the groups is found except that there are significantly fewer unremarkable maternal relationships in the homosexual group (Table 8.1). This is again reflected in Table 8.3, which shows that disturbance in both parental relationships is significantly more common in the homosexuals. Six of the 9 disturbed parental pairs in the homosexual group involved a weak father, though in only one of these was the mother dominating/controlling. Bieber *et al.* (1962) stressed the importance of the interaction of maternal and paternal influences in the development of homosexuality. These findings are consistent with this view. However, the presence of a disturbed paternal relationship appears to have no specific tendency to cause homosexuality but may be generally associated with sexual maladjustment, perhaps through its effect on gender identity development.

Disturbed maternal relationships may have more specific effects in producing homosexual orientation.

Similarly, physical factors of possible gender significance are common in both groups (56 per cent in each group, Table 8.4). This incidence needs to be compared with that in a sexually normal group, but it does suggest the possible non-specific contribution to sexual maladjustment, again via gender identity disturbance. Anxiety about the size of penis and transvestite tendencies are not significantly more common in the homosexual group. It is of interest that the incidence of the former factor in these two groups (44 per cent in the homosexual and 24 per cent in the sexually dysfunctional group) is strikingly similar to the incidence in Beiber's series (38 per cent in homosexuals, 28 per cent in heterosexual patient controls). In view of this the significance of this factor is difficult to assess but comparison with a sexually normal control group is again required.

Although there are few differences in individual factors, Table 8.5 shows that these factors accumulate more frequently in the homosexual group. This suggests the possibility that the more contributory factors that are present the more likely is it that homosexuality will become established rather than heterosexual dysfunction. It should be stressed, however, that the homosexual subjects studied here are those who have sought psychiatric help. It may be that in sexual maladjustment associated with homosexual preferences rather than the homosexuality *per se* that is determined by such factors.

CONCLUSION

We can summarize by postulating that factors which lead to gender identity disturbance have a non-specific effect in causing sexual maladjustment. Whether one particular type of sexual disorder develops rather than another may depend partly on the presence of specific aetiological factors. In sexual dysfunction, for example, specific physiological vulnerability may be all that is required for the problem to become established. In other cases, however, a relatively minor degree of physiological vulnerability may interact with psychological factors and result in severe difficulty. Transient erectile failure or premature ejaculation must be common in many sexual relationships. If it occurs, however, in a man who is sensitive about his gender identity it may lead to sufficient threat or anxiety to ensure its establishment. The possibility that gender identity disturbance may be linked with physiological vulnerability through a common cause must also be considered.

Homosexuality, or at least homosexual maladjustment, may have its specific aetiological factors also (e.g. appropriate maternal/paternal relationships) or it may be more likely to develop if non-specific contributory factors are sufficiently numerous or, alternatively, combined to form a specific aetiological complex.

These results are consistent with the hypothesis that gender identity problems contribute to sexual maladjustment of various kinds, including sexual dysfunction. Further work is needed to identify which factors related to gender identity are most important and most easily recognizable, and whether any particular constellation of factors is more likely to lead to a homosexual adjustment or maladjustment.

REFERENCES

BANCROFT, J. H. J. (1971). Sexual inadequacy in the male. *Postgrad. med. J.*, **47**, 562–71.

—— (1972). *The relationship between gender identity and sexual behaviour: some clinical aspects in gender differences.* (ed. C. Ounsted and D. Taylor). London.

BENE, E. (1965). On the genesis of male homosexuality. *Brit. J. Psychiat.*, **3**, 803–13.

BIEBER, I., DAIN, H. J., DINCE, P. K., DRELLICH, M. G., GRAND, H. G., GUNDLACH, R. H., CREMER, M. W., RIFKIN, A. H., WILBER, C. B., and BIEBER, T. B. (1962). *Homosexuality: a psychoanalytic study.* New York.

COOPER, A. H. (1969). Factors in male sexual inadequacy: a review. *J. nerv. ment. Dis.*, **149**, 337–59.

COPPEN, A. J. (1959). Body build of male homosexuals. *Brit. med. J.*, ii, 1443.

DONOVAN, B. T. (1963). *The timing of puberty.* Scientific Basis of Medicine Annual Review. London.

FENICHEL, O. (1945). *Psychoanalytic theory of neuroses.* London.

GREEN, R. (1969). Childhood cross-gender identification in transexualism and sex reassignment (ed. R. Green and J. Money). Baltimore, Maryland.

JOHNSON, J. (1968). Disorders of sexual potency in the male. Oxford.

MASTERS, W. H. and JOHNSON, V. E. (1970). Human sexual inadequacy. London.

MORAN, P. A. P. and ABE, K. (1969). Parental loss in homosexuals. *Brit. J. Psychiat.*, **115**, 319–20.

O'CONNOR, P. J. (1964). Aetiological factors in homosexuality as seen in R.A.F. psychiatric practice. *Brit. J. Psychiat.*, **110**, 381–91.

SIEGELMAN, M. (1974). Parental background of male homosexuals and heterosexuals. *Arch. sex. Behav.*, **3**, 3–18.

STAFFORD-CLARK, D. (1954). The aetiology and treatment of impotence. *Practitioner*, **172**, 397–404.

STOLLER, R. J. (1968). *Sex and gender.* London.

TANNER, J. M. (1962). *Growth at adolescence* (2nd edn). Oxford.

WEST, D. J. (1959). Parental relationships in male homosexuality. *Int. J. soc. Psychiat.*, **5**, 85–97.

9. SOME COMMENTS ON PREMARITAL SEX IN SCANDINAVIA

PREBEN HERTOFT

NOTES ON A PSEUDO-PROBLEM

A question such as 'Is there a relationship between pre-marital petting and marital success?' is, in my opinion, almost unanswerable. Usually the question is raised in connection with a case against premarital sex, or to convince us about what a recommendable game premarital sex is. I find it nearly unbelievable that anybody would be seriously occupied with such a problem. If the question were raised only very seldom, this would not be worth discussing; but, in for example, the United States several 'scientists' have tried to find a definite answer through complicated investigations.

William R. Reevy begins one of his articles (1972) by mentioning some of 'the technical problems' which have to be solved 'if one tries to establish by means of research what the relationship is or might be between premarital petting and marital happiness (or failure)'. And he continues:

A first difficulty is that to this date it has been impossible to quantify the exact accumulative incidence of each category of petting behavior in the life history of an individual at the time a questionnaire is administered or an interview taken.... A second technical difficulty encountered is that it is impossible to measure with exactness the number of times that, let us say, petting of the bare genitals, has occured in conjunction with the emotion of love or perhaps anxiety or disgust. It would be desirable to be able to gather such data with exactness so as to get the measure of the strength of the factor which might interact with petting, as petting which takes place in a context of love and affection might be predictive of marital success while petting which takes place in a context of disgust or anxiety, for example, might be predictive of marital failure.

Reevy enumerates some of the former investigations concerned with this topic and then describes a thorough investigation, published by himself in 1959, among unmarried college females. He asked them a number of questions which allow statistical treatment of the collected data, because in Reevy's opinion such a statistical treatment is a *sine qua non* for giving us the proper answer. The questions are of the type: 'Has the nipple of your breast ever been kissed?' 'Has the nipple of your breast ever been sucked (subjected to prolonged oral stimulation)?' A little surprising he does not try to distinguish between the left and the right breast (nipple). His conclusion from other statistical studies and his own study is:

The relationship between the independent variable petting (or 'spooning') and the dependent variable, marital success (or marital happiness prediction) pointed in the same direction — the less 'spooning' the greater likelihood of success. However, such a statistical relationship does not show a cause-effect relationship. There is no proof that absence of petting (or minimal petting) *causes* marital success.

And two pages later he continues:

With the little research that has been done to date further research is needed in order to establish causal relationships between premarital petting behavior and marital success. If further research were done it would undoubtedly reveal the totality of variables (and the proportion of each) which in combination or in interaction contribute to marital success. As yet, however, we do not know enough about the matter, and both chastising our unmarried clients for their 'untoward' behavior or urging them on to 'advanced' behavior seems irrational indeed. Likewise, chastising or praising our married counselees for what their premarital petting behavior may or may not have been seems indefensible scientifically speaking.

Nobody in Denmark would consider asking whether premarital sex benefits or harms a future marriage. The terrible truth is that everybody in the Scandinavian countries engages in premarital sexual relationships (not only petting, but premarital sexual intercourse) and our marriages seem neither poorer nor better than marriages anywhere else. Petting as an isolated phenomenon and as a consequence of a virgin-cult is hardly ever known. But of course petting is known as a sexual variation, an introduction to intercourse at the beginning of a relationship or as a reasonable substitute for sexual intercourse if contraceptives are not available, etc.

Confronted with articles such as Reevy's another question arises: who is listening to such advice? Do common people really care about what is expressed — 'scientifically' or not — regarding chastity or the contrary? Don't they do things their own way letting the wise scientists discuss such matters over their heads? But I fear the answer is not as simple as this; the discussion for and against premarital sex is obviously not only some theorists' other-worldly pastime, but is also of great importance for many people.

Therefore it might be of some interest if I describe the situation in Scandinavian countries, where such problems are not evident and where the explanation is not to be found — as some persons believe — in the culture's lack of moral, its obscenity, or lack of human dignity, but is indebted to a certain long tradition. Before I can do this, four questions have to be considered.

FOUR FUNDAMENTAL QUESTIONS

1. Why is it that although man is sexually mature at the age of 13–14 he usually has his sexual debut several years later? The mean age for the first coitus in Denmark and Sweden as in many other countries is 17 years for both sexes (Hertoft 1968; Zetterberg 1969; Eliasson 1971). It is not surprising that some youngsters engage in sexual intercourse very soon after they have reached their physical capability. But it is surprising that relatively few do start that early and that many youngsters wait 5–8 years or even longer after puberty before starting sex life with a partner. Part of the explanation might be that not only the physical maturation, but also a certain psychic maturation, a capacity for falling in love, is a necessary condition for many people before engaging in sexual intercourse — Money (1971) refers to this possibility in a survey article in a psychiatric textbook. I can only touch on the question here.

2. Is marriage such a fundamental, established institution as many people take for granted? Has the sharp distinction between married and unmarried persons always been a fact or is this differentiation a relatively new one? To answer this question a certain historical elucidation is necessary.

In the Scandinavian countries the laws regulating marriage have been altered from time to time, as I shall describe later in this chapter. In former days it was often quite impossible to distinguish between premarital and marital sex because there were no sharp limits between marital and non-marital relationships.

A third question is:

3. Why is the problem regarding premarital sex so irrelevant in Scandinavia, when it is obviously considered very important in many other countries? And why do so many persons outside Scandinavia believe that premarital sex and promiscuity are two sides of the same coin? For us there is no equality between premarital sex and promiscuity. (For many reasons I feel a little uncomfortable by using the word promiscuous, because it has so many unwanted overtones, but in lack of a better word I hope it can pass.) Of course some people in all age groups, unmarried as well as married, are promiscuous in our countries as in other countries. But it is a fact, often surprising also to ourselves, that a third of young Danish men and between a third and half of young Danish women marry their first sexual partner (Olsen 1968). And among the rest of the youngsters relatively few, approximately 10–15 per cent, have more than 3–4 premarital partners.

Finally a fourth question has to be raised:

4. Is it possible to reflect on the premarital traditions in a country without also taking account of all the background factors infuencing the daily life in that country? The answer is, naturally, no. But too often it is forgotten that human sexuality is part of a whole and therefore cannot be treated isolated or detached from life as such. And therefore it is not possible to export or import sexual norms from one country to another without also changing other parts of the society.

I shall now try, very briefly, to explain the development of premarital sex norms in the Scandinavian countries.

THE TRADITIONS FOR PREMARITAL SEX IN THE SCANDINAVIAN COUNTRIES

General remarks

The traditions of a nation may exist in their own obscure way, without many people being aware of them, or even admitting that they adhere to them. It may even happen that certain standards of contemporary behaviour are looked upon as breaks in tradition but that in fact, when studied more closely, they are seen to be rooted far back in ancient times. Paradoxically, it may be said that, occasionally, it is traditional to follow certain rules and, at the same time, to consider this traditional way of living as an expression of breaking with tradition: a deplorable decadence of the times. The fact that a tradition is old does not mean that it has any value, and a break with tradition does not necessarily imply a deterioration. The question is whether a break in tradition has in fact occurred.

As an example of an unheeded, traditional way of living with its roots far back in the past: it is perhaps not widely known that in the Scandinavian countries there is a centuries-old tradition for sexual intercourse before marriage. In the present century there is no lack of evidence that this custom continues to be common in all classes of the community.

Georg Hansen (1963) states that in the last century people were well aware of this tradition. With regard to conditions at the end of the eighteenth century he writes:

Other clergymen who wanted to teach the peasants that it was disgraceful for their daughters to enter into relationships with chance farm-boys, were regarded with distrust. They could not be in earnest. It had always been so. As long as the girl did not conceive, it was quite all right, but should she become pregnant, the young couple could marry. The parents had been similarly indiscreet, and what had been good enough for them, could also be good enough for their children. It was a peculiar idea for the priests to hold a different opinion, and people would not like it if their opinion found favour among the young people.

Hence, this is an unusual type of example of an older generation's distrust of new ways and habits. Furthermore, the quotation bears witness to a conflict between two culture groups who could not understand each other. Almost all investigations show that it was primarily the peasants and the common people in the towns who accepted premarital intercourse, whereas the middle classes and the nobility approved of such standards of behaviour to a far lesser extent.

In order to understand the tradition underlying pre-marital intercourse in Scandinavia, it is necessary to have some knowledge of the historical development of marriage in Denmark, Norway, and Sweden. Furthermore, brief mention must be made of the form of regular courtship which is known under the name of *'nattefrieri'* (night-courtship; *bundling, kiltgang*) and which, in the opinion of some research workers, has exerted an influence on the present sexual morality in the Scandinavian countries.

Night-courtship ('nattefrieri')

Many treatises have dealt with this peculiar custom which is known to have been common among many peasant communities in the Scandinavian countries and in neighbouring countries, England, and the eastern states in America (see e.g. Peters 1781; Hübertz 1834; Sundt 1855; Wikman 1937; Doten 1938).

In its most typical form, night-courtship was as follows: a group of young men visited young unmarried women in their sleeping quarters, late in the evening or during the night and often on specified times of the week. In most cases these sleeping quarters were isolated from the house as such, or were situated in a special house into which easy access could be gained. When the young men had entered, they had to behave decently and, only if the women agreed, one or more of them would be allowed to stay. This staying overnight did not imply that sexual intercourse was allowed. He who was allowed to stay had to comply with definite rules. The first time he had to keep his clothes on and lie on the blanket; later he was allowed to take off some of his clothes, but not more, etc. Gradually, a certain selection would occur among the young people and everybody would know who belonged to whom. Therefore, within the static peasant communities of the past there were hardly any problems as regards paternity where a relationship developed and had consequences. It is quite evident that industrialization and increased possibilities of communication would disturb this custom.

In Denmark *nattefrieri* does not seem to have followed quite the same pattern as in the other Scandinavian countries, but close interelationship between unmarried young people can be seen as far back as the middle ages.

In the middle of the last century, the custom was still very widespread in Norway and Sweden and it has been followed occasionally in remote districts of Sweden almost up to the present time. It is said to have been observed on the Orkney Islands as late as in 1941 (Jonsson 1951; Reynolds 1951).

Marriage

Throughout history, the rules governing the celebration of marriage in Scandinavian countries have changed considerably, and not until the eighteenth century were definite rules for marriage created. The present conception of marriage in the Scandinavian countries come from three not dissimilar origins: from old Northern law; from Christianity, as it appears from Canon Law; and also, later on, from the Lutheran religion.

Characteristic features of old Northern law were that the celebration of marriage was determined by two separate acts: the agreement of the parties prior to marriage, or betrothal, and the wedding ceremony, the marriage. The betrothal was a contract which was entered into before witnesses; at the wedding ceremony itself the bride was given to the bridegroom by her father or her guardian. Both acts were purely temporal. Apparently, there was no clear distinction between the betrothal and the wedding ceremony. If the betrothal was followed by actual union, the parties were considered to be validly married.

Gradually the influence of the Church on the establishment of marriage became more and more widespread. Formerly, the private temporal wedding ceremony was followed by a ceremony in church. The nature of this church ceremony changed at a later date from being voluntary to compulsory. Following the Lutheran reformation some confusion arose as to the actual time at which marriage was legally entered into. Gradually the rules became obscure and to a certain extent contradictory, and reform became necessary. In 1582 the authorities tried to clarify the position by making definite rules for the celebration of marriage.

It was laid down that all who wished to enter into matrimony should first be betrothed, this betrothal taking place before a priest and five witnesses and, furthermore, that the banns should be read from the pulpit on three consecutive Sundays prior to the solemnization of the marriage. Evidently, the intention was to suppress the more informal marriage agreements, so that betrothal followed by actual union no longer, in effect, made the marriage valid. Although it was not expressly said that a church ceremony was an absolute condition for a valid marriage, it was, however, laid down that betrothed couples should not live together before marriage. Not until a century later, in 1683, was a church ceremony made a condition for the validity of a marriage, but the betrothal ceremony was retained and, far into the eighteenth century, this resulted in a great proportion of couples living together immediately after betrothal without the church ceremony. In most cases the authorities accepted this practice tacitly, and children resulting from unions of this nature were almost always considered legitimate, particularly amongst the lower classes. Not until 1799 was the condition that a marriage should be preceded by betrothal abolished and rules necessary for a valid marriage established, rules very similar to those prevailing today.

Sexual union without the blessing of the authorities has always been known, as evidence the numerous premarital conceptions. We know from the Church Registers that, in the eighteenth century, when the betrothal ceremony was still valid, 30–35 per cent of first-born children were born so soon after betrothal that conception must have taken place before betrothal. It is not surprising, therefore, that almost 50 per cent of brides in rural areas were pregnant at the time of their marriage and that the percentage was even higher among the common people in the towns (Hansen 1957). A statistical study from the end of the nineteenth century shows that at two-thirds of the weddings the bride was pregnant or had borne a child before she was married (Rubin and Westergaard 1890). Similar figures are available from the present century, e.g. Auken (1953) found that 49 per cent of married women were pregnant when they entered into marriage and that 99 per cent of sexually experienced women had had sexual intercourse before marriage.

The official rules prevailing over the years did not have very much influence on the customs of the people in Scandinavia. Today it is accepted in our countries that young engaged couples have sexual intercourse, and this attitude represents a long unbroken tradition. The Scandinavian countries are not communities without rules, but communities which have developed their own rules and standards on the basis of their own premises, different from those observed e.g. in the United States or in the Mediterranean countries. But the situation in the Northern countries is not entirely an isolated phenomenon. It differs from that in other countries by degree rather than having absolute differences. Perhaps we have merely succeeded in our countries, assisted by a certain tradition, to establish a somewhat better agreement between the actual and the expected custom within certain sexual fields, including premarital intercourse, than in many other countries. In this field it had been a little easier for us to accept what people — to use on of Kinsey's expressions — really do.

CONCLUSIONS

As we have seen, there is a permissive attitude towards premarital sex in the Scandinavian countries and this attitude has a long tradition. But this has not caused the mean age for sexual debut to equal the age of physical maturation: the mean age of puberty is 13 years for both sexes, the mean age for sexual début is 17 years for both sexes.

The rules for entering into marriage are not as fundamental and established as one might think. Throughout history, at least in Protestant countries, the rules have been relatively confusing and it was often difficult to say whether a marriage was valid or not. The entering into marriage was originally purely temporal, but gradually became influenced by the Church. The distinction between unmarried and married people was blurred for centuries in the past and therefore it was not meaningful to distinguish between premarital and marital sexual life.

There is no special virgin-cult in the Nordic countries. Therefore, the special petting habits, which have been seen most pronouncedly in United States (and now, as far as I know, are declining) are not seen in Scandinavia. It is especially meaningless in Scandinavia to consider describing petting habits among youths, and through statistical procedures deciding whether there is a relationship between premarital petting behaviour and so-called marital happiness.

A permissive attitude to premarital sex is not the same as an acceptance of cohabitation with anybody. Promiscuous sexuality is hardly more common in the Scandinavian countries than in any other part of the world.

Because premarital sex is a common thing among our youngsters, young Scandinavian men very seldom have sexual relationships with prostitutes.

A number of laws protect the rights of unmarried mothers as well as children born out of wedlock.

Because certain sexual norms function in one country it does not follow that such norms function well in other societies with other background factors, traditions, and habits. It is to be expected, though, that the accelerating communication between countries will diminish the differences in regard to sexual behaviour and attitudes in different societies. One day studies regarding the possible relationship between premarital sex and marital happiness will be without much meaning and be abandoned in favour of more essential studies on human sexuality.

SUMMARY

A survey on the background factors for the tradition of premarital sex in the Scandinavian countries is given.

REFERENCES

AUKEN, K. (1953). *Undersøgelser over unge kvinders sexuelle adfaerd* (with an English summary: Investigation into the sexual behaviour of young women). Copenhagen.

DOTEN, D. (1938). *The art of bundling.* New York.

ELIASSON, R. (1971). *Könsdifferenser i sexuellt beteende och attityder till sexualitet* (duplicated copy: Sex differences in sexual behaviour and attitudes towards sexuality). Lund, Sweden.

HANSEN, G. (1957). *Saedelighedsforhold blandt Landbefolkningen i Danmark i det 18. århundrede* [Mortality situation among the rural population in Denmark in the eighteenth century]. Copenhagen, Denmark.

HERTOFT, P. (1968). *Undersøgelser over unge maends seksuelle adfaerd, viden og holdning* (with an English summary: Investigation into the sexual behaviour of young men). Copenhagen, Denmark.

HÜBERTZ, J. R. (1834). *Beskrivelse over Aerø* (Description of Aerø). Copenhagen, Denmark.

JONSSON, G. (1951). *Sexualvanor hos svensk ungdom* [Sexual habits among Swedish youth]. Official Report no. 41 from the Swedish Government. Stockholm, Sweden.

MONEY, J. (1972). Determinants of human sexual identity and behavior. In *Progress in group and family therapy* (ed. C. J. Sager and H. S. Kaplan). New York.

PETERS, S. (1781). *General history of Connecticut*. London.

REEVY, W. R. (1972). Petting experience and marital success. *J. Sex Research*, **8**, 48–60.

REYNOLDS, R. (1951). *Beds*. New York.

RUBIN, M. and WESTERGAARD, H. (1890). *Aegteskabsstatistik* [Statistics of marriage]. Copenhagen, Denmark.

SUNDT, E. (1855). *Om Giftermaal i Norge* [On marriage in Norway]. Oslo, Norway.

WIKMAN, K. (1937). *Die Einleitung der Ehe*. Acta Academiae Aboensis, Humaniora IX, 1. Åbo, Sweden.

ZETTERBERG, H. (1969). *Om sexuallivet i Sverige* (On sexual life in Sweden). Official Report no. 2 from the Swedish Government, Stockholm, Sweden.

10. FAMILY LAWS AND EQUALITY BETWEEN THE SEXES IN VARIOUS COUNTRIES: A SYNOPSIS

BIRGITTA LINNÉR

INTRODUCTION

Family law concepts cannot be considered in isolation, but are influenced by moral, ethical, and religious ideas, as well as sociopolitical and psychological attitudes prevailing in the country concerned. In Sweden there is a family law system with legal codes; but in some countries there is not even a praxis in the civil courts. Instead there are traditional rights with well-defined rules for family relationships. This is quite common in many of the developing countries. In other countries, different legal systems can exist side by side: federal and state laws; religious rules and traditional customary rights.

In the area of family life civil laws and traditional customary rights have often been closely tied to the religious philosophy of life. Religious philosophy has monopolized morality concerning marriage and divorce, sex life outside and inside marriage, the possibilities of planning a family, premarital sexual relations, the role balance between man and woman, subordination in family relations, etc.

SWEDEN

Sweden is a country which for many centuries has been influenced by the Judeo-Christian philosophy of family life. Moral principles based on religious teachings were clear and simple, but for many people unrealizable. These principles stemmed from teaching that considered all forms of sexual life immoral except for marital sex for reproductive purposes. No forms of contraception were accepted.

Sweden introduced secularization during this century and simultaneously introduced new secularized moral principles and a legal system which was rather more 'humane'. The basic philosophy of equality between man and woman extends into marriage, accepting the dual functions of sexual life; for purposes of reproduction, and for personal and mutual joy. This means that equal standards apply to both men and women. A direct consequence of this is equal rights for every child born, whether in or out of wedlock. It also means accepting marriage as a legal contract, which can be dissolved by mutual consent without a legal procedure, and acceptance of the availability of contraceptive techniques, therapeutic abortions, etc. (Linner 1972, 1975; United Nations 1976; Wallin 1972).

The realization of these new socio-psychological interrelations has taken about half a century and the process is still going on.

Some changes in family and sex laws in Sweden

1910. Parliament passed a law forbidding information on contraceptive methods.

1915. An old law punishing those who have sexual relations outside marriage was abolished.

1915–20. The legal institutions of marriage and family were changed from supporting a patriarchial system to a more democratic form of living together, with the basic assumption of equal responsibility of both spouses.

    (a) 1915. New divorce laws were passed, recognizing the possibilities of dissolving a marriage after a year of judicial separation, without guilt being assigned to either partner.

    (b) 1917. The term 'illegitimate' was abandoned from official use and the interests of children born outside wedlock were supported more actively by the legal profession.

    (c) 1920. The new marriage act was the last part of the renewal of the family laws, affecting both persons and property rights.

1938. Family planning through modern contraceptive techniques was legalized.
Therapeutic abortion laws were initiated.
Adultary was abolished from the Criminal Code.

1944. Homosexuality between consenting adults was no longer criminal.

1948. A law was passed making both parents custodians and guardians for the common children of their marriage.

1951. Marriage as such no longer affected a woman's nationality, since she was allowed to keep her Swedish citizenship.

1969. The legal marriage age was lowered for men and made equal for men and women, i.e. 18 years of age.

1970. A child born out of wedlock was given the same inheritance rights from its father and its father relatives as a child born in marriage.

1973. A family law reform put informal marriages on an equal footing with registered marriage in two respects: the custody of children and the common dwelling (Alexandersson 1973).

THE INTERNATIONAL SCENE

In many countries a shift from a traditional patriarchal and hierarchial family structure is taking place. The marriage structure with the dominant husband having a provider role and the subordinate woman a supported role is giving away to a new democratic type of family structure with more equality between the marital partners. Also emerging is a new interest of the welfare of the child in the parent/child relationship and a new outlook on the question of both personal and property rights in marriage.

There can never be basic equality between man and woman in a country that has male-dominated family laws, keeping women as 'second-class citizens'. The Commission on Status of Women in United Nations has given attention to this dichotomy in a report on Legal Status of Married Women, submitted by the Secretary-General 1958 (United Nations 1958).

In the field of private law, an unmarried woman enjoys generally the same rights as a man. Marriage, however, has in a great number of countries the effect of depriving the women of a number of important rights, personal rights as well as property rights. This is due to the fact that, traditionally and for centuries, the husband has been considered as the head of the family, vested with the exercise of marital and parental authority, over the person and over the property of his wife and his children.
… the material collected by the Secretary-General shows that the root of the discimination against women in private law still lies in the subordinate status of married women.

Or, as expressed by Folke Schmidt and Stig Strömbäck (1964), two Swedish experts on comparative family laws:

As anyone possessing even a superficial knowledge of the basic principles of Roman law will know, an almost fierce individualism in the relations between man and man is not necessarily incompatible with a system of strict subordination in family relations. Many legal systems based upon Roman principles still maintain the family as a dictatorial unit under the unchallenged leadership of the pater familias in the midst of otherwise democratic institutions.

During the 1960s the United Nations had seminars in co-operation with many governments in order to improve and renew marriage and family laws, but it was not until the 1970s that a noticeable change took place in the consciousness and attitudes towards the whole problem. This change was of course backed up by the new feminist movement, but also by a great number of non-governmental organizations as well as many governments. The new trend can be studied in documents published by the United Nations (*Newsletter on the Status of Women*; Spilä 1974; United Nations 1976, 1975), various governments and governmental agencies

(Alexandersson 1973; Linnér 1974), organizations like the International Planned Parenthood Federation (*IPPF News*), International Federation of Women Lawyers (*La Abogade Newsletter*), law schools (*Law and Population Newsletter*), etc.

I would like to give an example from Kenya showing the complex process of change: In 1967 a Presidential Commission on Marriage and Divorce was set up to study existing laws on marriage, divorce, and related matters, 'to make recommendations for a new law providing a comprehensive and, so far as may be practicable, uniform law of marriage and divorce applicable to all persons in Kenya, which will replace existing law on the subject comprising customary law, Islamic law, Hindu law and relevant Acts of Parliament and to prepare a draft of the new law; and to pay particular attention to the status of women in relation to marriage and divorce in a free democratic society.' The Commission reported in 1968 and appended a draft Bill to their Report. The Bill with a few amendments should be presented to the next Parliament in Kenya after the 1974 general elections to the National Assembly. The key-note of the enactment is justice both in the sense of the equality of men and women in matters of marriage and divorce and also in the sense of the equality among the different kinds of marriages in Kenya (Uche 1974).

Another example, taken from the United Nations, and showing the interrelationship between family law and the status of women is taken from a chapter ('The Family') in the *U.N. World Plan of Action* (United Nations 1975); 'Legislative and other measures should be taken to ensure that men and women shall enjoy full and equal legal capacity relating to their personal and property rights.… During marriage the principle of equal rights and responsibilities would mean that both partners should perform an active role in the home, and share jointly decision-making on matters affecting the family and children.

In the last few years increasing emphasis has been put on the fact that equality of the sexes can be obtained only if women can regulate their fertility, i.e. control their own bodies. Without this essential freedom, women are handicapped from benefiting from other reforms. In January 1974 the United Nations Commission on the Status of Women presented a comprehensive study and report bearing the title *The interrelationship of the status of women and family planning*, prepared by the Special Rapporteur, Ms Helvi Sipilä. Later the Commission submitted a draft resolution (Draft Resolution VI) to the United Nations Economic and Social Council, including the new classical words: 'The right to decide freely and responsibly on the number and spacing of their children is a fundamental right of individuals which facilitates the exercise of other human rights especially for women' (Sipilä 1974).

The traditional philosophy of *pater familias* regards the husband as the head of the family as well as the sole breadwinner. To change this philosophy, the value of the married woman must be upgraded through considering her work in the home as having an economic value. Thus, Italy has recognized in its new family code the work of housewives as a job. France is also considering putting an economic value on housework. Of interest in this connection is also that the 18-nation Council of Europe — a forum for all western European Nations — has called for recognition of the economic value of housework by according women the same kind of welfare protection as workers in cases of illness, maternity, and old age (IPPF 1976).

Much of what is said in these examples is little more than benevolent talk — feministic blueprint philosophy — this is true. But a trend is clearly discernible, a process of change toward equality between women and men.

REFERENCES

ALEXANDERSSON, B. (1973). *The 1973 family law reform.* Current Sweden No. 8. Stockholm.

IPPF NEWS. The International Planned Parenthood Federation, London.

IPPF (1976). Women's roles and rewards. In *People*, Vol. 3, No. 3. London.

LA ABOGADE NEWSLETTER. International Federation of Women Lawyers. New York.

LAW AND POPULATION NEWSLETTER. The International Advisory Committee on Population and Law. The Fletcher School of Law and Diplomacy, Medford, Massachusetts.

LINNÉR, B. (1972). *Sex and society in Sweden.* New York.

—— (1974). Social and legal aspects of the family. In *Second Seminar on Sex Education and Social Development in Sweden, Latin America and the Caribbean, April 1972* (ed. M. Holmstedt). Swedish International Development Agency, Stockholm; University of Stockholm; and International Planned Parenthood Federation, London.

—— (1975). *The case study session: Sweden.* Paper read at the Tribune of the International Women's Year, Mexico City, June 1975. (Mimeo)

NEWSLETTER ON THE STATUS OF WOMEN. The Commission on the Status of Women, the Secretariat General United Nations, New York.

SCHMIDT, F. and STRÖMBÄCK, S. (1964). *Legal values in modern Sweden.* Stockholm.

SIPILÄ, H. (1974). *The interrelationship of the status of women and family planning.* The Commission on the Status of Women, United Nations. New York.

UNITED NATIONS (1958). *Legal status of married women.* Commission on the Status of Women. New York.

—— (1975). *U.N. World Plan of Action. World Conferences of the International Women's Year, 1975.* New York.

—— (1976). *Status of Women and Law.* The United Nations has decided to publish a volume on laws affecting the status of women, covering all regions of the world. This material is being prepared by women jurists in 15 countries in observance of the International Women's Year, 1975. H. Sipilä, U.N. Deputy Secretary General, is writing the preface. A chapter on Status of women and law in Sweden by the author of this chapter will be included.

UCHE, U. U. (1974). *Law and population growth in Kenya.* Law and Population Monograph Series No. 22. Medford, Massachusetts.

WALLIN, G. (1972). The status of women in Sweden. *Amer. J. comp. Law*, No. 20.

SESSION 2

Potentially pathogenic psychosocial stimuli originating from, or interacting with, male/female roles and relationships

11.   STRESSOR ASPECTS OF SOCIETAL ATTITUDES TO SEX ROLES AND RELATIONSHIPS

PAUL H. GEBHARD

SEX ROLE AND MUSCULAR STRENGTH

'Sex role' may be operationally defined as the behaviour expected of the individual by society according to the individual's gender. Anthropology clearly demonstrates that humans are extremely plastic and that their thought and behaviour is powerfully conditioned by society — i.e., the behaviour and expressed thoughts of others. Consequently, a sex role is to be viewed as primarily a social phenomenon and, as such, it varies from culture to culture.

All human societies have clearly differentiated male and female sex roles. For at least 2 million years of human existence, Freud's statement that 'anatomy is destiny' has operated to dichotomize the behaviour of the two sexes. Sex role is based on two anatomic differences, that of reproductive function and of muscular strength. Of the two, strength is the more important. Until less than a century ago, strength was the chief factor in dominance hierarchies, political and individual, and the further back in history and prehistory one goes the more important was strength. If females were stronger than males, as is true in some life forms, the female would be the dominant gender despite the reproductive function.

Since strength has been so important for millennia and only recently minimized by technological advances, one can scarcely expect humanity easily to discard the idea that strength determines dominance and that 'might makes right'. Adjectives such as 'small', 'weak', or 'frail' all have a derogatory connotation, especially when applied to males, while the terms 'big', 'strong', and 'powerful' carry a prestigious significance. This is the legacy of our past which has become anachronistic in our technological world.

The human tendency to think in simplistic dichotomies has resulted in our viewing females as weak and small and males as strong and large. The next stop in this erroneous reasoning is to say that a female who is large or strong is somehow less feminine and that a small or weak male is less masculine. In other words, we have arbitrarily assigned certain attributes to each gender and then defined gender according to these attributes.

The result is that males strive to live up to the masculine ideal of strength, aggressiveness, initiative, and dominance and females try to conform to the ideal of dependency and passivity. A vast amount of individual and interpersonal stress arises from these efforts since the personalities and physiques of many humans are not suited to these culturally determined ideals. Even modern science has done little to remedy this situation.

Notice how our tests of masculinity and femininity depend upon traits which we assume are characteristic of the genders. An interest in art or music, for example, gives a male a higher feminine rating.

SEX ROLE AND REPRODUCTIVE FUNCTION

Although technology has largely counteracted the factor of strength in human relationships, until the last few years the reproductive factor has dominated females. Only a century ago there were no adequate contraceptive techniques and the life-span of many females did not extend much beyond the reproductive years. Now, with adequate contraception and vastly increased longevity, reproduction has become correspondingly less important in female life. Nevertheless, we still face the inescapable fact that child-rearing badly hampers the self-development and occupational careers of most women. Society continues to promulgate the myth that a female is somehow unfulfilled and something less than a woman if she has not produced a child. Moreover, society continues to insist that mothers should sacrifice their aspirations for the benefit of the children, and that virtually all mothers can rear their offspring better than any state nursery or public day-care centre. This is based on the optimistic assumption that the vast majority of mothers, and only mothers, are competent to rear children. This is at best a questionable assumption, but it has the support of society and religion. The woman with little maternal impulse or competence is disregarded, and the husband who wishes to devote himself to child care is considered deviant. Both are expected to conform to their sex roles.

Unfortunately, physicians, counsellors, and social scientists tend to reinforce this idea that women should be mothers, without making due provision for those who are disinclined to or who, despite their wishes, should not be mothers. Reproduction retains its sacred status and most persons still view it as an inalienable right despite the population crisis. This emphasis on reproduction only too often overshadows the other female capabilities, and the female is regarded, as one physician defined her, as a 'uterus with appendages'.

ALTERNATIVE ROLES

While in our society the primary role of the female continues to be that of wife and mother, we have greatly extended in recent decades the number of alternative roles for women. Whereas until recently in western civilization, the only alternatives were that of teacher, nurse, or nun, we now accept females in many careers and the role of the female as a worker outside the home has become the norm, even after marriage. This rapid proliferation of alternative roles has, like any rapid social change, engendered friction, confusion, resistance, and, consequently, stress. Some males resent their wives working, some wives resent having to work; and although females have massively infiltrated the lower echelons of employment, there is a powerful restraint upon their rising to high positions in business or the professions. This obviously involves a waste of human talent and education, and adversely affects male/female relationships.

Despite the proliferation of female roles, the female is seldom permitted to escape the conventional role of wife. A new bridegroom who as a bachelor took care of his own cooking, laundry, and housework generally assumes without discussion that his employed wife will take over these duties in addition to her work outside the home.

In addition to roles of employment, married females have in recent decades been assigned other role obligations by marriage manuals, magazine articles, newspapers, and television. Caring for the children and house is no longer sufficient. She must also be a companion, interested in and knowledgeable about her husband's business and recreational interests. She must be able to function as a practical nurse when illness strikes, and perform psychiatric therapy when her husband is distraught or depressed. She should be able to decorate and furnish the home and make certain repairs. Most importantly, she should retain her sexual attractiveness and be suitably responsive (or even initiative) in bed. On top of this, she should participate in worthy community affairs. Such a diversity of roles, and the agility necessary quickly to change roles, is beyond the ability of the average wife who, consequently, suffers from feelings of inadequacy, guilt, and resentment.

All this adaptation to the husband, children, and community is not considered a surrender of personality. Indeed, this adaptation is not only lauded, but has certain patronizing undertones: husbands must be cared for and managed without their being aware of it. In any case, such total and sometimes manipulative adaptation by the wife is a rather pathological substitute for what should be an egalitarian relationship between two humans.

AGE AND SEX ROLES

An examination of anthropological data as well as our own culture shows that while sex role is modified by various factors such as socio-economic status and ethnic group, a major determinant is that of age. Infants and children tend to be treated as though they were a single asexual gender and, in our society, the distinctions in dress are minimal. As children approach the age when reproduction is possible, all societies begin to differentiate the sexes strongly through establishing different ideals of behaviour and modes of dress. In many societies puberty rites dramatically signal the division of sex roles. Throughout the reproductive years, societies emphasize the male/female differences, but once the female reproductive span has passed, the artificial distinctions are lessened and the two genders once again become more similar. In various pre-literate societies, post-menopausal females, freed of the menstrual taboo, are allowed into organizations and rites previously denied them. In our own society aged males and females are increasingly exempt from the demands of sex roles and may perform the duties without regard to gender. Clearly much of the sex role distinction is based upon reproductive function.

SEXUAL ASPECTS OF SEX ROLES

Turning now to the specifically sexual aspects of sex role, one finds that Western European civilization inherited from the Judeo-Christian tradition the idea that there are but two classes of females: good and bad, the difference lying chiefly in their sexual behaviour. This polarity of thought is striking in the Old Testament wherein good women were extolled, but bad (i.e. sexual) women were the subject of repeated warnings. A few examples suffice: 'More bitter than death is the woman whose heart is snares and nets, and her hands as bands....', and 'The mouth of strange women is a deep pit: he that is abhorred of the Lord shall fall therein.' (Ecclesiastes 7:26 and Proverbs 22:14.)

The epitome of churchly denigration of females is found in a statement by St John Chrysostom: 'What else is woman but a foe to friendship, an inescapable punishment, a necessary evil, a natural temptation, a desirable calamity, a domestic danger, a delectable detriment, and an evil of nature painted in fair colours.' Even Spiro Agnew could not match this verbal display.

This biased view intensified in early Christian times when women and sin were judged synonymous. Even marriage was deemed an inferior way of life compared to sexual abstinence, and was only grudgingly accepted. While the early excesses such as self-castration and sexless marriage soon died out, a condemnatory image of women continued into Renaissance times. In the *Malleus Malificarum*, an official church book against witches, written in 1480–90, there is specific labelling of women as being inferior and prone to evil.

On the other hand, there were the good women: good dutiful wives, one's mother, one's sister, and above all, Mary. Such women were to be esteemed, treasured, and protected — preferably by cloistering them in the home.

Consequently, males categorized females into first, the good women, the rather sexless mothers whose world centred on the home and children, and the good girls whom one would convert into mothers; and secondly, the bad women with whom one had sex, but never married. This sharp distinction still exists in Latin America and portions of the Mediterranean area, and has not been wholly eradicated in North America.

The basic question is why did our ancient ancestors attribute these various characteristics to females and why did subsequent generations perpetuate such an obviously erroneous mythology? I believe that most of the explanation stems from the ambivalence men of Near Eastern and European cultures have felt toward women.

On the positive side, women were viewed as the givers of life and food. One's mother is the most important person in one's formative years and the mother/child relationship is one of the most intense. Later in life, males find females irresistable attractions and most men ultimately fall in love, one of life's most powerful experiences. Note that in early agricultural societies, the major deity was often female, the Earth Goddess, the Great Mother, etc. Late, with the advent of civilization, goddesses were still important and their sexuality was a vital part of religion (e.g. Isis, Astarte, and Aphrodite).

On the negative side were at least four items. First, men resented the power of female attraction. For the sake of a female, a man would risk his wealth, social position, friendships, and possibly his life. Such female destructive potential is noted in the Bible and in history: Cleopatra, Helen of Troy, Jezebel, Delilah, etc. Even good women often inadvertently caused disaster, as in the case of Juliet and Isolde.

Secondly, women were the enemy of spirituality and religion since they personify sexuality and the carnal side of life. The very presence of women distracts men from religious contemplation and prayer, hence they were often excluded from or segregated in religious rites.

Thirdly, because females could not compete with males in terms of strength, they were forced to pursue their goals through persuasion, subterfuge, nagging, and intrigue. This naturally gave them the reputation of being deceitful, nagging, and bad-tempered. Note that males have always reacted negatively to the female techniques of attaining goals: intrigue is worse than a good clean battle, and poison is far more evil than the sword. Lucretia Borgia suffers a poorer reputation than her more murderous brother, Caesare. It is interesting to observe that by Greco-Roman times when gods rather than goddesses were the most powerful, the goddesses were given the negative feminine characteristics such as spitefulness, vanity, deceit, and nagging.

Fourthly, men have always been concerned about the magical powers of females, these inexplicable creatures who give birth and who bleed and exhibit erratic behaviour in a cycle corresponding to the lunar cycle. There is, and has been, a universal fear of the magic potential of menstrual blood. Obviously, females have magical powers which are dangerous to men.

The ambivalence caused by these positive and negative feelings about females resolved into the simple dichotomy of good and bad women, a fallacious logic which has impeded male/female relationships to this day.

Although males may hold themselves superior to bad females, they suffer when compared to good females. The good woman is sympathetic and sensitive; men are tough and insensitive. Women are gentle and kind; men are aggressive and often cruel. Women are aesthetic; men are not. Women are faithful; men are promiscuous. Thus, a negative picture of masculinity developed, a view held by both sexes despite manifold evidence to the contrary.

The ultimate result of these attitudes discussed at such length is that each sex has an erroneous conception of the other, and that hostility is never far below the surface. Witness the anger and bias inherent in remarks such as, 'Isn't that just like a man!' or 'That's typical of women!'

THE MALE ROLE

Up until now I have talked chiefly in terms of the difficult role of the female since she has suffered the most in male-dominated society. However, males are not exempt from stress imposed by society, especially in recent times. The male role of provider, protector, and family head has been augmented, as in the case of the wife, by numerous other obligatory roles. He now should take a more active part in child-rearing, cultivate 'togetherness' with wife and children, and develop the sexual expertise necessary to insure his wife the sexual gratification which the mass media proclaim her due. This latter task is complicated by the contradictory demands made by the mass media and by marriage manuals. The male should be intuitive and gentle, yet the 'real man' is supposedly aggressive and bold. He is told that women want to be dominated by a masterful male and yet at other times resent it, and that women want to be treated as equals and yet given special consideration. To add to his confusion, females are not supposed to tell him what they want — he is to know what to do without instruction. In bed, he is weighed down by the statement that there are no frigid females, only clumsy males.

In keeping with our technologically oriented society, husbands often labour under the delusion that their sexual problems can be solved in a mechanistic fashion, knowing what parts should be stimulated for a given length of time and in proper sequence. This reduces love-making and coitus to mechanics with a resultant loss of emotion and abandon which, in turn, defeats itself.

ROMANTIC FALLACIES

As though the sources of male/female misunderstanding and stress were not enough, our society has exacerbated matters by promulgating various romantic fallacies. Some of these represent unattainable ideals which thereby cause guilt and feelings of inadequacy; others are so contrary to human inclination that subscribing to them guarantees trouble. A few examples will suffice:

'For each person there is only one true love in the world waiting to be discovered, and it is a mistake to marry anyone else.' 'A person can love only one individual at a time. Two simultaneous loves must inevitably involve competition and detract from one another. A person has only a limited potential for love which therefore must be bestowed on only one partner.' A common romantic fallacy of females is that love and sex are inseparable. Only love justifies sex which is otherwise coarse and animalistic.

Although romanticism is an integral part of male/female relationships and a pleasurable enhancement, its destructive potential should be recognized and avoided.

The picture I have thus far painted is rather bleak: two genders burdened with ignorance and bias floundering in a socially produced confusion in their attempts to achieve a mutually gratifying relationship without the benefit of honest communication and understanding. Fortunately, a number of recent trends justify some measure of optimism.

RECENT TRENDS

We now know that males and females are basically alike and that most of the troublesome differences have been culturally produced. While the artificial distinctions drawn between the sexes may have served certain social and economic purposes in hunting and agrarian societies, most of them are useless or harmful in our industrial civilization. Those artificial differences, such as some in dress and mannerism, which are pleasurable to both genders and not impediments should be retained, but the deleterious differences abandoned. We now know that the intellectual and emotional capacities of both sexes are equal. Even the Victorian myth that females are inherently less sexually responsive than males is being seriously eroded if not demolished. With each successive generation, thanks to the general emancipation of women and recognition that they are sexual beings with their own needs, females exhibit greater sexual response not only to tactile stimulation, but to visual and psychological stimuli as well. Indeed, there is good reason to believe that females far exceed males in one sexual respect: the ability to experience multiple orgasms.

The stresses on male/female relationships imposed by socially determined roles and concepts can be minimized by wider knowledge, by equitable division of labour and its rewards regardless of gender, and by freer and more honest communication. We must stop generalizing about gender differences and forcing individuals into preconceived categories. We must appreciate the vast range of individual differences and make appropriate arrangements in society to best accommodate and utilize the capacities and interests of individuals regardless of their sex. This remedy will be painful since it involves giving up or substantially modifying many of our most cherished and tenaciously held ideas and values. We must consider, as Margaret Mead and Judge Lindsey have, alternative forms of marriage. We must no longer hold up marriage as a goal in itself. Ultimately, we will be forced to realize that reproduction is not an inalienable right, but a privilege to be exercised within prescribed limits. Lastly, of course, we must abandon most of the artificial differences of sex roles so that individuals may be equals and humans first and secondarily males or females, to enjoy the real differences.

SUMMARY

Sex roles and relationships were based on differences in reproductive function and physical strength. From this grew dichotomous, stereotypic thinking of males and females being inherently and basically different, and of masculinity and femininity as being opposite ends of a scale. Such misconceptions are a source of trouble and stress since socially determined roles and values do not suit many individuals. The old Judeo-Christian division of women into good and bad, plus male ambivalence toward women has been a cause of stress. The perpetuation of sexual myths and unattainable expectations has occasioned additional trouble. Society must reappraise sex roles and relationships, and discard unrealistic stress-causing concepts and values.

12. UNMARRIED COHABITATION AND ITS RELATION TO PSYCHICAL AND SOCIAL CRITERIA OF ADAPTATION

JAN TROST

I would like to discuss two kinds of cohabitation: married and unmarried. They are defined and there are data on their frequency. Most of the analysis compares the unmarried cohabiting couples to the married couples. Examples are shown of how the law treats the two kinds of cohabitation. The effects of the different views held on the two states, and of the social environment are discussed — effects on the society, on the partners, and on the children — effects that are both directly and indirectly the result of the form of cohabitation.

This chapter is essentially a review of the subject as it was in 1972 and has been updated in 1976, primarily to take account of changes in the laws in Sweden concerning cohabitation and marriage since 1972.

DEFINITIONS

We shall limit ourselves here to *culturally defined* conditions because I shall be talking mainly about Sweden and only occasionally about other countries. And, for simplicity, we shall only take monogamous relations into account. I am fully aware that there are other marriage-like conditions in Swedish society. Alternative family forms are already being discussed and experimented with. But these other forms are either very few or very new (or do not exist), so that we have no data at all on them, which means that an attempt to analyse them would be an analysis with too many guesses and loose speculations. Thus, we will not discuss what are usually known group marriages, polygamous relationships, communes, or extended families with or without love-relationships or generational linkage, which are not at present clearly defined alternative forms of cohabitation.

Usually when one talks about marriage one has in mind some kind of a legal definition of marriage. The official statistics about marriages are almost always about legal marriages. However, it should be noted that the legal definition does not always represent the true state of affairs, i.e. all legal marriages are not dyads in a sociological sense. Some married couples do not cohabit; there is, for example, legal or actual separation (cf. Trost 1970, pp. 14–15) and there are casual or temporary separations (cf. Trost 1965, p. 171 *et seq.*). As an index of this we can point at the fact that between 85 per cent and 90 per cent of all divorces in Sweden have been preceded by either a legal separation for at least 1 year or an actual separation for at least 3 years.

However, of all legal marriages that exist only about 0·6–0·7 per cent divorce each year.

In official statistics and in many other connections non-cohabiting married couples are treated as if they were cohabiting. This problem of validity is only occasionally serious because there are so many cohabiting married couples compared to the few that are counted as cohabiting but are not. But this kind of validity problem is much greater for cohabiting unmarried couples. There is no legal definition behind which to hide, for each couple a decision has to be made as to whether they should be counted as cohabiting or not. One possibility is to let one or both members of the couple decide themselves whether they should be counted as a lasting cohabiting couple, i.e. living under marriage-like conditions. But there are at least two problems concerning the duration of the cohabitation: one has to define the length of time for which the two persons should have been living together in order to be counted as a *lasting* couple, and one has to decide what 'cohabitation' is. If the two potential 'spouses' have lived together regularly every week-end and have done so for a long time, they should be counted as a cohabiting non-married couple? Furthermore, what is really meant by 'marriage-like conditions'?

Sometimes it is feasible to talk about cohabiting married couples and cohabiting non-married couples as the same thing but usually it is necessary to deal with them separately, as we shall do here. In the former case, I prefer to use Löcsei's (1970) term, 'syndyasmos'. He defines syndyasmos as 'legalized and not legalized varieties of *lasting* living community between men and women'. Although Löcsei does not say so explicitly, it seems to me evident that he means only dyads with one member of each sex and not groups of men and women. There are two reasons for using the term syndyasmos. One is obvious, i.e. sometimes we need a common word for these two principal kinds of cohabitation which are prevalent in several societies. The other reason, as Löcsei says, and with which I fully agree, is that 'one can perhaps avoid ... certain comic or obscene overtones, which are often present in English expressions that refer to relationships within or outside marriage'. The same is true not only for English expressions but also for the same kind of problem in several other languages. Furthermore, it is often better to construct a new word for a complex social phenomenon than to try to use an old word that is burdened with many or diffuse connotations.

As late as in 1971, Cavan and Cavan (1971, p. 20) put prostitution and cohabiting unmarried couples in the same category. They define (p. 13) consensual or free unions, common-law marriage and concubinage as quasi-marriages. I shall return later to the curious views of Cavan and Cavan on various forms of 'quasi-marriages'.

THE FREQUENCY OF COHABITING UNMARRIED COUPLES

If we define cohabiting unmarried couples on the basis of their own perception, the number of cohabiting unmarried couples in Sweden in 1970 was about 105 000, which is equivalent to about 6·4 per cent of all the existing syndyasmos. A stratified probability sample of unmarried men and women were asked if at the time of data collection they had been living steadily together for a long time under marriage-like conditions with a person of the opposite sex (Näsholm 1972a). It is probable that this figure is an under-estimate since it seems reasonable to assume that non-response to the survey is selective. This means that we asume that more unmarried people that do live together under marriage-like conditions did not wish to answer the question than unmarried people who did not live under marriage-like conditions. There are several reasons for this, one of which is exemplified by the answers to a later question, in which the respondents were asked to give the name and the date of birth of the partner. In our opinion people should not be asked to give such information, as it furnishes perfect identification of the other person in the household, and especially since they are not classified in a legal way as family members. In such cases one is invading people's privacy or personal integrity, and this explains why for the first question the non-response is larger among the cohabiting unmarried couples than among the single unmarried.

According to another study (Näsholm 1972b) the estimate of the number of cohabiting unmarried couples in Sweden during 1969 was 135 000, which is about 6·8 per cent of the total number of syndyasmos. (The definition of the population is wider in this case.) In this study the definition of a cohabiting unmarried couple is any household listed in the official files that consists of two unmarried adults of different sexes. This means, for instance, that an unmarried mother living together with her unmarried son aged 20 years are defined as a cohabiting unmarried couple. But at the same time an unmarried person living together with a legally married but separated person of the opposite sex, who in reality constitute a cohabiting unmarried couple, are not included in this operational definition. It seems probable that these two kinds of situation are of about the same frequency and of fairly small importance, and that the estimate of 6·8 per cent is a fairly good estimate of the percentage of syndyasmos that is unmarried.

According to the experiences of the Central Bureau of Statistics in Sweden (personal communication) about 40 per cent of the one-parent families represent in reality cohabiting unmarried couples. The parents in the one-parent families are unmarried in the sense that either they have never married, or they have been divorced or widowed.

Since there has been an enormous decrease in the marriage rate in Sweden during the last few years (from 1966 to 1970 the marriage rate, defined as the number of marriages in relation to the number of unmarried inhabitants between 15 and 45 years old, has decreased by about 35–38 per cent), it is reasonable to assume that the frequency of cohabiting unmarried couples is higher today than it was in 1969 and 1970. The last available data indicates that 12–13 per cent of all syndyasmos in 1975 were unmarried — the age-specific rate is, however, different. Thus about 50 per cent of the syndyasmos in which the partners are around 25 years old are unmarried, compared to only 0–1 per cent in age over 50 (Trost 1975a). This means that this kind of syndyasmos is very common.

Sweden is not exceptional in this sense. The trend toward higher numbers of cohabiting unmarried couples is the same in the other Scandinavian countries, and 'engagement marriages' and 'cohabitation marriages' are very common in Iceland and have been so for a long time (Björnsson 1971). According to Hayner (1966, p. 113–14) the number of cohabiting unmarried couples in Mexico is about 20 per cent of all syndyasmos. Cavan and Cavan (1971, p. 13) say that 'consensual or free unions' (i.e., in our terms, cohabiting unmarried couples and common-law marriages) are like concubinage, 'semi-permanent in nature'. As far as we know there is no empirical evidence for this statement but, as Näsholm (1972a) has shown, the number of separation or 'divorces' is much higher among the cohabiting unmarried couples than among the cohabiting married couples or the legal marriages. The number of dissolutions among the unmarried couples is at least 10 per cent per year and among the married couples less than 1 per cent during any one year. Even if one takes into consideration the facts that the married couples are older, both in age and in duration of marriage, and that the divorce rate declines with age and duration of marriage, the rate of dissolution among the unmarried couples is still much higher than among the married couples. According to a study done in Malmö (the third largest city in Sweden) 12·6 per cent of the syndyasmos that received social welfare subsidies from the municipality of Malmö were cohabiting unmarried couples (Sjöström 1970, p. 67). (According to this study 8 per cent of the children in Malmö live in homes that get subsidies from the municipality.) Such a high figure could be explained by the fact that Malmö is a fairly large town with a higher population density and less social control than in Sweden generally. We know from Näsholm (1971a, p. 28) that the lowest social class is relatively over-represented among the cohabiting unmarried couples, and we know that the municipal subsidies tend to go to the lowest classes. These two facts constitute another explanation of the high number of unmarried cohabiting couples in Sjöström's investigation.

FORMAL AND INFORMAL NORMS

Cavan and Cavan (1971, p. 29) say that quasi-marriages 'may serve certain useful functions, not provided for in marriage-regulations. They break through the rigidity of endogamous and intermarriage rules and may lead to a re-definition of those rules.' This statement can be true where what Cavan and Cavan call quasi-marriages are outside the dominant cultural pattern. But it would be unreasonable to state, for instance, that in Iceland the large number of 'engagement marriages' or 'cohabitation marriages' break through any rules or norms, since these forms in Iceland can be classified as an informal cultural social institution.

Furthermore, it does not seem reasonable to say that the increase in what we here call cohabiting unmarried couples would have changed any endogamous norms or intermarriage rules, since Sweden has no formally or informally defined endogamous norms or intermarriage rules. But, at the same time, there are some informal endogamous norms that are not culturally defined but do in fact exist. It has been found (Trost 1974), for example, that there are endogamous or at least perceived norms that the spouses in marriage should be of about equal age and that the wife should not be older than the husband — at least not by more than a couple of years. But Näsholm (1972a) has shown that there is more of a tendency among cohabiting unmarried couples than among cohabiting married couples for the woman to be older than the man. This fact could, according to Cavan and Cavan, change the mentioned informal perceived norm that the wife may not be older than the husband. One (not very probable) explanation of the fact that there are more cases in which the woman is older than the man among the cohabiting unmarried couples is that if the woman is older than the man the couple is less likely to marry, because of the perceived norms, and instead prefer to cohabit unmarried. A more reasonable explanation would be that people who cohabit as an unmarried couple are more radical, non-traditionalist, or rebellious than the more conforming couples who marry. Cavan and Cavan (1971, pp. 21–1) say that what they call quasi-marriages result in certain dysfunctions for society. 'The unvalidated unions may place a strain on the social organization of the society. The individuals involved and their off-spring may be rejected by society and become personally demoralized. Children may be stigmatized as bastards and may be unable to inherit from their fathers.' In Sweden children born in cohabiting unmarried relations are legally looked upon as similar to children of all other kinds of unmarried mothers. Even if the cohabitation is steady the mother is the only one who is supposed to take care of the child, although there are some differences between the unmarried mothers living alone and those steadily together with the father of the child or children. The taxation law and some of the rules concerning social welfare subsidies treat the cohabiting unmarried couple as if they were married and this, of course, has indirect effects upon the children. It would be exaggerating to say that children of unmarried couples steadily cohabiting are stigmatized in the Swedish society. Some of them might feel or perceive that they are different from children in cohabiting marriages, since they are in some instances formally defined as children of an unmarried mother and not of a married mother and father.

Another statement by Cavan and Cavan (1971, p. 23) that does not hold for the increase in the number of cohabiting unmarried couples in Sweden is the statement that 'since all societies tend to be endogamous, intermarriage and quasi-marriage develop most rapidly during periods of social change when endogamous boundaries are borken.' The middle part of the sentence might be true, but not the first and the last parts. In Sweden the number of 'quasi-marriages' and cohabiting unmarried couples *has* increased most rapidly during a period of social change. But we cannot assume that this has occurred as a result of the change. It is hard to state exactly what social change has taken place in Swedish society during the last 5 or 6 years, when we have this increase in the number of cohabiting unmarried couples. There are many indicators that *something* has happened: the marriage rate has decreased (which might be the same as saying that the number of cohabiting unmarried couples has increased), the divorce rate has increased, fertility has decreased to a very low level (but is now increasing again, and will probably go on increasing for some years — the fertility rate goes in waves), the number of married women in the labour force has increased rapidly, etc.

Different kinds of norms and, especially, perceived norms are relevant when discussing cohabiting married couples in relation to cohabiting unmarried couples. These norms are particularly important in some cases, since there are so many kinds of reasons for, and types of cohabitation, even inside our two broad classes of cohabiting couples. We will now mention and discuss some of the existing and perceived norms that can affect the couple. For simplicity, and since there are no certain institutionalized norms concerning cohabiting unmarried couples, we will focus on such couples and examine them in relation to married couples.

Among the existing norms we can differentiate between formal norms, i.e. the law and the municipal and national regulations, and the informal norms, which come from the social environment — relatives, friends, and other social relationships.

Legal norms

It seems reasonable to start with family law. Swedish law states (GB 5:2) that the spouses must make contributions in relation to their abilities, in the form of money, activities in the home, or in other ways, to give the family that maintenance that can be seen as reasonable in relation to their present conditions. This rule is very seldom used in trials but, according to family counsellors, the rule is a very important guideline both in family counselling and in relationships inside the normal marriages. There is no equivalent to this formal rule for cohabiting unmarried couples, but it seems reasonable to assume that in most cases in which the spouses by free will live together without being married the rule is acting in the same way as for married couples, i.e. as some kind of guideline. One could say that this kind of rule is for most people an internalized social norm.

When there is a dissolution through the death of one of the partners or through 'divorce' there are, however, important differences between cohabiting married and cohabiting unmarried couples. The law says (GB 11:26) that when a couple is divorced and one of the spouses found by the court to be in need of a maintenance allowance, the court can order the other spouse to give such separate maintenance. In reality the court decides this in many cases in which the spouses have been living together for a fairly long time and have or have had children, and especially if the other spouse (normally the wife) has not been gainfully employed (cf. Trost 1975*b*). However, in the cases of 'divorce' among the unmarried cohabiting couples there is no legal rule about maintenance. This means that if in such cases the cohabitation has lasted for a long time, and if one of the spouses has been doing household work most of the time and if it is hard for him or her to go out into the labour force, he or she has no legal right to get a separate maintenance.

Another important part of the family law deals with the provisions concerning property. In legal marriages the property and the incomes of each of the spouses are his or her own, and he/she is allowed to do whatever he/she finds suitable with them, except for the limitations mentioned above. But, at the same time, unless the spouses have a marriage settlement to the contrary, each of the spouses owns half of the property, irrespective of who has earned it, has owned it before marriage, or has inherited it. This rule lies latent during marriage and becomes manifest in case of dissolution through death or divorce. If the spouses have a marriage settlement this division of the property is made as laid down by the marriage settlement. (Of course, the law is much more complicated, but this summary is adequate here, as an overall perspective).

There are no rules of this or a similar nature concerning cohabiting unmarried couples, which means that in cases of death or 'divorce' the two partners have no legal rules to lean on. It is evident that most persons who enter syndyasmos, independent of if they are legal or non-legal, do so with some kind of romantic love view. They do not think about a divorce or separation at the time and if they do they assume that in their case the divorce will be a nice friendly divorce with no aggression or hard feelings. In reality many legal marriages end in divorce (in Sweden now about 1/5) and a still higher proportion of unmarried couples separate (cf. Näsholm 1972*a*). For the legally married there are rules that can help them to solve many of the practical problems, but there are no rules for the cohabiting unmarried couples.

The legal problems in cases of dissolution through death of one of the partners/spouses are similar to the cases of separation or divorce. There are, however, two important dissimilarities. One of them is that in a separation at least one of the spouses want a separation, and very often both of them do, but in case of death normally neither of the partners wants the dissolution, and in practically all cases this is at least not overt. Another important dissimilarity is that in case of dissolution through the death of one of the partners only one of them remains, but in case of separation both partners remain. This means that in case of death in a married situation the law states how much of the household, etc. the widowed partner should get and how much the relatives should inherit, but in unmarried situations the laws do not take the remaining partner in consideration at all. This means that in principal the relatives will inherit all that the dead person had and the partner will get nothing of it (if there is no will).

An index of problems of this kind is an enquiry that was sent out to all Swedish lawyers. After half of them had answered the questionnaire it was found that during 1971 they had handled 541 cases of cohabiting unmarried couples who were 'divorcing', and 182 cases in which one of the partners had died. All these were cases with disputes of one sort or another. The lawyers had also handled 363 cases of disputes occurring during cohabitation (Lind *et al.*, personal communication).

A governmental commission was created in 1969 with the aim, *inter alia*, of giving suggestions of ways to solve some of these problems. Of course, it is reasonable not to treat the two kinds of cohabitation as absolutely equal from a formal point of view, since some of the unmarried cohabiting couples do not want to be treated as if they were married. The following list shows examples of situations in which, according to the law, marital status is of importance in Sweden (SOU 1972, p. 92, my translation):

Custody of children
Guardianship
Inheritance
Damages
Theft (larceny)
Defamation
Aiding and abetting a criminal
Action for recovery of property disposed of by a bankrupt by way of fraudulent preference of one creditor
Lawful disqualification
Obligation to appear as a witness
Right of action in court
Acquisition of land
Exercise of a right of pre-emption
Municipalities right of pre-emption

Tenant's right
Tenant ownership
Prolongation of a land lease
Fishing lease
Conditional sale
Insurance contract
Name
Copyright
Right to a trade name
A child's membership of the Swedish Church
Right of reindeer breeding
Official duty (duty of service)
Sterilization
Abortion
Service pension
Old age pension
Industrial injury insurance
Social assistance
War support
Social assistance to servicemen
Compensation to infection carriers
Liability to taxation
Registration of stockholders
Citizenship
Voting

The social environment

Near relatives and friends. Let us move now to the social environment and start with the near relatives of the two 'spouses' cohabiting in a marriage-like dyad. According to a case-study made by L. Alnebring (1973), it seems to be very uncommon for the near relatives (parents and brothers and sisters) to dislike or object to the unmarried couple's cohabitation. However, there is *some* evidence in the opposite direction. For instance, there are indications that cohabiting unmarried couples perceive that some of their near relatives do in fact dislike the cohabitation or prefer the two partners to consolidate their cohabitation through a legal marriage, or that their near relatives believe that they should marry legally if they have a child.

There are, as far as we know, no hard data in this derived from knowledge or experience. According to the author's experience it was relatively common a couple of decades ago for a man and a woman who were engaged or going steady with each other to live together but not admit it to others in their social environment, either in the immediate social environment or the more distant environment. Often, each of them had his own dwelling even though they actually lived together in one of the dwellings. The real frequency of cohabitation a couple of decades ago was therefore not zero in reality, although it was supposed to be at any rate very small. If a near relative knew that a cohabitation existed without marriage they tended not to admit it to other people, nor to let the two cohabiting partners know that the relatives knew it. This tendency has changed very much during the last ten years. Most cohabiting unmarried couples admit freely and to anybody who wants to know that they live together unmarried. Probably none of them feels ashamed of the cohabitation. Near relatives, such as parents and

brothers and sisters, do not hesitate to admit openly both to other persons and to the partners that they know about the cohabitation. This seems to be true even in social milieus or circles where 10 years ago it would have been impossible. The practice of unmarried cohabitation is now fairly common and openly discussed, so that it is perceived as quite natural for a son or a daughter to live together steadily with a partner of the opposite sex.

The openness that has existed for only the past few years has supposedly had two very important effects. One of these is, according to our assumption, that cohabitation among unmarried couples has become increasingly more common. Because of the verbal openness and the changed informal norms, many more couples cohabit now than if these changes had not occurred. The other effect is, or might be, that perceptions are now much more in accordance with social reality. According to the author's experience and perceptions and in accordance with Alnebring (1973), what was stated above concerning relatives seems also to be true for friends. Because of the high degree of geographical mobility in the society of today, especially among younger people, i.e. those in the mate-selection ages, it seems reasonable to assume that the perception of the informal norms of friends is more important for the behaviour of the norm receiver than the perception of the norms of relatives. It has often been said that we live in a permissive society, and this may be especially true concerning norms that have to do with the forms of marriage-like cohabitation. It can therefore be assumed that only in very few cases do cohabiting unmarried couples perceive themselves as norm-breakers or as deviant persons. They perceive cohabitation in an unmarried form as quite natural and common, so that there is no reason why, in this sense, they should have any problems with the cohabitation.

McDowell (1971) concludes that there are many indices that black/white intermarriages are subject to greater stress than intra-white marriages or intra-black marriages. Among the reasons for this are parental disapproval, job insecurity, and housing difficulties, which occur to a greater extent with the black/white intermarriages than in other kinds of marriages. It might be wrong to compare cohabiting unmarried couples with black/white intermarriages, but, at least to some extent, the couples are in the same kind of position. It seems reasonable to assume that in a social environment in which white couples cohabit unmarriedly in contradiction to the informal norms, these couples are subject to more stress than married couples. Less than 10 years ago cohabiting unmarried couples had great problems in getting apartments. The problems for them are still (in 1972) often greater than for married people.

Other factors in the social environment. First, we find that there are two sets of terms used to express the relationship inside a couple or a dyad. In married cases we talk about 'wife' and 'husband'. These terms cannot be used when an unmarried cohabiting person talks about the other group member to an outsider. People find it incorrect to talk about their husband or wife, fiancé/fiancée, or boy-friend or girl-friend. In many cases this is a problem, though it is not one of high intensity for most people.

Until a couple of years ago a woman had to change her surname to that of her husband when they married. Now it is possible for the wife to keep her maiden name but it is, however, very uncommon to do so; in most cases the woman takes the surname of the husband. So this tradition is very strong. This has the effect that for many of the cohabiting unmarried couples their different surnames are problematic, at least to some extent. They have to have two names on the door so the postman can find them, etc., and their children cannot have the same name as both the father and the mother. In titulation we still differentiate between married and unmarried women. Should a woman present herself as Miss or Mrs? What should other people say: Miss or Mrs?

THE CHILDREN

In many cases of cohabiting unmarried couples the partners claim (if they have no children) that when they have a child they will marry because otherwise the formal as well as the informal norms are negative, especially for the child. We have already mentioned the problem of surnames. It is generally assumed that the child could have problems and could feel stigmatized if he or she has a different name from his or her mother or father.

In unmarried couples only one of the parents, the mother, is the official care-taker of the child, but in married cases both parents are. It is commonly assumed that a child could suffer from the former arrangement; both the risk of the feeling of being stigmatized and directly practical problems could occur. For example if the child has to get the care-taker's signature, it is much easier if either of the parents are allowed to write his/her signature, as is the situation with married couples. Another reason why many people think that children in cohabiting unmarried cases perceive that they are treated as deviant is that they may find it curious that it is only his or her parents who are not married, when the parents of all their play-mates are married. There is a serious risk that the child will see himself/herself as a deviant person belonging to a deviant group. This is normally assumed to be really stressful for the child, since children have a very important need to feel that they are not different to other children in the neighbourhood.

INTERNAL STRESS

Let us now discuss the relationships between the unmarried cohabiting couple in relation to the married couple.

Kopreitan (1969, p. 13) claims that it has been shown that the 'normal family form' limits or totally destroys the possibilities for love and sexual satisfaction. He says that the unmarried family is in a better position, since it is not based on dutiful sexual, moral, and marital strength but on liberty, responsibility, and more spontaneous and free love. He goes on to say that in the married family the partners are bound together by a network of laws and norms that can give the man a feeling of bondage and the woman a feeling of security, the effect of which is stupidity. But (according to Kopreitan) since the partners in the unmarried family are not bound together by this network of laws and norms, the co-operation must be based on a steadily revived decision process.

Although we do not agree with what Kopreitan says this viewpoint should be mentioned. It is a kind of statement that is very often heard from people in favour of unmarried cohabitation. Alnebring (1973) has found that the kind of argument that Kopreitan uses is fairly common among the cohabiting unmarried couples that she has studied. She concludes that in many cases the partners assume that they are less secure when they know that they can separate any moment. But, at the same time, they see it as something positive that they cannot be too sure of each other. They assume that one more consideration is shown by partners in unmarried cohabitation.

This kind of view seems rather curious to a sociologist. It is reasonable from a family sociological point of view to say that all functions of the family have been changed. Many of its traditional functions have now been taken over more and more by society, which means that for most of the traditional functions the family is of little importance (economic or productive functions, socialization, reproduction, the sexual function, the religious function, the leisure-time function, and the material security function); but it is absolutely not true for what we usually call the emotive function or the primary group function. The family is the only institutionalized group that is a primary group. By a primary group we mean a face-to-face group that enjoys feelings of solidarity, and that is productive of the moral norms operating in our lives. The primary group is the one in which you can feel secure, and in which you can live out your emotions, where you can be angry, where you can show momentary hatred toward those who you love, etc., without being excluded from the group. The statement by Kopreitan and the findings by Alnebring are, as far as we can see, in contradiction to the idea of primary group function. They are saying that it is positive to belong to a group that is primary, but in which you do not necessarily feel secure or confident. If it is true that the partners in the unmarried cohabiting groups are less confident than in married groups the unmarried group is living under greater pressure due to the probability of dissolution of the group.

Another argument that is often used in favour of unmarried cohabitation is that in the unmarried union the partners feel less dependent on each other than they would feel if they had been married; instead of being dependent on each other they are self-dependent individuals. It is not clear if by dependency is meant a dependency as regards practical matters, or as regards values, interests, ideas, etc. If the idea of less dependency among cohabiting unmarried couples is true in reality, it seems reasonable that self-esteem and self-consciousness is higher in unmarried cases than in married ones. Today it is fashionable to see it as something positive to be personally independent, but as Kälvesten and Meldahl (1972) have shown, some degree of dependency is involving and important.

CONCLUSION

We can conclude that it is fairly common in many countries for unmarried couples to live together. However, this situation constitutes an unstable relationship. Because there is no pressure from the formal and informal norms towards stability of an unmarried group, a separation is easier to arrange than in the marriage situation with all its formal and informal norms.

As far as we can see the most important differences between unmarried and married cohabiting couples lie latent during the cohabitation but becomes manifest in a situation of dissolution. This seems to be true regardless of whether the group is dissolved by a separation or by the death of one of the partners. There is no doubt that there are often many problems when the spouses in a marriage separate or divorce. Andersson and Stenberg (1971), for example, have shown this in a very convincing manner. These problems also exist when the unmarried couples separate. But in the unmarried cases there are in addition further problems. In most cases there are no rules concerning the division of the household, finances, etc. At the beginning of a cohabitation people are convinced that he or she and his/her spouse/partner either will never divorce or separate, or that they will separate as friends. With only slight exaggeration it can be said that the most important reason for a cohabiting couple to get maried is that they will have the benefits of formal rules if the cohabitation should end in a separation. This means that, in relation to its goals, society should try to convince cohabiting couples to marry. This is not very easy to do. Those who marry do so not because it is good for them for rational reasons, but for traditional reasons; and those who do not marry do so to some extent because they dislike the formal norms. In fact, their cognition of the formal norms is wrong, which means that they believe that they know the formal norms but in reality they do not. But the sort of hypothetical reasoning we are undertaking here is however, too simple and too culture-bound to the existing marriage norms.

REFERENCES

ALNEBRING, L. (1973). *Sammanboende ogifta* [Unmarried cohabitation]. Research Report from the Department of Sociology, Uppsala University, Special Series: Family Research, FF 22.

ANDERSSON, M. and STENBERG, A. (1971). 'Om effekter av skilsmässa'[Effects of divorces]. Research Report from the Department of Sociology, Uppsala University, Sweden. Special Series: Family Research, FF 14.

BJÖRNSSON, B. (1971). *The Lutheran doctrine of marriage in modern Icelandic society.* Oslo, Norway.

CAVAN, R. and CAVAN, J. T. (ed.) (1971). Cultural patterns, functions and dysfunctions of endogamy and intermarriage. In a special issue on 'Intermarriage in a Comparative Perspective'. *Int. J. Sociol. Fam.*, **1**, 10–24.

HAYNER, N. S. (1966). *New patterns in Old Mexico.* Connecticut.

KOPREITAN, O. (1969). *Noen aspekt ved den ugifte families stilling i dagens Norge.* Oslo, Norway. (Mimeo)

KÄLVESTEN, A-L. and MELDAHL, G. (1972). *217 Stockholmsfamiljer* [217 Stockholm families]. Tidens förlag, Stockholm.

LÖCSEI, P. (1970). Syndyasmos in Contemporary Budapest. (Paper presented at the 7th World Congress on Sociology, Varna, Bulgaria, 1970.)

McDOWELL, S. F. (1971). Black-white intermarriage in the United States. In a special issue on 'Intermarriage in a Comparative Perspective.' *Int. J. Sociol. Fam.*, **1**, 49–58.

NÄSHOLM, A. (1972a). *Sammanboende gifta och sammanboende ogifta* [Cohabiting married and cohabiting unmarried]. In SOU 1972:41, pp. 355–71. Stockholm, Sweden.

—— (1972b). *Riksförsäkringsverkets föräldraundersökning* [A parent study made by the State insurance company]. In SOU 1972:41, pp. 372–7. Stockholm, Sweden.

SJÖSTRÖM, K. (1970). Fattiga barnfamiljer i Malmö [Poor families with children in Malmö]. In *Socialvård och samhällsförändrigg* (ed. Swedner). Stockholm, Sweden.

SOU (1972). 1972:41: *Äktenskap och Familj*, I. Stockholm, Sweden.

TROST, J. (1965). Äktenskapets upplösning [The dissolution of marriage]. In *Familjen i Samhället* [Family in society] (ed. G. Karlsson and J. Trost). Stockholm, Sweden.

—— (1970). *Utvecklingen i fråga om äktenskapets stabilitet* [Changes in marital stability]. Sociologisk Forskning.

—— (ed.) (1974). Dyad formation and received social norms. In *Miscellanea Sociologica.* Uppsala, Sweden.

—— (1975a). Attitudes to and occurrence of cohabitation without marriage. Paper presented at VI World Congress of Social Psychiatry, Jugoslavia, 4–10 October 1976.

—— (1975b). *Vårdnad och underhåll; en undersökning vid tingsrätter och allmänna advokatbyråer hösten 1973* [Custody and alimonies; a study at district courts and public solicitors during the Fall 1973]. In SOU 1975:24 pp. 33–120. Stockholm, Sweden.

13.   IS THE NUCLEAR FAMILY THE ANSWER IN A CHANGING SOCIETY?

RITA LILJESTRÖM

COINCIDENCE OF PRODUCTIVE AND REPRODUCTIVE ROLES

It would all be much simpler if one could beget one's children after being pensioned — the pension age could be lowered a little — or if, vice versa, one did not need to fully enter the job market until after one's children had passed the nursery school phase. In this second case, parents would have shorter working hours and other fringe benefits with regard to what society assumes that the child should receive from his or her parents. Parents would even be educated for their tasks. This would also help the parents develop those qualities of life which one receives from contact with children.

But let us not fly off into Utopia too quickly. My aim is to point out the risks of 'overloading' which arises because the heavy investments in reproductive and productive roles tend to coincide in time. It is noteworthy here that these investments tend not to coincide in space, i.e. the places for performance of the respective roles are segregated: to the home and the place of 'work'. Being tied to home and children, experiencing pressure from economic demands, and lacking any wide range of experience add up to a considerable load for the young parent just beginning his or her career. And the institutional unit that is to differentiate and make compatible the two roles generally consists of only two persons, one woman and one man.

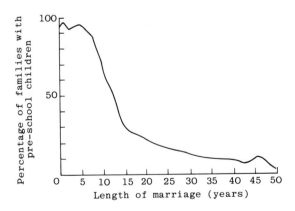

FIG. 13.1.

Fig. 13.1 (de Laval 1970, 1967), showing the distribution of families with preschool children and the length of marriage in Sweden, clearly indicates a concentration of youngsters in families that have been in existence for less than 15 years. If we assume that the average age for entering marriage is between the ages of 20 and 26 years, we can safely derive the conclusion that the reproductive age does in fact coincide with that of production and especially with those years when the young adult is trying *to establish* his or her place in the world of production.

Having to learn to manage two spheres of life at approximately the same time is an important cause of stress in the individual. However the situation becomes even more precarious when, as is the case today, the differentiation of roles is controversial and questioned.

How does one manage this heavy load? There seem to be two main alternatives in use:

(1) One specializes the above functions or roles — i.e. a functional differentiation takes place, creating independence and autonomy for the respective partners. Each one takes complete responsibility for his or her tasks.

(2) One pools or shares the relevant functions or tasks — i.e. a blending of functions takes place, creating interchangeability and the possibility for the respective partners to relieve one another.

I intend to look into each of these solutions, which occur side-by-side in today's families. The result of this investigation cannot be evaluated without taking into account the surrounding society. Obviously the role differentiation within the family has consequences for that of the labour market, especially its vertical differentiation. Institutional arrangements either encourage or discourage the husband and wife to choose or not choose a particular alternative. Last, but not least, there is the question concerning integration of the family in society and the possibility for the husband/wife configuration to transmit and exemplify the social patterns for the next generation. It is within framework (1) that I intend to identify the causes for stress.

ROLE SPECIALIZATION

The family can be studied as a small group, analogous to other small groups. In this way, one sees how roles come into being. On the one hand, all existing groups must expend some time and effort on internal relations: to preserve emotional cohesion, internal routines, and internal order. On the other hand, the group attempts to improve its adaptation to its environment: to main-tain integrity and autonomy in relation to the outside and to realize economic goals, the means of which lie outside the group. Both the 'internal' and the 'external' aspects must be dealt with by the group.

In the specialized family, the father attends to the external side of the family and the mother to the internal. The work role of the father is, according to Parsons and Bales (1955), the basis for his place in the family, i.e. his work role is the basis for his family role. By this role in production, the father becomes the instrumental (economic) leader of the family.

Again by analogy to small-group research, the main function of the father in today's family can be seen as the mediator or link between the family and the rest of society. As a worker and provider, his efforts are directed towards the more long-term economic and social goals (i.e. external goals) of the family. The mother on the other hand is mediator between the father and their children. Her function is to provide for the emotional outlets of the family, to interpret for the father the needs and reactions of their children, to mediate in conflicts, and to safeguard family cohesion.

In families where the mother is responsible for emotional functions and the father for economical, the children learn, through their daily interaction with their mother, an expressive technique which is especi-ally influenced by the wish to be liked and experience good personal relations. Interaction with their father transmits initiative, an orientation towards problem-solving and rationality, a suppression of expressive needs, and a psychological sensitivity in favour of goal-directed activities (Parsons and Bales 1955).

From a purely theoretical point of view, this func-tional specialization need not be coupled to sex — rather an insignificant number of parental duties are directly linked to gender — but could easily emerge instead on the basis of suitability and availability. In practice, however, specialization seems to maintain a traditional sex role differentiation which corresponds to what in Sweden is called the conservative sex role ideology. We have today quite an abundance of litera-ture on the *woman* as a parent and as a worker, but given our interest in the family it can perhaps be asked whether it is not the male who has the more differenti-ated role. Although men's work roles have undergone far-reaching functional specialization and differenti-ation in a social sense, mothers are expected to exhibit roughly the same emotions and talents in quite different social contexts and life conditions. I shall focus on the father attempting to illustrate his different commit-ments to the roles of reproduction and production. This perspective or focusing seems relevant since:

(a)   father represents 'society' and work life in the family,
(b)   father defines the social position of the family and thereby also the 'take-off status' of the children in society,

(c)   fathers are differentiated more than mothers, i.e. shaped by their specialized work roles and their highly differing working conditions,
(d)   conflicts that the transition from patriarchal to egalitarian society have created for men have been rather neglected, and
(e)   socially deviant behaviour (alcoholism, crime, suicide) is more frequent among men than among women, so that fathers consequently are in this sense a greater risk for the family.

Thus the responsibility of providing economically falls upon the man — and that at an age when his position on the job market is often uncertain. Invest-ments in his job occur to a large extent at the expense of investments in his role as father. These ideas are born out by the following investigation.

In his book, *The American male*, Myron Brenton (1967) discusses the paradoxes involved in fatherhood. He refers to a study carried out by Helena Lopata on slightly more than 600 married women, 30–49 years of age, living in Chicago and its suburbs. When asked to rank their life roles in order of importance, nearly all ranked their role as mother as number one. When asked to do a similar ranking of behalf of their hus-bands' roles, 65 per cent immediately put his role as provider at the top. The role of father came second and that of husband third. A large majority of the women having put their role as mother as number one ranked that of wife and home-maker as number two and three.

The father is in other words directed towards his work role as the basis for his self-esteem. Thus the work role is most central to the lives of most men. The masculinity of American men is based on their success as provider for the family. Their wives set up the same yardstick, thereby being loyal to the man's perspective of himself and conforming to the existing societal views on family roles (compare Parsons and Bales 1955).

But what consequences does this almost total depen-dence of the husband on his provider-role have for the emotional relationship between husband and wife? As Brenton points out, other roles, such as husband, father, or citizen, could have more importance for a man's self-esteem and identity. It is much easier for a woman to live with a low-status job because she builds her self-esteem on her work role only to a very small extent. Being a good mother and wife is what counts (and in that order). It is the quality of performances in these roles that is essential.

Today's disjointed attitude towards fatherhood is an ironic consequence of a patriarchal system. Compared with how girls learn mother-like behaviour, boys experience very little preparation for their role as father. The preparation for motherhood is a cumulative experience, starting at childhood and becoming more and more reinforced up to the day when the woman turns mother. Precisely because the father role does not have the same type of physical foundation (e.g. preg-nancy) as the mother role, one would expect boys to have a special need for knowledge or instruction in their parent-to-be role. Instead, many boys experience their own fathers as indifferent and helpless *as a father* in a personal or social sense, i.e. apart from their provider role. They have no chance to gain knowledge of their prospective father-role in any manner comparable to how girls are continuously psychologically prepared to become mothers. It is therefore little wonder that the role of father is included only very rarely in a boy's image of himself as a mature man.

To top this off, we have the cultural role models in mass-media, advertisements, family comedies, and comic strips which promote and picture father as a tragicomical figure. In comic strips the unmarried hero radiates virility and adventure while the married man is generally a compliant, harmless fellow — something of a blockhead, always outsmarted by his children, his wife and his dog. Family series on television are often a tiresome parade of situational comedy concerning the 'master of the house' who while heating his dinner almost sets the house on fire, or while fitting a new washer to the tap floods the house. Dad in suburbia is characterized as the village fool.

This characterization has a message: 'Not the work for a real man', 'Here is a man fooling around in a woman's domain.' To a boy this image of father involves a complete deheroization and ridiculing of fatherhood as a prospective life role. Many a young father encounters fatherhood with a feeling of inadequacy, a feeling that tends to grow strangers as he is also expelled from his central position in the world of his wife. When he looks for his wife, he finds that he is married to the mother of his children, with his main task being to provide for them. He is now free to become totally involved in his work and/or accept the place of a submissive, loving, easily manipulated extension of the symbiotic mother/child unit. Thus we arrive at the well-known family constellation composed of a dominating, over-protective mother and a passive, ineffective father.

The family constellation just mentioned is only one of the risks that the specialized family runs. Another potentially risky situation develops because the role of 'mum' does not have the same pull for all mothers. Many women are not prepared to accept this dominated family role. If they lack support from their husbands, they will reduce their own responsibilities. According to Brenton (1967) the sequence goes something as follows: the father is frequently not at home, the mother does not have the strength to carry the load of parenthood all by herself, both parents feel insufficient as authorities in the home, and so both withdraw from taking responsibilities. They leave behind a vacuum of power which is removed by someone else moving in and taking over. This 'someone else' is the children; the children and their peer groups. Since the children now hold the strong position, the parents turn to them for guidance, the result being a subversive, child-centered culture. The age-class has entered the stage and the 'generation gap' becomes quite considerable (compare Eisenstadt and Bronfenbrenner).

Paraphrasing Brenton, we can describe the dilemmas facing a modern father in the following way: if he commits himself to being friend to his children, he can reason, that once, in revolt against authoritarian patriarchism, it was considered that freedom and a permissive atmosphere would give children a healthy base for development. But something quite different happens. With no borderlines established, no rules upheld, and no punishment given, children are left without any experience in relating to authority. They receive no practice in self-control, having never encountered any resistance to test themselves against. This lack of authority creates both passivity and an unwillingness to take risks. Few fathers are willing to make the effort of setting borders as it is far easier to be a 'buddy'. Besides, if a man reveals the capacity for loving and looking after his children, this is turned against him as evidence of 'suppressed femininity'. If he buys his children things he never had, he is spoiling them and leaving them badly prepared for the realities of life; if he does not, he gets the reputation of a 'mean old man'. If he works hard all the week and tries to compensate to his family by planning to do something special with them at weekends, as thanks he learns from his wife that he is playing Santa Claus for his children instead of taking part in the more tiresome and tedious everyday activities. No matter what he does, it comes out wrong.

A sketch of the 'costs' of specialization

1. Childhood becomes a 'mother land'. Children have very little contact with their fathers.
2. The man is deprived of his influence in regard to socialization of his children, his father identity receives low esteem, and he is deprived of many of the life qualities that could be embodied in his reproductive role.
3. The family is vulnerable due to lack of reserves. Husband and wife are both irreplaceable if anything should happen.
4. There are disasterous consequences for men who fail in their role as provider or become unemployed. These consequences are a result of the one-sided anchoring of male identity (Grønseth 1970).
5. Women continue to have subordinate and low-paid positions on the labour market.
6. Women are isolated with low socio-political participation (Grønseth 1970).
7. An economical necessity to maintain marriage that has fallen apart emotionally may arise (Grønseth 1970).
8. The norms guiding family roles and work roles are so different that the family has difficulty transmitting to their children the social pattern of relations necessary for adult roles outside of the family (Dahlström and Liljeström 1967, p. 41–51).

ROLE SHARING

It has been suggested that married women seek employment in order to be able to indulge in what has been called surplus consumption, i.e. consumption that is luxurious rather than necessary. Gustaf de Laval in an analysis of census data arrives at the interpretation that the majority of working mothers feel that they are forced to work to help provide for necessary family expenses. It seems reasonable to assume that this necessity or at least feeling of necessity would be most acute among younger couples — when their households have just been formed and incomes are still rather low.

In somewhat simplified terms we can say that there are two basic ways for the above families to meet their economic demands:

(1) the wife can work and help bring in necessary resources; or

(2) the husband can seek extra employment and work overtime — in the long run this might also include adult education, full-time or at night school.

We have no knowledge of how Swedish fathers experience their roles, but one small exploratory study evokes curiosity and an interest in learning more. The study aimed at finding out how 12 young fathers perceived themselves in relation to different competitors for their time and effort: family, work, leisue, and society in general. The men all had working wives and one or two had pre-school children (Andersson and Andersson 1972).

There were some features and attitudes experienced by all the fathers in the study. For each one there was support for an equal division of work between him and his wife, an understanding for the demands put on his wife by her career, an interest and willingness to back up his wife in her work, and the experience of difficult mornings when children had to be fed and transported to day-care centres, and all other household chores had to be performed while getting ready for work. The family came before all other interests; and all free time was spent with the family. Nevertheless 8 of the 12 fathers, while stating their deep loyalty towards the family, expressed a desire to be able to spend some part of the year alone, away from the family, in order to avoid getting too tied down by their spouses, in order to renew and revitalize themselves and their marriages. They were willing to grant their wives the same kind of 'leave of absence'. In practice they advocated separate holidays.

Listing their different interests, society was always the last party to be mentioned. Nobody had any time for society, or had any political, union, or other society-geared interests.

The young fathers view on sex roles was rather undifferentiated and oriented towards equality, taking into account only what appeared most practical in the particular situation. Which solution was most practical was based on many factors. Advocating the practical implies an excuse for a not altogether unconditional pooling of household tasks. The fathers' own family background and upbringing had not prepared them for an equalitarian sharing of roles. Accordingly what was generally considered to be the most practical solution is that the wife took charge of the kitchen whereas the father devoted himself to the children. It was not yet altogether practical to take turns.

What is the most practical also depends on the relative educational level of the spouses, i.e. the level of education and competence of the wife compared to that of the husband. Antti Eskola conducted a survey of 450 Helsinki families and found the determining factor for role differentiation to be whether the wife was more, equally or less educated than her husband: the tendency to work was more strongly related to the wife's education as compared to that of her husband than to her education considered independently. In other words the relative position of the spouses strongly effected the differentiation of expressive and instrumental roles within the family. Eskola found that the husband's role in socialization increased as the wife shared the instrumental tasks. Or, to phrase it differently, we find a more equal sharing of emotional as well as economic input (Eskola 1960).

Rhona and Robert Rapoport made an intensive study of 5 families with children where both spouses had a professional career. This variant of a family with two providers is different from many two-provider families as the two careers are not primarily regarded as a necessary means for economical survival but as ends in themselves. Work makes possible efforts that are meaningful and promote a personal development. These dual careers are a source for satisfaction, but at the same time they can give rise to stress. All 5 couples were working under rather sophisticated and intense demands; they were all professionals of some standing. As individuals they gave the impression of being rational and goal-conscious. However, their family patterns seems to have grown out of along succession of choice situations that all appear to have been rather circumstantial. Things just turned out the way they are. Maybe we are functioning in a way that prevents a full insight of mechanisms involved in making choices.

Turning to the hardships inherent in dual careers, we find that all families had experienced five kinds of stress:

1. A feeling of being overloaded and overworked. Neither spouse had the services of a housewife, supporting and relieving the careerist of trivia. Household chores including child-care and social responsibilities, had to be redistributed or neglected.

2. Negative sanctions from the environment. There were as a rule housewives in the neighbourhood who expected the working wife to be a bad mother, a bad wife and, possibly, a selfish person. Sensitivity to criticism is heightened by one's own uncertainty as to how

to arrange for the children from time to time. The work situation can as a rule be planned and anticipated but the lack of day-care services severely limits the possibilities for planning. In this respect the families are left to luck or fate. Women experienced special exposure in work life, especially in high positions. Any slip or mistake runs the risk of judgements such as 'That's what to expect from a woman trying to do two things at once'.

3. Questioning of one's personal identity and worth. Given the fact that the spouses were themselves socialized some 30 years earlier, when sex roles were questioned to a lesser extent and models of new family patterns were non-existent, it is easy to realize how poorly equipped they were for the family structure they were trying to develop. The wives periodically turn depressive and self-dubious, with an increased sensibility for criticism. The husbands in turn have to deny themselves the usual male privileges in order to establish their solidarity with their wive's career interest. They go through periods of irritability and negativism when faced with the fact that self-denial is a necessary price to pay for a family with a successful career-wife — a price that might even include their own success.

4. Limited time for social contacts. Their friends as a rule were the people with whom they worked. The wife's colleagues help her support and keep her professional identity even when faced by her husband's colleagues. But there was a feeling of guilt with reference to the contacts for which there was just not enough time — for neighbours and relatives. Social energy was consumed when associating with people who rendered services to them and to the household, an association as thanks for rendered services.

5. Difficulties with co-ordination of career and family cycles. Roles tend to change over time in family life as well as work life. Attempting to co-ordinate demanding phases in the family and at work is a source of problems. Constant adaptation is necessary. The families had as a rule first established themselves professionally and later had children. In this sense they had established for themselves the economic conditions that appear necessary for the success of dual careers. Still, although faced with sanctions, mothers in these families found comfort in knowing that their husbands were actively involved with their children.

There seems to be little doubt that many of the difficulties experienced by these, in many ways privileged families, are created by conditions in society. The Rapoports (Rapoport and Rapoport 1971) give examples of possible improvements that are well-known in the Swedish debate: 'The need for housing service and different housing arrangements. Better child-care service. Jobs like day-care nurse and kindergarten teacher should be upgraded and better payed. A different planning and zoning of suburbia where, for example, work places could exist side by side with houses and appartment buildings. A more positive open-mindedness towards solutions of role differentiation in the family as well as at work....'

A sketch of the 'costs' of role sharing

There is a risk of overloading when both husband and wife invest in a career *and* parenthood at the same time in a society that presently lacks the institutional arrangements to support this variant of family. This inadequacy can be traced to the following 'costs':

1. Long working hours and travel for adults and consequently a long stay away from home and the children.
2. Childhood, although no longer a 'motherland' is usually still a 'womanland'.
3. Reduced services at home for everyone.
4. Reduction of possibilities for the parents to advance professionally because of responsibilities for their children.
5. No time for socio-political participation, either by husband or wife.
6. Self-doubt, role insecurity, role conflict, and disputes between husband and wife over who shall do what.
7. Criticism and sanctions from the environment.

If we were to assume that the costs were remarkably reduced by institutional arrangements and the liberation of human energy, we could safely expect conflicts and strains in the labour market due to the consequences of female intrusion into new work areas. This would probably lead to redefinitions and re-evaluations of the traditional male criteria for decision making in politics as well as economy.

COMPARISONS OF THE 'COSTS' OF ROLE SPECIALIZATION AND ROLE SHARING

Thus far, we have localized the points of stress surrounding the family with respect to how alternative role differentiations affect sex roles and life situations for men and women, especially at that period in life when they have children. Comparing the 'costs' for the two main alternatives that the young family has, one comes up with the following disheartening results:

1. Role specialization makes it more difficult for spouses to replace each other and a *lack of reserves* is felt, while role sharing gives *poorer service in the home* for both husband and wife.
2. Role specialization heightens the risk for a *strongly dependent relationship between mother and child*, and contact with the father becomes negligible, while with role sharing *contact with both parents tends to be reduced* (with present day working hours and travel time).
3. Role specialization means that both spouses anchor their identities on *skewed, traditional foundations*, while role sharing, in turn, brings with it *uncertain identity and role confusion*, at least in today's society.
4. Role specialization leads to *low socio-political participation for women*, while role sharing

causes both husband and wife to be so busy and tied down that they *both lack the time and energy for socio-political participation*.

5. Because parenthood comes relatively early in the life cycle, there are still a number of life-phases (taking up a number of decades) left over after the children are grown up. Some of the 'costs' of the two alternatives become apparent only during these later stages.

In the previous pages, I have intentionally given a somewhat sharpened description of present-day alternatives for the pair-family. My comparison shows that I am quite sceptical that there are any good solutions for reproductive and productive tasks within the framework of a pair-family with children. Neither do I believe that compromises between two untenable positions will lead to satisfactory solutions. The family is in need of complementary relations outward — and that at clearly defined points.

INTEGRATION OF THE FAMILY IN SOCIETY

The question of *distribution of tasks within the family* should be seen in relation to the *redistribution of functions between the family and society* which has taken place during industrialization. When sociologists have tried to see the nuclear family as a response to social change, they have referred to the 'good fit' between the nuclear family and the industrial system.

Geographical mobility is made easier and smoother with the small household group. *Social mobility* is increased when employment and promotion are based on merit instead of family ties. The individual becomes free to advance. The *new work organization* requires decision be made without the interference of family. The factory system removes old authorities, respect for old age, and interference from family or personal relations in favour of its own system of rules and standards.

The industrial system is based on impersonal relationships and achievement, which gives rise to psychological stress. Marriage and family make up an important complementary institution of individual emotional bands and competitive-free support. [Goode 1963]

But at the same time a redistribution of functions between the family and society occurs. Functions are differentiated and within each functional area, the individual is assigned a functionally relevant and *specialized role*.

For the most part, each function is carried out in, what for it, is a *specialized context*. By dividing up the functions, the integrated value system of which they were integral parts becomes relatively unintelligible. Individuals become members of several systems of functionally specialized roles. There are usually norms prescribing the stifling of all activity outside of the specialized role, in favour of a function-directed, function-efficient orientation within the narrow borders of the specific role.

After breaking up the previous working arrangements and turning many of the heavier functions over to society, the partial group that was left (i.e. the family) and the other activities in the interstices of the social structure were proclaimed private and free. Within the different functional areas the individual is 'fragmented' and accordingly only partially involved — but privately, in the border-land between the separated functions, the individual experiences a kind of illusive 'autonomy' (Luckmann 1967, p. 97, 112–14).

But what relationship does private life have to society? How is the family with children located in its environment? There are three overlapping tendencies in the relationship between family and society that are being talked about today, even if present documentation of them only gives clarification on specific points and a speculative perspective. Here, I am alluding to *geographical mobility*, with the resulting *changes in the family's total relationship to its social environment*, and the *privatization of the family*. Each of these phenomena has a connection with stress.

The politics of today's employment market builds on high geographical mobility. About 6–7 per cent of Sweden's population moves over district boundaries each year. It is mostly the young who are moving from their home communities. Mobility of the married employee on the employment market varies with the number of children in his family. It seems as if larger family size leads to a greater number of changes of employer. New additions to the family are a strong motive for moving (Rundblad 1971). Some families move only once, whereas others move many times in search of a better job and home.

How do those parents that, for example, become city dwellers as adults adjust? Researchers in Stockholm have separated out two main patterns.

(a) An attempt is made to hold onto the past, to shut out the strange city, to resist the new and pretend that one does not live in a modern suburb. This family type seems to dominate in the lower class and has been named the 'traditional farm-family in a city apartment' by Jonsson-Kälvesten. The possibilities of choosing, access to education, services, culture, etc., which are attributed to densely populated areas, lack reality for the newcomers who do not have the resources to make use of the city's possibilities, but who are affected by the city's disadvantages.

(b) The other pattern is to accept the new environment and adopt to its values: the wife begins to work, the children receive more schooling and family life becomes more embedded.

In cities, the neighbourhood, the domain of family life out of cities, is stripped of functions around which its occupants can congregate. The lack of a neighbourhood becomes, in other words, the basis for privatizing family life — not social life — and accordingly families with children are surrounded by a socio-cultural vacuum. Åke Daun has compared big city suburbia to smaller communities.

The adults' relation to their environment is completely different. Their knowledge of society is less. The ordinary suburb has a large number of multiple-family dwellings, some of which are apartment buildings, some row houses, others 'private homes', and a shopping centre. Suburbia has a large population that has arrived from practically the entire country as well as from abroad. The class and occupational structures are comparatively mixed. In other words, suburbia has a socially and culturally heterogenous population. Interaction is scarce. Neighbours usually do not meet at common work places. They do not drop in on one another. They rarely start a conversation if they bump into one another on the street. They do not co-operate in voluntary organizations. They do not become parts of the community's informal political structure. In newly developed housing districts there are hardly any concern that would initiate conversation between the renters. They have moved into a ready-made district and in general have no influence on the environment outside their own apartment — accordingly they do not fell any responsibility for the internal concerns of the district. They lack collective memories and mores. They do not know each other and can not approach one another in a collective local culture [Daun 1971].

British researchers describe a 'new working family', in *The affluent worker* (Goldthorpe *et al.* 1969). The family has few social ties in the local area. The type of 'solidarity' which is assumed to be established in working class districts, is lacking in the socially heterogeneous neighbourhoods without a community spirit. When the move has been made away from relatives to the new area lacking any sense of community, the home and the family of procreation are the only reference points available. It is not the job but the family which is the central interest in life for such people, suggest the researchers. A privatized social life and a purely economic relation to work are seen as two sides of the same coin — these seem to be two aspects of a way to live that mutually support another.

The workers' social life is also truncated by the persistence of shift-work and overtime. The wife works, unless she has young children. Add to this gardening and repair of the house, car, and other property. Time and energy have their limits and there is none left over to establish solidarity with society. One votes for the 'working-class' party and watches out for one's welfare. But solidarity involves only one's family. Feeling for collective interest, at work and in relation to society are in general weak or non-existent.

Having a family increases the pressure on the man to increase his income. Family responsibilities are in conflict with participation in unions, working-class clubs, and associations as well as any socializing with work friends during 'leisure-time'. The worker appears to give high priority to his family when dividing up time and energy. The majority of workers rank as their most important aim 'a steadily increasing standard of living in the home and possibilities to concentrate time outside of work on wife and children'. It should be noted that this research deals with highly-salaried workers with high geographical mobility (Goldthorpe *et al.* 1969).

The idealistic construction of the nuclear family must be viewed against the background of geographical mobility and socio-cultural homelessness. These factors, together with the process of urbanization, increase the importance of the primary groups as a fixed reference point for individuals. From society's viewpoint, we have a small family that fits into a highly mobile labour-market. Lacking strong ties to its environment, this family can easily be torn away and replaced in a new anonymous neighbourhood without any great effect on what goes on *within* the family (Berger and Kellner 1969, p. 48).

And from the child's viewpoint? What image of society can the nuclear family transfer to the children if the parents themselves are neither involved in any visible cooperative activities with other people nor have any collective expressions for social or value cohesion? Children growing up in the secluded world of such nuclear families are shaped by the social standards and attitudes of this small world. When as young adults they go out to live in the larger society they have a need for a 'little world of their own', since the manner in which they have been socialized tells them that this is the way to successfully make out in the big anonymous world that confronts them when they leave their parents. To be at home in society will, by definition, mean the formation of a 'small world' in marriage (Berger and Kellner 1969).

Modern suburban man is left on a little island of family life and private morality, surrounded by a society that contains on the one hand mass-loneliness, generational beings, or we can see it as an *urgent assignment* other, resource-concentration and the development of nearly autonomous specialized function areas (economic, political, and bureaucratic) where neither the 'private' nor the 'fragmented' personality experiences any real involvement or participation in the activities and events of society (Zijderveld 1971).

Many people no longer see the small family as the crowning achievement of freedom and progress — but rather as a fragment in a techno-economical rationalization process which transformed man's material conditions without regard for his social conditions. Now, we can guard that remnant as the last institution which undividedly recognized humans as total, socio-emotional beings, or we can see it as an *urgent assignment to re-integrate the reproductive unit with other social institutions and groups*. My argument favours the latter alternative.

What types of measures are needed to reintegrate the family into society? I shall suggest some that have to do with loneliness, generation gaps, other social problems, and the overloading which is inherent in the isolated nuclear family structure.

1. Day-care centres for children are a possible centre for suburbia's child-oriented activities and for contact between all those who are interested in children, both parents and other adults.
2. Recreation and youth centres in cooperation with school, parents, and other interested adults offer unexploited possibilities.

3. Gathering places and meeting rooms where confrontations with decision makers, parties, musical evenings other kinds of shows, night-classes, interaction with immigrants, discussion of social needs and local problems could be the basis for the building of bonds between the neighbourhood and society.

4. Restaurants and hobby rooms can be common contact points during leisure time, where people can talk with one another and begin the first steps towards new collective agreements on what they consider important and worth collectively guarding. This could be regarded as the beginning of a value-cohesion, while it is also a basis for collective organized action.

5. Local initiative for open health-care service to serve old people as well as the handicapped and sick is necessary. Search activities to find isolated individuals and involve them in some interaction can be important here.

6. Social workers, voluntary groups, and laymen can organize activities for young people with problems, for alcoholics, outcasts, and other deviants.

7. Cultural activities promote social life.

A rich social life can prevent social problems and rebuild the relationships between groups that are so important to society. The Swedish federal 'service-kommission' has introduced an extended conception of 'service'. This conception includes the more *technical* aspect of service (food, apartment up-keep, laundry service, distribution of goods, etc.) as well as a more *social* service (child care, help to old people, help to

sick and disabled, free-time activities and the distribution of cultural products, etc.). The commission has initiated an ideological debate on the goals of different kinds of services, meeting-places and equipment with emphases placed on the ideas of equality and cohesion (Boendeservice 2, 1970, p. 11–14).

Social workers and groups that initiate the breakdown of isolation, that create contacts and new relationships, that develop free-time activities and social responsibility will find a complicated array of needs related to labour market, the school system, etc. These needs demand cooperation from other organizations in society, both voluntary and official. In extending these lines of change, one has begun social planning of social change in a broad and important sense.

SUMMARY

The very fact that the heavy investments in the roles of reproduction and production tend to coincide in time given rise to stress. Two adults, a man and a woman, try within the framework of a nuclear family to fulfil their different tasks while at the same time society is experiencing vast disagreement concerning the distribution of these tasks. Today, families are trying out two principally different alternatives, role specialization and role sharing, both of which are receiving heavy criticism and distrust. Workable solutions are questionable *within* the framework of the nuclear family.

The obvious familism found by researchers is interpreted as socio-cultural homelessness and as an indicator of the weak integration of the nuclear family in society.

REFERENCES

ANDERSSON, A.-G. and ANDERSSON, S. O. (1972). Rollen som far och andra roller [The institute of sociology]. University of Gothenburg, Sweden.

BERGER, P.-K. (1969). Marriage and the construction of reality. In *Artikelsamling i familjesociologi*. Student-litteratur, Lund, Sweden.

BOENDESERVICE 2, SOU (1970), **68**, 11–14.

BRENTON, M. (1967). *The American male*. New York.

DAHLSTRÖM, E. and LILJESTRÖM, R. (1967). The family and married women at work. In *The changing roles of men and women*, pp. 41–51.

DAUN, Å. (1971). Social struktur på mikronivå. *SOU*, **28**.

DE LAVAL, G. (1970). Familjecykeln och den gifta kvinnans förvärvsarbete, 67.

ESKOLA, A. (1960). Some factors influencing the differentiation of the roles of spouses. Publikation No 9, The institute of sociology, University of Helsinki, Finland.

GOLDTHORPE, J. H., LOCKWOOD, D., BECHOFER, F., PLATT, J. (1969). *The affluent worker*. Cambridge, England.

GOODE, W. (1963). *World revolution of family patterns*. New York.

GRØNSETH, E. (1970). *The dysfunctionality of the husband provider role in industrialized societies*. Oslo,

JONSSEN. G. and KÄLVESTEN, A.-L. (1964). *222 Stockholmspojkar*. Stockholm, Sweden.

LUCKMAN, T. (1967). The invisible religion, pp. 112–14. London.

PARSONS, T. and BALES, R. (1955). *Family, socialization and interaction process*. Glencoe, Scotland.

RAPOPORT, R. and RAPOPORT, R. (1971). *Dual career families*, pp. 278–296. Harmondsworth.

RUNDBLAD, B. (1971). Inflyttad arbetskrafts anpassning i en expanderande arbetsmarknad. In *Arbetslivet i kris och förvandling* (ed. C. V. Otter). Stockholm.

ZIJDERVELD, A. (1971). *The abstract society*. New York.

14. INSTITUTIONALIZED SEXISM AS A SOCIAL CONSTRAINT IN MALE/FEMALE INTERACTION

JAMES A. GOODMAN

DISCRIMINATION AND FAVOURITISM

The notion of male superiority is closely linked to acts of discrimination against women in the society. As Levitin *et al.* put the issue: (Levitin 1971)

The concept of discrimination is inextricably linked to a particular ideology or set of values. Ideologies delineate desirable social conditions; discrimination refers to departures from ideological prescriptions. More specifically, discrimination may be defined as the withholding of rewards or facilities on the basis of allocative criteria inconsistent with a particular ideology. Discrimination refers to providing individuals with fewer rewards or facilities than are deserved; favoritism, to providing more rewards or facilities than are legitimately deserved.

At issue here are the responses women make to their position as well as the consequences for the rest of society.

DISENGAGEMENT AND ALIENATION

Recent research suggests that when individuals feel unable to influence their environment, they may develop a sense of powerlessness and accompanying feelings of apathy, fatalism, and general disengagement from society's demands. This disengagement phenomenon can be conceptualized as alienation. Hayda (1961) views alienation as

an individual's feelings of uneasiness or discomfort which reflect his exclusion or self-exclusion from social and cultural participation. It is an expression of nonbelonging or non-sharing, an uneasy awareness of perception of unwelcome contrast with others. It varies in its intensity and scope. It may be restricted to a few limited situations, such as participation in a peer group, or it may encompass a wide social universe including the participation in the larger society.

Dean (1961) has described the major components of alienation as powerlessness, normlessness, and isolation. Powerlessness is the individual's belief that his own behaviour cannot determine the educational, political, economic, or other important social outcomes he seeks. Normlessness refers to the process issue: the individual's belief that socially approved means are not available to attain the social ends he has in view. Isolation is his sense of being separate and apart from the group or from the standards of a high valence group.

WOMEN'S RESPONSES

The individual's inability effectively to interact with his environment may, in many instances, preclude the effective utilization of internal resources. These notions are particularly significant when viewed against the current status occupied by women in our society. A recent report by the U. S. Department of Health, Education, and Welfare (1972) notes:

Modern women are remarkably resilient — considering the conflicting expectations in women's roles, the traditional designation of women, the fear of physical attack, and the backlash against the women's movement. But these conditions have taken their toll — in mental illness, drug usage, alcoholism, and a general undercurrent of unhappiness. Many problems are ignored when they primarily affect 'only' women. Women are traditionally taught not to complain, not to react aggressively, not to blame others; and as a result they frequently withdraw from and internalize their problems — but the latent distress eventually erupts.

ROLE OF INSTITUTIONS

When we consider the social and cultural aspects of personality, in so far as they reflect the statuses and roles that the individual achieves or is assigned, we are reminded that most of these elements are related to one or more institutions, whether the parental, the church, or the school. The individual initially functions as a member of only one such pattern of interaction, the family unit. His first role is that of dependent infant, who is warmed, fed, clothed, and otherwise kept alive and reasonably comfortable by others in their parental roles. The individual's language development, moral valuations, and attitudes toward other persons and toward himself are interpreted to him in this way (Winch 1950). As he grows older, other institutional patterns begin to influence him. His personality gradually assumes more complete characteristics until he becomes an adult, with a wider range of responses reflecting his position in the status structure.

The family, however, is a micro-statement of the larger society and as such must be viewed in relationship to other social institutions. It must be viewed as an evolutionary system which adapts to societal demands in order to preserve not itself but the society of which it is representative. As indicated earlier, for example, the socialization of children is the most exclusive domain of the family. It is within the life space of the family that the child develops his personality, his intelligence, his aspirations, and indeed his moral character. After all of this is done, the child is placed in the broader society.

Even here, however, the family does not act unilaterally, but as a subsystem of the wider society. The mandates from the larger society are translated into explicitly expressive acts in the family constellation. The child is therefore socialized into institutional structures which incorporate the family as a contributing subsystem. These include the schools and peer groups as well as what some sociologists refer to as anticipatory roles of the future.

It is generally held that for females, socialization is responsive to a repressive system of stratification with respect to opportunities for personal growth and development. Moreover, as a consequence of being denied a full range of anticipatory socialization, women are taught to have an exceedingly limited view of their potential to succeed in certain areas of the society.

During the past few years there has been an increasing awareness on the part of most segments of the society that women suffer as a consequence of their lack of access to the full range of socially sanctioned roles in the society. The specifics of this suffering await delineation in clear research findings that posit cause-and-effect relationships between structured inequality and women's responses to this inequality.

SEX-LINKED STRESS-INDUCING SITUATIONS

The potential range of perceived stress-inducing situations that are sex-linked creates a demand for a comprehensive, multivariate research model that accounts for the overt and subtle interactional possibilities inherent in sex-linked patterns of discrimination. However, the exploration of the issue need not wait for these research models to be developed. There

is a range of data that suggests that women suffer later stresses as a consequence of their inability to actualize aspirations which are culturally induced. The potential damage related to failure to achieve culturally induced aspirations has been described by the alienation theorists. Merton (1957), for example, suggests that 'aberant behavior may be regarded sociologicaly as a symptom of dissociation between culturally prescribed aspirations and socially structured avenues of realizing these aspirations.' Aside from the question of opportunity to achieve their full potential, women are given multibonded messages with cultural valuation operating to their disadvantage.

Beginning with toddlers, children are trained in behaviours that are considered appropriate to their sexual identification. Although the physical differences at this stage are minimal, cultural expectations focus on and exaggerate these differences. Hunt (1962) further suggests that:

At the very time when girls are learning to identify themselves with traditional female roles, they are also learning to prefer masculine roles which they think inappropriate for themselves. This is conflict built into the foundations of the female character; thus is the future woman made uncertain of her worth, hesitant about her abilities, fearful of trying roles other than those of tradition, and anxious if she succeed in them.

DIFFERENTIAL OUTCOMES BETWEEN WOMEN AND MEN

Relatively little effort is required to uncover trends in various studies dealing with differential outcomes

TABLE 14.1

Sex ratios in utilization of psychiatric facilities in the U.S.A. 1969 (males per 100 females)

	State and county hospital admissions	Private mental hospital admissions	General hospital inpatient psychiatric service discharges	Outpatient psychiatric service terminations	Community mental health centres admissions
Age	137	68	62	101	88
<18	157	85	81	178	145
18–24	170	83	72	85	81
25–44	137	55	56	70	73
45–64	133	77	64	73	79
65	104	62	54	74	74
Select diagnoses					
Alcoholism	537	262	242	286	317
Organic brain syndrome	114	73	81	135	110
Schizophrenia	91	55	59	81	77
Depressive disorders	48	45	35	37	41
Psychoneurosis	67	42	47	62	49
Drug disorders	225	129	161	202	176
Personality disorders	219	77	81	114	110

Source: U.S. Department of Health, Education, and Welfare (1972).

between women and men in connection with any number of stress-producing events. The National Institute of Mental Health statistics indicate that 125 351 more women than men were hospitalized for psychiatric problems and/or treated on an outpatient basis for the period between 1964 and 1968. Chesler (1971) states that:

Most female neuroses are a result of societal demands and discrimination rather than the supposed mental illness of the individual.... The statistics on the mental health of women are startling, because they flaunt the common myth of female 'privilege' and happiness. It seems logical, after all, that men, must daily live with achievement stresses, business competition, work pressures, and super-highways, should be the most likely to succumb to physical and mental disease.

In the report compiled by the United States Department of Health, Education, and Welfare (1972) a further piece is fashioned into the mosaic in the following statement:

It is extremely difficult to make flat statements about the distribution of mental illness by sex. Interpretation is greatly complicated by the interaction of many factors including age, race, socio-economic status, demographic characteristics, and inconsistencies in statistical reporting methods. Nevertheless, recent studies of admissions to the variety of mental health service facilities (including State and county mental health hospitals, private mental hospitals, community mental health center services) suggest differences in male and female utilization of the various types of facilities and in patterns of diagnoses.

Table 14.1 summarizes the sex differences in the utilization of psychiatric facilities by age and by selected diagnoses for five major types of disabilities. The three leading diagnostic categories for males aged 15–24 were schizophrenia, personality disorders, and drug abuse. For women in the same age group, the top diagnostic category was neurosis, with schizophrenia second, and mental retardation and personality disorders third.

Comparisons of admissions to State and county mental hospitals for white and non-white females between ages 18 and 44 showed that non-white females had much higher admission rates. While schizophrenia appeared to be the most frequent diagnosis for both non-white females and white females, the proportion termed schizophrenic was far greater among non-white females. This finding may reflect the double jeopardy associated with non-white female status in the society.

DISCRIMINATION IN THE JOB MARKET

Data generated by the United States Department of Labor (1970) indicate that women are subject to discrimination in the job market. These and related problems have created a surge, a feminine thrust for equality in the society. Perhaps there is a real shift towards a recognition of the human quality — the duality of 'woman' — that should characterize the relationships between the sexes. Implicitly, men and women view data, experiences, and the world within the context of

their own knowledge of what constitutes survival modes. These survival strategies, however, are based upon the assumption that biological description should make a difference in social interaction. On the other hand, the feminine surge may itself be the locus of current tension and stress between men and women in the society.

SEXUAL POLARIZATION

Beliefs and behaviours that lead to sexual polarization and conflict reflect the utilization by men and women of an either/or explanatory model in male/female interaction. This model is consistent with the primary mode of thinking in the Western world. It is an Aristotelian (Aristotle 1952) position: 'it is impossible for the same thing at the same time to belong and not to belong to the same thing and in the same respect; and whatever other distinctions you might add to meet dialectional objections, let them be added. This then is the most certain of all principles....'.

This thought process is taken for granted in the Western world. It flows from the law of identity that states that A is A; the law of contradiction, that A is non non-A; the law of the excluded middle, that A cannot be A and non-A, neither A or non-A. Therefore, a position that B is A and not A at the same time and in the same particular evokes defence system activities.

In male/female interaction, females fall into the category non-male and male falls into the category of non-female; therefore the either/or habit of mind easily allows one to conceive of male and female as mutually exclusive opposites (Dixon 1971).

NEED FOR INTERVENTION

Given the nature of these socially induced perceptions, one is struck with the need for intervention in those social institutions that are of prime importance in the formation of sex-linked attitudes. Institutions of general public control such as schools, the media, and secondary organizational associations such as lodges, fraternities, etc., should be viewed as appropriate first entry-points.

No argument is made for specific methodology. Rather, the point is that human experience is viewed on a continuum with multiple points at which spiralling can occur. In specific terms, the labels male and female are social conveniences; we need to be free of the social responsibility of limiting social behaviour to these labels.

SUMMARY

Women in Western society appear to suffer a higher degree of emotional illness than do men. Stresses generated for women are partly attributable to their relative lack of access to high-status roles in the society. Meaningful change must emanate from intervention in the primary institutions that socialize men and women into their expectations of what is normative.

REFERENCES

ARISTOTLE (1952). *Metaphysics* (trans. R. Hope). New York.

CHESLER, P. (1971). Men drive women crazy. **5**, 18.

DEAN, D. (1961). Alienation: its meaning and measurement. *Amer. sociol. Rev.*, **26**, 753–8.

DIXON, V. (1971). *An alternate America: beyond black or white.* Boston, Massachusetts.

HAYDA, J. (1961). Alienation and integration of student intellectuals. *Amer. sociol. Rev.*, **26**, 758–7.

HUNT, M. M. (1962). *Her infinite variety*. New York.

LEVITIN, T. (1971). Sex discrimination against women. *Amer. behav. Scient.*, 237–54.

MERTON, R. K. (1957). *Social theory and social structure.* Glencoe, Illinois.

U.S. DEPARTMENT OF HEALTH, EDUCATION, AND WELFARE (1972). *Report of the Women's Action Program*. Washington, D.C.

U.S. DEPARTMENT OF LABOR (1970). *Background on women workers in the United States.* Washington, D.C.

WINCH, R. F. (1950). The study of personality in the family setting. *Social Forces*, **28**, 310–16.

15. MARITAL STRESS

PAUL H. GEBHARD

In the interviews conducted by the staff of the Institute for Sex Research, Bloomington, Indiana between 1938 and 1960, every ever-married respondent was routinely asked, 'What troubles or problems have there been in your marriage?' If in the course of the interview the respondent had recounted marital problems (which were recorded at once), the question was rephrased as, 'What *other* troubles or problems have there been in your marriage?' A second question was asked to ascertain the extent of arguments, fights, separations, and divorces which resulted from marital problems. The information derived from these two questions was ordinarily noted in very brief form. For example, trouble concerning the husband's relatives might simply have been recorded as 'male's relatives' regardless of the nature of the trouble, and a lengthy account of a wife's jealousy would have been compressed to 'female jealous'. This information has not been previously tabulated or published, and seemed particularly appropriate for that section of this book dealing with stress resulting from, or associated with, relationships between males and females.

METHODS AND SAMPLE

In order to avoid the complexities which would result from including in the sample persons of different ethnic groups and socio-economic classes, the sample was restricted to white residents of the United States who had at least some college education. In addition, anyone convicted of a crime (felony or misdemeanour) other than a traffic violation was excluded from the sample. Only the data pertaining to first marriages were utilized.

In view of the time available for completing this study, only percentages were calculated. Correlations and measures of statistical significance were not made. Despite this parsimony, the study engendered a large amount of computer printout, since we controlled two variables. It was anticipated that marital troubles might vary according to the duration of marriage and the age at which marriage took place; consequently, both of these variables were simultaneously controlled. Since there were five categories of duration of marriage (under 1 year, 1–5 years, 6–10 years, 11–20 years, and over 20 years) and four categories of age at marriage (under 21, 21–25, 26–30, and over 30), even a simple 'yes/no' tabulation resulted in 40 cells (20 category cells × 2 possible responses). Most items analysed were not of the simple 'yes/no' variety, but consisted of a number of possible responses so that the number of resultant cells was correspondingly large.

There was no direct control of the age of the respondent at the time of the interview, but this omission is

TABLE 15.1

Sample size by age at marriage and duration of marriage

Age at marriage	Duration of marriage in years									
	<1		1–5		6–10		11–20		>21	
	M	F	M	F	M	F	M	F	M	F
<20 years old Total M: 89 Total F: 327	16	45	47	133	7	70	18	57	1	22
21–25 years old Total M: 810 Total F: 744	100	72	344	252	141	154	159	183	66	83
26–30 years old Total M: 547 Total F: 273	38	18	154	83	143	62	140	85	72	25
31 and over Total M: 161 Total F: 101	7	3	58	39	49	28	32	26	15	5
Totals M: 1607 F: 1445	161	138	603	507	340	314	349	351	154	135

unimportant since (1) we are not concerned only with current marital troubles, but with all troubles regardless of when they occurred, and (2) some indication of the effect of age may be inferred from the combined duration-of-marriage and age-at-marriage categories. For example, a person who has been married over 20 years and who married after age 30 must be at least age 52.

The sample consists of 1607 males and 1445 females. Only a minority were married to one another. This sample size is adequate for determining the incidence of particular types of trouble, but sometimes inadequate for ascertaining the relationship between the controlled variables and an uncommon type of trouble. For example, if a given trouble is reported by only 2 per cent of the males, that means there are only 32 individuals to occupy, or fail to occupy, 20 category cells. In such cases, sample vagary is inevitable and one can speak only in generalities or in terms of trends. The number of individuals in each category cell is given in Table 15.1

Only 5·5 per cent of the males married before age 21, but 22·7 per cent of the females did so. The most common age at marriage for both sexes was between 21 and 25 (males 50·4 per cent, females 51·7 per cent). Marriage between ages 26 and 30 accounted for 34·1 per cent of the males, but only 18·7 per cent of the females. Lastly, smaller numbers married after age 30: 10·0 per cent of the men and 6·9 per cent of the women.

With regard to duration of marriage, the figures given by both sexes are in close accord. Some 10·1 per cent of the males and 9·6 per cent of the females had first marriages of less than 1 year; 37·8 per cent of the husbands and 35·1 per cent of the wives had marriages of from 1 to 5 years' length; 21·2 per cent of the men and 21·7 per cent of the women had marriages of from 6–10 years' duration; and 21·9 per cent of the males and 24·3 per cent of the females had had marriages lasting between 11 and 20 years. Only a few, 9·0–9·3 per cent, had marriages enduring over two decades.

In the interview, there were no preconceived categories for types of marital troubles, which are potentially infinite. Instead, the respondents were simply asked to enumerate whatever troubles beset their marriages. Subsequently, we categorized these as best we could into major groups, each of which consisted of further subdivisions. The major groups of sources of marital stress were as follows:

Economic: Extravagance or carelessness with money, inadequate financial contribution, employment troubles.

Relatives: The respondent's and spouse's relatives, including the spouse's children by any former marriage.

Household duties: Inadequate performance of duties and insufficient help offered the spouse.

Religion: Differences in type of religion or in degree of devoutness.

Children: Differences in the desire for children, involuntary sterility, and discord over rearing children.

Differing interests: This broad category included discord arising from differing interest, educational attainment, tastes, and philosophies. In addition, a separate category was made for difference in sociability, as where one spouse desires to socialize with others and the other spouse is more reclusive.

Alcohol and drug use: This category proved to be almost wholly a matter of alcohol consumption; drug usage (including barbiturates and amphetamines) was uncommon.

Physical attributes: This included age discrepancies sufficient to cause trouble as well as unpleasant physical traits such as ugliness, obesity, and body odour.

Health: In addition to poor health as a source of trouble, chronic fatigue was included.

Involuntary separation: Living apart because of military service, employment requirements, institutionalization, etc.

Poor reason for marriage: This included forced marriage, marriage to escape the parental home, marriage to spite someone, marriage for material reasons only, and impetuous, ill-considered marriage.

Personality traits: This category was so large and diverse that it was necessary to treat its subdivisions separately. Some 17 subdivisions, including one residual category and one unspecified category, were necessitated. Each trait was identified as being that of the respondent, the spouse, or of both.

Sexual troubles: Again, this large and varied category merited separate treatment of its constituent subdivisions which were: (a) sexual jealousy; (b) extramarital petting or coitus; (c) duration of foreplay; (d) petting techniques; (e) coital frequency; (f) coital positions; (g) coital circumstances (e.g. time, place, nudity, etc.); (h) coital duration; (i) female orgasm; (j) general sexual responsiveness (including lack of sexual attractiveness); (k) male sexual difficulties (e.g. impotence, premature ejaculation); (l) female sexual difficulties (e.g. dyspareunia, inadequate lubrication); (m) male sexual deviation (chiefly homosexuality); (n) female sexual deviation (chiefly homosexuality); (o) fear of pregnancy.

Miscellaneous or unspecified troubles Lastly, we tabulated some of the results of marital stress in terms of arguments, physical violence, desire for separation or divorce, and separation or divorce.

Contrary to expectation, neither age at marriage or duration of marriage had any marked effect upon the presence of marital trouble. Only 8 per cent of the males and an equal percentage of the females reported trouble-free marriages. Obviously, with a latitude of only 8 percentage points, the two variables can show little. About all that can be said is that the reporting of marital trouble tends to increase with greater duration of marriage and that fewer persons who marry after age 30 report trouble than those who marry at younger ages. Both of these trends are quite small and only the consistency of the trends among both males and females suggests their validity. Nevertheless, both trends conform to rational anticipation: the longer a marriage, the greater the exposure to factors contributing to marital discord; those who marry late are presumably more mature, financially more secure, have more reasonable expectations concerning matrimony, and are less inclined to impetuous marriage.

MARITAL TROUBLES

Economic troubles

Difficulties over the management of money constitute the second most common source of marital discord reported by both husbands and wives: 29·5 per cent of the males and 31·2 per cent of the females complained of this. In the majority of cases the respondent did not specify who was chiefly at fault. In the few cases where one person was blamed, it was generally the spouse and not the respondent. Males were more inclined than females to blame themselves; this is understandable since financial matters are often controlled by the husband. While age at marriage seems unrelated to economic trouble, duration of marriage is a factor for persons married before age 26: there is a tendency for the trouble to increase as marriage continues. Among persons married at age 26 or older, the economic trouble decreases after 26 years of marriage — i.e. in middle life, when the husband is apt to be at the zenith of his earning power.

Inadequate income was an insignificant problem according to the husbands (1·2 per cent so reporting), but was more important to the wives, 5·5 per cent of whom complained. Inadequate income was primarily the problem of those who married before age 21; those marrying at older ages were, as one would expect, in better financial situations. This is especially true of those marrying after age 30: none of the husbands mentioned inadequate income as a problem.

Marital difficulty because of employment was ranked ninth by wives (14·6 per cent) and twelfth by husbands (9·8 per cent). The nature of the trouble was generally not specified; the record often merely said 'male job.' No trends were observed in the male data, but wives reported an increase in this trouble with increased age at marriage and greater duration of marriage. The wife being employed caused some trouble: 2·2 per cent of the women disliked having to work, 1·7 per cent felt their husbands resented it, and 1·4 per cent resented not being employed outside the home. Interestingly, the equivalent figures reported by the husbands were lower.

In the female data there was an increase in the percentage of women with increasing age at marriage who said their husbands resented their working, the figures beginning at about 1 per cent among those married young (when a wife's employment is often necessary) and grading up to 3 per cent among those who married after age 30 (when males feel they should be able to sustain the household). This trend was not visible in the male data.

Trouble because of relatives

Friction caused by relatives proved to be a common source of marital discord among both males and females. Husbands ranked trouble over their wives' relatives in fourth place (18·9 per cent) and wives ranked trouble over their husbands' relatives also in fourth place (22·1 per cent). Unfortunately, the relatives involved were not always specified, but when they were, it is clear that the mother-in-law was the primary offender. Trouble over relatives was least among the older individuals, presumably because the relatives had been reduced in number by death.

Both sexes ranked trouble over their own relatives as important, but considerably less important than the difficulties caused by their spouses' relatives. Wives said their relatives occasioned trouble in 14·8 per cent of the cases (ranking eighth) and 16·6 per cent of the husbands reported their relatives were a source of discord (ranking fifth in the male list of complaints). Again, the mother was the major difficulty, and again the trouble is least among the oldest couples.

The folklore concerning the disruptive mother-in-law seems validated by scientific data.

Trouble over household duties

Despite the impression that husbands grumble about their wives' cooking and neglect of the household and that women perpetually nag their husbands to perform chores and repairs, rather few people reported this trouble. Female deficiency in the discharge of household duties was mentioned by 2·8 per cent of the husbands and 1·7 per cent of the wives agreed with this complaint. The husbands had a high opinion of themselves: less than 1 per cent acknowledged deficiency on their own part, but the wives had a different verdict — 1·5 per cent of them said their husbands were derelict in their duties.

Religious trouble

Differences in religion or degree of devoutness were also unimportant in the sample. Only 1·7–1·8 per cent of the spouses stated that differences in religion caused discord and 2 per cent named differences in devoutness. The only trend noted was small: the husbands reported more trouble over devoutness after the tenth year of marriage.

This unimportance of religion stems from the fact that the sample was largely Protestant, where differences in denomination are generally minor, and there were very few cases of marriage between persons of different faiths.

Trouble because of children

The matter of begetting children caused marital discord, according to 5·7 per cent of the wives, but only 3·6 per cent of the husbands. This was not a common trouble since it ranked twenty-fifth and twenty-seventh. However, there were interesting differences in the reporting. Some 4·3 per cent of the wives stated they wanted a child, or more children, and that their husbands did not. Only 1·4 per cent of the husbands said they did not have this desire, but that their wives did. This reproductive disagreement was most common in the fifth to tenth year of marriage.

The male and female reports again differed with respect to the husband desiring a child, or more children, and the wife not. While 1·7 per cent of the husbands mentioned this, only 0·9 per cent of the wives did so.

A correlation between age at marriage and this reproductive problem was visible only in the male data. Among those who married young (before age 21), the tendency is for the wives to want children more than did their husbands during the first decade of marriage. Among those who married between ages 21 and 25, disagreement was minimal — evidently both spouses felt they were ready for offspring. Among those who married at older ages, there was a reversal of the former picture: now the trend was for males to be more desirous of children than their wives were. One assumes that these wives were older and that their lateness of marriage reflects a relative disinterest on the part of some of them in procreating.

Involuntary sterility on the part of either spouse constituted only a tiny problem: less than 1 per cent listed this as a source of trouble.

It would appear that most couples have a sufficiency of children, but that if any spouse perceives a lack, it is generally the wife.

Trouble over child-care and rearing was quite important to males, ranking seventh (14·5 per cent), but was of somewhat lesser importance to females, who ranked it in twelfth place (13·1 per cent had this complaint). Despite the difference in rank order, the similarity of the percentages is noteworthy and shows that child-rearing is a rather common source of marital friction. It increases with duration of marriage, which one would anticipate since more children are being produced and some children are in the difficult adolescent period. In some groups, between one-fifth and one-third of the individuals list this as a complaint. One would expect that among older individuals, whose children were presumably grown, there would be much less reporting of this problem, but such is not the case. Indeed, a third of the women who married in their early twenties reported this trouble even after 20 years of marriage, and slightly over a quarter of the men who married after age 30 reported the trouble after 20 years of marriage. Some of these high figures must be the reporting of former rather than current discord, but if this is so, it demonstrates that the problem was serious enough not to have been forgotten.

There is also an inexplicable trend for problems of child-rearing to increase with increased age at marriage, at least up to age 30. This trend is seen in both the male and female data. One can only speculate that older parents may be more rigid and dogmatic in their ideas as to how to rear children. However, among those married after age 30 — who should be the most dog-

matic — the problem ameliorates. Perhaps these persons have fewer offspring to quarrel about. The solution to the enigma would be to do an analysis according to number of children.

Trouble over differing interests
This is an important source of difficulty for both husbands and wives; almost identical percentages (16·6 per cent and 16·4 per cent) reported it.

Relatively little (under 3 per cent) of the problem of differing interests stems from persons from different socio-economic classes marrying. There were relatively few such marriages in our sample. The male data show an interesting trend: the trouble decreases both with age at marriage and duration of marriage. The decrease accompanying greater length of marriage is probably the result of adaptation, but the decrease seen with successively older ages at marriage is more puzzling. Perhaps the older a person is, the less likely he or she is to marry someone of a markedly different socio-economic class.

Most of the discord over differing interests and tastes is not due to differing social class. It increases with age at marriage. For example, for the four age-at-marriage groups, the male percentages steadily increase: 9·0, 13·3, 15·5, and 16·1 per cent. The female percentages increase only in the first three groups. Persons who delay marriage are inclined to be more resistant to changing established habits and preferences. It is possible they have higher expectations with regard to a spouse — which would explain their delaying marriage. No trends were seen regarding duration of marriage except that the first year of marriage had the least number of persons reporting this problem.

Trouble over sociability
One often hears of the couple wherein one spouse is reclusive while the other delights in parties and interaction with other people. However, in our sample, this situation seldom caused a problem. Only 4·1 per cent of the females and 3·6 per cent of the males had this complaint. The husband was the least sociable member of the couple. No trends were noted except that the older the woman was at marriage, the more likely she was to complain of her husband's lack of sociability.

Trouble over alcohol or drug use
So few of the respondents mentioned drug use that these figures pertain almost wholly to drinking, which constituted a problem ranked seventeenth (8·3 per cent) by the wives and twentieth (5·4 per cent) by the husbands. The male was the chief offender. One per cent of the women admitted their own drinking was a problem, but 7·4 per cent said their husband's drinking was a problem and caused trouble. The female data reveal a tendency for the husband's drinking problem to increase with age at marriage up to age 30, rising from 5·5 to 10·6 per cent, a trend less clearly evident in the male data. Alcohol problems do not seem to

correlate with duration of marriage except that they were least during the first year of marriage.

Trouble over physical attributes
Age difference rarely disturbed the marriages: only 1·0 per cent of both the husbands and wives listed this. It is, however, interesting that males said their wives were too old and females said their husbands were too old; fewer felt their own age was the problem. Those who married after age 30 were more prone to report trouble resulting from age discrepancies: as many as 3·0–3·7 per cent did so.

The appearance or odour of the spouse also seldom caused trouble: only 1·2 per cent of the males and 1·1 per cent of the females mentioned this.

The major difficulty concerning physical attributes centred on the health of the couple. The husbands ranked this thirteenth (7·8 per cent) and the wives sixteenth (8·4 per cent). The most common complaint concerned the poor health of the spouse, not of the respondent. Some 4·0 per cent of the males said their wife's poor health caused trouble while 3·4 per cent of the females said the same of their husbands. Both genders reported, logically enough, an increase in health problems with increased age at marriage. Duration of marriage correlated with poor health chiefly in marriages of over 20 years. Among those long-married persons the proportion of individuals listing the health of a spouse as being a problem naturally increased, reaching as much as 16–20 per cent.

Both men and women stated that female fatigue was the second most common physical problem (1·6 per cent of the males and 2·0 per cent of the females). As one would guess, fatigue increased with increased age at marriage, reaching 3 per cent. Oddly enough, duration of marriage did not seem a factor; perhaps age took its toll equally from both spouses.

Trouble over involuntary separation
Lengthy separation has long been known to weaken marriage and lead to extramarital liaisons. The involuntary separations endured by our sample of spouses caused marital trouble in from 4·2 per cent (male data) to 6·3 per cent (female data) of the cases. Husbands ranked involuntary separation twenty-third on their list of trouble sources, and wives rated it in twenty-fourth place. Most of these separations were due to military service, and consequently the problem was more prevalent among younger couples, as shown by the decrease in percentages with increased age at marriage. The problem also tended to be confined to couples married 5 years or less, where as many as 8·4 per cent of the wives spoke of it as causing trouble. Marriages of longer duration were less likely to have husbands of military age and more likely to have husbands who were exempt from service because of children.

Separation due to employment, education, and institutionalization was numerically inconsequential. However, there was a residual category of separation which consisted chiefly of spouses living apart for other reasons — 1·9 per cent of the wives and 1·0 per cent of the husbands said this caused trouble. The reasons must have been economic since this trouble was concentrated in the first years of marriage and was particularly evident among those who married before age 21. Presumably the newly married couples were financially unable to establish their own homes.

Trouble because of inadequate reason for marriage
A number of persons felt that marital stress arose from their having married for inadequate reasons, such as marrying to escape the parental home, marrying to spite someone else, marrying because of pregnancy, marrying because of impetuous impulse, etc. An identical percentage, 4·4, of the males and females reported this, but the husbands ranked it twenty-second in their list of marital troubles while the wives ranked it twenty-ninth.

No trends were apparent in the female data except that such trouble was most common among those who married before age 21. In the male data, however, there were correlations. Trouble because the marriage was forced by pregnancy was reported by 7·9 per cent of those husbands who married before age 21, by slightly over 1·0 per cent of those who married between 21 and 30, and by no one who married after age 30. This particular trouble was most common in the first year of marriage. Males evidently resent forced marriage more than females: a total of 1·4 per cent listed this as a source of trouble, whereas only 0·6 per cent of the wives did so. A similar age-at-marriage trend was reported with regard to marrying too impetuously, the percentages ranging from 5·6 per cent for those marrying young to about 0·5 per cent among those marrying after 30. Lastly, for the category of unspecified poor reasons for marriage, the trouble was commonest among those marrying young.

Personality troubles
Marital difficulties resulting from unpleasant personality traits were not grouped together as a unit and percentage calculated. Had this been done, such a total category would rank very high in the list of troubles. Instead, we subdivided personality troubles into seventeen categories designed to include the variety of responses given since we were interested in the specific sort of personality conflict. Wives were somewhat more inclined than husbands to cite personality difficulties: in their lists of the thirty commonest troubles, women named three personality items not in the male list, whereas the males named only one item not on the female list.

The commonest trouble listed by wives (10·7 per cent) and one which ranked fourteenth was the feeling that there was insufficient love and affection. Males gave this a similar rank, seventeenth, but only 6·2 per cent reported it. The complaint was primarily that the respondent rather than the spouse was the one who did not have sufficient affection for the other marital partner. This was true of both husbands and wives. Some 6·6 per cent of the wives said they lacked such affection for their husbands, whereas only 2·7 per cent complained their husbands did not love them. The equivalent male figures were 3·4 per cent and 1·6 per cent. Length of marriage seems to have had no effect, but age at marriage did among females. The younger the bride, the more apt she was to lack affection for her new mate: the percentages were 10·7 for those marrying young, 5·8–5·5 for those marrying before 30, and 2·0 per cent for those who wed after age 30. This was an unanticipated finding, and one suggesting that those who marry young are more subject to subsequent disillusionment. Conversely, the older a bride at marriage, the more likely she was to complain that her husband did not love her sufficiently. Less than 2.5 per cent of the wives who married by age 25 had this complaint, but the figure rose to 3·7 per cent among those married between ages 26 and 30, and reached 4·0 per cent among those women marrying after 30.

In brief, we have a curious situation in which the women who marry young say, 'I don't love him' while those who marry later in life are inclined to say, 'He doesn't love me.'

Unspecified personality troubles (generally recorded ambiguously on the case histories as simply 'spouse's personality' or 'personality trouble') ranked fairly high: fifteenth among males (7·4 per cent) and also fifteenth among females (8·7 per cent).

According to husbands, bad disposition and bad temper was the fourth most common personality trouble (5·7 per cent) and one they ranked eighteenth; wives ranked this twenty-first even though more (6·8 per cent) complained. Both sexes predominantly blamed the spouse rather than themselves. No age-at-marriage effect was noted, but there was a tendency for this trouble to be more common among those married longest. Evidently, disposition does not improve with age.

The personality category which annoyed males most was that of being over-emotional, hypersensitive, and temperamental — traits which they generally attributed to their wives. No less than 9·8 per cent of the husbands had this complaint and ranked it twelfth in importance among all marital troubles. This is in keeping with our cultural myth that females are by nature far more emotional and sensitive. Despite this cultural stereotype, more women accused their husbands of these characteristics (4·7 per cent) than blamed themselves (2·6 per cent), the total (including another 1·0 per cent where both spouses shared the defect) being 8·3 per cent and seventeenth in rank order. The older the wife at marriage, the more apt she was to find her spouse with these undesirable traits.

A category was made for descriptions such as selfish, egotistical, vain, inconsiderate, and spoiled. Again, these attributes were usually claimed for the spouse rather than the respondent. Husbands ranked this trouble twenty-fifth (3·8 per cent) and the wives ranked it twenty-third (6·5 per cent). Duration of marriage had no effect, except that this trouble was less often reported by those married less than 1 year. In the male data the troubled increased with increased age at marriage from 1·1 per cent to 4·3 per cent.

Being too domineering was a complaint of 3·7 per cent of the husbands and 4·6 per cent of the wives. Both ranked it low: twenty-sixth and twenty-eighth. As usual, the spouse was generally labelled the domineering partner. The older the husband or wife was at marriage the greater the percentage who found his or her spouse overbearing and domineering. Since duration of marriage showed no trends, it is unlikely that age alone exacerbates this particular trouble. The more likely explanation is that the longer a person waits to marry the more resistant he or she is to changes the spouse wishes to make and hence the spouse is viewed as domineering.

Near the bottom of the list of thirty marital troubles were miscellaneous other personality difficulties which did not warrant separate categories. Some 6·6 per cent of the women (twenty-second in rank order) and 3·5 per cent (twenty-eighth in rank) of the men mentioned these. There were no significant trends.

Three per cent of the men felt they or their wives were too ambitious, critical, and overly demanding. This ranked last on the list of 30 male complaints and is the only personality complaint which does not also appear in the female list of 30. It is interesting to note that the men held themselves almost as guilty as their wives of these traits, 1·6 per cent blaming the wife while 1·4 per cent blamed themselves. The men married after age 30 were more likely to assume the blame, whereas males who married younger were more apt to blame their wives. A few more wives (3·6 per cent) reported this marital trouble and, unlike the husbands, generally felt the male was at fault. In keeping with the male reports, the women found this trouble with their husbands increased with age at marriage. Older husbands evidently are prone to overly high expectations and often recognize this trait in themselves.

The wives had on their list of the 30 commonest sources of marital discord a number of personality traits which did not appear on the husbands' list. One consisted of immaturity and unreliability, which ranked eighteenth, with 7·3 per cent of the wives so reporting. This was usually attributed to the husband and, strange to say, the trouble increased with age at marriage. The percentages who found their husbands immature grew from 4·9 per cent among those married young to 9·9 per cent among those women who married after 30 despite the fact that their husbands were generally of corresponding age. This growth in alleged immaturity despite increasing age suggests that the older the wife at marriage, the greater degree of maturity and reliability she expects of her husband. Few men (1·9 per cent) found their wives immature enough to cause marital problems, and there were no age-at-marriage trends.

A second complaint made by 5·4 per cent of the wives was that feelings of inferiority and inadequacy handicapped the marriage: 3·5 per cent said their husbands felt inadequate and 1·5 per cent said they themselves felt so; 0·5 per cent said they both suffered from inferiority feelings. Perhaps because a facade of competence is vital to male self-image, less than 1·0 per cent of the men stated that their inferiority feelings constituted a marital problem.

Third from last on the female list (4·6 per cent) was marital trouble resulting from nervous breakdown, including psychosis. The women reported this chiefly of their husbands (2·6 per cent) and less often (1·5 per cent) of themselves. Fewer men (1·4 per cent) said their wives had such difficulty and less than 1·0 per cent reported a breakdown for themselves. Such mental troubles were correlated to some extent with age at marriage, being most common among those married after age 30. Duration of marriage had less effect, but breakdowns were rare prior to the fifth year of marriage.

Other troubles stemming from personality traits were quite uncommon, and the rarity of some is rather surprising. For example, very few spouses accused one another of laziness or stupidity, although such derogatory adjectives are supposedly used frequently in heated arguments. Even stubbornness, a common characteristic, was listed as a source of discord by less than 1·0 per cent.

Sexual troubles

Among males sexual troubles were more important than any other type: the list of ten most common troubles includes five of a sexual nature. Among females the ten most common difficulties include four sexual items, also sufficient to make sexual troubles the most frequent type of marital stress.

Sexual jealousy ranked ninth in the husbands' list and eleventh in the wives', but more females (14·0 per cent) than males (12·4 per cent) made this statement. As usual, more jealousy was attributed to the spouse: 7·2 per cent of the husbands said their wife's jealousy was the source of friction, but only 3·2 per cent blamed their own jealousy. The wives were somewhat more inclined to acknowledge their own jealousy: 6·9 per cent reported the husband's jealousy and 4·6 per cent reported their own jealousy. Only 2·0–2·5 per cent of either sex stated that both husband and wife were jealous enough to constitute a marital problem. No clear trends were noted except that among males mutual jealousy decreased with greater age at marriage.

Extramarital petting or coitus was treated separately from jealousy although the two categories overlap. Males ranked stress over extramarital activity eighth (14·4 per cent), and an equal number of females (14·3 per cent) reported the same, although among females this item ranked tenth in their list of sources of stress. Both males and females agreed that the most frequent trouble was the wife being upset by her husband's extramarital activity (reported by 7·8 per cent of the males

and 8·0 per cent of the females). The husband being distressed over the wife's activity was less common (4·0 per cent and 4·1 per cent), and stress because of mutual extramarital behaviour was least common (1·3 per cent and 1·5 per cent). The agreement of the males' and females' figures is remarkable. A few persons (1·3 per cent males, 0·6 per cent females) said that their own guilt feelings created marital stress even though their spouses were ignorant of, or unconcerned about, their extramarital behaviour.

The male data show a decrease in concern over extramarital petting or coitus, with increased age at marriage. For example, distress over the husband's activity steadily declined from 9·0 per cent among those married before age 21 to 3·1 per cent among those married after age 30, and a similar decrease (from 5·6 per cent to 1·9 per cent) was seen in stress occasioned by the wife's behaviour. This trend was only partially corroborated by the female reports wherein the minimum percentages were always among those married after age 30. Duration of marriage had a less pronounced effect, and one can only say that the problem was most acute in the sixth to twentieth years of marriage, particularly in the eleventh to twentieth years.

The duration of pre-coital petting constituted a problem for 5·0 per cent of the husbands and 6·9 per cent of the wives, but it was not an important source of discord since it placed twentieth and twenty-first in rank order. The problem consisted almost wholly of the wife desiring more protracted foreplay than the husband provided. The number of both sexes reporting this tended to increase with increased age at marriage, which is rather surprising since one would assume that younger, and hence presumably less experienced, wives would be most in need of protracted foreplay. This reversal of the anticipated trend is confirmed by the female data in that those married less than 1 year had the lowest percentage of wives complaining of brief foreplay.

Stress arising from disagreement over petting techniques was somewhat more important. Some 10·6 per cent of the men reported this, earning it eleventh place in rank order. Fewer females were concerned (7·1 per cent) and they ranked this problem in nineteenth place. The controversy was primarily over mouth/genital contact.

The most important source of marital stress for both husbands and wives, ranking first in the lists of both, was disagreement over frequency of coitus. Almost equal numbers complained: 30·4 per cent of the males and 32·1 per cent of the females. The difficulty was chiefly that of the husband desiring more coitus: 20·2 per cent of the males said they wished more and 15·2 per cent of the wives stated their husbands wanted more. The female data reveal that this particular problem decreases with increased age at marriage, dropping successively from 16·5 per cent to 10·9 per cent. The male data show no such clear trend, but the smallest percentage does occur among those married latest which offers some confirmation of the trend reported by wives. Duration of marriage evidently has little influence, but the problem seems more prevalent after the fifth year of marriage.

A smaller, but still substantial, number of wives desired more coitus. Although it is difficult for husbands to admit this, 5·6 per cent did so and, naturally, a larger proportion of wives (8·7 per cent) had this complaint. As one might have predicted, the problem increases with age at marriage: in the female data the figures steadily increase from 6·7 per cent among those married before age 21 to 12·9 per cent among those married after 30. The male data show only that the problem is commonest among those married after age 30. Duration of marriage is naturally involved in this matter which appears to be that of lessening male activity: wives most often reported the problem after 11 years of marriage and the highest figures (as much as 22 per cent are among those married over 20 years. No corroborative trend was visible in the male data.

Discord because the wife wished less coitus than the current rate was reported by 1·8 per cent of the husbands and 4·1 per cent of the wives. The husbands of some older women found this more of a problem, for example it was reported by 6·7 per cent of men who married after age 30 and who had been married over 20 years. However, these women are outweighed by a contrary trend: the older the woman at marriage, the less likely she was to desire less frequent coitus. The proportion of wives desirous of lower coital frequency steadily declined in successive age-at-marriage categories from 4·9 per cent to 2·0 per cent. For some reason, this trend does not appear in duration of marriage. Perhaps duration is not a factor, whereas with increased age at marriage one has more sexually experienced brides whose sexual desires match or exceed those of their husbands.

Differing wishes for coital positions were listed as a problem by 6·3 per cent of the men and 3·5 per cent of the women. This problem was ranked sixteenth by husbands, but it does not appear in the list of the thirty commonest complaints of wives.

The circumstances in which coitus was had — the time, type of contraception, degree of nudity, place, etc. — constituted a source of contention according to 5·5 per cent of the males and 3·8 per cent of the females. Both reported this friction increased with increased age at marriage.

The duration of coitus, which one might have thought would be a moderate problem, proved to be an inconsequential matter for both sexes, less than 1·0 per cent of whom mentioned it as causing difficulty.

On the other hand, lack of, or difficulty in achieving, female orgasm posed a substantial problem, being ranked tenth (12·0 per cent) by husbands and seventh (16·3 per cent) by wives. There were no trends with regard to age at or duration of marriage other than one: the older the age at marriage, the fewer the number of men reporting that they were upset over the lack of female orgasm. Whether this is because they had more responsive wives or whether older males are less concerned is a moot question. Unfortunately, the majority of responses were so phrased that we were unable to ascertain which spouse was disturbed about the problem or whether both were.

This brings up the subject of general sexual responsiveness, which constituted a major problem according to men, who ranked it third, with 22·5 per cent mentioning it. Among women it was also important, being ranked fifth (17·0 per cent). According to husbands, the problem was the wife: 19·7 per cent said she was not responsive enough, and only 1·2 per cent admitted that they themselves were not responsive enough to suit their wives. The wives presented a somewhat different report: 10·5 per cent acknowledged their own unresponsiveness, but 5·2 per cent complained of this same problem in their husbands. The male and female data contain contradictory trends. In male reports, complaints of female unresponsiveness increased with increased age at marriage up to age 30, but the females reported a steady decrease in this problem.

A few individuals (under 2·0 per cent) of both sexes stated that the unresponsiveness involved was due to one of the spouses not being sexually attractive to the other. It is interesting that each sex perceived the problem to be chiefly the spouse's, rather than their own, unattractiveness.

Male sexual difficulties involving impotence or too-rapid ejaculation were noted by 7·6 per cent of the husbands (fourteenth in rank order) and 10·8 per cent (thirteenth in rank order) of the wives. The problem was mainly that of the male reaching orgasm too quickly. This common problem is not, as some believe, confused to youth. The percentages of both sexes reporting the difficulty tend to increase with increased age at marriage. For example, only 3·7 per cent of the wives married before age 21 complained about premature ejaculation, but this figure successively increased to 7·9 per cent among those women who married after age 30. The male data confirm this trend up to age 30, with percentages of 4·5 (for those married before 20), 5·2 (those married from 21 to 25), and 6·0 (for those married from age 26 to 30). Only 1·7 per cent of the husbands reported erectile impotence as a problem, but 3·9 per cent of the wives did. Both agreed that such impotence increased with increased age at marriage, and no less than 7·9 per cent of the women who married after age 30 made this complaint. This figure is more than twice that reported by the males who married after 30. Ejaculatory impotence was very rare.

Female sexual difficulties of a physical nature were reported by 4·0 per cent of both husbands and wives. The most common complaint was of dyspareunia, painful coitus, which was noted by 2·6 per cent of the wives and corroborated by 2·4 per cent of the husbands. Such painful coitus is not confined to early marriage nor does it seem linked with youthfulness. On the contrary, the female datá suggest a gradual small increase in dyspareunia with increased age at marriage. Insufficient vaginal lubrication was mentioned by less than 1·0 per cent of either sex. Other female physical sexual troubles such as vaginal infections, episiotomy scar tissue, retroverted uterus, etc., were described by about 1·0 per cent of both sexes.

Sexual deviations played a small role in marital stress. One per cent of the wives reported their deviation caused trouble and 0·7 per cent of the husbands complained of their wives' deviation. The deviation was almost wholly homosexuality. Male deviation provided a somewhat more substantial, though still small, problem: 1·9 per cent of the wives noted this and about the same percentage (1·7 per cent) of husbands listed their own deviance as a source of trouble in the marriage. The deviation was usually homosexuality and the problem increased with increased age at marriage.

Fear of pregnancy was listed as a cause for marital stress by 2·3 per cent of the women and 3·2 per cent of the men. This problem does not appear in the wives' list of the 30 most common troubles and barely makes the husbands' list where it ranks twenty-ninth. The surprising unconcern over pregnancy is the result of confining our sample to persons with at least some college education, i.e. persons who would be more knowledgeable about contraception than the average person. Moreover, our sample was above average in income so that an unwanted pregnancy would not be as disastrous as it would be to a lower-income family. Probably, a substantial proportion of both husbands and wives were concerned about the possibility of an unwelcome pregnancy, but did not feel their concern caused marital stress and consequently, did not report it. The wives' reports show that trouble resulting from fear of pregnancy increased with increased age at marriage, going from 1·2 per cent to 4·0 per cent. Older brides usually desire fewer children, a trend previously described under troubles involving children.

Miscellaneous troubles
Various miscellaneous and unspecified marital troubles were cited by 15·9 per cent (sixth in rank order) of the men, but by no less than 23·8 per cent of the women (third in rank order). This difference was due to the wives having more unclassified complaints; the percentage of persons with unspecified troubles was the same for both sexes. Although no trends were observed in the males' data, one can see in the females' data a steady trend for such troubles to increase with increased age at marriage, rising from 14·7 per cent to 21·8 per cent.

RESULTS OF MARITAL STRESS

Although we have no data on the psychosomatic consequences of marital stress and were unable to measure the effects upon the personalities of the spouses and children, we do have some information regarding arguments, violence, separation, and divorce.

An almost equal proportion of men (33·9 per cent) and women (34·5 per cent) listed arguments when asked what marital difficulties they had experienced. One may assume that nearly all married couples argue, but only this smaller number found the arguments stressful enough to be specifically mentioned. Most of the males and females (about 14 per cent) said the arguments were infrequent; about 5·0 to 6·0 per cent reported occasional arguments, and 7·0 per cent of the males and 9·0 per cent of the females stated there were frequent arguments. The remaining persons did not specify the frequency. Duration of marriage appears to have little effect on the frequency of arguments, but there is some evidence that they are progressively fewer among those who marry at older ages. For example, the percentages of those women complaining of frequent arguments decline in each successive age-at-marriage group thus: 11·0, 9·4, 8·1, and 7·9 per cent. Arguments of unspecified frequency similarly dwindled from 5·8 to 3·0 per cent. Infrequent to occasional arguments showed no trends in the female data.

Physical violence was reported by 1·8 per cent of the husbands and twice as many (3·6 per cent) of the wives; males of this social level are obviously reticent about confessing breaking the taboo on violence toward females. However, the male and female reports agree in some respects: 0·2–0·3 per cent reported female violence upon a non-retaliating husband, and 0·4–0·5 per cent stated there was mutual violence. The discrepancy is found in the proportions reporting male violence upon the non-retaliating wife: only 1·0 per cent of the husbands confessed to this, but 3·0 per cent of the wives stated they had experienced such aggression. While the husbands said that mild violence (e.g. a slap or a shaking) exceeded severe violence (e.g., a blow with a fist or with an object) by a considerable amount (0·7 per cent–0·3 per cent), the wives reported far more violence: 1·3 per cent mild and 1·7 per cent severe. Some of this discrepancy is due to interpretation. Males are more accustomed to violence and hence minimize it. Also, the disparity in size and strength influences the assessment of the degree of violence.

A desire by one or both spouses at some point in their marriages for separation or divorce was expressed by 29·2 per cent of the wives and 19·0 per cent of the husbands. In most instances it was not possible to ascertain who desired the separation or divorce.

In general, there was a decrease in the desire for separation with increased age at marriage. For example, taking the largest category (unspecified as to who desired separation), the women reported lesser percentages in each successive age-at-marriage group: 25·6, 14·3, 11·2, and 8·1 per cent. Where the wife was specified as the only one who wanted separation, there was a similar decline: 2·2, 1·5, 1·1, and 0·6 per cent. The male data are less clear, but in general confirm this trend.

Calculating the effect of duration of marriage upon the desire for separation or divorce is more difficult, due to our analysis format and to the fluctuations in the percentages which tend to obscure overall trends. However, it is clear from the reports of both husbands and wives that the desire to terminate marriage decreases with length of marriage. The first year was the most critical. During that time, different age-at-marriage groups had from one-eighth to nearly half of their members wishing for separation. From the first year of marriage to the tenth the situation ameliorated considerably, the proportion desirous of separation ranging from about one-eighth to two-fifths. Among those married 11–20 years, the figures are lower still, running from 6·0 to 25·0 per cent. Finally, of those married over 20 years, no more than 0·0–12·0 per cent reported a wish for separation.

The wives generally reported higher percentages of persons, specified or not, being desirous of separation or divorce. Females not only reported a higher percentage of women wishing separation than the males had estimated, but females thought a larger number of husbands wanted separation than the husbands themselves reported. It is clear that wives are generally the most dissatisfied spouse; however, one exception must be made to this generalization. Both sexes agreed that among those who married after age 30 more husbands than wives desired separation. The figures are small, but the differences are great. The males reported 1·2 per cent for themselves and 0·6 per cent for their wives, while the females reported 1·0 per cent for themselves and 4·0 per cent for their husbands.

The actual occurrence of separation or divorce was reported by 16·9 per cent of the husbands and 27·5 per cent of the wives. These figures cannot be compared to census data since even a brief separation was sufficient

TABLE 15.2.

Rank order of sources of marital stress

Rank	Per cent	Item	Rank	Per cent	Item
		Husbands' reports			Wives' reports
1	30·4	Coital frequency	1	32·1	Coital frequency
2	29·5	Economic: extravagant, careless	2	31·2	Economic: extravagant, careless
3	22·5	General sexual responsiveness	3	23·8	Miscellaneous and unclassified troubles
4	18·9	Wife's relatives	4	22·1	Husband's relatives
5	16·6	Husband's relatives	5	17·0	General sexual responsiveness
	16·6	Differing interests			
6	15·9	Miscellaneous and unclassified troubles	6	16·4	Differing interests
7	14·5	Child-rearing	7	16·3	Female orgasm
8	14·4	Extramarital petting or coitus	8	14·8	Wife's relatives
9	12·4	Sexual jealousy	9	14·6	Employment
10	12·0	Female orgasm	10	14·3	Extramarital petting or coitus
11	10·6	Petting techniques	11	14·0	Sexual jealousy
12	9·8	Over-emotional, temperamental	12	13·1	Child-rearing
	9·8	Employment			
13	7·8	Health	13	10·8	Male sexual difficulties
14	7·6	Male sexual difficulties	14	10·7	Lack of love or affection
15	7·4	Unspecified personality troubles	15	8·7	Unspecified personality troubles
16	6·3	Coital positions	16	8·4	Health
17	6·2	Lack of love or affection	17	8·3	Over-emotional, temperamental
				8·3	Alcohol and drug use
18	5·7	Bad temper, bad disposition	18	7·3	Unreliable, immature
19	5·5	Circumstances of coitus	19	7·1	Petting techniques
20	5·4	Alcohol and drug use	20	6·9	Duration of foreplay
21	5·0	Duration of foreplay	21	6·8	Bad temper, bad disposition
22	4·4	Poor reasons for marriage	22	6·6	Other personality troubles
23	4·2	Involuntary separation	23	6·5	Selfish, egotistical
24	4·0	Female sexual difficulties	24	6·3	Involuntary separation
25	3·8	Selfish, egotistical	25	5·7	Having children
26	3·7	Domineering	26	5·5	Inadequate financial contribution
27	3·6	Sociability	27	5·4	Inferiority feelings
	3·6	Having children			
28	3·3	Other personality troubles	28	4·6	Domineering
				4·6	Nervous breakdown
29	3·2	Fear of pregnancy	29	4·4	Poor reasons for marriage
30	3·0	Overly demanding, perfectionist	30	4·1	Sociability

for the inclusion of an individual in our percentages. However, it should be noted that our sample contained somewhat more divorced persons than did the general white population. The problem which confronts us is the discrepancy between the figures of the males and the females. This same discrepancy exists even when one takes cognizance of all marriages, and not merely first marriages, and notes the incidence of divorce for the white college-educated which was 15·7 per cent for males and 28·8 per cent for females. The only explanation I can offer is that our sampling was generally obtained through the co-operation of organized groups and businesses; thus, we were apt to encounter more career and employed women than we would have had we had a random sample. In brief, we tended to miss the presumably contented *hausfrau* at home and interviewed her divorced sister who was out in society earning her living and joining organizations.

At any rate, both the male and female data indicate that there is a decrease in separation or divorce with increased age at marriage and increased duration of marriage. The most vulnerable are the first years of marriage, particularly if the couple married before age 20. Of the wives who married before 20, nearly half (44·8 per cent) reported a separation or divorce. Among those married later, this figure fell to about one-fifth (22·1 per cent for those married at ages 21–25; 23·4 per cent for those married 26–30; and 21·8 per cent for those married after age 30).

Fortunately, the purpose of this chapter is not to ascertain the incidence of separation or divorce, but to investigate the more common sources of marital stress. For this purpose, an unduly high proportion of divorced respondents is an advantage.

COMPARISONS

The rank orders of frequency of marital troubles reported by husbands and wives are in substantial agreement. The 30 most common troubles were tabulated separately for men and for women (see Table 15.2) and the combined list comprised only 39 items — i.e. there were only nine items not included in both lists.

Three items were given identical ranks and it is noteworthy that both sexes agreed that the commonest trouble was over coital frequency and the second commonest involved economic matters.

Five items were only one rank apart, six items differed by two ranks, and seven items by three ranks. In summary, 54·0 per cent of the items were within three ranks of agreement, 36·0 per cent were within two ranks of one another, 21·0 per cent differed by one rank or less, and 8·0 per cent were identically ranked. Even greater agreement exists among the items listed as the ten commonest. Both husbands and wives agreed on nine of the ten items. The husbands had two items not on the wives' list, and the wives had one item not on the husbands' list. However, these three items are found in eleventh and twelfth ranks.

Of the nine items that appeared on one list, but not on the other, males provided five and females four. These discrepant items were in the lower half of each list, all but one ranking eighteenth or lower. It is interesting to note that of the five items listed by males, but not by females, four concerned sex: coital positions, female sexual difficulties, fear of pregnancy, and coital circumstances. The four items listed by females, but not by males, consisted of three items dealing with personality and one concerning financial support. In general, sexual matters were perceived as more important by the husbands: twelve of the items which comprised their list of the 30 commonest sources of marital stress were specifically sexual whereas the wives had but eight sexual items.

For each rank, regardless of the item involved, the wives invariably have a somewhat larger percentage figure than the husbands. I do not think that this should be interpreted to mean that wives are more prone to marital dissatisfaction than husbands, but merely that our sample of wives contained more divorced individuals than did our sample of husbands.

In comparing these reports of men and women, one must continually bear in mind two qualifications. First, these individuals in general represent the older generations; the great majority of respondents were born before 1930. Consequently, the findings cannot be said to reflect marital stress among younger married persons today. However, it is likely that the marital troubles of the younger people do not markedly differ from those which afflicted their parents. Personality conflicts, trouble over relatives, economic problems, and sexual difficulties seem to have been inescapable throughout human history.

The second qualification to be remembered is that the sample contains only a minority of spouses married to one another. Someday, we will compare the marital troubles of paired spouses, and it is possible that the findings would differ in some respects from those presented here. The fact that our sample of females contains more divorced individuals than does our sample of males undoubtedly accounts for the larger percentages of women reporting stress. Nevertheless, the close agreement in rank order of stress-producing problems indicates that the male and female samples can be fruitfully compared and that the effects of sample bias are not great.

CONCLUSION

The purpose of this chapter was to describe the various stress-producing situations in marriage, with particular attention to the sexual aspects, and to evaluate in this connection the effect of age at marriage and duration of marriage.

The findings are based on interviews conducted with 1607 college-educated white married males and 1445 college-educated white married females, the great majority of whom were born before 1930. The data derive only from first marriages.

Various categories and sub-categories of marital troubles were formulated and the percentages of males and females reporting such troubles were calculated. The troubles were then arranged in rank order according to their degree of commonness. While the percentages reported by males and females for the same item differed to varying degrees, there was close agreement in the ranking of the troubles. In the two lists of the 30 most common sources of marital discord compiled separately for husbands and wives, there were only a few items which did not appear on both lists.

The major categories of sources of stress were sexual problems, economic and employment difficulties, differing interests, relationships with relatives, and unpleasant personality traits.

The sexual problems in early and middle marriage stemmed from the discrepancy between husbands and wives in terms of sexual drive and responsiveness. Generally, the husbands desired coitus more frequently than the wives and both were disturbed by the lesser sexual responsiveness of the wives and their difficulty in achieving orgasm. This discrepancy in sexual interest involved some subsidiary problems regarding coital positions and petting techniques. Both sexes ranked trouble over coital frequency as the most common source of marital stress with nearly one-third of the husbands and wives reporting this difficulty. General sexual responsiveness, chiefly the wife's, constituted a problem for 23·0 per cent of the males and 17·0 per cent of the females, earning it third and fifth rank. Trouble over female orgasm ranked seventh (16 per cent) among women and tenth (12 per cent) among men.

These problems seems less among those who married at older ages. This is probably the result of women losing their inhibitions through experience and becoming more responsive, and also the result of age diminishing the male's sexual drive. It is curious that duration of marriage seems to have little effect. This may be because the respondents were not reporting on just their current marital problems, but listing as well those of previous years. This would result in masking the effects of duration of marriage. Whereas trouble over coital frequency, female orgasm, and general responsiveness decreases with increased age at marriage, some other troubles tend to increase with age. Male sexual difficulties, such as impotence and premature ejaculation, grow as the males ages, and with the passing of years, an even larger percentage of wives desire coitus more often than their husbands.

Sexual jealousy ranked ninth among males (12 per cent) and eleventh among females (14 per cent); each tended to label the spouse rather than himself or herself as being the jealous individual. Jealousy does not seem to be affected by age at marriage or duration of marriage. Stress because of extramarital activity, chiefly that of the husband, ranked eighth (14 per cent) among men and tenth (14 per cent) among women.

There is a trend for persons marrying at older ages to be less concerned over extramarital behaviour.

Other sexual problems, although numerous, were less common than those just described.

Marital stress resulting from economic problems was the second commonest trouble reported by both sexes: 29·0–31·0 per cent reported this problem, which was generally described as the spouse being extravagant, improvident, and careless with money. Trouble over actual earnings was surprisingly seldom cited, but complaints about employment were ranked ninth by wives (15 per cent) and twelfth (10 per cent) by husbands. The major complaint concerned the husband's job, which seems to have conflicted with his marital and family responsibilities.

Stress resulting from the spouses having different interests was important, being ranked fifth (17 per cent) by men and sixth (16 per cent) by women. This problem seemingly increases with increased age at marriage, which suggests that older individuals are progressively less adaptable and are more fixed in their tastes and interests.

Discord because of relatives, particularly mothers-in-law, was ranked high. Males placed their wives' relatives in fourth rank (19 per cent) and their own in fifth (17 per cent). Females ranked their husbands' relatives in fourth rank (22 per cent) and their own in eighth (15 per cent).

Stress arising from unpleasant personality traits was important, but not treated as a unit. The unfortunate trait was generally attributed to the spouse and only infrequently admitted by the respondents. Both husbands and wives agreed that three sorts of traits were most common: (1) over-emotional and temperamental, (2) bad temper and bad disposition, and (3) selfish and egotistical. Wives more often than husbands accused their spouse of being unreliable and immature, ranking this eighteenth in their list. Interestingly enough, although disagreeable personality traits are important in the aggregate, comprising between a quarter and a third of the 30 most common complaints, no single item ranked higher than twelfth.

The age of the respondent at marriage was more influential than the length of time married, and the effects are more marked among females than males. Increased age at marriage seemingly intensifies troubles over personality traits, differing interests, child-rearing, health, and many sexual problems. On the other hand, the older a person is at marriage, the less likely is discord over coital frequency and sexual responsiveness, and there are fewer arguments and less desire for separation or divorce. One has the impression that two opposing factors are involved: on one hand the older person is less adaptable, but on the other hand, more mature and rational. Increased age does not allow one to escape problems, but does make one more able to endure them.

The effects of the duration of marriage were largely concealed by the respondents reporting past as well as present sources of stress. However, some trends are seen. Marriages improve as persons improve their economic status and as their relatives die, but the passage of time exacerbates problems of child-rearing, health, and bad temper. The overall picture is more one of improvement than deterioration, since the desire for separation or divorce declines with the years as both spouses become accustomed to the inevitable stresses involved in a close relationship with another human.

SUMMARY

White ever-married males and females with college education were asked what troubles and problems they had experienced in their marriages. The percentages of males and females reporting these various sources of marital stress were calculated and put in rank order. The commonest stresses involved sexual problems, economic and employment difficulties, differing interests, relatives, and personality traits. There was much agreement between the reports of the males and females. The effects of age at marriage and duration of marriage were investigated.

16. MENTAL REACTIONS OF WOMEN AND OF HOSPITAL STAFF TO PERINATAL DEATH

JOHAN CULLBERG

INTRODUCTION

Stillbirth or the death of a newborn child are catastrophes not only to the mother but also to her husband (if she has one) and any older children who have been waiting for the newcomer, ambivalently but eagerly, all of whom are other important parts of the family in crisis.

The staff at the maternity clinic also find this experience very painful (Bruce 1962) and try to deal with its emotional impact on the family in what are often rather unsuccessful ways.

Literature on the psychological aspects of this rather common event has been sadly lacking until recent years. Kennel *et al.* (1970) have pointed to the higher degree of mourning in the mothers who touched their baby before its death, and in those who have not talked with their husbands about the loss.

Since I had observed several cases of this trauma preceding long-standing grave mental insufficiencies, I performed an investigation to get an idea of the impact of perinatal death as a crisis-releasing event in a 'normal population'.

THE STUDY

In order to get an unbiased sample, one year's registered cases of perinatal death at a Stockholm maternity clinic, comprising 62 women (i.e. 2·5 per cent of the total births) were collected for investigation.

A follow-up interview was arranged 1–2 years after parturition to get information on the women's mental reactions to the trauma. Fifty-six of the 62 women could be interviewed. Four had moved away from the city and 2 could not be contacted. In most cases the interview was performed and tape-recorded at the clinic and lasted 1–2 hours. There were no serious difficulties about contacting the patients, and most of them expressed their gratitude for the opportunity of discussing their feelings about the death of their child — for several of the women it was their first discussion with a doctor about the matter.

RESULTS

The main reactions in all mothers (except in nine, who denied any reaction) were grief, apathy, feelings of emptiness, and inadequacy. These reactions developed a few hours to some days after an initial shock reaction. During the second or third month most women had returned to their usual life situation and at the time of the interview most of them seemed to have regained their mental stability.

Table 16.1 shows the main symptomatology in 19 of the 56 women (one-third of the total material). These 19 reported more serious mental symptoms than the rest.

TABLE 16.1

Main symptoms in 19 women after perinatal child death (n = 56).

Main symptom	Number of women
Psychosis	2
Anxiety attacks	9
Cancer uteri phobia, etc.	3
Obsessive thoughts	2
Deep depression, etc.	3
Total	19
('No reaction')	9

In 9 cases, attacks of acute death anxiety dominated. Psychotic delusions of an impending castration were present in one case and in another a grave psychosis with pseudocyetic fantasies developed. Another woman believed that she was to be sterilized. Phobias of uterine cancer developed in two cases and two women became obsessed by the thought that the rest of their families were going to die. Twenty-six of the women reported more or less outspoken guilt feelings.

The symptoms usually culminated a few months after the death of the child. Subsequently most of them subsided while some persisted as chronic maladaptive behaviour.

There is little pre-crisis information, and no definite conclusions can be drawn regarding the final outcome of the crisis.

The intensity of the reactions was not clearly correlated to age, civil status, parity, or to earlier miscarriages. The grief reactions tended to be shorter in connection with premature birth. Malformation was often accompanied by a prolonged grief period or by symptom formation.

One third of the women reported marital conflict or other social complications after partus. Unfortunately their husbands could not be interviewed except in a few cases. Initial suppression or denial of feelings were expressed by 11 women. This attitude seemed to have been supported by hospital staff members or by relatives. In those cases, open grief reactions were felt

TABLE 16.2

Initital suppression of feelings and late reactions

	Number of women	Grief		Back to work	
		Less than 3 months	More than 3 months	Before 3 months	After 3 months
Initial suppression	11	4	7	6	5
No suppression	45	33	12	38	7

$$\chi^2 = 5 \cdot 39 \qquad\qquad \chi^2 = 4 \cdot 69$$
$$\text{D.F.} = 1, p < 0 \cdot 05 \qquad \text{D.F.} = 1, p < 0 \cdot 05$$

to be taboo, and the patient frankly told to 'pull yourself together', or to 'be brave', or to 'think about something else'. Table 16.2 shows that the period of the mental symptomatology was longer in these cases than in the others ($p < 0 \cdot 05$).

In addition to a woman's relationship with her family, and how she is treated at the maternity clinic, two aspects seem to be of specific importance for understanding the reactions in this emotional catastrophe, namely the object loss, and the challenge of her own sexual identification.

A deep feeling of physical inadequacy long since forgotten was revived in many women. This made them feel that they had been punished and that they deserved further punishment, often in the form of some genital injury. The well-known concept of the child as a magical repair for the infantile castration seems to fit well into many mother's consious guilt feelings and deeper reactions.

THE DOCTOR/PATIENT RELATIONSHIP

The patients seemed to have been extremely sensitive as to what the doctor had said or had not said after the delivery, his facial expressions when he was speaking, whether he showed signs of approval or disapproval, etc. These were often given hidden meanings, far beyond that which the doctors possibly could have imagined.

Nine of the women seemed to have been given reasonable opportunities for emotionally working through what had happened, (in 4 of these cases thanks to a nurse). The following are reports of some typical examples of the disturbed communication between doctor and patient, in the patient's words.

'Nobody would mention the subject'
This was a very common statement. One woman remembered that 'the doctor just stared at me when he entered my room. He never said anything to me'. Another said 'I would have talked to a doctor, but nobody seemed to touch upon my problems. I used to wonder why I should be punished in this way. These feelings lasted about half a year'.

The doctor was perceived as angry
'Afterwards I asked some questions, but the doctor seemed to think that I was accusing him. He just told me that no mistake had been made.' 'During the last part of labour everybody became silent and serious. The doctor got angry when I asked him if there was anything wrong with the child.'

The accusing doctor
'He asked if I really had wanted my child. I was terribly hurt and I felt that I would like to slap his face.' An unmarried journalist was asked by the chief of service (whom she had never met before) in the presence of some medical students, if several men could be father to the child: 'When I saw my private doctor he said that I had really behaved bravely. Why did I have to be so brave?' Four months later she was able to cry for the first time, when she was kindly questioned by an 11-year-old boy about what had happened.

Soothing
'Soothing' often seemed to be more helpful to the doctor than to the patient. In several cases the mother was advised to forget about what had happened by becoming pregnant again. Another method was to show the woman that her grief was inadequate: ' "It's all for the best", he said. I never understood what he meant.' — 'I was down and apathetic and they told me not to feel bad about it.'

On discharge the patients were often prescribed large doses of sedatives.

DISCUSSION

Stillbirth and allied conditions provoke a sense of guilt in the staff on a maternity ward. One could observe three principal ways of handling anxiety: (1) avoidance of the situation, (2) projection of personal feelings on the patient in the form of aggressive or accusing behaviour, and (3) denial and magical repair ('forget it', 'have another child', heavy doses of sedatives). Most doctors are not theoretically or emotionally prepared to act in a more realistic and conscious manner, and they often feel inadequate and awkward in these situations.

Adequate psychotherapy includes meeting some of the emotional needs by understanding the impact of the situation in the specific case. Of course, this requires basic knowledge of psychodynamics and also some ability of self-knowledge.

This makes it possible to let the patient accept and work through her grief and anxiety and also her feelings of protest and anger, which often are overlooked. She should also talk about her conceptions and misconceptions concerning her labour and the child's death in order that she can receive adequate information. This should be given by her obstetrician, and during two periods: first in the period after she has been told about the child's death, and secondly one or two months later, during the symptom phase of the crisis. If possible her husband should be present at these occasions. If the reaction is unduly intense, the patient should be referred to a psychiatrist.

REFERENCES

BRUCE, S. J. (1962). Reactions of nurses and mothers to still-birth. *Nursing Outl.*, **10**, 88–91.

KENNEL, J. H., SLYTER, H., and KLAUS, M. H. (1970). The mourning response of parents to the death of a newborn infant. *New Engl. J. Med.*, **283**, 344–9.

17. THE PSYCHOLOGICAL ASPECTS OF CONTRACEPTION

LARS ENGSTRÖM and MEREDITH TURSHEN

INTRODUCTION

Contraception — especially since the advent of new, highly effective methods of birth control — has been hailed as a great boon to mankind by people fighting for human rights, for improved health, for population control, and for economic and social development. But in many countries, the acceptance and practice of contraception have not matched the enthusiasm of family planners. There are, of course, many reasons for this; for example, contraceptives may not be readily available, or they may be beyond the purchasing power of poor people, or the necessary health services may be lacking. But even in areas where all of the facilities and resources exist, contraception is not universally practised, or is tried and dropped, or is practised with disagreeable side-effects. We believe that one of the reasons lies in the psychological significance of contraception, which is so complex, so little understood, and has been so little researched.

This chapter explores the psychological aspects of contraception. Psychological aspects comprise all of the positive and negative behavioural reactions — including physical ones that may be psychogenic — of men and women to contraception. In this chapter, contraception refers to any of the traditional and clinical, non-surgical methods and agents used to prevent conception. Abortion and sterilization will not, therefore, be discussed. It was our intention to include the attitudes of men as well as women, and the attitudes of people in a variety of cultures and societies, but this wish was for the most part thwarted by the dearth of studies on these subjects.

All contraceptives have some psychological significance for men and women since their use interferes with conception, which may be thought of as the natural outcome of sexual intercourse. In addition, particular methods of contraception have specific psychological side-effects that depend, for example, on their mode of action, the degree to which they are believed to endanger the physical health of the user, and whether the user is a man or a woman. Since most of the relevant literature deals with oral hormonal contraception, and since much of the discussion of this method applies to contraception in general and to other specific methods, we shall begin our discussion with the pill.

THE PILL

The pill has been the subject of increasing attention in research on the psychological aspects of contraception in recent years, partly because mood and behavioural changes are known to be associated with hormonal medication. Although some authors, noting the positive effects of the pill, have mentioned the psychological benefits accruing from almost 100 per cent certainty of temporary infertility, few have taken this as a starting point in their investigation, and fewer still have made any comparisons of the pill to the intrauterine device — the next most effective contraceptive in terms of preventing pregnancy — or of the pill and IUD to any other method of contraception. Yet it might be supposed that these two methods — unique in separating the act of coitus from the technique of contraception — would have an important psychological impact on attitudes and behaviour with respect to sex and intimate, interpersonal relationships between men and women.

Psychopharmacological effects

What has primarily been studied is the incidence, frequency, or severity of unwanted side-effects such as depression, nausea, headache, weight variation, breakthrough bleeding, changes in libido, fatigue, tension, cramps, breast tenderness, etc. — all of which may have a psychological component. Fawcett (1970) notes that 'the scattered research in this area has been conducted from a variety of theoretical and methodological perspectives ... and thus tends to be non-cumulative.' Two findings that have not been taken into consideration by later investigators will serve to illustrate the non-cumulative nature of the research.

1. Pincus (1966) reported the impact of admonitions concerning possible side-effects: the reaction rate in women given the pill who had not been admonished was much lower than that of users who had been warned, and there was a definite occurrence of breakthrough bleeding in women given placebos who were warned to expect side-effects. No recent studies mention what was said to women at the time the pill was prescribed.

2. Hines *et al.* (1967) in a very large series in 27 maternal health and university centres found that nausea in the first cycle varied from 1 per cent to 33 per cent between centres. 'Since the same preparation and the same report forms were used by all centers, the variations among centers must be due to some combination of different patient populations and different attitudes and questioning technics at the different centers.' With few exceptions, no control for these variables is reported in recent studies.

Finally, before turning to the investigations in question, we would caution that the majority of studies have been carried out in highly industrialized countries, often among middle-income women. The conclusions drawn about the unwanted effects of the pill may, therefore, not necessarily be applicable to women outside Europe and the United States. Comparability among studies is further limited by the fact that both the compounds and the amounts used have continuously been altered over the years. The investigations reviewed here are selected as examples of the conflicting findings that one encounters in the literature on the side-effects of hormonal contraception.

The effect of the pill on depressive mood changes was studied by Grant and Pryse-Davis (1968). A total of 797 women receiving one or more of 34 types of pill were observed over a 6-year period. The incidence of depression and loss of libido ranged from 28 per cent of women on combined oestrogen/progestogen preparations to 5–7 per cent of women on sequential regimens. This study concluded that the progestogenic component causes more depressive side-effects and loss of libido than does the oestrogenic component of the pill. Psychotic reactions have also been reported: Daly et al. (1967) described two cases, both of which had a previous history of post-partum psychiatric disturbance. In these cases sequentials were given. Hussain and Murphy (1971) report a case of psychosis in a woman using a sequential pill who had no previous history of psychiatric disability. Herzberg et al. (1970), in a careful study of 251 women, found little correlation between the type of pill and the general incidence of depressive symptoms. They suggest that 'depressive side-effects result from a situation which is probably more complex than alterations in a theoretical oestrogen/progestogen balance.'

On the other hand, Murawski et al. (1968) followed for 15 months 72 patients using a combined pill and found no increase in depression as measured by a variety of tests and scales. Bower and Altschule (1956) used progesterone successfully in the treatment of post-partum psychosis. Bakker and Dightman (1966) used questionnaires, psychological tests, and personal interviews to study 100 patients over a 4-year period; they found no basic changes in libido. Patients reporting relaxation in sexual activity and freedom from fear of pregnancy have sometimes been classified under 'increased libido' (e.g. Wearing, 1963).

Although Mears (1967) has grouped symptoms according to the oestrogenic or the progestogenic content of the pill, surprisingly no one has attempted to find clusters of side-effects that might be expected to occur together; instead investigators have attributed each effect individually to the pharmacological properties of the pill and have not considered whether one effect (e.g. depression) might be the cause of another (e.g. decreased libido).

Inadequacy of research design probably accounts for some of the conflicting results of the studies that have been carried out. One indication of inadequacy is that certain investigators always find the same side-effects

in their studies, while others consistently note an absence of these effects or find opposite effects occurring. Poor research design includes statistical considerations such as small size of samples and lack of control groups; faulty techniques of data acquisition that permit investigator bias; and problems of reliability and validation of data as in the use of suggestive questionnaires and the non-use of sensitive and specific instruments to measure behaviour. As Goldzieher (1968) notes, 'probing — that is, inquiring as to the presence or absence of particular symptoms — has great drawbacks, in that such inquiry sensitizes patients with regard to specific symptoms, and repeated inquiry has a powerful suggestive effect.' There is also often an absence of detailed knowledge of other, relevant disciplines; for example, public opinion research could contribute to studies of reactions to oral contraceptives. In fact, almost no study takes account of the impact of mass media or hearsay on subjective reports of side-effects.

Probably the most interesting data come from the few double-blind, placebo-controlled and/or cross-over studies that have been carried out. A recent study of this type by Goldzieher et al. (1971) of 398 women† through a total of 1523 cycles found that the 'pre-treatment cycle' had a higher incidence of side-effects than the placebo cycle. 'Complaints such as headache, nervousness, depression, weight gain, even nausea and vomitting occur with some frequency to normal women....' The authors conclude that the incidence of complaints during a pre-treatment cycle cannot be used as a control for subsequent cycles or as a substitute for placebo cycles. The only symptoms that occurred consistently more often in drug users than in the placebo group were gastrointestinal complaints, which were correlated with the oestrogen level of the oral contraceptive. 'A significant increase in nausea and vomiting, headache and nervousness could be demonstrated statistically only in the 1st treatment cycle with high-oestrogen agents; the frequency of all other symptoms in all other cycles fell within the placebo range.'

Aznar-Ramos et al. (1969) gave contraceptive placebo tablets to 147 low-income Mexican women 'who had a recent spontaneous abortion and were interested in becoming pregnant' during 424 months of observation. The investigators, using questionnaires that did not suggest any symptomatology, found in a large variety of side-effects, the most frequent being decrease in libido, headache, pain and bloating in the lower abdomen, and dizziness. They conclude that 'we cannot attribute all side effects to [contraceptive] medication but [the findings] do not permit us to state that the use of oestrogens and progestogens for contraception is free from adverse reactions.' An interesting finding in this study is that of reduced libido. Apart from the difficulties of defining libido, which is variously used to indicate the frequency of intercourse or the amount of sexual desire, the absence of data on the

† The women were told it was uncertain when the pill would be effective and they were requested to use cream or foam.

117

male attitude complicates interpretation of the data. The implication in many studies is that women who report lower frequency of intercourse have less desire for sexual relations. But it may be that the male has less desire. Some of Gluckman's patients complained, after starting on the pill, that their husbands lost interest in them. He suggests that 'perhaps the hazard of pregnancy compelled the male to greater interest in the partner to rouse her to a high level of emotional desire. The pill may make intercourse very casual and matter of fact (Gluckman 1969).

Goldzieher (1968) administered a questionnaire designed for oral contraceptors to 1064 users of IUD in a single random sample in order to assess the frequency of general symptoms. He notes that 'the "placebo" level of nausea in IUD users suggests that any experiment designed to detect nausea causally related to the oral contraceptive will have to discriminate against a background of non-drug related incidence of about 1%.'

We conclude from this review of the literature on the pill that the presence and frequency of adverse psychological effects as causally related to the compounds are not established. In general, such effects are less than reported by investigators, who did not take into account general reactions to new medication or the host of other psychological factors that may be activated when the pill is used. Further, carefully designed investigations should be carried out on the effects of hormonal steroids in different geographical areas and in different groups of the population subdivided, for example, according to socio-economic status, educational background, and marital status. Positive as well as negative effects should be examined: for example, psychological benefits from the use of the pill to treat certain menstrual disorders, including premenstrual tension and physical and psychic disorders of the post-ovulatory phase of the cycle.

Underlying psychological factors

The underlying psychological factors, as opposed to subjective reports of symptoms, in the selection and use of almost 100 per cent effective[†] contraceptives have been described in the literature, but rarely systematically investigated, by a number of psychologists, psychiatrists, and psychoanalysts. In the few investigations carried out, attempts were made to identify personality traits by means of psychological tests, scales, and questionnaires, and to correlate personality traits with behaviour related to contraception. For example, Bakker and Dightman (1964) in a much-cited study, concluded that women who forget to take contraceptive pills are deficient in their ability to assume responsibility, control impulses, and appreciate long-range goals. Pohlman (1969a), commenting on this study, notes that because of the small numbers of women compared and the fact that the number of significant comparisons[†] was quite close to chance expectation, 'Bakker and Dightman seem to have little justification for their assertion that women with such-and-such personality factors (the 3 of 92 that were significant) are more likely to forget pills than the mature ones.'

Ziegler et al. (1968) studied 39 middle-class couples by means of interviews, psychological tests, and questionnaires over a 4-year period that began just before first use of oral contraceptives. Fifteen wives used the pills throughout the study, while 9 discontinued them permanently. Within the group of 15 couples that continued, they found the wives more responsible and more intellectually and socially effective than the husbands; husbands of women who discontinued were more concerned about propriety and reputation than were husbands of women who continued to take the pill. In another analysis of the same data, Rodgers and Ziegler (1968a) examined social role theory, the marital relationship, and the use of ovulation suppressors. They conclude that husband/wife dynamics are highly predictive of which couples will effectively utilize pills and which will not. They found that couples in which the husband was ascendant (which they define as more dominant, effective and responsible, older, higher preferred rate of intercourse, and a history of using primarily masculine methods of contraception) discontinued oral contraception, whereas couples in which the husband and wife were approximately equal in dominance or in which the wife was clearly dominant continued oral contraception. Since this series is small, and there is no indication of how the couples were selected, one cannot generalize from these observations. Studies on random samples should be carried out to test the hypothesis before any conclusions are drawn.

One aspect of behaviour that is much commented upon in relation to the pill is promiscuity,[‡] which is thought by some to have increased since the introduction of this method of contraception and by others to be independent of it. One argument against the belief that the pill will encourage promiscuity runs like this: if fear of pregnancy has in the past interfered with sexual adjustment, an effective contraceptive may be expected to remove that obstacle. Better sexual adjustment between partners may, in turn, remove one reason for frequent change of partners, namely, the search for satisfaction of sexual needs. Thus, far from increasingly promiscuity, the pill could strengthen the bonds between partners and stabilize relationships. However, it is also true that if there is no love between the partners, an effective contraceptive may remove fear of pregnancy as a constraint on sexual relations outside the pair bond.

[†]We refer, throughout the text, to theoretical effectiveness, not use-effectiveness.

[†]Pill-forgetters and other women were compared on 46 scales, as were complainers and others. Of the total of 92 comparisons, only 3 showed differences significant at the 0·05 level.

[‡]Promiscuity is variously defined as premarital or extramarital relations, or intercourse with more than one partner.

Black and Sykes (1971) analysed several studies of the changing incidence of premarital sexual intercourse and concluded that use of the pill is not a major factor. Juhlin and Liden (1965) investigated 250 women and found that the ones using the pill had a significantly higher number of sexual partners per year and a higher frequency of intercourse, suggesting increased promiscuity. However, this may be a self-selected population of women who prefer or have partners who prefer a higher frequency of intercourse; this hypothesis should be tested. Engström (1971) points out that other changes are taking place in society which may influence attitudes toward sexual relations, and which are independent of the advent of the pill.

The pill may be used by a younger population of women than are IUDs and, if so, age may be a factor in the frequency and type of side-effect reported. Cullberg *et al.* (1969) suggest that disappointment and frustration among the sexually inexperienced, especially those whose expectations of the pill were that it would improve sexual relations, may lead to negative effects which are assigned to the pill. This may apply not only to young inexperienced partners, but also to older couples with jaded sexual appetites. A number of authors note the tendency to use the pill as a 'scapegoat' for problems that existed long before its use began (e.g. Gottleib *et al.* 1970).

Zell and Crisp (1964) studied a group of 250 private patients who started taking the pill, 31 of whom had been receiving psychotherapy. The initial fears of the women in therapy were related to any harmful effects the drug might exert (e.g. cancer, masculinization); to the control of sexual impulses or changes in libido (e.g. frigidity and sexual aggression, promiscuity, and prostitution no longer contained by the fear of pregnancy); to the effectiveness of the method (stemming from ignorance of the mechanism of action); and to its effect on future fertility and later menopause. The authors found that 'a response to the drug by a decrease in sexual impulses and sexual behaviour indicated a rather intense conflict in the sexual area.' Perhaps such conflict accounts for some of the decreased libido and lower frequency of intercourse in women usually attributed to the pharmacological properties of the pill.

Gluckman (1969) accounts for other side-effects of the pill by exploring women's desires for pregnancy that are repressed in deference to the wishes of their partners. He suggests that women hit back with both physical and emotional symptoms including weight gain, irritability, depression, and frigidity. 'All of these symptoms have a punishing quality. Obesity may be indirectly symbolic of pregnancy and directly annoying to the husband.... Temper, depression, loss of libido, all punish the husband by interfering with the interpersonal relationship.' Gluckman does not elaborate on why the male partner may wish to avoid a pregnancy, but Pohlman (1969*b*) suggests that one reason among the unmarried may be that men fear pregnancy as a way of forcing them into an unwanted marriage.

None of the studies cited this far attempts to answer such basic questions about the psychological aspects of oral contraception as: how do fertile men and women react when they know that intercourse *cannot* result in pregnancy? Does this knowledge affect the sexual experience or the interpersonal relationship for either partner or both, for married and unmarried couples? Are there men or women who need to risk pregnancy in order to enjoy sexual relations, although they say they do not want a child? The clinical impressions of psychiatrists and psychoanalysts give some interesting insights into these questions.

Sandberg and Jacobs (1971) studied 4000 patients seeking abortion and tried to schematize the explanations given for the misuse and rejection of contraception. They suggest that some people invoke the mechanism of denial; they deny the possibility of pregnancy, the effectiveness of contraception, or any personal responsibility for contraception. Flugel (in Pohlman 1969*a*) attempts to explain this in several ways: because sexual gratification is desirable people tend to ignore any situation that limits or conditions this gratification; reducing potential reproduction through contraception may symbolically threaten potency; also, if an individual represses sexuality, he or she may find it necessary to oppose birth control, ignore the need for contraception, and maintain the imagined 'penalty' for sex — children.

Sandberg and Jacobs suggest that even love may be given as a reason to avoid contraception, when it is believed that the willingness to risk pregnancy is a demonstration of love, although pregnancy is not wanted. Perhaps this is a rationalization of deeper guilt feelings. The impression of Sandberg and Jacobs with respect to guilt is that there are individuals — taught that sexual activity is permissible for procreative purposes but is highly immoral and sinful if indulged in for pure sensuality — who feel greater guilt with contraceptive use than with no protection. In a study of premarital contraception, Pohlman (1969*b*) found that Roman Catholic female university students believe it is more sinful to use contraceptives in a premarital sex relationship than not to use them and have a pregnancy as a result. With traditional, nonclinical methods of contraception, protection may be perceived as minimal and pregnancy may still be thought of as a real risk; the much-bruited 100 per cent reliability of the pill eliminates this doubt. The use of the pill may result in an increased desire or demand for coitus by one partner; in such circumstances, the sensual aspects of coitus may be accentuated and may increase guilt beyond the other partner's capacity to compensate for guilt feelings.

Fear of pregnancy may be used by either the male or the female partner to hide impotence or frigidity. This sense of sexual inadequacy may be well-founded or groundless — the point is that a 100 per cent effective contraceptive may reveal unsuspected psychosexual problems. Meldman (1964) reports that three husbands became impotent after their wives started using pills. It is important for the physician who suggests that a couple use the pill or switch to it from some other method to look for latent problems or for a fragile balance in the male/female relationship that might be upset by use of the pill.

Sandberg and Jacobs note that 'contraceptive use must be considered to be synonymous with coital preparedness. This realization may arouse considerable guilt in some through its implication of promiscuous behaviour....' The latter is of special interest in the case of extramarital relations, but in general it would be interesting to know the attitudes of men to women who practise reliable contraception, as well as the women's self-image. No doubt these attitudes are conditioned to some extent by the status of women in a given society, a question that is discussed later in this chapter.

Again, if traditional methods are viewed as unreliable, the guarantee of certainty connected with the pill may interfere with what Eric Berne (1971) describes as sexual games. In power struggles between partners, a contraceptively protected woman may no longer be able to control the frequency of sexual activity by invoking the fear of pregnancy as an excuse. Similarly, a man might resist oral contraception for his partner if he believes that maintaining fear of pregnancy is a way of controlling her.

Some authors discuss the special relation of the pill to sexual pleasure and freedom. They assert that whenever there is important scientific progress promising increased enjoyment of sexuality, 'psychosomatic, neurotic, behavioural, and even psychotic disturbances can be theoretically expected as the *quid pro quo* for this advance' (Orchard 1969). Gluckman (1969) states that 'there was opposition to anaesthesia in childbirth, because it was believed mothers who conceived in sin should be delivered in pain. Dissemination of knowledge about contraceptives has been a major offence in many societies. Education about venereal disease has been opposed on the grounds that such education would promote promiscuity.'

Sandberg and Jacobs point out the importance of sexual identity conflicts. For the woman with low self-esteem — whether this is an internal problem or one created by prevailing attitudes in her culture — pregnancy may be regarded as a compensation, a means of being creative, of producing something, of being worthwhile, and motherhood is a means of achieving respect, deference, and attention. In these circumstances, 'contraception may be regarded as tantamount to sterility and viewed as producing a degrading lack of femininity. Women with low self-esteem are not likely to do well with any of the contraceptive methods as the prevention of fertility is too threatening.... Depression, impotency, and innumerable other symptoms or dysfunctions may result....' Latent sexual identity conflicts in men may be exposed when their partners being using the pill, especially when the woman's fear of pregnancy has been a real reason, and not a rationalization, for low frequency of intercourse. According to Erikson (1966), the resolution of sexual identity conflicts is a prerequisite for psychosexual maturity. Orchard maintains that 'on general psychiatric grounds, it can be stated that psychosexual maturity in general is an indication of ability to tolerate oral contraceptives.'

This raises an interesting question for research. In all societies women are identified with child-bearing, but alternatives to motherhood that are compatible with feminine identity are greater in industrialized societies and more limited in primitive cultures (Mead 1949). To what extent does oral contraception interfere with stereotyped sex roles? To what degree are alternative roles for women a prerequisite for successful contraceptive practice? The importance of understanding these psychological factors for successful stabilization of world population growth cannot be over-emphasized.

Much of what has been said about the pill applies in some degree to contraception in general. Psychological factors specific to other contraceptives are discussed below.

INTRAUTERINE DEVICES

In comparison to the literature on oral contraception, there are relatively few studies on the psychological aspects of IUD contraception.

Peel and Potts (1969) note that 'pain is the primary complaint leading to removal in 2 to 3 per cent of patients. Sometimes pain is associated with an anxious personality or with religious beliefs that do not accept contraception freely.'

Among religious groups that forbid intercourse during menstruation, prolonged bleeding may make the IUD unacceptable and lead to requests for removal of the device. Khan and Wishik (1965) note that in Pakistan the removal of the IUD is requested because prolonged bleeding interferes with a woman's daily prayers, which are forbidden during menstruation. Failure to secure permission from husbands for insertion of the IUD may also lead to requests for removal if they protest; we assume that the same objections men have to the pill as mentioned above (e.g. fear of infidelity) apply to the IUD.

In addition, according to Peel and Potts (1969), 'some men appear to be aware of the presence of cervical threads and one member of the couple, by accident or design, may pull on the threads and remove the device.' They would appear to recommend devices without threads. However, Pohlman (1969a) notes that the threads provide continued reassurance that the device is in place and may help overcome fears that it will get lost somewhere inside the body. Since the tolerance level of unwanted effects is a relative value, it would be interesting to learn whether threads really interfere with intercourse or whether this is an excuse masking an underlying rejection of the device on other grounds.

Metzner and Golden (1967) investigated attitudes toward IUDs in a random sample of 100 women considering contraception at the obstetrics service of a university medical centre. A standardized interview was used. When asked which contraceptive method was preferred, 26 specified the IUD; and, following persuasion by the interviewer, 51 said they would be interested in trying the IUD. Comparisons of interview responses in this group of 77 with the group of 33 women who could not be persuaded to try the IUD revealed no difference in socio-economic and educational background; more enthusiasm about contraception generally among those pro the IUD; and significant differences in sexual attitudes and experiences — there was a greater amount of 'sexual inhibition' in the anti-IUD group as compared with the relative 'sexual freedom' of the pro-IUD group. The authors suggest that 'a practical application of these findings might be in the guidance they should provide for prescribing the IUD to patients seeking birth-control information.'

King (1967), in an attempt to establish criteria for the selection of IUD contraceptors, discusses some psychological factors involved. On the basis of 3 years' experience with 240 private patients, he suggests that one basic problem in women who could not use the IUD satisfactorily seems to be conflict over femininity.

Saxton and Pike (1969) made a long-term study of IUD acceptability in Uganda, comparing the experience of 99 European women and 122 Asian women with that of 699 African women. They conclude 'that African women in Kampala continue to expel IUD's at a constant significant rate even in the second year after insertion.' It would be interesting to investigate whether this is due only to some physical factor or also occurs because of differences in the psychological acceptance of contraception among the three groups.

Pohlman also notes that 'IUD's may be perceived as hard foreign objects, and dangerous in that they may tear or damage one's insides or produce cancer or other diseases.' The insertion of the IUD may be equated with intromission and be problematic for women who view the penis as a 'dangerous, tearing, explosive thing.'

King (1967) suggests that 'except for tubal ligation, the IUD is the only contraceptive technic ordinarily beyond the power of the woman to give up immediately if she happens to change her mind.' In cases of ambivalence about contraception, this may be an important drawback, although family planners rate it an advantage in that it eliminates 'patient idiosyncrasy', e.g. forgetting to take pills.

Rainwater (1960) sees as an important psychological aspect of contraceptive effectiveness the general disposition to plan ahead. Reluctance or inability to do so is seen as one major cause of lower class difficulties with contraception. This was thought to be eliminated with the introduction of the IUD. Polgar (in Pohlman 1969a) disagrees with Rainwater, noting that poor people and those living in non-Western cultures are not necessarily unwilling to plan. However, willingness to plan in the examples cited by Polgar is not evidence for willingness or ability to plan families.

The IUD is used throughout the world because it is a reversible method; it does not require the user to take any further action after the device is inserted; it is inexpensive; and it is divorced from the sexual act. Considering its widespread use, the lack of psychological studies is regrettable. Psychological aspects of this method of contraception may relate to the role of rumours and adverse publicity, the fear of pain and irregular bleeding, the fear of having a foreign body in the uterus, and the decision to use the IUD because the pill is feared. Since trials of new shapes and types of IUD continue to be carried out in many countries, we would recommend that investigations of the psychological aspects of acceptability, including side-effects, to be linked to those trials.

DIAPHRAGMS AND CERVICAL CAPS

Psychological problems associated with the use of the diaphragm are said to be linked to a complex of sexual taboos, including masturbation and such social customs as the dictate that man is the sole initiator of intercourse. Since we found no scientific studies on the subject, most of the discussion in this section is anecdotal, or at best based on reports of interviews.

Genital contact is necessary to insert the diaphragm each time it is used. Pohlman (1969a) notes that touching the genitals may be associated with the guilt of forbidden masturbation and the arousal of banished feelings and conflicts. Some women, uncertain whether the diaphragm has been inserted properly or afraid that the 'violence' of intercourse might dislodge it, doubt that they could ever feel sure about its effectiveness. Rainwater (1960) suggests that many people in the lower socio-economic groups fear that the diaphragm can be lost inside the woman, or become so firmly lodged that it cannot be removed without a physician's assistance, or that it might hurt the woman's body in some way. Some of these fears may be found among members of every socio-economic group.

Peel and Potts (1969) note that many women abandon use of the cap because they find it messy. This reaction would also be a disadvantage associated with the use of creams, jellies, and foams. In some instances the real target of this complaint may be the sex act itself, which some women may reject as messy.

One very important point raised by Rainwater (1960) is that, when a diaphragm is prescribed and fitted by a physician, there comes into play the whole complex of physician/patient relations, which not only vary according to social class, but may be different for racial and ethnic minority groups within a society. Rainwater notes that the contacts of many lower-class people with physicians are often frightened and tenuous. The impact of doctor/patient relations on the use of contraception and the incidence of side-effects is recognized, but has not been carefully studied. This problem arises not only with the diaphragm, but also with the methods already discussed — the pill and the IUD. In pressing for the use of the IUD in a national family-planning programme, one group of physicians (Zipper *et al.* 1965) has said, 'We believe that the so-called "cafeteria choice" is not advisable — in our opinion the medical profession rather than the patient must ultimately decide on the efficiency of any procedure in the light of all the relevant factors, and accommodate one or several techniques to the specific conditions of a country.' Such a paternalistic attitude demonstrates lack of training in psychology and human relations.

Traditions in many societies dictates that man should be the initiator of sexual relations. The fact that the diaphragm — like the pill and IUD — is a 'woman-controlled' method may be disturbing to men on the grounds that initiative is seen to be passed to the woman. Pohlman (1969*a*) notes that if the diaphragm is inserted in advance, the woman must admit to herself and later to her partner that she is willing to make love. 'Some women complain that they are then irritated when spouses do not initiate intercourse.' Both partners may feel that the spontaneity of sex relations is ruined by advance preparations. When the diaphragm is not inserted in advance, it acts as a longer interruption to intercourse than does putting on a condom.

In conclusion, there is clearly a need to undertake scientific studies of the psychological aspects of this method of contraception.

MALE ATTITUDES AND METHODS

So far we have examined female attitudes and methods of contraception and male reactions to them; we turn now to male attitudes and methods and female reactions.

It will be remembered that Rodgers and Ziegler (1968*a*) in the study on oral contraception cited above correlated the use of primarily masculine methods of contraception with male ascendancy in relationships and with male dominance, effectiveness and responsibility, higher age, and higher preferred rate of intercourse. The question of responsibility for contraception is indeed an important one; female responsibility may be associated with recent technological development of new contraceptives, which coincides with new and more independent roles for women in modern society. Thus male control of contraception may be symbolic of male superiority in the minds of some men.

Hall (1970) questioned 960 men in Chile on contraceptive use. An analysis of men's opinion of each marital partner's responsibility in matters of family planning revealed that 60–72 per cent of men in the sampled rural area and three socio-economic groups stated that in their own family both partners were equally concerned about the number of children. No psychological factors were investigated in this study. The author's conclusion is that a majority of men in all socio-economic groups felt they had an active role in birth-control decisions.

The literature on the psychological advantages and disadvantages of condoms is based on clinical impressions and is not verified by research. Thus the condom is said to interfere with sexual pleasure by reducing sexual sensation during intromission and by interrupting intercourse when the man stops to put it on. Further, Pohlman (1969*a*) suggests that the check on ejaculation imposed by the condom may be seen as a limitation of male potency or even as a threatened castration. Information obtained by Masters and Johnson (1966) would seem to dispute this; they state that concepts of male potency are linked to penile erection and not ejaculation.

Advantages of condom use are said to include security associated with protection from venereal disease, simplicity and ease of use, and anonymity in procurement (for instance, when obtained through vending machines). Another advantage, cited by Peel and Potts (1969), is that the condom may be used by men 'as an alternating technique for couples who wish to share the responsibility for birth control'.

Female reactions quoted in the literature are more often positive than negative. Pohlman (1969*a*) suggests that for women who want to be insulated from sex and the intimacies of intercourse, who want their role to be as passive as possible, who resent sex or feel ambivalent about it, the condom may represent a symbolic barrier, separating male from female genitalia. Gluckman (1969) characterizes such attitudes vividly:

there is a type of woman psychosexually and emotionally immature. She often has a history of leucorrhoea, frigidity, menstrual disorder, ill-defined pelvic pain and dyspareunia. She feels positively dirty both physically and mentally following intercourse. To her semen is filth. In the past she has found protection with the condom, diaphragm or with coitus interruptus. The pill leaves her defenseless and as one would expect is badly tolerated.

Of coitus interruptus or withdrawal, Rodgers *et al.* (1965) say that it is judged, even by wives, as relatively difficult, inconvenient, uncomfortable, crude, embarrassing, unsuccessful, and undesirable, although inexpensive. Peel and Potts (1969) note that it is widely used in all societies around the world but that the aesthetic biases of middle-class western commentators have encouraged condemnation of the practice 'not merely on hygienic grounds but also on grounds of reliability and psychological hazards'. They go on to say that 'in the past a variety of disturbances has been attributed to its use including prostatic hypertrophy and impotence in men and pelvic congestion and frigidity in women.' No studies have been carried out to demonstrate whether a causal relationship exists between methods and symptoms. To the advantage of no cost, one might add that of coital preparedness without the psychological difficulties sometimes associated with contraceptive purchases. The objection that coitus interruptus interferes with orgasmic satisfaction is questionable since orgasm may be achieved in other ways. For example, Rodgers and Ziegler (1969b) found among pill users that 'non-coital methods of stimulation to orgasm (mutual masturbation, oral-genital contact) increased appreciably, indicating that such procedures are used primarily for sexual pleasure.' In summary, while couples should be warned that coitus interruptus is not a reliable method of contraception, there seems to be no reason to discourage its use unless one of the partners explicitly objects to it.

RHYTHM

The rhythm method has many names (e.g. periodic abstinence, Ogino-Knaus method) and several variations (e.g. calendar method, basal body temperature method); but the salient feature having a psychological impact is the period of coital abstinence required each month. Considering that this method of birth control was sanctioned by the Roman Catholic Church in 1930 and remains the only method approved by the Church, one would expect many studies of psychological aspects to appear in the literature. This is not the case.

Rhythm is the only method of birth control that requires the active co-operation of both partners, and would seem to offer an interesting opportunity to study at least some aspects of the dynamics of male/female relationships as regards contraceptive behaviour. Since motivation is such an important factor in the successful use of the rhythm method, it would seem that psychological studies could contribute to our knowledge of this aspect of contraceptive practice in general. For example, motivation is one variable in tolerance levels of unwanted effects. A study of the basal body temperature method by Marshall and Rowe (1970) revealed that the great majority of both men and women found abstinence difficult, yet reported that the method was satisfactory in general and 'were of the opinion that it had helped their marriage'.

Some self-discipline is required with all contraceptives, except the IUD; but the self-control related to abstinence is particularly emphasized in the literature. Peel and Potts (1969) opine that 'the self-discipline required for the correct use of the safe period is unlikely to impair a healthy marriage' and may even improve sexual adjustment. 'On the other hand a poor marriage ... can be wrecked by the frustration and failures of the rhythm method.' Rainwater (1960) suggests that the 'rhythm ritual' symbolizes allegiance to the church, and this may help bind the believer to both the method and the church.

Since the rhythm method will continue to be used by certain groups, we would suggest that more research be carried out on the psychological aspects of this form of contraception.

MALE/FEMALE ROLES AND RELATIONSHIPS

We would like to end this chapter with a general discussion of male/female roles and relationships from the viewpoint of the psychological aspects of contraception.

There is presumed to be a link between the practice of contraception and the status of women. It is believed that family planning may help women as individuals and that lack of it may hinder them; that the exercise by women of their various rights may influence fertility; and that there may be an interrelationship between population growth and the status of women.

Improvement of the status of women in a community — so long as status is defined according to traditional values — will not, by itself, bring about psychological change in contraceptive acceptance. A woman's status may be high, but if no alternative roles to child-bearing are open to her, she may still be unable psychologically to practise contraception. For example, among the Tiv of Nigeria, women were highly prized and had high status, although they were not equal to men by Western standards. 'A Tiv married to get children. A man without children was sneered at and called useless, however successful he might be in his other undertakings. A woman, however excellent otherwise, would be despised if she was childless' (Mead 1955).

Similarly, social or economic independence for women will not, by itself, bring about a change in contraceptive behaviour, if other factors in the culture impel women to bear children because child-bearing is the accepted norm. For instance, in Burma 'women were actually fully equal to men, handling their own property, acting in their own right, negotiating family matters, making decisions. They were not dependent on men, except incidentally, in so far as there was interdependence among all members of a family' (Mead 1955). But everyone in Burma did want to have children and childless couples were considered unfortunate; there was a marked preference for male children and failure to have at least one son was very disappointing. Presumably, couples would continue to have children in the hope of producing a son. 'For a woman to bear a son is equivalent to her achievement of full existence as a human being' (Mead 1955). In these circumstances, a decision not to have more children, if one already has one or more daughters, might create a psychological conflict.

Kingsley Davis (1967) suggests that 'changes basic enough to affect motivation for having children would be changes in the structure of the family, in the position of women, and in sexual mores.' The pill — because it is theoretically almost 100 per cent effective — offers the possibility of effecting those basic changes, but cannot bring them about. Thus, because of the pill, new options exist for women — a career with marriage and without children; a career with both, since the number and timing of births can be regulated; a career without marriage, with or without children, and with a full sexual life. A few societies are experimenting with these options, but they are not widely accepted.

Davis notes that no modern society has restructured both the occupational system and the domestic establishment to the point of modifying permanently the old division of labour by sex. This would entail an alteration of the complementarity of the roles of men and women. 'Men are now able to participate in the wider world yet enjoy the satisfaction of having several children because the housework and child care fall mainly on their wives. Women are impelled to seek this role by their idealized view of marriage and motherhood and by either the scarcity of alternative roles or the difficulty of combining them with family roles.' Women are also influenced by the conflict that the choice of career or children may present. In some countries, where both possibilities exist, a compromise has psychological implications that will affect contraceptive acceptance.

CONCLUSIONS

From the foregoing survey it is concluded that there are psychological aspects to the practice of contraception *per se*, as well as of specific methods of contraception. Unwanted side-effects, in the case of the pill, may be induced by the pharmacological effects of hormonal compounds; in the case of other methods, such effects may be related to the contraceptive technique employed. Psychological side-effects may also be due to the presence of conflicts in and between men and women, and the use of highly reliable contraceptives may reveal these conflicts. In general, the psychological side-effects of specific methods seem to be less important than the psychological aspects of contraception as such; negative reactions to contraception result in non-acceptance of methods, discontinuation of use, unwanted pregnancy, or abortion. There is a lack of research on the psychological aspects of contraception, as understood in this sense.

Changes in male/female roles and relationships, and the resolution of problems in intimate, interpersonal relations between men and women, seem to be important for the promotion of psychological acceptance of contraception and the ability to practise it adequately. Emancipation from marriage and motherhood gives equal opportunities to men and women for participation in all social and economic activities. Sexual, social, and economic independence for women is made possible by contraception. On the other hand, this freedom generates conflicts, as it assigns women a double responsibility for career and family in modern society or offers them a choice between the two which, in itself, implies a conflict. The development of new and improved methods of contraception will probably not be sufficient to remedy the psychological problems already described. It seems to us essential that, in clinical trials of new methods, the psychological aspects of acceptability be investigated. Abortifacients in particular would seem to pose special psychological problems, yet we know little about the impact of legal, easy, accessible abortion procedures on the use of contraception, and even less why individuals select one contraceptive as opposed to any other.

REFERENCES

AZNAR-RAMOS, R. et al. (1969). Incidence of side effects with contraceptive placebo. Amer. J. Obstet. Gyn., 105, 1144–9.

BAKKER, C. B. and DIGHTMAN, C. R. (1964). Psychological factors in fertility control. Fertil. Steril., 15, 559–67.

—— and —— (1966). Side effects of oral contraceptives. Obstet. Gynec., 28, 373–9.

BERNE, E. (1971). Sex in human loving. London.

BLACK, S. and SYKES, M. (1971). Promiscuity and oral contraception: the relationship examined. Soc. Sci. Med., 5, 673–43.

BOWER, W. H. and ALTSCHULE, M. D. (1956). Use of progesterone in the treatment of postpartum psychosis. New Engl. J. Med., 254, 157–60.

COLES, R. (1964). Children of crisis. Boston, Massachusetts.

CULLBERG, J. et al. (1969). Mental and sexual adjustment before and after six months' use of an oral contraceptive. Acta psychiat. Scand., 45, 259–76.

DALY, R. et al. (1967). Psychosis associated with the use of a sequential dual contraceptive. Lancet, iii, 444–5.

DAVIS, K. (1967). Population policy: will current programs succeed? Science (N.Y.), 158, 730–9.

ENGSTRÖM, L. (1971). Socio-economical and medical aspects of planned parenthood. Stockholm, Sweden.

ERIKSON, E. H. (1966). Eight ages of man. Int. J. Psychiat., 2, 281–307.

FAWCETT, J. T. (1970). Psychology and population. New Haven, Connecticut.

GLUCKMAN, L. K. (1969). Psychiatric aspects of failures with oral contraceptives. New Zealand Med. J., 70, 10–13.

GOLDZIEHER, J. W. (1968). The incidence of side effects with oral or intrauterine contraceptives. Amer. J. Obstet. Gynec., 102, 91–4.

—— et al. (1971). A placebo-controlled double-blind cross-over investigation of the side effects attributed to oral contraceptives. Fertil. Steril., 22, 609–23.

GOTTLIEB, A. et al. (1970). Psychological aspects of contraception. J. reprod. Med., 5, 45–7.

GRANT, E. C. G. and PRYSE-DAVIS, J. (1968). Effect of oral contraceptives on depressive mood changes and on endometrial monoamine oxidase and phosphatasis. Brit. med. J., iii, 777–80.

HALL, M.-F. (1970). Male use of contraception and attitudes toward abortion, Santiago, Chile, 1965. Milbank Mem. Fd Quart., 48, 145–66.

HERZBERG, B. N. et al. (1970). Depressive symptoms and oral contraceptives. Brit. med. J., iv, 142–5.

HINES, D. C. et al. (1967). Side-effects in a large-scale study of an oral contraceptive agent. 5th World Congress on Fertility and Sterility. International Congress Series No. 133. Amsterdam, Holland.

HUSSAIN, M. Z. and MURPHY, J. (1971). Psychosis induced by oral contraception. *Canad. med. Ass. J.*, **104**, 984–6.

JUHLIN, L. and LIDEN, S. (1969). Influence of contraceptive gestogen pills on sexual behavior and the spread of gonorrhoea. *Brit. J. vener. Dis.*, **45**, 321–9.

KHAN, A. and WISHIK, S. M. (1965). The national intrauterine contraceptive device evaluation program of Pakistan. *Intrauterine contraception*. International Congress Series No. 86. Amsterdam, Holland.

KING, A. G. (1967). Selection of patients for the intrauterine contraceptive device. *Obstet. Gynec.*, **29**, 139–41.

MARSHALL, J. and ROWE, B. (1970). Psychological aspects of the basal body temperature method of regulating births. *Fertil. Steril.*, **21**, 14–19.

MASTERS, W. H. and JOHNSON, V. E. (1966). *Human sexual response*. Boston, Massachusetts.

MEAD, M. (ed.) (1955). *Cultural patterns and technical change*. New York.

——— (1949). *Male and female*. New York.

MEARS, E. (1967). Side effects of oral contraception. *5th World Congress on Fertility and Sterility*. International Congress Series No. 133. Amsterdam, Holland.

MELDMAN, M. J. (1964). Behavioural changes in the husbands of women treated with oral contraceptives. *Psychosomatics*, **5**, 188–9.

METZNER, R. J. and GOLDEN, J. S. (1967). Psychological factors influencing female patients in the selection of contraceptive devices. *Fertil. Steril.*, **18**, 845–56.

MURAWSKI, B. *et al.* (1968). An investigation of mood states in women taking oral contraceptives. *Fertil. Steril.*, **19**, 50–63.

ORCHARD, W. H. (1969). Psychiatric aspects of oral contraceptives. *Med. J. Aust.*, **56**, 872–6.

PEEL, J. and POTTS, M. (1969). *Textbook of contraceptive practice*. Cambridge, U.K.

PINCUS, G. (1966). Control of conception by hormonal steroids. *Science (N.Y.)*, **153**, 493–500.

POHLMAN, E. (1969*a*). *Psychology of birth planning*. Cambridge, Massachusetts.

——— (1969*b*). Premarital contraception: research reports and problems. *J. Sex. Res.*, **5**, 187–94.

RAINWATER, L. (1960). *And the poor get children*. Chicago, Illinois.

RODGERS, D. A. and ZIEGLER, F. J. (1968*a*). Social role theory, the marital relationship, and the use of ovulation suppressors. *J. Marr. Fam.*, **30**, 584–91.

——— and ——— (1968*b*). Changes in sexual behavior consequent to use of noncoital procedures of contraception. *Psychosom. Med.*, **30**, 495–505.

RODGERS, D. A. *et al.* (1965). Comparisons of nine contraceptive procedures by couples changing to vasectomy or ovulation suppression medication. *J. sex. Res.*, **1**, 87–96.

SANDBERG, E. C. and JACOBS, R. D. (1971). Pscyhology of the misuse and rejection of contraception. *Amer. J. Obstet. Gynec.*, **110**, 227–42.

SAXTON, G. A. and PIKE, M. C. (1969). Long-term effectiveness and acceptability of IUCD's in Uganda. *East Afr. med. J.*, **46**, 107–20.

WEARING, M. P. (1963). The use of norethindrone (2 mg) with mestranol (0·1 mg) in fertility control. *Canad. med. Ass. J.*, **89**, 239–41.

ZELL, J. R. and CRISP, W. E. (1964). A psychiatric evaluation of the use of oral contraceptives. *Obstet. Gynec.*, **23**, 657–61.

ZIEGLER, F. J. *et al.* (1968). Ovulation suppressors, psychological functioning, and marital adjustment. *J. Amer. med. Ass.*, **204**, 849–53.

ZIPPER, J. *et al.* (1965). Intrauterine contraception with the use of a flexible nylon ring: experience in Santiago de Chile. *Intrauterine Contraception*. International Congress Series No. 86. Amsterdam, Holland.

18. PSYCHOSOMATIC PROBLEMS ASSOCIATED WITH ORAL CONTRACEPTION

JOHAN CULLBERG

THE TWO UNCONNECTED ASPECTS OF ORAL CONTRACEPTION

To the individual consumer, the pill represents two different things which are very loosely connected: On one hand it is a synthetic hormone compound (usually a progestagen in combination with an oestrogen) with certain molecular structures, pharmacological properties, and physiological effects. On the other hand it is something which prevents sexuality from being followed by an unwanted child.

This means that there are two main questions in any discussion of mental problems of the pill, the differentiation of which is too often forgotten. First: do the hormones influence the mental state via pharmacological (endocrinological, physiological) actions in the organism? Secondly: what does it *mean* to a woman to take a pill cathected by the following promises: (1) sexual enjoyment and procreative function will be definitely separated; (2) sexual intercourse will be undisturbed by mechanical troubles (pessaries, condoms, etc.); (3) freedom to govern the personal future development and female role is made possible — at least in theory.

These two main aspects, the endocrine and the psychological, have only *one* thing in common — the round pill. Most of the literature on the mental effects of the pill, however, deals with a conglomerate of mental symptoms without separating them, which makes symptom frequencies vary from one investigation to the other.

The pitfalls of this lack of analysis are serious. They can perhaps be better understood if we take an example from quite another area. Take for example the analysis of the symptom of fainting in connection with watching television. The symptom could either be analysed within a neurological frame of reference, namely as caused a flicker-released epileptical seizure, or it could be caused by what the subject feels in connection with the particular programme, e.g. executions, torture scenes. The only common agent in these two causes is the television-apparatus and a very superficially described symptom, namely fainting.

I will here try to analyse mental reactions in connection with the pill from the three main viewpoints, beginning with the biological viewpoint and then discussing certain social and psychological aspects of taking the pill.

PHYSIOLOGICAL ACTIONS OF THE PILL UPON MENTAL FUNCTIONS

In order to study the mental effects of female sex hormones *per se*, three combinations of gestagen/oestrogen compounds and placebo tablets were given to 320 female volunteers in a randomized double-blind design (Cullberg 1972).

The medication was taken during 2 months, and the subjects mental status was investigated before and after the medication period. The subjects, who used non-oral contraceptives during the investigation, were all told that they were receiving either a weak 'female hormone' or a sugar pill. Thus the tablets were not introduced as oral contraceptives.

In the placebo group, comprising 76 women, the frequency of adverse mental symptoms was 18 per cent. Another equally large group which was given identical hormones as in a commercial pill showed a frequency of adverse mental symptoms of 32 per cent. This difference of 14 per cent is statistically significant ($p < 0.05$). The symptoms as a rule were quite mild, the most common complaints being irritability and a dysphoric mood. No difference of sexual drive was found between the groups.

The mental and somatic side-effects of the pill were generally reported to pass in 2–3 months. This is also illustrated in a prospective investigation on 100 women on the pill during 6 months, which showed that the frequency of mental symptoms at 6 months was not higher than before starting medication (Cullberg et al. 1969). This could partly also be explained by 6 per cent dropping out due to mental symptoms during the first months.

Several authors (Petersen 1969; Grant and Pryse-Davies 1968; Lewis and Hoghughi 1969) have reported their clinical impressions and also given some experimental evidence for regarding the progestagen component of the pill as responsible for the depressive reactions.

Several hypotheses have been advanced concerning the mental actions of oestrogens and progestagens. One of these hypotheses discusses the interference of oestrogen with abnormality in tryptophan metabolism (possibly through a Vitamin B_6 deficiency) after ingestion of an oral contraceptive (Price et al. 1967). (Tryptophan is a precursor to serotonin, which acts as a transmitter substance in the central nervous system.) In a double-blind crossover trial, it has also been possible to show that a group of depressed women on oral contraceptive responded clinically to the administration of Vitamin B$_6$ and not to placebo (Adams *et al.* 1973).

The described hormonal effects of the pill upon mental functions are usually mild and of a low frequency. There are clinical reports, however, that describe dramatic severe depressions, suicidal attempts, psychoses, etc. which are attributed to the pill. Such strong reactions might also have been caused by hormonal factors but occur so rarely that they were not registered in the investigation cited above.

I feel that the symbolic 'mental ingestion' usually gives a better clue towards the understanding of these mental reactions than the hormonal ingestion. 'The pill' very often becomes a scapegoat for emotional problems, either released by the specific problems connected with this contraceptive method, or existing before the pill but now displaced upon it. These aspects will be discussed later.

SOCIOLOGICAL ASPECTS OF THE PILL

I will here discuss the sociological aspects of the pill in Sweden only, since my knowledge about the problems in other countries is too small. The Swedish figures are probably representative for many other Western countries, with the possible exception that unmarried women use the pill to a higher degree in Sweden.

A report (Appelgren *et al.* 1972) was a part of a large '1968 level-of-living survey' of the Swedish people, gives some important information about differences between the pill-consumers versus the non-pill-consumers: 1808 women of fertile age, comprising a representative sample of the Swedish population, were asked, among many other questions in the interview, whether they had used the pill during the last 14-day period; 249 answered yes (14 per cent).

Some of the differences between the pill-using group and the non-using group are given below.

Social grouping. Higher social group showed a higher frequency of pill consumption. Social group 1 had one-third, group 2 one-fifth, and group 3 has one-seventh pill-consumers irrespective of age classes.

Urbanization. The more urbanized, the higher frequency of pill-use, except for social group 1 where no differences were found.

Civil status. As large a proportion of unmarried as of married women use the pill (i.e. about 14 per cent of each).

Religion. Pill-consumers go less frequently to church. This may also be an age-bound phenomenon, younger ages being more secularized.

Age. The pill is most used in the ages of 20–29 years, and accordingly it has been called 'the contraceptive of the young generation'.

Smoking. There is a large difference, with 22 per cent more smoking in the pill group. (This association with smoking is also reported in a large British survey (Kay *et al.* 1969).

Mental symptoms. Four per cent more respondents report 'nervous troubles' in the pill group (the difference is not significant) during the last 14-day period. There is no difference regarding depression or fatigue.

Headache. Sixty-three per cent complain of headache in the pill group against 54 per cent in the other group ($p < 0.05$). The difference lies mainly in the group 'severe headache'.

These findings tell us that pill consumers probably are not representative for the total group of fertile women in the society. They could, according to the authors, be said to be more inclined towards innovations of all kinds.

The figures regarding mental troubles in this sociological survey generally seem to be somewhat low (11 per cent reporting nervous troubles), and minor complaints might have passed unnoticed.

It is noteworthy that no clear differences regarding mental symptoms (tiredness, depression) could be found in the two groups.

The differences in frequency of headache and of general well-being are difficult to interpret. They could be regarded either as a consequence to the pill, or as a consequence to the smoking habits or other life habits among the pill consumers.

One conclusion is, however, that the pill consumers as a group differ from non-consumers in several respects. Reported differences regarding mental symptom in a population of pill consumers must therefore be interpreted carefully.

INTERPERSONAL ASPECTS OF THE PILL

A large interview survey of parents of boys in the latency age in Stockholm (Jonsson and Kälvesten 1964), showed that around 30 per cent of all mothers reacted negatively towards having sexual intercourse with their husbands. For these women and probably also their husbands, as for many other women and men, sexuality is a source not only of pleasure, but also, and sometimes more, of anger and anxiety. Here the troubles around a preoccupation with pessaries, condoms and other mechanical devices is a 'legitimate' way to escape from sexuality or at least to lessen the frequency of intercourse.

These hypotheses are supported by a prospective study (Cullberg *et al.* 1969) where those women who for different reasons stopped treatment, and who reported mental and sexual side-effects, were characterized by a lower sexual interest from the onset, and also by a lower feeling of security with the pill. This group must be vulnerable to the emotional challenges of the pill. One of these challenges is that the frequency of intercourse is raised, which is showed by many investigations.

Lidz (1969) and others have also pointed to the importance of interpersonal factors in marriage for understanding many of the cases of stopping using the pill or report of adverse mental reactions.

INTRAPSYCHIC ASPECTS OF THE PILL

Many authors agree about the importance of considering the unconscious fantasies evoked in individual women by the pill. Psychoanalysts are familiar with these problems which have been thoroughly discussed by Molinsky and Seiff (1967), Wittkower (1971), and others. I will not here go into any great detail discussing the different kinds of symbolic values which can be attributed to the pill. Only one rather common feature will be dealt with; the challenge against the sexual identity of certain women, which can not be called primarily neurotic in its clinical sense.

These women have a somewhat dramatic personal connection with their own body and with their bodily functions. They are rarely quite happy with the pill since the method is predominantly looked upon (quite correctly) as an act of chemical sterilization. This takes away their deeper feeling of legitimacy of sexuality and the separation between sex and procreation is perceived as a threat. They also feel 'castrated' by the contraceptive method. The pill here unconsciously becomes an enemy, evoking depression, sexual unresponsiveness, and also aggressiveness against the partner, who is looked upon as the deeper cause of the conflict. These women often experience an adverse reaction almost immediately after having swallowed the first tablet, and they feel great relief at the end of the medication period.

The severity of these psychological reactions can be quite impressive, but of course one can never say in the individual case that this is the only explanation for the reaction.

FINAL COMMENTS

In combination with the somatic side effects of the pill all the mental problems discussed here contribute to make the pill unsatisfactory for many women. (The so-called low-dose gestagens may be an alternative, though a disturbance of the menstrual rhythm will probably not be accepted.) The pill is also for several reasons not an acceptable method for many teenagers and for women with a low frequency of intercourse.

There is one final aspect of oral contraception which, as far as I can see, must seriously limit its use in under-privileged cultures. Probably every woman is somewhat anxious about what happens in her body when she takes the pill. She knows that she ingests something which blocks important physiological systems, but yet she wants to take the risk because of the advantages inherent in the method. Many women deny their fears. This conflict is not present with conventional, locally applied contraceptive methods. These act from the 'outside' and are never assimilated by the body which also never makes them important part of the individual's psychic system. In most cultures, 'oral incorporation' is deeply interwoven with the possibilities of magic influences upon the individual, in harmful or good directions. The oral contraceptive thus becomes an integrated part of the individual's psychological system (self-identity system) in the same time as it is a part of her physiological system. As was discussed in the introduction, these non-pharmacological effects are an integral part of taking the pill, and probably never quite disappear even with a high degree of sophistication in the consumer. Naturally these aspects must be even more accentuated in underprivileged parts of the world, where the tendencies towards superstition are probably greater than in our culture. This being the case, large-scale oral contraception programmes will for this and for other reasons probably never be completely successful, and 'external' contraceptives such as the IUD might become the contraceptive of choice for many women.

REFERENCES

ADAMS, P. W., ROSE, D. P., FOLKARD, J., WYNN, V., SEED, M., and STRONG, R. (1973). Effect of pyridoxine hydrochloride (Vitamin B₆) upon depression associated with oral contraception. *Lancet*, 897–904.

APPELGREN, B. and OLENMARK, U. (1972). 'Socialmedicinsk undersokning om P-pillerkonsumtionen i Sverige.' Social-medicinska Institutionen vid karolinske Institutet, Stockholm, Sweden.

CULLBERG, J. (1972). Mood changes and menstrual symptoms with different oestrogen/gestagen combinations. *Acta psychiat. Scand.*, Suppl. 236.

——, GELLI, M., and JONSSON, C.-O. (1969). Mental and sexual adjustment before and after six months' use of an oral contraceptive. *Acta psychiat. Scand.*, 45, 259–76.

GRANT, E. and PRYSE-DAVIES, J. (1968). Effect of oral contraceptives on depressive mood changes and on endometrial monoamine oxidase and phosphatases. *Brit. med. J.*, iii, 777–80.

JONSON, G. and KÄLVESTEN, A.-L. (1964). *222 Stockholm-*

spojkar. Uppsala, Sweden.

KAY, C. R., SMITH, A. and RICHARDS, B. (1969). Smoking habits of oral contraceptive users. *Lancet*, ii, 1228–9.

LEWIS, A. and HOGHUGHI, M. (1969). An evaluation of depression as side effect of oral contraceptives. *Brit. J. Psychiat.*, 115, 697–701.

LIDZ, R. (1969). Emotional factors in the success of contraception. *Fertil. Steril.*, 20, 761–71.

MOLINSKY, H. and SEIFF, M. (1967). Einige psychische Reaktionen bei der Einnahme von Ovulationshemmern. *Z. Psychother. med. Psychol.*, 17, 202–10.

PETERSEN, P. (1969). *Psychiatrische und psychologische Aspekte der Familienplanung bei Oraler Contraception.* Stuttgart, Germany.

PRICE, J. M., THORNTON, M. J., and MUELLER, L. (1967). Tryptophan metabolism in women using steroid hormones for ovulation control. *Amer. J. clin. Nutrit.*, 20, 452–6.

WITTKOWER, E. D. (1971). Some selected psychosomatic problems of current interest. *Psychosomatics*, 12, 21–9.

19. EQUALITY OF THE SEXES: SOCIAL AND PSYCHOLOGICAL IMPLICATIONS

BIRGITTA LINNÉR

INTRODUCTION

In Sweden, where the goal of equal sex roles for men and women has the endorsement of the Government and the backing of public opinion, new individual and family life styles are emerging. This chapter examines changes in the legal, political, economic, and social situations in Sweden, and explores the psychological problems and possibilities of a life in which men and women are equal. Special attention is given to the problems of men in the struggle to go beyond divided sex roles and achieve a new human role.

Within the context of three possible sex role systems—patriarchal, complementary, and equal — this chapter will describe Sweden's current climate of change, and explore the new family and life styles taking shape as the nation moves closer to equality between the sexes. Contributing to this climate are legal, economic, and social policy, government and education, and public attitudes.

Although the goal of sex equality in all areas of life is now widely accepted in Sweden, there is still a long way to go. Since no real changes can occur among women in isolation, the focus has broadened to include the situation of men and the question of 'men's emancipation'. The aim in Sweden is not for a male role or a female role, but for a basically human role.

The steps already taken in Sweden toward equality between the sexes have, of course, produced changes in the psychological relationship between men and women. These changes will be discussed in the areas of marriage and family life, divorce, child-rearing, the men's situation, and sex.

THE THREE SEX ROLE SYSTEMS

Patriarchal

In the traditional system, men are the providers of the family's needs, and as such are usually considered superior; women are economically dependent on — and supplemental to — men. Although such a system may be efficient within a family, it carries negative consequences for society.

Complementary

Men and women are regarded as equal, but emphasis remains on their basic differences: they polarize each other. It is a system to which many psychologists cling: Erik Erikson's concept of inner and outer space would seem to be an example. On the other hand, as Johan Cullberg (1970) a young psychiatrist at Stockholm's Karoline Hospital, has pointed out:

the stereotyped sex roles in our Western culture mean ... that masculinity implies activity, strength, emotional restraint, and dominance. Femininity is defined as passivity, weakness, sentimentality, and submission.... The man or woman who makes high demands on himself or herself to fulfill these role stereotypes, runs the risk of feeling chronically threatened in self-esteem and possibilities for sexual happiness.

Equality (the human role sytem)

This system acknowledges that differences between the sexes exist, but sees them as secondary, and rather uninteresting, and hold the view that human beings are much more alike than they are different. Thus, it should be possible not merely to balance male and female sex roles, but to create a new, flexible human role in which the same possibilities are open to men and women within the family, in the labour market, and in all other social situations.

LAWS AND SOCIAL POLICY

Sweden, in her legal recognition of equality of men and women within the family, stands in contrast to the astonishing number of countries that, although basically democratic, still embody the traditional leadership of the *pater familias* within their systems of law. It is impossible for a people to attain economic and emotional equality as long as the subordinate status of married women is maintained in their nation's laws.

The great changes in the structure of Swedish marriage and divorce laws occurred in the first decades of this century. The Marriage and Family Acts of 1915–20 abolished ties between church and civil laws regarding marriage and sex, and laid the groundwork for the more advanced reform efforts of recent years. They permitted a shift from the male-dominated, hierarchical family toward a family structure based on social and economic equality between husband and wife. Thus, today, if one partner stays at home, he or she is legally regarded as providing economic support for the family. Further, the law makes no distinction as to sex, so that the *hemmaman*, or house-husband, has been legally established in Sweden. Similarly, both partners are equally responsible for the guardianship of their children, and couples may voluntarily agree to divorce without guilt being assigned to either partner.

There have been no illegitimate children in Sweden since 1917, when that term for children born out of wedlock was banned from official usage. Every child born is legitimate. In 1970, the last vestige of discrimination against out-of-wedlock children was wiped out when they were granted equal paternal inheritance rights with other children. Social attitudes have kept pace with these legal advances. A 1969 report of a government survey (Swedish Department of Education 1969) showed that 99 per cent of the population feels that all children, born in or out of marriage, should have equal rights; 98 per cent feels that the community should treat unmarried mothers exactly as it treats married mothers; and 16 per cent further declares that since unwed mothers often face greater difficulty in child-rearing, they should be accorded special benefits.

Family planning has been a part of Sweden's public health and welfare programme since 1938. It is considered that couples have the right to decide whether and when to have children, and the duty of the government to provide counselling and information on contraceptive methods, as well as a fertility programme for those who want children. Also in 1938, therapeutic abortion was made legal (Trygg-Hansa/Swedish Institute 1975). (Today Sweden has one of the lowest rates of abortion in the world.)

Homosexuality between consenting adults has not been a criminal offence since 1944, and there is increasing social tolerance and understanding of divergent forms of sexual behaviour. In 1962, a new penal code allowed equal and open acceptance of sexuality for men and women, providing it is not damaging to either partner. Premarital sex has been legal for women as well as men since 1915, when a law dating from 1686 was abolished that had required women engaging in premarital sex to pay a penalty of two silver dollars, which went to maintain church property.

Sweden's legal and social policy contains a number of other provisions important to the establishment of equal sex roles. These points, which I have discussed in greater detail elsewhere (Linnér 1972), include an extensive programme of prenatal and postnatal care, as well as free delivery. The traditional 6 months' maternity leave with pay was changed in 1973 to include fathers, in a new parental insurance system (Millgårdh and Rollén 1975). Municipal day care, intended not as a substitute for the mother, but as an enrichment for the child; free public schools; equal pay for equal work (although this has not yet been accomplished in practice); and an individual income tax system that has supplanted the former joint, family tax system were also included.

PUBLIC ATTITUDES AND ACTIVITIES

Despite the enlightened laws enacted early in the century to improve the status of women and create equality in marriage, those in control of the institutions of society — the politicians and many of the religious leaders — were successful in maintaining the traditional family role system and the public's adherence to it. It was not until the 1960s that real debate, research, and reform exploded. In 1961, Eva Moberg opened a somewhat confused and emotional debate with the publication of an essay claiming that

as long as society demands a double role (work outside and inside the home) from women and a single role from men, equality can never be achieved. Responsibility for home and children must be shared by mother, father, and society, she said, calling for the introduction of the 'human role'. At the same time, the concept of 'sex role', originally used only by sociologists, was taken up by Swedish and Norwegian psychologists and other social scientists (Dahlström 1967). During the early 1960s, the 'woman question' was abandoned and replaced by the 'sex role question' that embodied the idea that the role of women could not be viewed separately from that of men.

In Sweden, it was not only the angry young rebels who challenged the validity of the traditional family system in the 1960s. Questions such as those explored in recent research by Harriet Holter (1970) on biological as opposed to cultural roots of sex differences, were taken up early and seriously by newspapers, magazines, radio, and television. Further, all major labour unions and political parties take the position that there should be equality between the sexes in all areas of life (Report 1971), and all agree that it is not a question of single reforms but of restructuring society.

In the mid-1960s, consideration was first given to the concept of male emancipation. Due to the imbalance in the traditional role system, men have taken on the entire burden of supporting the family, have been deprived of emotional contact with their children, and are weighed down with responsibility that often leads to serious physical and psychological disturbances. Men have a higher rate than women of ulcer problems, heart disease, early death, suicide, crime, and alcoholism.

The debate on equality between the sexes has become to some extent a political issue. Some believe that capitalism and the patriarchal society are close companions; one leading spokesman for this view maintains that the sex role movement of the 1960s has become watered down ideologically and has stagnated. Eva Moberg (1971) replied to this position as follows:

I have never claimed that there is no connection between capitalism and male-dominated society! There are ... many threads between them. But I do not believe that the one is a direct consequence of the other, or that socialism is any guarantee whatsoever against sex discrimination.... I believe that social conditions and the human psyche are interwoven into one another and ceaselessly influence one another reciprocally. That's why I also believe that — in the case of such a relatively open and free society as Sweden nonetheless is — society can be changed in crucial and profound ways through continuous reform work. A revolution on the other hand must wage constant warfare, after its dear victory ... *to preserve itself.*

For my part, I think it is unfortunate that the sex role question, an issue of basic human rights, be made mainly a political issue.

Group 8
Among Sweden's women's organizations currently striving for equality, one of the more prominent is

Group 8. It might be interesting to compare the goals and demands of Group 8 with those of women's liberation groups in the United States, in order to get some indication of the stages of development of the movement for equality in the two countries.

The Group 8 manifesto, which maintains that 'even if women manage to gain equality with men, they will not be free ... before men are also free', calls for: (1) the legal right to the same working conditions as men; (2) unemployment insurance and free adult education for all women who apply for but do not get work; (3) educational assistance for adult students, regardless of spouse's level of income; (4) laws protecting part-time personnel; (5) day care for all children between 6 months and 7 years old, backed by unemployment insurance for mothers who cannot work because of lack of nurseries; (6) free abortion, with the right — but not the obligation — to consult a social worker, and free contraceptives for men and women; and (7) the assignment of 25 per cent of all new housing to collectives.

GOVERNMENT

The Swedish government is quick to absorb and promote new attitudes arising out of public debate and economic, social, and medical research (Sandberg 1975). For example, the idea of men's emancipation was stressed by the government in a 1968 report to the United Nations on the Status of Women in Sweden (Sandlund 1968), probably the first time a government has taken the men's situation, as well as the women's, into official consideration:

A decisive and ultimately durable improvement in the status of women cannot be attained by special measures aimed at women alone; it is equally necessary to abolish the conditions which tend to assign certain privileges, obligations or rights to men. No decisive change in the distribution of functions and status ... between the sexes can be achieved if the duties of the male in society are assumed *a priori* to be unaltered. The aim of reform work in this area must be to change the traditional division of labour which tends to deprive women of the possibility of exercising their legal rights on equal terms. The division of functions ... between the sexes must be changed in such a way that both the man and the woman in a family are afforded the same practical opportunities of participating in both active parenthood and gainful employment.

Or, as expressed by the Prime Minister of Sweden in a speech about the emancipation of men (Palme 1970):

In modern society boys grow up practically wholly in a female world. At home they are as a rule taken care of by the mother. During the early school years their teachers consist entirely of female teachers. There is a risk that the boys, by means of TV, comic strips, and other mass media, create a false and exaggerated picture of what it means to be a man: Men are tough and hard-boiled wild-west heroes, agents, supermen, soldiers. Boys compensate for their lack of contact with ordinary men by looking upon the men of massmedia as their ideal. It should be possible to counteract these problems. Men should from the beginning have just as much contact with

their children as the women. And we should have both men and women as child nurses, kindergarten teachers, and primary school teachers.

The involvement of the marriage and family lawmakers in the present reforms to establish equality was admitted officially in August 1969, when the Minister of Justice, in a directive to the governmental commission established to overhaul the present family law (Kling 1969) said:

... legislation is one of the most essential instruments which society possesses for meeting ... people's desires or for channelling development into new paths.... The transition from old to new should be made with care and consideration for individual people, but there is no reason to abstain from using marriage and family legislation as one of several instruments in reform efforts toward a society where every adult individual can take responsibility for himself without being economically dependent on relatives and where equality between men and women is a reality.

There is interest in the equality process on the municipal, as well as the federal level. In my home town, Uppsala, Sweden, the programme of the Social Democrats includes improvement of child care facilities because (*Uppsala Nya Tidning* 1972):

A speedy expansion of childcare is an important means for increased equality between children from different home environments, between single and two-parent families, between high and low wage-earners, and between women and men.... A speedy expansion of day-care centers, led and controlled by the community, is needed to further guarantee all children security and stable care and to enable all parents, especially single and low income parents, to fend for themselves and to increase their standard of living by their own work.

EDUCATION

The educational system is one of the most important instruments in creating equality between the sexes, as it is in creating equality between different social, economic, and geographical groups. Sweden's 9-year comprehensive school, coeducational as is all other education and training (except military training), incorporates the ideas of emancipation from traditional sex roles. Since 1962, when the new school system was introduced, boys have been taught such traditionally feminine, role-dividing subjects as home economics, sewing, and childcare. Girls learn modern manual handicraft and other once exclusively masculine skills.

Textbooks are continually being revised and updated to promote the concept of equal sex roles in all areas of life. The latest curriculum, promulgated by the National Board of Education for the 1970s, is even more positive and progressive in regard to the sex role issue. Information on sex role questions will be provided in all grades and in various subjects. Pupils will be encouraged to discuss and question differences between men and women in terms of influence and salary, as well as in family life. This emphasis on equality will, of course, be included in teacher training (Vestin 1975).

In discussing these questions with students in the schools, I have found that boys and girls enjoy these themes; they feel the injustices that exist in society, and they are open for re-orientating themselves, both in professional life and in family life. In addition, the boys seem to be showing a new concern for the care of children.

RESEARCH ON EQUALITY

At a Scandinavian seminar for sex role research in the 1960s, sex differentiation and the effects of sex roles were studied in collaboration with colleagues from the other Scandinavian countries (Dahlström 1967). Various government agencies and universities are also conducting surveys (Liljeström, Fürst–Mellström, and Liljeström 1975).

At the university level, an extension course on sex roles at Uppsala University offers classes in, 'The fight for franchise in Sweden: in reality and literature', 'Men's roles in some modern Swedish literary works', and 'Is there sex discrimination in our academic textbooks?' In regard to the last, medical texts in obstetrics and gynaecology might well be singled out for their prejudices against women.

At Gothenburg University Library, there is a Woman's History archive, where research on the history of women and on modern sex role problems is collected and catalogued. University research projects in such areas as social anthropology, economic history, church history, literature, psychology, law, and sociology are included in the archive, as are labour union research and projects devoted to the sex role question.

NEW LIFE STYLES

Various types of family and co-operative living arrangements have become accepted in Sweden, including one-parent families, communes, and weekend marriages. A new trial marriage has evolved, in which a couple sets out to see if they can co-operate in everyday life, and if their relationship is emotionally solid enough for them to have children. Other young people may choose either legal or 'loyalty' marriages, whichever seems most suitable to their needs (Trost 1974).

Sweden's social welfare programme accepts different patterns of co-living and various family styles. In civil law, however, only registered marriages have been valid. Since many young people have adopted one of the new informal marital relationship patterns, a government commission was appointed to find forms for legalizing different marital and family styles. According to Sweden's Minister of Justice, 'The function of legislation in this connection is to solve practical problems, not to privilege one form of living together above others.' The Family Law Reform Commission suggested reforms and Parliament took certain steps in 1973 (Sandberg 1975). The Family Law Commission is still working to revise and improve family laws.

Since the new family concepts are of wide general interest, they are given cosiderable space in the nation's mass media. However, there are some who feel that more attention is needed. In a 1969 interview in the Stockholm newspaper *Expressen*, a woman who characterized her experiences in communal living as 'more love, less fear, less egoism', went on to say:

The practical problems are legion. No one builds communal family flats ... even though it would be economically profitable for society to invest in [them].... The communal family is simply not a common alternative yet, just as adoption is not a common alternative ... despite the fact that there are hundreds of thousands of children without parents. This is where the mass media have a responsibility, which they of course have shirked. A constructive debate, information and analysis could have made the communal family alternative of interest [to] city planners and architects, building firms, social scientists, and the ordinary man in the street.

PSYCHOLOGICAL ISSUES

With our society paving the way for equality, we must consider what a high degree of equality means for the psychodynamics of interpersonal relationships. I will discuss some aspects of the changing content of the man/woman relationship from the viewpoint of my experiences as a marriage counsellor.

MARITAL PROBLEMS

In the traditional marriage, the wife lives through her husband, demanding that he make her happy and give her status. He must be the breadwinner for the family. This unbalanced economic structure can easily create an unbalanced psychological structure, particularly observable at critical moments in the relationship.

For a couple with legal, economic, philosphical, and practical equality, there is available a new type of dynamic process with which to work through an emotional crisis. Each partner has his or her identity, and there is no need to place blame on one partner, as there tends to be in a superior/inferior relationship. The more role-fixated and unbalanced a relationship is, the more tempting it is to project one's own faults and frustrations onto one's partner, and to create guilt feelings. When there is equality and self-esteem, it is easier to accept one's own responsibility in a conflict and to find solutions humiliating to neither party. Of course, all problems do not disappear, but the possibilities of working them out are greater when the man and woman are equal.

Divorce

False dependency easily leads to neurotic crisis situations, especially in divorce, where there is often much bitterness, aggressiveness, anxiety, and guilt. With equality between the spouses and with a rational law system that accepts divorce between consenting adults, the possibilities for psychological destruction during the divorce proceedings are greatly reduced.

If the divorce occurs between equals, the children have a better chance of being able to love both parents. Though the marriage has failed, there is no need for the partners to point at each other as guilty, cruel or unfaithful. If marriage is to be a meaningful psychological relationship, not merely an economic arrangement, simpler divorce laws entailing less dramatic proceedings are a definite requirement. When divorce is no longer considered a crime, but merely a rational means of dissolving a contract, then there will be possibilities for mature dissolutions of bad marriages.

Children

Female and male identity, long tied rigidly to the bearing and supporting of children, is finally being freed from these traditional roles. In fact, young people today often decide not to have children, or to adopt them, rather than add to an already overpopulated world. But what about the effects of the new, equal family upon the children? Is the child made insecure when the father does the housework and the childcare? Or when the parents share the duties, both at home and in the labour market? Will there emerge a new sex-identity, or a lack of such identity, among the children of these modern parents? There are many such unanswered questions. But, as one child psychologist recently put it to me, it is difficult to believe that identification with more harmonious and mature adult personalities will not have positive consequences for the children. We may get new personality types, but why be afraid of that?

Since young people today openly accept equal sexuality, they are better able to make candid and reasoned decisions as to whether or not to have children. Married women are no longer under the social pressures they once were to have children, more or less automatically. Modern contraceptive techniques also help to realize this healthier and more mature approach, in which having a baby is now more often an accurate reflection of mutual emotional desire on the part of the couple concerned. This freedom of choice is an indication of greater maturity, and children are less likely to be used as outlets for marital frustrations.

Men

What happens to the man as the new equality threatens the bastion of his supremacy? What happens when the decision-making positions in business and politics are no longer reserved exclusively for men, but are open to the qualified regardless of sex? When it is no longer taken for granted that the man is the erotic initiative-taker, and the one who makes the important family decisions and is thereby released from common household chores? How will he manage, how will he take it emotionally?

Certainly, in this transitional stage, there are problems for men. Having been brought up in a male-oriented society, men do not dare to share emotions and closeness with women on equal terms. The solu-

tion lies in women and men together conceptualizing what mutuality in a personal relationship means. We have to remember that, as women have been deprived of responsibility in society, men have been deprived emotionally, and have therefore been prone to stagnate as emotional beings.

It is interesting to observe how young men absorb the new male emancipation, as the society begins to move in a direction in which it will not be demeaning to the man to do housework or childcare. Expectant fathers are now taking part in childcare courses. More and more hospitals are allowing fathers to be present and assist in the delivery of their children, and many of these young fathers are experiencing new depths of emotion during the experience. There is also the new parental insurance system (Millgårdh and Rollén 1975), giving fathers the opportunity to share the responsibility at home for the baby in its first 6 months of life, and also for a sick child who needs one parent to stay at home for a few days. Thus, increasingly, men seem to like taking part in childcare and the practical and emotional responsibility of bringing up children.

Family life

One of the most frequent questions raised is whether the new equality will destroy family life. It is important to emphasize that flexibility does not mean a break-down of family structure. As one couple living as a new 'equality-family' put it, if family structure means that the woman cleans the house and caters to the man, then our family has broken down. But, they add, for us this new family style means more harmonious and creative interrelations, wider range of common interests and communications, and greater chance for fulfilment in family life (Linnér 1975).

Thus, with the emphasis of family life on full, all-around development of the individual, the new equality offers better grounds for a healthy start in life for children, and for enriched stable relations between man and woman.

Sex

Masters and Johnson have given scientific validity to facts that were hidden or ignored for centuries, as society denied women the rights to their own sexuality. The demonstration that women are capable of sexual pleasure and satisfaction to the same degree as men will be very important in changing the rigid attitudes toward women's sex life, and meaningful in leading to more harmonious, equal relationships in the future (Linnér 1973).

Under the new equal role system, sexual satisfaction carries less guilt and becomes more meaningful and enjoyable than previously. When a couple has good sex relations, infidelity becomes correspondingly less interesting and tempting. A publication (Report 1971) of the government's Commission for Sex Education proposed as a basic sex education ethic that men's and women's sex behaviour must be judged equally, and that all reasoning based on women not being equal to men must be dismissed.

CONCLUSION

Sweden found a champion for the cause of women's emancipation as early as 1793 in the poet Thomas Thorild, whose essay on 'The natural dignity of the female sex' upheld women's right to be regarded, first of all, as human beings, and only secondly as females.

Now, nearly 200 years later, there is still much to be done. But a dynamic process of change is under way. What I have tried to show, if only sketchily, is that this movement toward equality between man and woman is to noone's detriment, and to everyone's benefit. The aim is for a new role-balance allowing greater personal independence and integrity, and opening new possibilities for mature and harmonious relationships. As men and women continue to free themselves from misconceptions about the other sex, we will begin to evolve a more human society for both.

REFERENCES

CULLBERG, J. (1970). 'Medical aspects of gender identity.' Paper presented at seminar on Planned Parenthood and Sex Education in Sweden, April 1970. Division of Population and Family Welfare, Swedish International Development Authority, Stockholm.

DAHLSTRÖM, E. (ed.) (1967). *The changing roles of men and women.* London.

HOLTER, H. (1970). *Sex roles and social structure.* Oslo.

KLING, H. (1969). Statement by the Minister of Justice for the Family Law Reform Committee. Ministry of Justice. Stockholm.

LILJESTRÖM, R., FÜRST-MELLSTRÖM, G., LILJESTRÖM, S. G. (1975). *Sex roles in transition.* A report on a plot program in Sweden. Advisory Council on Equality between Men and Women/Swedish Institute, Stockholm.

LINNÉR, B. (1972). *Sex and society in Sweden.* New York.

—— (1973). *Equality — in society, in family, in bed.* In Advances in the Biosciences 10. Oxford.

—— (1975). 'Equality and the psychodynamics of interpersonal relationship.' Paper delivered at the International Women's Year Tribune in Mexico City. (Mimeo)

MILLGÅRDH, M. and ROLLÉN, B. (1975). Parent's insurance. *Current Sweden*, No. 76. Stockholm.

MOBERG, E. (1971). *VI-Magazine* No 3. Stockholm.

SANDBERG, E. (1975). *Equality is the goal.* A Swedish report to the U.N. International Women's Year 1975. Advisory Council on Equality between Men and Women, Stockholm.

SANDLUND, M.-B. (1968). *The status of women in Sweden.* Report to the United Nations.

REPORT (1971). *Towards equality. The Alva Myrdal report to the Social Democratic Party.* Stockholm.

TRYGG-HANSA/SWEDISH INSTITUTE (1975). *Social benefits in Sweden.* Stockholm.

SWEDISH DEPARTMENT OF EDUCATION (1969). *Om sexuallivet i Sverige* [on sex life in Sweden]. Sex Education Commission Offical Reports, SOU 1969:2

TROST, J. (1974). *Married and unmarried cohabitation: the case of Sweden, with some comparisons.* Department of Sociology, Uppsala University, Sweden.

PALME, O. (1970). The sex role problem. An extract from a lecture entitled 'The emancipation of man.' Hertha 1975:2. The Fredrika Bremer Association, Sweden.

UPPSALA NYE TIDNING (1972). 2 April.

VESTIN, M. (1975). *A free choice.* Sex roles studies — equality programme for schools. The National Board of Education, Stockholm. (Mimeo)

20. SEX DIFFERENCES IN REACTIONS TO PSYCHOSOCIAL STRESSORS AND PSYCHOACTIVE DRUGS

MARIANNE FRANKENHAEUSER

BIOCHEMICAL EVENTS, STRESS, AND ADJUSTMENT

Man, as other living organisms, shows remarkable plasticity in adjusting to his physical and social environments. Today's knowledge of the mechanisms underlying this plasticity firmly supports the conclusion that behaviours of all kinds are related to the dynamics of an organism's internal biochemical environment. Accepting this concept, it is still a most difficult task to specify which among the thousands of biochemical changes that characterize every moment of the individual's life are involved in any aspect of behaviour, and what the mechanisms of involvement really are. The task becomes even more complex when it is related to problems of 'biochemical individuality', i.e. differences between individuals with regard to specific biochemical changes induced by different stimuli in the physical and psychosocial environment. This chapter is concerned with one particular aspect of interindividual differences in biochemical changes, namely sex differences in adreno-medullary function as related to various factors in the external and internal environment.

In healthy individuals, exposure to conditions involving stress and strain is generally accompanied by an increased release of adrenalin from the adrenal medulla. The rise in circulating adrenalin brings about a series of changes in, for example, cardio-vascular and metabolic functions, all of which serve to mobilize the organism's resources so as to increase effectiveness under conditions which require intense physical effort. Recent research (reviewed by Frankenhaeuser (1971a, 1971b, 1975)) shows that adrenalin does not act only as an 'emergency hormone' under conditions involving physical challenge but, in addition, this hormone plays an important part in psychological stress and coping behaviour. In general, adrenalin facilitates psychological adjustment and enhances behavioural effectiveness. Noradrenalin, a transmittor substance which is chemically closely related to adrenalin, is also influenced by conditions affecting behaviour, although in a less consistent way.

The greater part of the investigations concerned with relationships between adrenalin secretion and behavioural functions has been carried out on male subjects. Therefore, currently accepted views concerning the role played by adrenalin in stress and adjustment have been based mainly on data obtained in the study of male subjects.

It has generally been assumed that — when adrenalin excretion is expressed in relation to body weight —
there is no difference in excretion rate between the sexes (e.g. Kärki 1956; Lambert et al. 1969). However, the data reported in this chapter show a somewhat different picture, suggesting that differences do in fact exist between males and females with regard to adrenalin release during certain psychosocial and psychopharmacological conditions. In view of the important part played by adrenalin in stress and adjustment a possible difference between the sexes is of considerable interest.

THE TYPICAL PATTERN OF ADRENALIN SECRETION IN MALES

Studies of healthy male subjects show that the rate of adrenalin secretion, as measured by its urinary excretion (Euler and Lishajko 1961), is generally low during rest. Under ordinary daily activities these measures of biochemical activity are about twice as high. During moderately stressful conditions the levels rise to between three and five times the resting levels, while severe physical and mental stressors may induce even more pronounced increases.

In male subjects, situations characterized by novelty, anticipation, uncertainty, and change produce a rise in adrenalin excretion, the magnitude of which is closely related to the intensity of the subjective stress reactions evoked. It is of special interest that this relation is typical only of situations in which the subject acts as a passive recipient of stressful stimuli. By contrast, when a subject is trying to cope actively with the stressor the intensities of both his emotional and endocrine responses are influenced by his success in mastering the situation (Frankenhaeuser and Rissler 1970). Although adrenalin excretion provides a sensitive index of the intensity of an emotional reaction, it is not related to the quality of the emotion: both pleasant and unpleasant emotions are accompanied by increased adrenalin output (Levi 1965, 1972; Pátkai 1971). It is significant that when relations between adrenalin output and personality variables are studied, individuals who secrete relatively more adrenalin tend to be emotionally and socially better adjusted than those who secrete less.

Experimental analyses of human performance have also been revealing. Male subjects who excrete relatively more adrenalin perform better under conditions of understimulation, while those with lower excretion rates are superior when overstimulation occurs (Frankenhaeuser et al. 1971). High rates of excretion are also associated with better performance in terms of speed, accuracy, and endurance when working under low or moderate stimulation, while the opposite tendency holds with high stimulation. Relationships between noradrenalin and performance are similar although less consistent. Thus, there appears to be an inverted-U relation between behavioural efficiency and bio-catecholamine arousal.

ADRENO-MEDULLARY REACTIVITY IN FEMALES

Systematic studies of adrenalin excretion in females are scarce, and the results obtained so far permit only tentative conclusions. However, some characteristic features are beginning to emerge. One reason why males are generally preferred as subjects in experimental research is the variability of biological processes related to the menstrual cycle in women. Some endocrine and metabolic functions, for example, show pronounced variability during different phases of the cycle and these physiological changes are accompanied by changes in mood and general arousal. In view of these fluctuations in functions associated with arousal level one would expect adrenalin excretion — which in males has proved to be a sensitive indicator of sympathetic and behavioural arousal — to vary during the different phases of the cycle. However, results from recent studies (Pátkai et al. 1974; Silbergeld et al. 1971) suggest that adrenalin as well as noradrenalin excretion remain relatively constant in one and the same subject during the different phases of the menstrual cycle. Self-reports showed that pre-menstrual tension was not reflected in adrenalin excretion. Hence, the data now available show that adrenalin excretion is not a particularly sensitive indicator of the fluctuations in mood and arousal occurring during the menstrual cycle.

Another interesting example of low adreno-medullary reactivity in females in different emotional states is provided in a study reported by Levi (1972) in which different film programmes, e.g., sexually arousing films, and films dealing with different forms of violence, and with romantic themes, were used to induce different emotional states. The assumption that strongly arousing films would produce an increase in adrenalin excretion was supported in some cases, while on other occasions a rather surprising lack of adreno-medullary response was noted.

The overall picture may be tentatively interpreted as indicating that adreno-medullary activity is a less sensitive indicator of behavioural arousal in women than in men.

SEX DIFFERENCES IN RESPONSE TO PSYCHOSOCIAL STRESSORS

In some recent studies of biochemical stress reactions, males and females have been examined under the same conditions, which makes possible a direct comparison. The outcome of these studies, which will be reported below, supports the assumption that men and women differ in their adrenalin response to psychosocial stressors. Consistent sex differences in noradrenalin output have not been demonstrated.

It should be noted that, when body weight is taken into account, there is no indication of a difference between males and females in adrenalin excretion under conditions of inactivity and rest (e.g. Lambert et al. 1969). The fact that adreno-medullary function in men and women tends to be the same under resting conditions may have contributed to forming the generally prevailing view that there is no difference between the sexes in this particular function. However, data are now available which show that a different picture is obtained when the sexes are compared under psychosocial conditions involving mental strain.

An investigation was performed on a group of 12-year-old boys and girls, sampled from a longitudinal study on behaviour and adjustment (Magnusson, Dunér, and Zetterblom 1975). The children's adrenalin excretion was measured under a 'passive' period and an 'active' period (Johansson, Frankenhaeuser, and Magnusson 1973). The passive period was spent by the children viewing a non-engaging and emotionally 'neutral' film on iron-ore mining. During the active period the children performed an attention-demanding arithmetic task. In the group of girls the adrenalin excretion was only slightly higher in the active as compared with the passive condition. The boys, however, excreted significantly more adrenalin during the active than during the passive period (Fig. 20.1). Thus, the difference between the sexes was slight and nonsignificant in the passive condition, but during work the boys excreted significantly more adrenalin than the girls (for a detailed report, see Johansson (1972)).

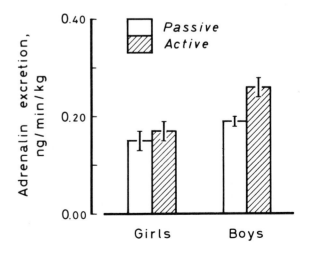

Fig. 20.1. Means and standard errors for adrenalin excretion, expressed in relation to body weight, in 12-year-old girls and boys during a passive and an active period. (Johansson 1972.)

Among both sexes, adrenalin 'increasers', i.e. those who increased their secretion during work as compared with the preceding passive period, performed better than adrenalin 'decreasers' throughout the work session. The girls' performance in the task was significantly better than the boys' in the terms of accuracy.

The next step was to compare adult men and women employees in a Swedish metal industry (Johansson and Post 1974). Measurements of adrenalin excretion were obtained while the subjects were engaged in their ordinary routine activities, and while they performed an intelligence test. The subjects' routine jobs were of different kinds, office work or work of assembly-line type being the most common. Intelligence was measured by a factor test of verbal, spatial, inductive, and numerical ability. The results were similar to those obtained in the study of children (Fig. 20.2). In the group of women adrenalin excretion was about the same when they performed the intelligence test as during daily routine activity. In contrast, the male subjects increased their adrenalin output significantly when they were required to perform the intelligence test. Thus, the men excreted significantly more adrenalin than the women in the test session. There was no sex difference in noradrenalin excretion. Nor did the sexes differ in their performance on the intelligence test. There was, however, a significant sex difference in neuroticism, as measured by Eysenck's personality inventory, women having higher scores than men. This is in agreement with results from other investigations in which neuroticism has been assessed by the same inventory.

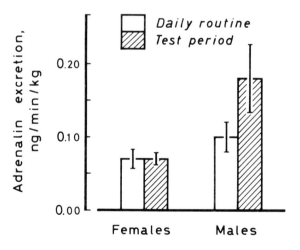

FIG. 20.2. Means and standard errors for adrenalin excretion, expressed in relation to body weight, in adult female and male subjects during daily routine activities and during intelligence testing. (Johansson and Post 1974.)

In view of the fact that the females performed equally well or slightly better than the males in both these studies, it did not appear likely that the larger

adrenalin release of the males was associated with a more intense effort. Nor is there any empirical support for the commonly held view that the prevailing sex-role pattern would tend to make mental work under time pressure a more challenging experience for males than for females (cf. Maccoby and Jacklin 1974, p. 135 *et seq.*). A possibility which should be examined is that females tend to respond by adrenalin release to specific stressors only, whereas in males this is the common response to *any* kind of stressor.

To examine this possibility, a study was designed (Frankenhaeuser, Dunne, and Lundberg 1976) in which males and females were compared under conditions which differed with regard to the nature of the stressor to which they were exposed. Interest was focussed on male and female reactions to two situations, in one of which the subject played a passive, in the other an active role. In the passive situation stress was induced by repeated venipuncture, a procedure which is generally considered moderately stressful by members of both sexes. In the active situation, the subjects performed a cognitive task (based on Stroop's colour/word conflict test), which is known to elicit arousal reactions in males (Frankenhaeuser and Johansson, 1976). Catecholamine excretion, heart rate, and subjective reactions were measured. Control values were obtained under conditions of relaxation in the laboratory.

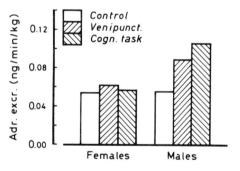

FIG. 20.3. Mean adrenalin excretion, expressed in relation to body weight, in female and male university students during a control condition, during repeated venipuncture, and during a cognitive task. (Frankenhaeuser, Dunne, and Lundberg 1976.)

The results showed that subjects of both sexes responded to both stressors by increased heart rate and feelings of unpleasantness and distress. The pattern of adrenalin excretion, however, differed between sexes as shown in Fig. 20.3. In the male group both stressors induced a significant adrenalin increase, whereas in the female group excretion remained on the same level under the two stress conditions as during relaxation. Noradrenalin excretion was not systematically affected by either stressor in either sex group. With regard to performance on the cognitive test, the female group was slightly, but not significantly, superior.

SEX DIFFERENCES IN REACTIONS
TO PSYCHOACTIVE DRUGS

In view of the important part played by adrenalin in adjustment to everyday stress situations it is interesting that drugs in common use modify the rate of excretion. In general, barbiturates and tranquillizers, taken orally in clinical doses, decrease adrenalin excretion while, for example, caffeine, nicotine, and alcohol have the opposite effect. At least in respect of reactions to alcohol there appears to be a sex difference.

In a recent series of experiments (Myrsten, Hollstedt, and Holmberg 1975) reactions to *alcohol* in male and female students were compared. It was shown that a moderate dose of alcohol, 0·72 g per kg body weight, taken as whisky (2 ml per kg), produced significantly higher peak blood alcohol values in females. This sex difference is probably related to the higher percentage of body fluid in males (cf. Wallgren and Barry 1970).

Self-estimates of wakefulness and mood during intoxication differed between the sexes. Thus, pleasant mood effects generally associated with moderate alcohol intake such as feeling happy and relaxed, were more pronounced among the male subjects while negative effects such as feeling irritated and tired were more pronounced among the females (Fig. 20.4).

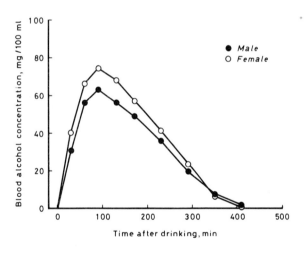

FIG. 20.4. Self-estimates of wakefulness and mood during alcohol intoxication in male and female subjects. (Myrsten, Hollstedt, and Holmberg 1975.)

Measures of catecholamine output showed that adrenalin excretion was significantly higher in female subjects in a control condition, which was identical with the alcohol condition except for alcohol intake (Fig. 20.5). In the alcohol condition, however, adrenaline excretion was significantly higher in female subjects. There was no marked difference in nor-adrenalin output between the sexes in either condition.

It is likely that the females' higher blood alcohol level as well as their more intense feelings of unpleas-

antness both contributed to the relatively larger adrenalin release in the female group. It is also possible that there is a sex difference in effects of alcohol *per se* on adreno-medullary activity. On the basis of the present experiments it is not possible to choose between these alternative interpretations. It is interesting to note that results from earlier studies (Frankenhaeuser *et al.* 1974; Wallgren and Tirri 1963) indicate that psychological stress may reduce alcohol intoxication and that more aroused subjects tend to show a greater resistance to alcohol-induced impairment of performance than less aroused subjects. Thus, the greater resistance to alcohol of female as compared with male subjects which has been demonstrated in animal experiments (Wallgren 1959) may be associated with a higher level of behavioural arousal in females. The suggestion has been made (Leikola 1962) that the decreased sensitivity of the central nervous system to alcohol during stress might be mediated by the release of adrenalin from the adrenal medulla.

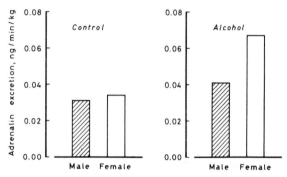

FIG. 20.5. Mean values for adrenalin excretion, expressed in relation to body weight, in male and female subjects after alcohol intake and in a control condition. (Myrsten, Hollstedt, and Holmberg 1975.)

Nicotine acts as a stimulant when taken in small and moderate doses, whereas large doses may have depressant effects. It is commonly believed that people use the nicotine in tobacco to produce either an increase or a decrease in their arousal level. The increase in arousal induced by smoking is reflected in elevated levels of adrenalin excretion. There appears to be no sex difference in adreno-medullary reactions to nicotine (Myrsten and Frankenhaeuser, unpublished).

In general, people tend to have a greater desire to smoke in low-arousal situations, which is consistent with nicotine acting as a stimulant. However, a marked sex difference in the tobacco-smoking habit has been demonstrated, indicating that men tend to have the highest desire to smoke in situations inducing boredom and tiredness, while women experience their most intense craving for cigarettes in stress-inducing situations. This sex difference was first demonstrated by Frith (1971) in a study of British men and women, and has later been verified in a study of Swedish male and female students (Elgerot, in preparation). It appears that tobacco smoking provides a tool by which arousal level can easily be modified, and that women and men tend to use this tool to obtain different — sometimes even opposite — effects.

COMMENTS AND CONCLUSIONS

The studies outlined in this chapter serve to illustrate how the problem of sex differences in reactions to psychosocial stressors and psychoactive drugs may be approached by experimental methods in the laboratory. By such methods it has been possible to examine interactions between the organism's biochemical state and exposure to specific psychosocial or psychopharmacological influences. On the one hand we find a close similarity in the adreno-medullary function of males and females — both adults and children — under conditions of rest, relaxation, and routine activity. On the other hand there is a distinct sex difference in adrenalin release under psychosocial stress conditions, males being more reactive than females. With regard to drug effects, our data suggest a greater susceptibility of adreno-medullary activity to alcohol in females.

It is interesting to speculate about the implications of the data from many different sources indicating that females do not show the same degree of readiness as males to respond by adrenalin release to emotionally arousing stimuli. This appears to be true regardless of whether the situation requires active effort or passive acceptance. The data so far available show no indication of reduced adaptive capacity in females under conditions of low adreno-medullary reactivity. This suggests that the endocrine mechanisms involved in coping are to some extent different in males and females. Studies of individual differences among women may throw light on the mechanisms underlying this sex difference. Such studies are under way (Frankenhaeuser and Collins, in preparation). We have already obtained some striking data from female members of our research team, showing a very high adrenalin release under conditions of intense examination stress.

A tentative hypothesis, on which ongoing investigations are based, is that the tendency to respond by adrenalin release to requirements of the psychosocial environment is linked, not to sex *per se*, but to a behaviour pattern which is more common in males in Western Society. Type-A behaviour, i.e., a behaviour pattern which is implicated in the aetiology of coronary heart disease (Friedman 1969) seems to answer this description. Its characteristic features — hard-driving competitiveness, a sense of time urgency, involvement in multiple activities having deadlines, a strong need to be in control of life events — are all likely to be products of attitudes, expectations, and pressures of the early environment. Hence, one might speculate about the possibility that the current change in sex-role patterns will lead to a growing proportion of type-A women. This, in turn, may lead to a decrease of the sex difference in catecholamine secretion and a concomitant decrease in the difference between the sexes in their susceptibility to diseases associated with the action of peripheral catecholamines.

By and large, readiness to respond to threat and strain by increased adrenalin secretion appears to bring short-term gains and long-term risks. The fact that women do not appear to mobilize adrenalin with the same readiness as men might mean that women live more 'economically'. These and other differences in the biochemical mechanisms mediating stress reactions might contribute to the longer life-span of women.

It still remains to be determined under what conditions adrenalin secretion in males and females, respectively, should be regarded as a desirable adaptive function and when it should be considered a potential harmful response. The answer may depend partly upon the time course of the secretion. A rapid return of adrenalin output to baseline values after cessation of the stressor is probably indicative of good adjustment, while a slow return means poor adjustment in the sense that the organism 'over-responds' by mobilizing resources that are no longer required to meet the demands of the environment. We already know that there are large interindividual differences in the time taken for adrenalin output to return to baseline level after exposure to stress (Johansson and Frankenhaeuser 1973), but we do not yet know whether males and females differ in this respect.

SUMMARY

In this chapter experimental approaches to the problem of sex differences in reactions to psychosocial stressors and psychoactive drugs are illustrated by data from studies of the adreno-medullary function in healthy males and females under different conditions. The outcome of these studies suggests that while adrenalin secretion in males and females does not differ under conditions of rest, relaxation, and routine activity, males show a greater readiness to respond by adrenalin release when exposed to different stressors. It therefore appears that the biochemical mechanisms involved in the coping process are at least partly different in men and women. Possible short-term advantages and long-term risks associated with adrenalin mediated adjustment to the psychosocial environment are discussed.

REFERENCES

EULER, U. S. V. and F. LISHAJKO, F. (1961). Improved technique for the fluorimetric estimation of catecholamines.

Acta physiol. scand., **51**, 348–55.

FRANKENHAEUSER, M. (1971a). Experimental approaches to

the study of human behaviour as related to neuroendocrine functions. In *Society, stress, and disease* (ed. L. Levi), Vol. I, pp. 22–35. London.

—— (1971*b*). Behavior and circulating catecholamines. *Brain Res.*, **31**, 241–62.

—— (1975). Experimental approaches to the study of catecholamines and emotion. In *Emotions — their parameters and measurement* (ed. L. Levi), pp. 209–34. Raven Press, New York.

—— and RISSLER, A. (1970). Effects of punishment on catecholamine release and efficiency of performance. *Psychopharmacologia (Berl.)*, **17**, 378–90.

—— and JOHANSSON, G. (1976). Task demand as reflected in catecholamine excretion and heart rate. *J. Human Stress*, **26**, 15–23.

——, NORDHEDEN, B., MYRSTEN, A.-L., and POST, B. (1971). Psychophysiological reactions to understimulation and overstimulation. *Acta Psychol.*, **35**, 298–308.

——, DUNNE, E., BJURSTRÖM, H., and LUNDBERG, U. (1974). Counteracting depressant effects of alcohol by psychological stress. *Psychopharmacologia (Berl.)*, **38**, 271–8.

——, ——, and LUNDBERG, U. (1976). Sex differences in sympathetic-adrenal medullary reactions induced by different stressors. *Psychopharmacology*, **47**, 1–5.

FRITH, C. D. (1971). Smoking behavior and its relation to the smokers' immediate experience. *Brit. J. soc. clin. Psychol.*, **10**, 73–8.

JOHANSSON, G. (1972). Sex differences in the catecholamine output of children. *Acta physiol. scand.*, **85**, 569–72.

—— and FRANKENHAEUSER, M. (1973). Temporal factors in sympatho-adrenomedullary activity following acute behavioural activation. *Biol. Psychol.*, **1**, 63–73.

—— and POST, B. (1974). Catecholamine output of males and females over a one-year period. *Acta. physiol. scand.*, **92**, 557–65.

——, FRANKENHAEUSER, M., and MAGNUSSON, D. (1973). Catecholamine output in school children as related to performance and adjustment. *Scand. J. Psychol.*, **14**, 20–8.

KÄRKI, N. T. (1956). The urinary excretion of noradrenalin and adrenalin in different age groups, its diurnal variation and the effect of muscular work on it. *Acta physiol. scand.*, **39**, Suppl. No. 132.

LEIKOLA, A. (1962). Effect of stress on alcohol intoxication in rats. *Quart. J. Stud. Alc.*, **23**, 369–75.

LAMBERT, W. W., JOHANSSON, G., FRANKENHAEUSER, M., and KLACKENBERG-LARSSON, I. (1969). Catecholamine excretion in young children and their parents as related to behavior. *Scand. J. Psychol.*, **10**, 306–18.

LEVI, L. (1965). The urinary output of adrenalin and noradrenalin during pleasant and unpleasant emotional states. *Psychosom. Med.*, **27**, 80–5.

—— (1972). Stress and disease in response to psychosocial stimuli. *Acta. med. scand.*, **191**, Suppl. No. 528.

MACCOBY, E. E. and JACKLIN, C. N. (1974). *The pscyhology of sex differences.* Stanford, California.

MAGNUSSON, D., DUNÉR, A., and ZETTERBLOM, G. (1975). *Adjustment: a longitudinal study.* Stockholm, New York.

MYRSTEN, A.-L., HOLLSTEDT, C., and HOLMBERG, L. (1975). Alcohol-induced changes in mood and activation in males and females as related to catecholamine excretion and blood-alcohol level. *Scand. J. Psychol.*, **16**, 303–10.

PÁTKAI, P. (1971). Catecholamine excretion in pleasant and unpleasant situations. *Acta Psychol.*, **35**, 352–63.

——, JOHANSSON, G., and POST, B. (1974). Mood, alertness, and sympathetic-adrenal medullary activity during the menstrual cycle. *Psychosom. Med.*, **36**, 503–12.

SILBERGELD, S., BRAST, N., and NOBLE, E. B. (1971). The menstrual cycle: a double-blind study of symptoms, mood and behavior, and biochemical variables using Enovid and placebo. *Psychosom. Med.*, **33**, 411–28.

WALLGREN, H. (1959). Sex differences in ethanol tolerance of rats. *Nature (Lond.)*, **184**, 726–7.

—— and BARRY, H. III (1970). *Actions of alcohol.* Amsterdam.

—— and TIRRI, R. (1963). Studies of the mechanism of stress-induced reduction of alcohol intoxication of rats. *Acta pharmacol. toxicol.*, **20**, 27–38.

SESSION 3

Psychiatric and psychosomatic diseases possibly associated with male/female roles and relationships

21. PATHOGENIC ASPECTS OF SEX ROLES AND RELATIONSHIPS: EPIDEMIOLOGICAL CONSIDERATIONS

AUBREY KAGAN

INTRODUCTION

In Chapter 1 I discussed and defined the parts of a concept of how social situations can give rise to psychological stimuli which, according to the individual's psychobiological programme, may give rise to mechanisms that will lead to precursors of disease or disease (Fig. 1.1, p. 3). In that chapter, I speculated that social change in sexual relations, reproduction, child-rearing, mutual care, and work and community roles, interacting with aspects of the psychobiological programme common to most human beings — high sexuality, strong tendency to pair bonding and male dominance — were likely to produce psychobiological stimuli that might lead to disease.

Psychological stimuli likely to be important, as mentioned in Chapter 1, are threat, ambiguity or difference between expectation and perceived situation in relation to:

(1) physiological needs and safety of the individual family, or community;
(2) sense of belonging;
(3) self-esteem and status;
(4) sense of purpose and self-realization.

In this chapter I speculate further and give evidence for the notion that such stimuli arising from change in male/female roles and relations may give rise to precursors of disease and disease.

DISEASES AND PRECURSORS

The diseases and precursors (P) that arise in male/female roles and relationships and that will be discussed here are as follows:

(1) venereal disease;
(2) unwanted pregnancy;
(3) suicide;
(4) interpersonal problems;
(5) diminished pair bonding;
(6) individual ill health;
(7) family ill health.

Venereal disease
Methods of spread, prevention, and treatment for these diseases are well understood, yet even in communities where understanding is high and facilities for treatment are available, incidence rates are high, and rising. The rise is particularly high in adolescents, and young, unmarried adults. (For example, at age 15–19 years in

Sweden, the incidence is approximately 1 per cent per annum in males, and 1·5 per cent per annum in females.)†
It is associated with permissive social attitudes to premarital intercourse and promiscuity, coupled with high, natural sexuality. When sexual relations take place between people who do not know each other's name and address, or with numerous fleeting acquaintances, it is difficult to stop the spread of disease. The psychosocial reasons may be a perceived threat to individual physiological needs, safety or status. The result is a real threat to community safety.

Spread is further encouraged by the frequency with which infected individuals neglect to obtain adequate treatment. The latter is sometimes due to ignorance, but often not. The reason then may be a perceived threat to the individual's sense of belonging and status, and this is likely to be enhanced or diminished by society's attitudes and manner of providing curative services.

Ignorance, of course, plays a large part in the spread of venereal disease, but when this is reduced, the main problem is due to motivational and behavioural factors.

Unwanted pregnancy
This is probably a precursor of disease. There is strong, but inconclusive evidence suggesting that it is associated with high infant mortality, child behavioural disorders, and adolescent psychological disturbance (Forssmann and Thuwe 1966). These risks are probably increased when the mother is unmarried, and the chances of the latter have increased with increased permissiveness with regard to premarital and promiscuous intercourse.

Society's approach to prevention of unwanted pregnancy is through education and provision of family planning facilities. Its approach to prevention of disease, once pregnancy has taken place, is through provision of facilities for abortion, or care of children. None of these approaches work very well at the moment. This is probably more often because the remedies are inadequately applied than because the remedies are inadequate. This may be because society and individuals rightly or wrongly perceive these remedies as a threat to safety.

Suicide
There is an association between high risk to suicide and breaking of the pair bond. This may happen in its formative stage, and be unilateral or bilateral. Thus, jilting

---

†There is some associated evidence that the main rise is in a 'high-risk group' of school drop-outs, delinquents, etc.

(unilateral) or forced separation (bilateral) of young lovers may be the crisis event that impels those of suicidal tendency to make the attempt. The stimuli that arise from the social situation are probably threats to sense of belonging, status, and self-actualization.

The pair bond may also be suddenly broken at a well-established stage by the death of a spouse. Incidence of suicide is high in young widowers and in young or old widows. Several theories have been put forward to explain the high suicide rate, and mortality from other causes, in the bereaved spouse, e.g. grief manifesting as the death wish; high risk because of loss of mutual care; deprivation of sense of belonging; intensive life change due to having to deal with new problems.

Interpersonal conflict

When persons entering into a social arrangement have different expectations of the outcome, and these conflicts cannot be resolved, they are liable to become precursors of disease in so far as mental or physical dysfunction occurs and risk to personal or family ill health follows.

For example, partners in sexual intercourse may have an unresolvable conflict over the nature of the relationship, e.g. superficial and fleeting, versus deep and long-term, or promiscuity versus fidelity; or there may be dissatisfaction with sexual performance. These conflicts may threaten safety, or physiological needs; sense of belonging; status or self-esteem; or self-actualization; and be associated with high risk of suicide or, through weakened pair bonding, with individual or family ill health.

Irreconcilable conflicts on the role of partners in child-rearing, mutual care, or other domestic duties, by producing the same threats, may also affect pair bonding and individual family health.

Similarly, threats to safety, sense of belonging, status or self-esteem, or self-actualization may arise at work because dominance of men to women or women to men differs from expectation, or because some women enjoy advantageous treatment because of their charms. Although this does give rise to dissatisfaction, high risk to disease is entirely theoretical.

Diminished pair bonding

I have indicated above that there is some evidence for the hypothesis that severance of an established pair bond, or a developing one, may be associated with suicide, and perhaps other forms of ill health, and that diminution of the pair bond may lead to individual or family ill health. Here I only wish to point out that if and when this is the case, diminished pair bonding can be regarded as a precursor of disease.

Individual ill health

I have indicated above that individual ill health may result when the pair bond is severed or diminished by high interpersonal or social conflict. In the case of suicide, this notion is not proved but is fairly well supported by associative evidence. There is less

TABLE 21.1

Rank	Life event	Mean value
1	Death of a spouse	100
2	Divorce	73
3	Marital separation	65
7	Marriage	50
9	Marital reconciliation	45
12	Pregnancy	40
13	Sexual difficulty	39
19	Change in number of arguments with wife	35
26	Wife begins or stops work	26

evidence, and the relationship is less plausible, in the case of morbidity or mortality from all causes of specific diseases. Nevertheless, there is some evidence for the idea, and if it were true, it might be of greater importance than the problem of suicide which is not very common. I will therefore take a closer look at it.

Rahe and others (Rahe and Arthur 1968; Rahe *et al.* 1967, 1970) have listed 42 'life events', ranked them in order of perceived importance by several groups of people, and given each a weight. A life-event unit score is obtained by summating event, multiplied by its weight over a period of time. They have found that general morbidity over a period of 6 months is correlated to life-event unit score over the preceding 6 months.

Of the 42 life events referred to by Rahe, 9 are concerned with sex roles and their relationships. Their ranks and weights are given in Table 21.1 (Rahe 1969a). Five of these (including the top 3) are directly related to pair bonding.

This is no more than a 'straw in the wind' because direct association between these life events and general morbidity has not yet been shown and no causative relationship has been tested. It is worth noting, however, that Rahe (1969b) has found a high rank order correlation of the same life events in people of different nationalities and culture.

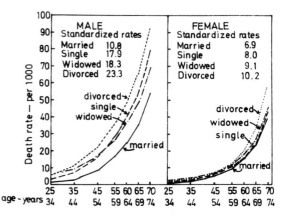

Fig. 21.1. Death-rates, by all causes, by marital status, in the United States (1949–51).

TABLE 21.2

Deaths per 10 000 for the period 1886–95

	Males, aged:			Females, aged:		
	20–39	40–59	60 and over	20–39	40–59	60 and over
France						
Married	77	153	583	80	121	456
Single	103	246	794	78	166	730
Widowed or divorced	211	293	1,148	145	198	930
Prussia						
Married	71	175	582	79	128	497
Single	84	231	806	59	179	729
Widowed or divorced	201	346	1,091	101	172	805
Sweden						
Married	53	114	453	66	96	364
Single	83	204	690	61	120	528
Widowed or divorced	104	190	856	98	132	698

Data showing that married people have a lower mortality rate than widowed or divorced have been published from time to time since William Farr first pointed this out in 1858. Berkson (1962) published a thoughtful paper in which he shows a table (see Table 21.2) of mortality rates for France, Prussia, and Sweden for the years 1886–95 from Lucian March. He goes on to examine data from the United States for the years 1949–51 (see Fig. 21.1) for total mortality and from New York State for disease-specific mortality for the same period.

He shows that the high mortality rate for single and divorced compared with married is true for many causes of disease, for example, tuberculosis, syphilis (except in single women); cancer of the digestive tract, bronchus, genito-urinary tract, breast; benign neoplasm; cerebral haemorrhage (except in single women); arteriosclerotic heart disease; peptic ulcer; cirrhosis of the liver (except for single women; nephritis; hyperplasia of the prostate; accidents; suicide; homicide (except for single women). He considers that because mortality is increased for so many different causes in the unmarried, that this supports the view that the unmarried are constitutionally weaker. This may be so but his data also support the hypothesis that there is an environmental factor common to the unmarried that imparts a risk to many kinds of illness. Thus, his data also support our hypothesis that absence or breakage of the pair bond or lack of mutual care is a risk factor for a broad variety of illness.

This latter view is supported by Young et al. 1963. They showed that the excess of mortality of widowers over married men of the same age occurs almost entirely in the first 6 months of widowhood for men aged 60 and over, although it extended into the second year for men aged 55–59.

The main excess of mortality in these widowers was due to suicide and arteriosclerotic heart disease. Rees (1969) showed that the relative excess of mortality was greater in young widowers than old and, again, may be due to suicide, tuberculosis, vascular lesions of the central nervous system, and arteriosclerotic heart disease. Although suicidal tendency and tuberculosis in the widower may be related to the cause of death of his wife (though there is no evidence that this is so) it is unlikely that this would be so for cerebrovascular and arteriosclerotic heart disease deaths. It is more likely, though again, strong evidence is absent, that these diseases were triggered by the death of the spouse.

In Chapter 1, p. 5, I referred to the possibility that men were innately more in need of care from their women than women from their men. Fig. 22.1 (from

TABLE 21.3

'Proportional benefit from marriage' for males and females compared in two epochs

	Ratio Mortality divorced (or widowed)/mortality married			
	1886–95†			1949–1951‡
Sex	France	Prussia	Sweden	United States
Male	2·2	2·2	1·9	2·0
Female	1·8	1·4	1·6	1·4

†Average figures based on Berkson (1962), age 20 years +
‡Standardized rates, from Berkson (see Fig. 22.1) age 25–74 years

Berkson 1962) supports this. The mortality rates for men are higher than those for women for each type of marital status, reflecting the innately higher risk of death for men. But the excess of mortality of unmarried men over married men is much greater than the excess for unmarried women compared with married women. Indeed, the risk for the single woman is scarcely greater than that for the married.

Table 21.3 compares Berkson's data from the United States for 1949–51 with March's data from France, Prussia, and Sweden for 1886–95. The 'proportional benefit from marriage' is remarkably similar for the four countries and the two epochs, and the 'benefit' for men is clearly greater than that for women.

It is possible that other environmental factors explain these findings, but it is difficult to think of any which would remain constant or balance out over a period when great environmental change has taken place.

A dozen years or so ago, when national differences in coronary heart disease mortality were being explained in terms of diet and plasma cholesterol level, I pointed out that the geographical differences might also be associated with differences in male/female marital roles in mutual care. The rates ranking from high to low in males in the United States, United Kingdom, Holland, and Japan suggested an inverse relationship to the care given to the husband by the wife. More recently, I understand Medalie *et al.* (1973) have found supporting evidence in a large follow-up study in Jerusalem for the notion that happy marriage in men is associated with less risk for coronary heart disease than unhappy marriage or divorce, widowhood, or being single.

There is no direct evidence, even of an associative nature, of a change in male/female mutual care roles. However, indirect evidence of a somewhat speculative nature is available from analysis of data in the World Health Organization's National Mortality Register.

We have to make two assumptions:

(1) that the majority of men and women in most countries at age 30–50 or so are not living singly;
(2) that in most countries the trend in recent years has been for women to give less care to their men;

then, if we compare male/female mortalities within countries over 10 recent years, we shall, if our hypothesis is correct, find that in most countries the ratio will have increased and that this will be greatest in those countries where male/female roles are likely to have changed most during the 10 years under study, and least in these countries in which the changes were most marked prior to the years of study.

Table 21.4 compares the ratio of male/female mortality for the years 1956–8 with the years 1966–8 for twenty countries from the World Health Organization Mortality Register. These countries were selected solely because age/sex specific mortality was available for both periods. The table refers only to men and women aged 40–44. Results were not very different at other ages, but I chose 40–44 because at this age, child-bearing mortality affects females least and war injury and coronary heart disease minimally affects males.

In all countries except one (Northern Ireland) the ratio increased from 1956–8 to 1966–8. The average increase was 15 per cent. The four countries with the least increase were Belgium, United States, New Zealand, and England and Wales (2, 4, 6, 8 per cent increase respectively). The four countries with the greatest increase were Ceylon, Israel, Finland, and Japan (33, 32, 30, and 25 per cent increase respectively).

In conclusion, though all these data fit in with our notion that psychosocial stimuli arising from reduction of mutual care enhances mortality in males to a considerable extent, the evidence is not conclusive but does indicate that the hypothesis ought to be tested.

Family ill health

I have referred on numerous occasions to the possibility that psychosocial stimuli arising from social situations such as sexual intercourse, child-rearing, mutual care, and home roles may cause family ill health. Conflict or threat arising from these situations is probably associated with 'broken homes' and there is considerable literature associating this with behaviour disorders in children, need of psychiatric attention, suicide, tuber-

TABLE 21.4

Ratio of male/female mortality: all causes age 40–44. 1956–8 compared with 1966–8† in twenty countries

| | 1 | 2 | 3 |
Country	1956–8	1966–8	Percentage increase 2/1
Ceylon	0·94	1·22	33
Israel	0·99	1·33	32
Finland	2·03	2·60	30
Japan	1·28	1·58	25
Austria	1·50	1·82	20
Switzerland	1·51	1·81	20
Sweden	1·35	1·58	18
West Berlin	1·25	1·54	17
France	1·77	2·00	14
Australia	1·45	1·65	14
Canada	1·53	1·72	13
Netherlands	1·30	1·47	13
Scotland	1·36	1·53	13
Norway	1·68	1·85	10
Portugal	1·76	1·94	10
England and Wales	1·34	1·44	8
New Zealand	1·31	1·39	6
United States	1·65	1·71	4
Belgium	1·57	1·60	2
Northern Ireland	1·35	1·32	—
Average	1·45	1·65	15

†From Analysis of data from World Health Organization Mortality Register

culosis, schizophrenia, alcoholism, etc. It is very likely that there is a condition short of the 'broken home' in the sense that none of the family members are absent, but in which a continuous state of disruption and conflict exists, and that this may be associated with ill health of members of the family. It is certainly associated with unhappiness.

INTERACTING VARIABLES

The discussion above on disease arising from male/ female roles and relationships is set at a simple level so that the ideas expressed may be clearly seen.

The real situation must take into account more factors and seems more complicated. Part of this is because of our ignorance — cause-and-effect relationships in the cycles of events leading from social situation via psychological stimuli to disease have not been proven. But much of the complexity is due to the role of interacting variables which may predispose to or protect from disease at each stage of the pathway.

Levi and Kagan (1974) have classified interacting variables as shown below. They are predisposing or protective:

Predisposing variables
(1) *Psychosocial* — combinations of noxious psychosocial environmental stimuli.

(2) *Physicosocial* — physical environmental stimuli — heat, noise, chemical hazards, altitude, malnutrition, overcrowding, etc., alone or in combination. These often have a psychosocial element.

(3) Lack of 'protective' intervening variables.

Protective intervening variables
(1) *Mental processes*:
habituation;
adaptation;
coping;
substitution — other ways of satisfying need;
increasing tolerance of ambiguity;
learning; critical period (implanting);
reinforcing by painful association;
conditioning.

(2) *Psychosocial factors*:
belonging to a group;
available acceptable substitute activities;
source of advice;
availability of someone to talk to about own troubles;
education.

(3) *Physicosocial factors*:
nutrition, clothing, housing, health services.

The effect of those predisposing or protective factors will depend on the individual's psychobiological pro-

gramme (Box 2, Fig. 1.1, page 3), e.g. individual variability in production of adrenalin when subjected to similar non-symbolic stimuli (Frankenhaeuser); similar changes with adreno-cortical secretion (Hamburg). Certainly not all subjects who are exposed to adverse social situations develop precursors of disease or become ill.

In some, this may be because their psychobiological programme is such that the social situation does not give rise to pathogenic stimuli. For instance, children brought up to speak freely, to understand and to know how to obtain guilt-free advice on problems arising from sexual intercourse, are probably less likely to suffer from venereal disease, unwanted pregnancy, or interpersonal conflict because by the time adolescence is reached, they will either be restrictive in sexual practices, or, if not, will not feel guilty or threatened by taking preventive measures and will know how to obtain them.

Some may divert pathogenic stimuli into other ways of satisfying their needs, e.g. some young people, though greatly upset by an unfortunate love affair, may, instead of committing suicide, deviate their energies into becoming proficient as an artist, poet, or scientist.

Interpersonal conflict arising from male/female sexual relations or roles may be resolved by interacting factors such as having someone to talk to about the problem or learning how to cope with the differences of opinion and thus preventing interpersonal conflict reaching the stage of a precursor of disease.

When high blood-pressure has developed and there is risk of coronary heart disease — perhaps as a result of interpersonal conflict — interacting variables such as understanding the cause of the conflict or changing the mode of life may reduce the risk. Similarly, one could think of interacting variables that will augment the risk of ill health for any potentially pathogenic social situation.

Though all this is speculative and unproven, it is of the utmost importance if it is true. Knowledge of which interacting variables are protective or promotive might very well provide the clues to identification of those at risk and the appropriate protective health action. Studies are therefore required that will test existing hypotheses and show relationships of the parts of the complex system of disease causation or prevention so that the whole may be better understood. Some suggestions for this, relevant to male/female roles and relations, are made in the last chapters of this book.

SUMMARY

I have postulated that changes in social situations, such as male/female relationships in sexual intercourse, and male/female roles in child-rearing and mutual care, at home and at work, may give rise to psychological stimuli which, in the presence of a psychobiological programme including high sexuality, tendency to pair bonding, and male dominance, will set off mechanisms that may lead to ill health.

I have speculated, and provided some evidence, that stimuli such as threat, ambiguity, or difference between expected and perceived situation in relation to basic needs may give rise to precursors of disease, such as unwanted pregnancy; interpersonal conflict; diminished pair bonding; and disability, such as venereal disease, suicide, and individual and family ill health.

In particular, I have cited old and new evidence to support the notion that social changes in male/female mutual care may place the male — already subject to higher mortality risks than the female — to still greater disadvantage.

REFERENCES

BERKSON, J. (1962). Mortality and Marital Status. *Amer. J. Public Hlth.*, **52**, 1318.

FORSSMANN, H. and THUWE, I. (1966). One hundred and twenty children born after application for therapeutic abortion was refused. *Acta Psychiat. scand.*, **42**, 71–88.

KAGAN, A. R. and LEVI, L. (1974). *Health and environment — psychosocial stimuli: A Review.*

MENDALIE, J., KAHN, H. A., NEUFELD, H. N., RISS, E., and GOLDBOURT, U. (1973). Five-year myocardial infarction incidence — II. *J. chron. Dis.*, **26**, 320.

RAHE, R. (1969a). *Psychotropic drug response. Advances in prediction*, p. 97. Illinois.

—— (1969b). Multi-cultural correlations of life change scaling: America, Japan, Denmark, and Sweden. *J. psycho-som. Res.*, **13**, 191–5.

—— and ARTHUR, R. J. (1968). Life change pattern surrounding illness experience. *J. psychosom. Res.*, **11**, 341–5.

——, MCKEAN, J., and ARTHUR, R. J. (1967). A longitudinal study of life change and illness pattern. *J. psychosom. Res.*, **10**, 355–66.

——, GUNDERSON, E. K. E., and ARTHUR, R. J. (1970). Demographic and psychosocial factors in acute illness reporting. *J. chron. Dis.*, **23**, 245–55.

REES, D. (1969). Mortality among widowers. *Brit. med. J.*, ii, 825–8.

YOUNG, M., BENJAMIN, B., and WALLIS, C. (1963). The mortality of widowers. *Lancet*, ii, 454–6.

22. THE STRESS FACTORS IN SEXUAL INADEQUACY

JOSEF HYNIE

I shall use the term 'sexual inadequacy' in a wider sense than Masters and Johnson, to mean inadequacy both in sexual relations and in the genital organs and their functions. It is probable that such inadequacy can more often and more easily be caused by stress situations than can heart and gastrointestinal diseases. I would like to discuss here our experiences and work at the Sexological Institute in Prague, Czechoslovakia. Some of our experiences have yielded data that could be evaluated statistically; others were interesting single observations.

I would like to consider a few examples of stress factors, grouped as (a) problems of physical abnormalities and abnormalities of development, (b) problems connected with the dynamics of sexual activity, and (c) other stress factors.

PHYSICAL ABNORMALITIES AND ABNORMALITIES IN DEVELOPMENT

Genital development

First I would like to give examples to show how real and imagined abnormalities in the development of genital organs can become stress factors to an individual.

For many years we have followed a group of so-called hermaphrodites, some of which are true hermaphrodites, but most of which are pseudo-hermaphrodites (more of the latter group are male than female). When such people come to us for advice, our current policy is to recommend they retain their originally determined sex. But this is not always possible.

Male pseudo-hermaphrodites, who have a small penis, vagina, and testicles, are often determined as girls at birth, especially if they have a small penis fixed down like a clitoris, and can only urinate like girls. But, sometimes in childhood, and particularly at the beginning of puberty, these people may feel different from other girls. A stress situation is created: these people are anxious to be thought the same as other girls and may try to hide abnormal characteristics. One male pseudo-hermaphrodite lived as a girl until she was 12 years old. At the beginning of her premature puberty she developed a stutter and her male characteristics, beard, broad shoulders, and growth of the down-fixed penis and testicles became pronounced. We first informed the patient's father, then the patient, that it would be better to change her sex, which had been falsely determined, and to correct the genital organs towards 'maleness'. Both were apprehensive at first, but soon came to see that the change was necessary.

Some years after the correction the young man seemed completely to have forgotten that he had ever been a girl.

In another case a young patient of 15 herself asked for a change of sex — she did not want to live as a girl. Her genital organs were developed like a male's, although they were defective. Routine preparation for the sex change included a change of the patient's domicile and school. After the patient's sex had been changed in the register and the operation performed, I asked the patient about his domicile and school. I found out that he had changed neither and that nobody in his school had the courage to remind him that he was once a girl. Today he is a happily married engineer-geologist, his only disappointment being that he is not able to have children; sexual life is perfectly possible. In this case adaptation to the change of sex was excellent, without difficulties or stress.

Of the other problems of development I would like to mention hypospadias, a condition in which urethral opening is not at the top of the gland, but below it. The corpus spongiosum urethrae is maldeveloped and in erection the penis is bent down, so that copulation is impossible. Our plastic surgery clinic has been routinely correcting this defect for 50 years and after operations the patients are usually fully capable of sexual relations. But when we conducted a survey on the patients who had been operated on we were surprised to discover that only about 30 per cent of them had married afterwards and 50 per cent did not engage in any sexual activity at all. These people had been stressed many years ago by the knowledge of their deficiency and the effect remained with them even after the deficiency was corrected.

Similar stress can occur in men with a small penis. In fact even men whose penis is a normal size may believe it is too small and suffer the same stress.

Transsexualism

The first sexual differentiation is known to take place in the third month of intrauterine life. In the past 15 years researchers have found a second sexual differentiation which occurs in the second trimester of pregnancy, at the same time as the brain structures are differentiated, and occurs chiefly in the hypothalamus (Dörner 1971). In a few cases it does not agree with the previous differentiation of the genital organs.

In both male and female special structures are formed in the front of the nucleus ventromedialis. The function of these is the tonic regulation of gonadotropin production. In the female there are formed in addition other structures, more ventrally, for the cyclic production of FSH in the area hypothalamica anterior and of LH in the area praeoptica. Dörner (1972) also distinguishes centres for male and female erotic (sexual) activity: in the area praeoptica in the male and in nucleus ventromedialis hypothalami of the female. Stereotactic destruction of these centres can be used to treat sexual deviation, mainly in homosexuals and sadist aggressors (Roeder *et al.* 1971).

Evolution of these areas in the brain is dependent on the level of androgens in the blood at the time of this second differentiation. High levels in the female induce male behaviour; a low concentration in males causes sexual insufficiency or transsexualism. Such individuals have been experimentally produced in animals. During the second period of differentiation the male organism was insufficiently supplied with androgens or the female organism was supplied with a surplus of androgens. In the human being we suppose these conditions result in transsexualism; and some observations testify to this theory, especially the cases in which the mother of a female transsexual is known to have taken androgens in late pregnancy.

Transsexuals (Hynie 1970*a*, 1974), who 'feel' they are of different sex to that suggested by their genital organs, constantly live in a stress situation. People with whom they come into contact, particularly their parents, cannot understand that a person with female genital organs wants to be transformed into a male, to live as a man, and finally to marry as a man. The stress situation is so severe that out of a sampled studied by Wålinder (1967) 60 per cent suffered pronounced depression, accompanied in 8–20 per cent of cases by suicide attempts. In our experience this figure is slightly lower.

We have had more experience with, and collected more statistics on, female transsexualism than has any other centre in the world. We have 67 female transsexuals under observation at present, but only 18 male transsexuals. We cannot explain this difference in frequency. Female transsexuals in most cases look virile — sometimes very virile. One such case was arrested ten times and charged with being a man in female dress; and women drove her out of women's cloakrooms. Clearly, help was needed in this case.

We proceed as follows in such cases: first we change the patient's name to a neutral one. In Czechoslovakia the names and forenames of men and women are usually different, but there are some forenames that can be used for both sexes. With such a name, and dressed in men's clothing, female transsexuals are not easily identifiable from men, and some are contented for a period with this. In cases where they work with men and wash with them they often ask for breast-correction. Menstrual bleeding can be weakened by androgens or by hysterectomy, without castration. It is, seldom, necessary to form an artificial penis — a cylinder without urethra or cartilage. Alternatively the oversized clitoris can be transformed into a small penis. But this is always only an imitation without sensibility

or reactivity. The last step that can be made to help female transsexuals is transcription of the sex in the register. We prefer not to recommend this because it gives the patient the right to marry as a man. This can lead to situations such as where, for example, the mother of a child wishes to be known as her child's uncle. Whatever is done for transsexuals cannot entirely rid them from difficulties, conflicts, and stress situations. Such people can also bring stress to others.

I have sometimes spoken to women who want to marry a male transsexual. These people are often surprisingly determined, even when I try to convince them that it will not be possible to have children or to live regularly as man and wife in such a marriage.

In one week I met two cases in which a girl had fallen in love with a man who had made her pregnant, then persuaded her to have an abortion and afterwards abandoned her. This caused the girl great stress which affected her whole life, and resulted in her becoming a transsexual.

Other physical abnormalities, defects, and disease
Other bodily defects can assert themselves as stress factors. I examined a man who was lame in one leg, and therefore was convinced that he could not count on marriage. He remained single, although he was not without sexual desires. He had a niece of 6 years old and once, as though accidentally, he touched her genitals. This was agreeable to the girl and afterwards she often asked him to play with her in such a way. In the end her parents took the matter to court. This man's physical defect caused him stress which resulted in his resorting to abnormal sex relations.

In another case physical and mental defects combined caused a 16-year-old dwarf with low intellect to commit a sexual crime, and murder. For their amusement his fellow workers encouraged him to touch women's breasts and touch them below the skirts. The dwarf was thus sexually excited without the possibility of real sexual relations. Once he met a girl of 13 in a deserted mill, and struck her down with a blow on the head and copulated with her. Afterwards, when she did not awake, he put her in the brook in the conviction that she was dead.

There can be a very strong stress factor for the wife where her husband suffers from premature ejaculation, or practises coitus interruptus. Before the wife has an orgasm her husband has finished, and over a period of time she will become very frustrated. It is not surprising if a woman refuses such a sex life.

In Graves's disease excitability is much increased, the patient is exhausted and, in severe conditions, sexual desires are sometimes increased, but activity is very weak and connected with anxiety.

Hypothyroidism on the other hand results in indolence and incapability to participate in sexual activity which is sometimes accompanied by unhappiness and efforts to compensate this lack. Tuberculosis also results in a decrease in sexual acitivty (Raboch 1967*a*).

The effect of stress during childhood

We have also studied (Raboch et al. 1967b) how inadequate environment in childhood can later evoke unfavourable tension and troubles in sexual function. We compared 600 men with sexual inadequacy with a control group of 600 normal men; and 300 pathological cases in women with a normal group of 300 women.

In the pathological group of men and women we found more frequent (highly significant at 0·1 per cent level) unsatisfactory marriages between parents, whose quarrels had provoked anxiety in their children, resulting in their forming unfavourable assumptions about sexual life and marriage. Also, in the pathological group (significant at 1 per cent level) it was more likely that one of the parents had been absent during childhood. About one half of the pathological group had had parents who were divorced, or were illegitimate children. Life up to about 12 years old without one or other of the parents to provide a model of the male or female role in life can cause difficulties in fitting into an accepted sex role later on.

Only, or eldest, sons showed a tendency for failure in the earlier phases of sex life. But this was not significant in the case of an only or the eldest daughter. The explanation is probably that the acquisition of sex information, very important for men, is more difficult for an only or eldest son.

Some mothers speak fearfully about pregnancy and the dangers of childbirth in the presence of their daughters, which can result in fear and anxiety. Girls are also warned against the wickedness of sexual contact before marriage, against possible pregnancy, dangers of abortions, etc. This upbringing can influence the girl's future relations with the opposite sex.

THE DYNAMICS OF SEXUAL ACTIVITY

A very common trouble in marriage is differences in sexual appetite. If mutual adaptation is not possible, one partner is continually hungry and the other is condemned to self-sacrifice. This is a severe stressing factor and cause of many divorces. It is not possible to evoke readiness for sexual activity and feeling at will; and a couple's sexual life can be disturbed by every stress situation: diseases, pains, overloading with work and cares, etc.

From the reports of people who have been in concentration camps we have learnt that starvation decreases sexual appetite; in many cases menstruation disappears in women (probably due to lack of gonadotropins). Potency can decrease when a man's diet is deficient in proteins and lipids. Too much work and too little sleep, for example during the care of sick children or old parents, have the same effect and cause matrimonial disharmony. Depression can also decrease or even suppress sexual activity. We have seen parents who, after a loss of a child, wish to find compensation in a further child, but are not able to continue their sexual

life. Again, it is possible that the production of gonadotropins is temporarily suppressed. Depression can originate from widely varying factors: failures at work, in love, or in society can reflect in sexual life. It is interesting to note the consequences of jealousy; when a man most wishes to demonstrate that he is better than his rival, he may find himself impotent.

At the time of the World War II Stieve (1952) performed autopsies on the testicles of men who had been executed. In the seminal vesicles he found remnants of spermatozoids dating from the time before the men knew their sentence. But production of sperm cells had ceased when they knew their sentence, many months before their death. So this very strong stress was capable of stopping spermatogenesis because it reduced the release of gonadotropins via the hypothalamus.

The genitalia are capable of being excited and giving pleasurable feelings very early in life (years before a proper sex life is possible), chiefly through onanism. But children are often very severely punished by their parents for doing this. The children are confused and bewildered by this and become stressed. This stress may then accompany all future manipulations with genital organs. Such anxiety can hinder erection or provoke disordered reaction such as premature ejaculation when the time comes to start a real sex life. Unfortunately this parental attitude persists, also applying to sexual activity during puberty. At puberty young people are capable of having sexual relations, but it is still not socially acceptable for them to do so. Their instinctive reactions are suppressed and substitutive activities such as masturbation takes place. In such people the habit of suppression is not lost easily and they may be inadequate when the time comes to make love. This lack of success is a further stress which induces depression and more failures.

In Czechoslovakia a population exists with very different traditions — the gipsies. They begin a full sexual life at sexual awakening and then have as many children as possible. We have never seen impotency in gipsies although they do come to our public consulting rooms, e.g. for sterility. These people are not stressed in puberty through restrictive morals: masturbation is nearly unknown.

Another critical period in sex life is growing old. some men of about 50 years old enter in to relationships with young women of 20–30. The man strives to prove that he can compete with young men in sexual prowess. But this is not possible over a long period of time, which can create stress for him, leading to his consulting a doctor.

OTHER STRESS FACTORS

Planned parenthood

Complete social maturity also represents readiness to found a family. Before this, or when planned parenthood is accomplished and no further children are desired, sexual life continues, but with care to prevent conception. The pill and the IUD have reduced the necessity to concentrate on contraception during copulation. But some women dislike these methods or fear adverse side-effects and live constantly under tension, which can influence their sexual life.

Other women are distressed at their failure to become pregnant and every menstruation depresses them very severely. I have known women who refused sexual relations when after some time they still had not become pregnant.

Fear of sterility

In some cases a couple may adopt a child supposing their marriage to be sterile; and when the stress of childlessness is thus lifted then have their own child.

Abnormal sexual tendencies

In other cases there are difficulties when sexual tendencies and activities of one person in a family do not conform to those acceptable to society. This happens in the case of homosexuality. When parents realize that their son is a homosexual, all his family are suddenly against him. They cannot accept the idea that he is abnormal and try to have him treated, usually with dubious results. Public opinion is almost as hostile to homosexuality as it is to criminality. Even if homosexuality is not punished in a particular country, homosexual tendencies have to be hidden, and these people live under constant tension.

The environment, chiefly, his family, may persuade the young homosexual man to marry. He will probably not be happy if he does even if he is capable of marital relations with his wife and of having children. Sooner or later homosexual tendencies break through and when they are recognized, still more stress is created. Once a homosexual man came to me to ask for treatment. He loved his daughter very much and was afraid that she would overhear that her father was a 'fairy'. This type of worry condemns the homosexual married man to live in a constant stress situation. The wife in these cases will also be discontented.

I have also known divorce to be caused by the husband's fetishism. As a young boy, one man I saw had suffered nocturnal enuresis, night urination. This would not be cured, and it was necessary to use rubber or plastic napkins. Later he learned to masturbate with the help of these napkins. As an adult he married, but after a misunderstanding with his wife he brought himself to ejaculation using a plastic napkin and was seen by his wife. She asserted that she was so disgusted that she could no longer live with her husband.

In another case a woman told me that before coitus she had to play the part of a severe school-teacher who chided and caned her husband for some small matter. Only after such a scene was he able to copulate; he was a masochist. This was so distressing for his wife that a divorce was necessary.

Personality differences

Leary (Mellan 1970) evaluates personality by asking a number of questions about the patient, his partner, his parents, and his ideals, and plots dominancy/submissiveness on the y-axis and hostility/love on the x-axis (Fig. 22.1). Using this system, slight variations of personality are found near the origin, but a personality with characteristics distant from the origins of the axes would probably be neurotic and very hard to live with.

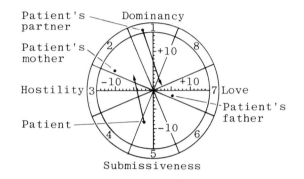

FIG. 22.1.

Natural male and female characteristics are known to be different. Generally speaking men have more initiative, aggression, and force, and women possess finer reactivity and adaptation. But a man or woman over-endowed with these typical characteristics could be very hard to live with. Mellan (1969) studied more than 1000 men and 400 women by the modified Leary Method and related personally to sexual troubles.

USEFUL STRESS FACTORS

I would like to mention that some stress factors can be useful; moderate stressing can sometimes help sexual relations. Travel, taking part in competitive events, moderate hunger, or even slight jealousy can result in more-than-usually stimulating sexual relations. This type of stress factor will be discussed further in Chapter 33.

SUMMARY

This chapter is mainly about the experiences and studies at the Sexological Institute in Prague, with reference to the stress factors that can weaken or disturb sexual function. Problems of real or imagined inadequacies in sexual equipment, other physical abnormalities, problems with the dynamics of sexual activity, problems of incompatible personalities, and the problems imposed by certain life-styles are discussed. Some stress factors can also be beneficial to a couple's sex life.

REFERENCES

Dörner, G. (1971). The differentiation of the hypothalamus produced by sex homones and its effect on sex function. *J. neuro-visc. Relations*, Suppl. X, 287–95.

Farkaš, G. L. (1967). *Hypospadias*. Prague, Czechoslovakia.

—— and Hynie, J. (1969). Some aspects of sexual life of men who were in their childhood operated on for hypospadias. *Symposium Sexuologicum Pragense*, pp. 286–7. Prague, Czechoslovakia.

Hynie, J. (1969). Lékařská opatření při transsexualismu. *Čslka Psychiat.*, **65**, 295–9.

—— (1970a). Behandlungsmöglichkeiten bei Transsexuellen. *Ars Med., Liesthal*, **60**, 719–22.

—— (1970b). *Lekárska sexuológia* [Medical sexology]. Martin, Czechoslovakia.

—— (1974). Feminine Transsexualism. *International Congress of Medical Sexology*. Paris.

—— and Šípová, I. (1963). [Personality of patients with inadequately developed male genitals, particularly with hypospadias.] *Acta Chir. plast.*, **5**, 220–6.

Kinsey, A. C. and Gebhard, P. H. (1953b). *Sexual behavior in the human female*. Philadelphia.

——, Pommeroy, W. B., and Martin, C. E. (1953a). *Sexual behavior in the human male*. Philadelphia and London.

Masters, W. H. and Johnson, V. E. (1970). *Human sexual inadequacy*. London.

Mellan, J. (1969). Sexual disorders in men and interpersonal relations estimated by the Leary Method. *Symposium Sexuologicum Pragense*, pp. 129–34. Czechoslovakia.

—— (1970). Interpersonal relations of sexological patients according to Leary test. *Čas. lék. česk.*, **109**, 613–16.

Nedoma, K. and Mellan, J. (1966). Syndrom transsexualism. *Čslka Psychiat.*, **62**. 42–7.

Neumann, F., Elger, W., and Steinbeck, H. (1971). The importance of androgens in imprinting patterns in the brain. *J. Neuro-Visc. Relations*, Suppl. X. 296–312.

Raboch, J. (1970). Female sexual response and marital life. *J. Sex Res.*, **6**, 29–35.

—— and Šípová, I. (1961a). Sexuální poruchy a rodinné prostředí. *Čslka Psychol.*, **57**, 246.

—— and —— (1961b). Sexualstörungen und Familien-milieu. *Psychiatrie Neurol. med. Psychol.*, **13**, 137.

—— and Barták, V. (1968). Das Sexualleben frigider Frauen. Psychiatr. Neurol. u. Psychol., **20**, 368–73.

—— and Lábus, I. (1968). Die sexuelle Reaktivität tuberkulöser Frauen. Prax. Pneumol. Tuberk., **22**, 251–7.

——, Barták, V., and Luksch, F. (1964). Ein Beitrag zum Dyspareunie-problem bei Frauen mit chronischen Genitalentzündungen. *Zentbl. Gynk.*, **86**, 979.

——, Šípová, J., and Barták, V. (1967a). Sexuální poruchy u žen a rodinné prostředí. *Čs. Psychiat.*, **63**, 397–401.

——, Ryšavý, J., and Scholz, W. (1967b). Die Potenz bei Turberkulösen. Prax. Penumol. Tuberk., **21**, 95.

Roeder, F., Müller, D., and Orthner, H. (1971). Further experiences in the stereotactic treatment of sexual perversions. *J. Neuro-Visc. Relations*, Suppl. X, 317–24.

Stieve, P. H. (1952). *Der Einfluss des Nervensystems auf Bau und Tätigkeit der Geschlechtsorgane des Menschen*. Stuttgart, Germany.

Walinder, J. (1967). *Transsexualism*. Göteborg, Sweden.

23. PSYCHOLOGICAL AND PHYSIOLOGICAL RESPONSES TO SEXUAL STIMULI IN MEN AND WOMEN

JOHN BANCROFT

The recent intensification of the public debate on the effects of pornography has highlighted our ignorance of normal sexual psychophysiology. The work of Masters and Johnson (1966) has greatly increased our understanding of the anatomy and physiology of sexual responses but this has been confined to that part of sexual behaviour which involves direct physical stimulation leading usually to orgasm, and what might be termed the 'action phase'. Paradoxically, less is known about the phase preceding this, when sexual drive may be heightened and sexual approach behaviour initiated. The implications of this phase for sexual adjustment are as great, if not greater, than those of the action phase. This review will concentrate on this 'pre-action phase' and will consider the following questions:

What are the characteristics of a sexually desirable person? How does the behaviour of that person affect his or her sexual desirability? How do visual stimuli compare with literature and fantasy in producing an erotic response and how do men and women differ in their responses to such stimuli? To what extent does .exposure to erotic stimuli such as pornography affect overt sexual behaviour? What are the physiological responses to erotic stimuli and what happens to these responses with repeated exposure to such stimuli? Is there a typical pattern of psychophysiological change involved in sexual arousal? What is the relationship between sexual arousal and anxiety?

A substantial amount of research relevant to these questions has been sponsored by the U.S. Commission on Obscenity and Pornography. Most of these studies have been mentioned in the Report of the Commission (Barnes 1970) but with insufficient detail to enable proper assessment. These studies will only be dealt with briefly, the review focusing mainly on other published results.†

WHAT CONSTITUTES A SEXUALLY DESIRABLE PERSON?

When one considers the amount of money spent on pictorial representations of sexually attractive people, it is surprising how little systematic research has been carried out in defining the relevant characteristics of such people.

Wiggins *et al.* (1968), by using silhouettes as their experimental stimuli, investigated the relative importance of size and shape of breasts, buttocks, and legs, varying these three characteristics separately in an otherwise unchanging female silhouette. A principal components analysis showed that subjects did use these dimensions in determining their choices. In addition, clear-cut personality 'syndromes' were associated with the preference for large breasts and large buttocks. In the first case a 'playboy' image was involved reflecting a tendency to date frequently, to have masculine interests, and to read sports magazines. In the second case personalities were of the 'orderly/frugal/obstinate' type appropriately labelled 'the anal character'.

Mathews *et al.* (1972) used photographs of actual women to investigate sexual preferences in males. Their 75 subjects included 15 psychologists, 15 psychiatrists, 15 soldiers, 15 porters, and 15 homosexual patients. Subjects were asked to rate each of 50 photos on a 10-point scale for sexual attractiveness ('how attractive as a short-term sexual partner is she?'). These ratings were subjected to a principal components analysis. This revealed a general factor of attractiveness (accounting for 27·3 per cent of the variance), on which all individuals loaded positively and the five groups (including the homosexuals) did not differ significantly from one another in their loading on this component. The second factor or component (accounting for 16·8 per cent of the variance) did distinguish between groups. This was described as a 'sexy-sexless' factor with at one pole pictures of sexually inviting, mainly nude women, and at the other pole sexually uninviting, mainly fully dressed women. Here the homosexuals differed significantly from all the other groups except psychiatrists in disliking the 'sexy' pictures, but there were also many individual heterosexuals whose scores were similar to the homosexuals on this component. This factor seemed to indicate, not sexual attractiveness, but sexual availability. The third component (which accounted for 7·6 per cent of the variance only) suggested a 'conventional-unconventional' dimension, with pictures of conventional 'old-fashioned' women at one end and unconventional 'with-it' women at the other. Here the porters differed significantly from all other groups in preferring the 'conventional' women. The only social class difference, therefore, was the slight but paradoxical preference for upper-class women by working-class men.

These findings, though limited, do suggest that it is possible to select pictures of women which will have some sexual appeal to the majority of males irrespective of social class or age. Where the pictures contained

†Since this review was written full reports of these studies have been published in *Technical Report of the Commission on Obscenity and Pornography*, Vols. 6 and 7. U.S. Government Printing Office, Washington, D.C. 20402.

cues of sexual 'availability' or social class, however, differences between individuals may be more marked.

A further study (Bancroft et al., unpublished) has investigated the sexual preferences of women in the same way. Fifty photographs of men in varying degrees of undress or fully dressed were rated by 60 women forming four groups comparable to the non-patient male groups. These were 15 psychiatrists, 15 psychologists, 15 nurses, and 15 hospital domestics.

Here again, a general factor of attractiveness was evident (accounting for 25·3 per cent of the variance) on which all of the subjects loaded positively. No naked men were found at the attractive pole of this component, however. The second component (representing 12·7 per cent of the variance) was of some interest. This clearly discriminated between groups with the domestics being significantly different from the psychiatrists and psychologists. The nurses came in between, being significantly different from the psychologists, but not from the other two groups. The pictures preferred by the domestics not only included men in varying degrees of undress but also various social-class cues (suggesting lower socio-economic class) such as hair style, facial appearance, and dress. Thus when compared to the men much more striking social class factors were evident. In addition, the mean ratings of sexual attractiveness were lower in all female groups.

At the present time, therefore, our understanding of what constitutes a sexually desirable person is very limited. However, the available evidence does suggest that, particularly in males, there is sufficient consistency in this respect to allow more detailed analysis of these essential 'stimulus' properties. The evidence also suggests, particularly in females, that sexual attractiveness is frequently compounded with other non-sexual forms of attractiveness such as desired or compatible social status. Further experimental work in this area will therefore usually need to control for these factors if the sexual component is to be more clearly understood.

WHAT CONSTITUTES AN EROTIC STIMULUS?

However sexually attractive an individual may be, the sexually arousing effect of that individual on another may vary considerably depending on the activity or attitude of the individual, the characteristics of the person responding, and the situation in which both are involved. A sexually attractive girl may most excite one male by acting demurely and another by acting in a sexually provocative way. For some people the fantasy of a sexual situation may be more arousing than the real thing.

The study by Mathews et al. (1972) suggested a variable relationship between sexual availability and sexual attractiveness. An uncertain association between sexually arousing properties and sexual attractiveness was further demonstrated by Schmidt et al. (1969), who in analysing the ratings of a series of photographs either of attractive women or of sexual activity, found a negative correlation between ratings for sexual arousal and favourableness. This negative relationship was not a simple one, as pictures portraying particularly tabooed acts (e.g. oral/genital contact) were especially unfavourable whilst only generating moderate sexual arousal.

Clearly, therefore, a sexually arousing stimulus may produce negative reactions in some people, particularly in certain situations such as the experimental one. This aspect was looked at by Byrne and Sheffield (1965) who took a group of 'sensitizers' and a group of 'repressors' as defined by the Repression/Sensitization scale derived from the Minnesota Multiphasic Personality Inventory. The subjects were asked to read some erotic literature and then to give various self-ratings. Sexual arousal was significantly correlated with ratings of anxiety, entertainment, and lack of boredom amongst the 'sensitizers', and with disgust and anger amongst the 'repressors'. Schmidt et al. (1969) found differences in favourability and sexual arousal ratings of their pictures of sexual activity according to the 'conservatism' of the subjects; the 'conservatives' finding the pictures less favourable and less sexually arousing than the 'liberals'. This difference was absent in the ratings of pictures of women not depicting sexual activity. It does not, of course, follow that similar feelings or reactions would be experienced in the non-experimental situation or in private. This factor has to be taken into consideration in all experiments involving responses to sexual stimuli; individuals may not only vary in how they react to such stimuli, they may also vary in how they react to being exposed to such stimuli in an experimental situation.

With this important qualification in mind what evidence is there for the relative effectiveness of different types of erotic stimuli and how do they differ between males and females? At this point it is appropriate to list the main types of erotic stimuli that may be involved:

(a) observation of a sexually desirable person;
(b) observation of sexual activity;
(c) appropriate olfactory stimuli;
(d) pictorial representation (either still or moving) of (a) and (b);
(e) erotic literature (read or spoken);
(f) erotic fantasy.

So far experimental work has been confined to the study of the last three categories.

The effectiveness of different types of visual erotic stimuli in males has been investigated by Levitt and Brady (1965) and Schmidt et al. (1969). In the first study photographs depicting 19 different sexual themes were rated by 68 male students. These themes included normal heterosexual coitus, heterosexual petting, oral-genital contact, homosexuality, both male and female, masturbation both male and female, and nude partly clad male and female figures. The themes rated most sexually arousing were normal coitus, heterosexual petting, and heterosexual fellatio. The nude female came next in the ratings and was hence considered more sexually arousing than a number of clearly pornographic if relatively tabooed scenes.

In the study by Schmidt et al. (1969) a comparable series of pictorial themes was shown to 99 males. The rank order of sexually arousing effect was similar to the previous study. Coitus and petting were most stimulating and semi-nudes and kissing scenes were least so. Nude females and oral-genital acts came in between. It is of some interest that the close-up of female genitalia had the lowest arousal rating. Other studies in agreement with these findings are those by Amoroso et al., Wallace et al., Mann et al., and Mosher (all reported in Branes (1970)). Cook and Fosen found a similar pattern in sexual offenders also (Barnes (1970)).

The relative efficacy of erotic fantasy compared with erotic visual stimuli and erotic literature has been investigated by Byrne and Lambeth (Barnes 1970). In this case imaginary situations were more effective than either photographs or literary descriptions of the same situations in producing sexual arousal. In a study by Bancroft and Mathews (1971), on the other hand, self-ratings of sexual interest were significantly higher for slides of 'pin-ups' than for erotic fantasies. However, when the slides were again presented with instructions to avoid any fantasy and simply to observe, ratings were significantly lower and no different from the ratings for fantasy alone. Thus it seems possible that visual stimuli of a sexually attractive but non-pornographic type may act to facilitate erotic fantasy and that any sexual arousal is dependent on the fantasy rather than any direct effect of the visual stimulus.

In a further study evaluating effects of libido-reducing drugs on sexual offenders (Tennent et al. 1974; Bancroft et al. 1974) the erectile response and self-ratings of sexual arousal were significantly greater to pornographic film than either erotic still pictures or fantasy alone (Bancroft 1974). Although the design of the experiment did not permit firm conclusions on this point, the difference between the three types of stimuli was considerable. It is thus also possible that observing a pornographic film is sexually arousing without the mediation of fantasy and the importance of fantasy in the case of still pictures is to bring the picture to life.

The differences in the response of males and females to erotic stimuli was first investigated systematically by Kinsey et al. (1953); in their survey of several thousand men and women they included questions about the subjects' response to a variety of erotic stimuli. The results of this enquiry are shown in Table 23.1. Their findings led Kinsey and his co-workers to conclude that there were basic differences in the responsiveness of the two sexes, with women being less responsive to the majority of such stimuli, though they were unable to offer any explanation why this should be so.

The results of some later studies have thrown further light on this problem. Jakobovits (1965) presented two types of erotic literature to two groups of 20 men and 20 women. The two types of literature were described as 'erotic realism' and 'pornography', the latter sacrificing realism for the sake of sexually stimulating effect, and containing much less non-sexual detail than the 'realistic' stories. Self-ratings of the sexually stimulating properties of the various stories were collected. Men and women did not differ in their response to the 'erotic

TABLE 23.1

Erotic responses to different types of stimuli in males and females (from Kinsey et al. 1953)

	Definite and/or frequent erotic response		Some response		Never responds	
	Males (per cent)	Females (per cent)	Males (per cent)	Females (per cent)	Males (per cent)	Females (per cent)
Observing opposite sex	32	17	40	41	28	42
Observing own sex	7	3	9	9	84	88
Pictures of nude figures	18	3	36	9	46	88
Observing genitalia of opposite sex	Many	21	Many	27	Few	52
Observing own genitalia	25	1	31	8	44	91
Commercial films	6	9	30	39	64	52
Pornography (pictures of sexual action)	42	14	35	18	23	68
Fantasies concerning opposite sex	37	22	47	47	16	31
Erotic literature	21	16	38	44	41	40

realism' stories, whereas women were stimulated to a significantly greater extent by the 'pornographic' tales. This is inconsistent with the findings of Kinsey and his co-workers (Table 23.1) but may reflect selection factors in the later study.

Sigusch *et al.* (1970) reported a study in which male and female responses to erotic photographs were compared. This followed the procedure reported in their earlier study of males (Schmidt *et al.* 1969). The photographs of sexual activity were the same for the two groups, other pictures were matched for content and showed members of the opposite sex in various poses and degrees of undress.

Ratings of sexual arousal and favourability were made. These showed much variation with considerable overlap between the groups. Differences between the sexes were most marked in those pictures simply showing members of the opposite sex, the women rating these significantly lower. Women were higher than the men (though not significantly so) in their ratings of pictures of sexual activity involving affection (e.g. kissing and embracing). For the other scenes depicting activity women gave slightly lower ratings than men, but again not significantly so. It was also noticeable that the differences in favourability ratings were greater than those in sexual arousal ratings.

These workers (Schmidt and Sigusch 1970) went on to compare the effects of pornographic films on males and females. The films were of two main types: one showing normal love play, and the other more intensive and unorthodox activity such as oral-genital contact and variations of coital position. There was no difference between the sexes in their ratings of sexual arousal for the 'orthodox' films, but whereas the women rated the 'unorthodox' films about the same, the men rated them more arousing and in this case the groups were significantly different at the 5 per cent level. Similar findings were obtained in the studies by Mosher, involving students and Mann *et al.*, involving married couples between the ages of 40 and 50 (Barnes 1970).

An earlier study by Levi (1969) also explored the effects of pornographic films on groups of 50 males and 50 females. An important difference in this experiment was that all subjects watched the film at the same time (i.e. as in the cinema with a mixed audience). In addition the main measure of change in this study was urinary catecholamine excretion (see below), though subjective ratings of sexual arousal were also collected. On this latter measure both groups showed a significant increase in sexual arousal in response to the film when compared with before and after scores, but the male group's increase was significantly greater than that of the female.

The evidence therefore suggests that the difference between males and females in their response to erotic stimuli is not as general as the results of Kinsey *et al.* (1953) implied. Where sexual activity between heterosexual pairs is involved, particularly of a reasonably conventional kind, there is very little difference between them. The difference is more obvious when the erotic stimulus is simply a picture of an unclothed or partially clothed member of the opposite sex. Caution is needed in generalizing on this latter point, however, which is based on studies involving students only. The findings of Bancroft *et al.* (unpublished) suggesting that working class women are more likely than professional women to find pictures of nude and semi-nude men sexually attractive is relevant here.

WHAT EFFECTS DO SUCH STIMULI HAVE ON THE INCIDENCE OF OVERT SEXUAL BEHAVIOUR?

This is a question crucial to the purpose of the U.S. Commission on Obscenity and Pornography. Is there evidence to show that exposure to erotic stimuli increases the likelihood of overt sexual behaviour, in particular behaviour of a socially unacceptable or psychologically harmful kind?

This question was directly considered in the studies by Schmidt *et al.* (1969), Sigusch *et al.* (1970), and Schmidt and Sigusch (1970). In each case sexual activity in the 24 hours after the experiment was compared with that of the same period before the experiment. There was a significant increase in the number of total orgasms, although this was largely due to an increase in masturbation.

Similar findings were obtained by Amoroso *et al.*, Byrne and Lambeth, Davis and Braucht, Kutchinsky, Mann *et al.*, Mosher and Cook and Fosen (all cited in Barnes 1970) involving subjects of varying ages, married and single and, in the last study, sexual offenders. The occurrence of a particular form of sexual behaviour for the first time following these experiments was very unusual and, when deviant erotic stimuli were shown, there were no reported cases of such deviant sexual behaviour being provoked by the experiment. Although it is possible that subjects' reports of sexual behaviour would be influenced by social desirability, it seems likely that the most predictable short-term effect of exposure to erotic stimuli is an increase in sexual arousability leading to a transient increase in the form of sexual outlet normally available (e.g. masturbation in those with no partner currently available).

Some studies reported an association between prior exposure to pornography and higher levels of sexual arousal in the experimental situation (Abelson *et al.*, Davis and Braucht, Kutchinsky, Mann *et al.*, all cited by Barnes (1970)). Other studies have found that previous exposure to such stimuli is associated with experience of sexual intercourse at an early age, higher current rates of sexual intercourse and more sexual satisfaction (Berger *et al.* and Zettenberg, both cited in Barnes (1970)). However, as pointed out in the Commission's Report (Barnes 1970) early sexual experience could make exposure to erotic stimuli more likely and vice versa, and both factors could stem from a common cause such as involvement with certain peer groups.

WHAT ARE THE PSYCHOPHYSIOLOGICAL RESPONSES TO EROTIC STIMULI?

Studies of this question have either involved asking subjects to describe physiological changes or have used physiological measures of various kinds.

In the first case reported reactions have included erections, pre-ejaculatory emission and ejaculation in the male, and genital sensations (warmth, pulsations and 'itching'), vaginal lubrication and orgasm in the female. Sigusch *et al.* (1970) and Schmidt and Sigusch (1970) found that more than 80 per cent of their males reported erections in response to erotic stimuli and 65–70 per cent of their females reported genital sensations in the experimental situation. Ejaculation in the male and orgasm in the female occurred in only one or two cases, although pre-ejaculatory emission was reported by 30 per cent of the men and vaginal lubrication by 24 per cent of the women.

Similar findings in students were obtained by Mosher (Barnes 1970) whilst Mann *et al.* (Barnes 1970) reported a 57 per cent incidence of erections and 59 per cent incidence of genital responses respectively in their 40–50 year-old males and females exposed to pornographic films.

A variety of autonomic measures have been used to indicate an arousal response to erotic stimuli. These include skin conductance, heart-rate, blood-pressure, forearm blood-flow, skin temperature, finger volume, and pupil dilation. Studies using such measures have been well reviewed by Zuckerman (1971) and will not be considered further in detail. In general the findings indicate that all such measures are non-specific and do not individually discriminate between sexual arousal and other forms of arousal, such as anxiety or responses to novel or exciting stimuli.

There has been disagreement in the literature over the specific nature of pupil dilation as an indicator of sexual interest or arousal. The conflicting results are well described in Zuckerman's review, but a more recent report by Bernick *et al.* (1971) claims that pupil dilation may be used to discriminate between sexual arousal and anxiety. This is based on a significant correlation between pupil size and the subjective ratings of erection. There was no significant difference in pupil size in response to erotic film and a suspense film, however, and from the evidence presented these workers are not justified in making their particular claim.

The autonomic response which is most clearly sexual in nature is penile erection in the male. Erection is readily measured by standard plethysmographic techniques, the most convenient of which are the mercury-in-rubber or solid-state strain gauges (Bancroft *et al.* 1966; Johnson and Kitching 1968) Freund (1965, 1967) and Freund *et al.* (1965), using a relatively cumbersome volumetric plethysmography, showed that penile volume changes discriminate between more and less effective erotic stimuli of a simple kind (i.e. slides of females and males of different ages). Bancroft and Mathews (1971) found that measurement of erectile changes discriminate between weak 'erotic' stimuli (e.g. slides of 'pin-ups') and non-sexual stimuli, whereas skin conductance, heart-rate, and forearm blood-flow fail to do so. Bancroft (1971*a*) has also found a high correlation between penile erection and subjective ratings of sexual arousal, providing that the erectile changes involved were of a degree likely to be noticeable to the subject. This raises the possibility that, in some males at least, subjective ratings of sexual arousal are based on, or certainly influenced by, awareness of the degree of erection.

In the male, therefore, measurement of erection is clearly the most specific autonomic measure of sexual arousal currently available.

A comparable measure in the female presents greater technical as well as interpretative problems. A technique for measuring vaginal blood-flow has been briefly reported by Shapiro *et al.* (1968) and Cohen and Shapiro (1971). As yet there is insufficient data to assess the value of this technique.†

Apart from measures of autonomic activity the only other physiological indicators of sexual arousal that have been investigated have involved biochemical changes. Levi (1969) measured adrenaline and noradrenaline excreted in the urine in 50 males and 50 females before, during, and after a pornographic film-show. As mentioned previously, both groups showed significant increases in subjective ratings of sexual arousal, though the increase in the males was significantly greater than in the females. Adrenalin and noradrenalin excretion also increased significantly in both groups but, whereas the increase in noradrenalin was similar for the two sexes, the increase in adrenalin in the males was greater to a highly significant extent ($p = < 0.001$). A further intriguing finding was the absence of correlation between subjective ratings of sexual arousal and changes in either adrenalin or noradrenalin secretion in the males, whilst the correlation with changes in adrenalin secretion in the females was significant. No adequate explanation of these interesting findings was given (see below). As a measure of sexual arousal catecholamine excretion must again be considered to be non-specific although the sex difference in the pattern of excretion deserves further study.

Bernick *et al.* (1971) measured 17-OHCS changes in response to erotic and suspense films but found no significant increase in the majority of their subjects to either type of stimulus.

The excretion of acid phosphatase in the urine was first suggested as a measurable response to sexual stimulation by Clarke and Treichler (1950). Some evidence in support of this was reported by Gustafson

---

†Since this review was written several studies have been reported using photoplethysmographic measurement of vaginal blood-flow as a correlate of sexual arousal in the female (e.g. Greer *et al.* 1974; Wincze *et al.* 1976).

et al. (1963) and its validity as a measure of sexual response has been assumed in a recent study by Reifler *et al.* (1971) (see below). A recent study by Barclay (1971), however, suggests that the relationship between acid phosphatase secretion and sexual arousal is far from straightforward and as yet this should not be assumed to be a valid indicator of a sexual response.

WHAT IS THE EFFECT OF REPEATED EXPOSURE TO EROTIC STIMULI?

This is a further question of importance to the U.S. Commission enquiry. The study by Reifler *et al.* (1971) paid particular attention to this question. These workers exposed their 23 experimental subjects to a wide variety of pornographic material for 90 minutes a day, 5 days a week for 3 weeks. They assessed the effects of this exposure in two main ways: first by comparing the experimental group with a control group (of 9 subjects) in their response to pornographic film before the 'exposure' experiment started and after it was completed. Penile erection and urinary acid phosphatase were the two principal measures involved. Secondly, after each exposure period the experimental group completed a series of self-rating scales and the acid phosphatase excretion for the period was measured.

Results showed that the experimental group produced less erection and excreted less acid phosphatase than the controls in response to the second film session (i.e. at the end of the intensive exposure period). In addition the amount of time looking at pornography rather than neutral material declined during the exposure period as the experiment continued. These findings, it was suggested, supported the hypothesis that repeated exposure to pornography results in decreased responsiveness to it. This report is open to criticism, however. Although measurement of erection was used, the strain gauge was not apparently calibrated. Results were analysed in terms of amount of pen deflection and yet were presented graphically in the report as millimetres increase in penile circumference. No test of the significance of the difference between the experimental and control groups on this measure was reported and no indication of how similar the two groups were on initial testing was given. The method of measuring acid phosphatase involved the subject wearing a condom. It seems probable that, for many subjects, wearing a condom would have a sexually arousing effect, far more so than a mercury-in-rubber strain gauge which is not only less stimulating but has less obvious sexual connotations. In this study the experimental group wore a condom daily for 3 weeks, whereas in the control group this happened on only two occasions. Habituation to the condom could, therefore, have contributed to less erectile response as well as lower acid phosphatase secretion in the experimental group.

Finally, the practical conclusions from this study seemed to be limited. Such concentrated exposure may indeed lead to some degree of satiation, but would

satiation occur if the exposure was repeated at longer intervals rather than in such an unusually intense manner? In the study by Mann *et al.* (Barnes 1970) middle-aged couples were shown erotic films at weekly intervals. However, no information on the occurrence of satiation in this group was given in the Commission's Report. In a drug study of sexual offenders in which erectile response to pornographic film was one of the measures of change (Tennent *et al.* 1974; Bancroft *et al.* 1974) the films were shown at 6-weekly intervals. There was a tendency for erections to increase with repeated exposure, though not to a statistically significant extent. This may have been partly due to decreasing inhibition in the experimental situation but there was certainly no evidence of satiation.

WHAT IS THE PHYSIOLOGICAL NATURE OF 'SEXUAL AROUSAL'?

There is now considerable evidence to show that a variety of physiological changes may occur in response to psychic erotic stimuli. Do these changes constitute a predictable pattern which can be called 'sexual arousal' a unitary concept? Until recently it has been generally assumed that physiological changes occurring in the pre-action phase are a milder version of those accompanying the sexual behaviour itself which reach a peak at the point when orgasm occurs (e.g. Kinsey *et al.* 1953). This is an assumption, however, based on little evidence. It is helpful at this point to consider the concept of general arousal. Over the past 20 years or so this concept has undergone various changes. Early attempts to identify characteristic patterns of physiological response associated with particular emotions, such as anger or anxiety, by people such as Ax (1953) were not very successful and gave way to the unidimensional concept of arousal as a continuum ranging from coma to disorganized excitement. In this view the subjective quality of the arousal, whether anxiety, anger, or sexual arousal, would not be indicated by the pattern of physiological change which is essentially non-specific. This view has now been effectively criticized and modified by Lacey (1967) who points out first that there are different types of arousal (e.g. behavioural, cortical, autonomic) which though they usually occur together are, in fact, independent of one another; secondly that the interrelationship of physiological responses accompanying arousal will vary according to the nature of the arousing stimulus, an example being the slowing of heart-rate with outwardly directed attention compared with the increase accompanying inwardly directed attention. Thirdly, that predictable patterns of response to certain stimuli will occur within individuals but would tend to vary from individual to individual; the concept of response specificity.

Two studies are relevant to this issue. Wenger *et al.* (1968) followed the approach of Ax and set out to identify a characteristic autonomic pattern of sexual arousal across individuals distinguishable from other states such as anxiety. They demonstrated significant differences in the electrodermal activity and blood-pressure changes between the responses to erotic and neutral stimuli but they failed to demonstrate that their reported pattern would distinguish sexual arousal from other types of arousal and they did not include any measure of erection.

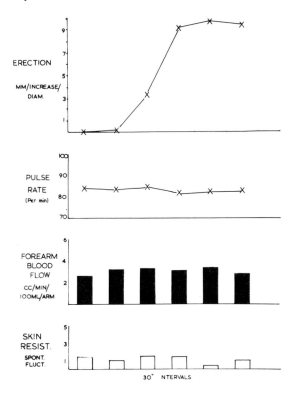

FIG. 23.1. *Association between erection and autonomic arousal* This Figure shows the mean values for three successive erections in a normal male in which no evidence of autonomic arousal occurred during full erection.

Bancroft and Mathews (1971), on the other hand, examined the correlation between non-specific autonomic changes and penile erection in response to erotic stimuli and fantasies. In a pilot study they found that normal subjects varied in the relationship between erection and other autonomic variables. (See Figs. 23.1 and 23.2.) They then systematically studied 10 further normal subjects, measuring in addition to erection, skin conductance, heart-rate, and forearm blood-flow. Six subjects showed a significantly positive correlation between erection and at least one of the other physiological measures; one subject showed a negative correlation. These correlations were based, however, on the total testing situation and in only one subject in the main experiment was the association clearly observable during the development of full

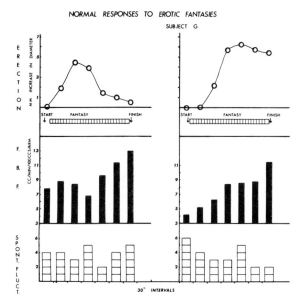

FIG. 23.2. *Association between erection and autonomic arousal* This Figure shows two separate erections in a normal male. In both cases evidence of autonomic arousal, as reflected in the forearm blood-flow measurement (F.B.F.), accompanies erection but is more obviously associated with the presence of an erotic fantasy than the erection *per se*.

erection and this was in the subject showing a *negative* correlation with all three non-specific measures. (Two subjects in the pilot study had shown obvious 'negative' associations during full erections.)

These findings, though preliminary and limited, suggest that Lacey's modification of unitary arousal theory should apply also to the unitary concept of sexual arousal. Sexual arousal as it is generally understood is probably composed of several different types of response which, though they usually accompany one another, are in fact independent. Penile erection is one of these and is probably the only specifically sexual response in the male. Which responses occur will depend partly on the nature of the arousing stimulus and partly on how the individual subject appraises it. But it also seems possible that, at least in some people, the pattern of autonomic response accompanying erections would be relatively predictable showing response specificity and, if such patterns involved a negative association between erection and autonomic arousal, then this would be of possible clinical relevance. It may be, for example, that such people are particularly vulnerable to the effects of anxiety.

In order to test this hypothesis, it is necessary to carry out repeated measurements of erections and other autonomic meaurements in varying conditions. Such an experiment is possible but has not yet been carried out. Some evidence, which is of relevance but of limited value, was obtained in a study of behaviour therapy of

160

homosexuals (Bancroft 1971*b*). Seven patients, receiving systematic desensitization of their heterosexual 'phobia', had their skin conductance and erections monitored throughout treatment, involving 30 sessions. All 7 patients produced erections on several occasions, the lowest number in any one individual being 12; in most of it was many more. These patients were divided into three groups on the basis of the pattern of skin conductance activity accompanying their erections; first those that showed consistent increase in skin conductance activity accompanying erections, whether the patient was relaxed or not, secondly those who showed a consistent absence of or reduction in skin conductance activity accompanying erection, and thirdly those in whom the amount of skin conductance activity varied from occasion to occasion and there was no particular pattern; in other words, those patients who were predictably aroused when getting an erection, **those who were predictably calm when getting an erection, and those that varied.** Of those 7 patients 4 were in the consistently calm category and 2 were consistently aroused; 1 showed a variable relationship. (See Figs. 23.3 and 23.4.) This rather circumstantial data does support the possibility that response specific patterns may occur in some individuals and further investigation should be carried out to explore this possibility.

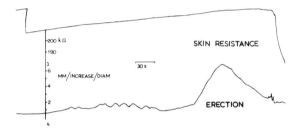

FIG. 23.3. *Erection and skin conductance* This polygraph tracing is taken from a subject who consistently showed erections unaccompanied by skin conductance activity.

It will be clear that up till now most of the relevant physiological data refers to males; we know even less about the concept of sexual arousal in females. One important difference between the sexes is the occurrence of penile erection in males. This is a readily observable response which is usually interpreted as sexual in nature and which may have arousing properties of its own in a 'positive feed-back' sense. Most women are aware of physiological changes in their genitalia but are possible less likely to interpret them as sexual responses. This point may have some bearing on the sex differences in correlation between catecholamine excretion and self ratings of sexual arousal reported by Levi (1969). If females base their self-ratings on generalized physiological changes which are likely to be accompanied by increased catecholamine excretion the correlation will be high. If males, on the

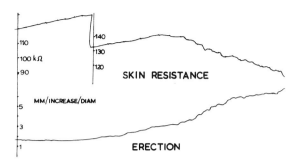

FIG. 23.4. *Erection and skin conductance* This polygraph tracing is taken from a subject who consistently showed erections accompanied by increased skin conductance activity.

other hand, base their ratings predominantly on awareness of erection which, as has been shown, is not necessarily accompanied by generalized arousal (Bancroft and Mathews 1971), the correlation will be less high.

Further work is needed to clarify the psychophysiological relationships in sexual arousal in both males and females.

WHAT IS THE RELATIONSHIP BETWEEN SEXUAL AROUSAL AND ANXIETY?

Anxiety as an emotional state is widely held to be the crucial factor in determining neurotic behaviour, acting in at least three ways. One behaves to avoid or reduce anxiety; the presence of anxiety indicates that a problem exists or acts as a cue for danger; physiological accompaniments of anxiety may interfere with performance. Anxiety is also generally held to play a central part in the causation of many forms of sexual dysfunction in men and women. Its effects have been most clearly implicated in the case of premature ejaculation and erectile impotence. The presence of anxiety, it is assumed, is sufficient to inhibit erection, presumably due to its sympathetic activating effect.

It is now clear that the sympathetic-parasympathetic dichotomy is a misleading oversimplication, though it tends to linger in relation to sexual physiology. The physiology of erection is complex and sympathetic mediation may be involved in both the production and inhibition of erection (Bancroft 1970). Inhibition of erection cannot, therefore, be assumed to be an invariable peripheral manifestation of the state of anxiety. Ejaculation is more predictably associated with states of high arousal and may, therefore, be precipitated by either anxiety or excitement. What then is the relationship between anxiety and erection?

There is experimental evidence from animals, of which Horsley Gantt's dogs provide the best example (Gantt 1944) that anxiety-provoking situations sometimes lead to erection. Ramsey (1948) reported that a considerable number of boys between the ages of 10 and 12 experience erections to a variety of non-sexual stimuli many of which are basically frightening. What is lacking is good experimental data on this relationship. Because of this lack some further circumstantial evidence from the author's behaviour therapy experiments may be worthy of consideration.

In homosexuals receiving systematic desensitization of their heterosexual anxiety, it became clear that whether or not erections occurred in the presence of anxiety depended on their cognitive appraisal of the situation. One patient, for example, reported anxiety when erections occurred in response to heterosexual stimuli but no anxiety with homosexual responses. As treatment continued the relationship reversed, heterosexuality becoming less threatening, whilst homosexual responses posed a threat to the success of treatment. There were two other patients receiving desensitization who reported intense anxiety accompanying erections outside the treatment situation. In one this was when homosexual thoughts intruded into his masturbation fantasies and the other reported a homosexual incident which resulted in an erection and high levels of anxiety (Bancroft 1974).

Further interesting observations were made during aversion therapy (Bancroft 1971*b*). The method used involved giving a shock when an erection developed to a particular level in response to photographs of attractive males. This was a level of which the patient was only just aware. If anxiety predictably inhibits erections it would be surprising if any shocks were delivered at all in such a situation. However, not only were shocks frequently given but they were associated with a paradoxical facilitation of erections to heterosexual stimuli which became greater at the end of the aversive sessions than at their beginning.

If anxiety tends to inhibit erections then one would expect that in this aversive situation it would lengthen the response latency, i.e. the time taken for the erection to develop to the criterion level. One would therefore predict that the higher the level of anxiety in the aversive session, the longer the response latencies would be. This relationship was examined in 10 cases. In 8 there was no significant correlation, the remaining 2 showing significant negative correlations. One of these men, showing a correlation of -0.78, gave an interesting account that since his early teens he would get slight erections whenever he was feeling anxious such as on the verge of a row, before interviews, or when about to play sport, particularly if he was captain. He also experienced this when reading about fight sequences or any sadistic or masochistic literature.

Thus it does seem that in some individuals, if not all, anxiety may be accompanied by erection. In some of these cases the erection may lead to anxiety.

A further interesting observation suggests a rebound type of phenomenon. Three patients having aversion complained that they received shocks if they allowed their minds to wander off the erotic fantasy. In other words whilst they were trying to produce the response nothing happened, but when they stopped trying it did happen and they were shocked. Most patients showed a comparable effect at the end of aversive trials; the instruction to stop trying would be followed by transient slight erection. This suggests a Sherringtonian type of rebound effect in which excitation temporarily outlasts inhibition (Bancroft 1974).

These observations raise the possibility that inhibition of erection is a very specific physiological response of which the subject is not aware and cannot control. On occasions such inhibition can be sudden and extreme leading to virtual disappearance of the penis into the scrotum (Bancroft and Mathews 1967; Masters and Johnson 1966).

Let us, therefore, reconsider the relationship between anxiety and erection. Available evidence is insufficient to draw firm conclusions but it does suggest three types of hypothetical relationships which may co-exist.

1. Appraisal of threat may occur in a sexual situation. This leads to anxiety as well as neurophysiological inhibition of erection, though each may occur independently. The inhibition of erection may serve in some cases, to reduce the threat hence lowering anxiety whilst in others, it may increase the threat so raising the anxiety.

2. Erection probably depends on cognitive mediational processes involved in the response to erotic stimuli or fantasies. A worried, preoccupied person may not be able to respond to such stimuli, the effect of anxiety being to disrupt these mediational processes.

3. Some individuals may require an optimal level of autonomic arousal for erection to occur. Anxiety may increase arousal above this point thus interfering with the erectile process.

Individual variation in the relationship between anxiety and sexual responses such as erection is potentially important in attempting to understand sexual inadequacy and its treatment. Up to now individual variation has been assumed to operate at the psychological level, people varying in the level of sexual conflict or anxiety involved. Perhaps in many the variation is at the physiological level rendering some individuals particularly vulnerable to the effects of psychologically threatening situations (Bancroft 1971*c*). Certainly this is a further area in which clarification of psychophysiological mechanisms is needed.

SUMMARY

Experimental evidence of the normal range of psychological and physiological responses to psychic erotic stimuli has been considered. Understanding of the essential characteristics of a sexually desirable person is still very limited, though further research in this area should be possible. Responses to erotic stimuli involve a wide variety of physiological changes most of which are non-specific. Very little is known about the pattern of such responses involved in sexual arousal and, in particular, individual variations in response specificity.

This could have an important bearing on the relationship between anxiety and sexual response. Hypotheses relevant to this relationship are suggested.

REFERENCES

Ax, A. F. (1953). The physiological differentiation between fear and anger in humans. *Psychosom. Med.*, **15**, 433–42.

Bancroft, J. H. J. (1970). Disorders of sexual potency. In *Modern trends in psychosomatic medicine* (ed. O. W. Hill). London.

—— (1971a). The application of psychophysiological measures to the assessment and modification of sexual behaviour. *Behav. Res. Ther.*, **9**, 119.

—— (1971b). A comparative study of aversion and desensitisation in the treatment of homosexuality. In *Behaviour therapy in the 1970's* (ed. L. E. Burns and J. L. Worsley). Bristol.

—— (1971c). Sexual inadequacy in the male. *Postgrad. med. J.*, **47**, 562–71.

—— (1974). *Deviant sexual behaviour*. Clarendon Press, Oxford.

—— and Mathews, A. M. (1967). Penis plethysmography; its physiological basis and clinical application. *Acta med. Psychosomat.* (Proceedings of 7th European Conference, Rome).

—— and —— (1971). Autonomic correlates of penile erection. *J. psychosom. Res.*, **15**, 159–67.

——, Jones, H. G., and Pullen, B. R. (1966). A simple transducer for measuring penile erection, with comments on its use in the treatment of sexual disorders. *Behav. Res. Ther.*, **4**, 239–41.

——, Tennent, G., Loncas, K., and Cass, J. (1974). The control of oestrogens and antiandrogens. *Brit. J. Psychiat.*, **125**, 310–15.

Barclay, A. M. (1971). Urinary acid phosphatase secretion in sexually aroused men: some response parameters, *Psychophysiology*, **8**, 252.

Barnes, C. (1970). *The report of the Commission on Obscenity and Pornography*. New York.

Bernick, N., Kling, A., and Borowitz, G. (1971). Physiologic differentiation of sexual arousal and anxiety. *Psychosom. Med.*, **33**, 341–52.

Clark, L. C. and Treichler, P. (1950). Psychic stimulation of prostatic secretion. *Psychosom. Med.*, **12**, 261–63.

Cohen, H. D. and Shapiro, A. (1971). A method for measuring sexual arousal in the female. *Psychophysiology*, **8**, 251–2.

Freund, K. (1965). Diagnosing heterosexual pedophilia by means of a test for sexual interest. *Behav. Res. Ther.*, **3**, 229–34.

—— (1967). Diagnosing homo- and heterosexuality and erotic age preference by means of a psychophysiological test. *Behav. Res. Ther.*, **5**, 209–28.

——, Sedlacek, F., and Knob, K. K. (1965). Simple transducer for mechanical plethysmography of the male genital. *J. exp. Anal. Behav.*, **8**, 169–70.

Gantt, H. (1944). *The experimental basis of neurotic behaviour*. New York.

Greer, J. H., Morotoff, P., and Greenwood, P. (1974). Sexual arousal in women: the development of a measurement device for vaginal blood volume. *Arch. sex. Behav.*, **3**, 559–64.

Gustafsen, J. E., Winokur, G., and Reichlin, S. (1963).

The effect of psychic and sexual stimulation on urinary and serum acid phosphatase and plasma non-esterified fatty acids. *Psychosom. Med.*, **25**, 101–5.

Jakobovits, L. A. (1965). Evaluational reactions to erotic literature. *Psychol. Rep.*, **16**, 985–94.

Kinsey, A. C., Pomeroy, W. B., Martin, C. E., and Gebhard, P. H. (1953). *Sexual behaviour in the human female*. London.

Johnson, J. and Kitching, R. (1968). A mechanical transducer for phallography. *Biomed. Eng.*, September, 416–18.

Lacey, J. I. (1967). Somatic response patterning and stress: some revisions of activation theory. In *Psychological stress* (ed. M. H. Appley and R. Trumbull). New York.

Levi, L. (1969). Sympatho-adrenomedulary activity, diuresis and emotional reactions during visual sexual stimulation in human females and males. *Psychosom. Med.*, **31**, 251–68.

Levitt, E. E. and Brady, J. P. (1965). Sexual preferences in young adult males and some correlates. *J. clin. Psychol.*, **21**, 347–54.

Masters, W. J. and Johnson, V. E. (1966). Human sexual response. London.

Mathews, A. M., Bancroft, J. H. J., and Slater, P. (1972). The principal components of sexual preference. *Brit. J. soc. clin. Psychol.*, **11**, 35–43.

Reifler, C. B., Howard, J., Lipton, M. A., Liptzin, M. B., and Widmann, D. E. (1971). Pornography: an experimental study of effects. *Amer. J. Psychiat.*, **128**, 575–82.

Ramsey, G. V. (1943). The sexual development of boys. *Amer. J. Psychol.*, **56**, 217.

Schmidt, G., Sigusch, V., and Meyberg, V. (1969). Psychosexual stimulation in men: emotional reactions, changes of sex behaviour, and measures of conservative attitudes. *J. Sex. Res.*, **5**, 199–217.

—— and —— (1970). Sex differences in responses to psychosexual stimulation by films and slides. *J. Sex. Res.*, **6**, 268–83.

Shapiro, A., Cohen, H. D., Di Bianco, P., and Rosen, G. (1968). Vaginal blood flow changes during sleep and sexual arousal. *Psychophysiology*, **4**, 394.

Sigusch, V., Schmidt, G., Reinfeld, A., and Wiedemann-Sutor, I. (1970). Psychosexual stimulation: sex differences. *J. Sex. Res.*, **6**, 10–24.

Tennant, G., Bancroft, J. H. J., and Cass, J. (1974). The control of deviant sexual behaviour by drugs: a double-bind controlled study of benperidol chlorpromazine and placebo. *Arch. Sex. Behav.*, **3**, 261–71.

Wenger, M. A., Averill, J. A., and Smith, D. B. B. (1968). Autonomic activity during sexual arousal. *Psychophysiology*, **4**, 468–78.

Wiggins, J. S., Wiggins, N., and Conger, J. C. (1968). Correlates of heterosexual somatic preference. *J. person. soc. Psychol.*, **10**, 82–90.

Wincze, J. P., Hoon, E. F., and Hoon, P. W. (1976). Physiological responsibility of normal and sexually dysfunctional women during erotic stimulus exposure. *J. psychosom. Res.* (In press)

Zuckerman, M. (1971). Physiological measures of sexual arousal in the human. *Psychol. Bull.*, **75**, 297–329.

24. PSYCHOSOCIAL FACTORS AND VENEREAL DISEASES IN DIFFERENT CULTURES

MALCOLM TOTTIE

CLASSIFICATION OF VENEREAL DISEASES

For centuries past, diseases have been classified as venereal diseases if they are nearly always transmitted through sexual contacts. The most important venereal diseases of today are gonorrhoea and syphilis. There are two other venereal diseases, soft chancre and climatic bubo, and various other diseases, i.e. scabies, which can be transmitted in the same way. The two main diseases are quite different in mode of transmission, clinical picture, and severity.

Gonorrhoea

Gonorrhoea is a disease that is mainly localized in the genital tract and is, in adults, practically always transmitted through intercourse or direct contact between the sex organs. The incubation period, i.e. time from infection to diagnosis, is relatively short — up to 1 month. Complications occur in 10–20 per cent of the cases and are also localized to the reproductive organs. These may cause sterility both among men and women. In rare occasions, the disease can cause arthritic symptoms or infection of the heart valvule or septicaemia. The gonorrhoea of today is mainly cured by penicillin treatment. Some cases, however, show increased resistance to penicillin and require higher doses or a change of drug. On the whole, treatment is successful.

Syphilis

Syphilis, on the other hand, is a general infection; the germ can enter the body by any microscopic rupture of the body surface. The entrance is usually in the genital area but can be in the oral region, on the fingers, the nipples, or anywhere else on the body. The incubation period is within 2 months. On the other hand, visible symptoms can be delayed and the first clinical reaction may therefore not be observed until 10 years or more after the infection.

At the place of the primary infection, there may be a local ulceration followed by enlarged lymph glands. This ulceration may heal spontaneously and can be followed by different types of rash, fever, pain in the joints, loss of hair, etc. during the first years after the infection. Later, there may be symptoms detected from the valvule of the heart, the big vessels, the brain, and the spinal cord, which may progress and if not treated, lead to invalidity or death.

A pregnant woman with syphilis may transmit infection to the foetus through the umbilical cord. The baby may die or be born with syphilis, giving rise to symptoms of a very serious nature which may manifest themselves at any stage in life.

The treatment of syphilis is now very promising and, from the medical point of view, 100 per cent effective. There has up to now been no proof of any resistance to penicillin. The only problem is to get the patient to treatment as early as possible to cure the disease early and thereby to prevent the germs to cause serious damage which might be irreversible.

PROSTITUTION

In older times, the venereal diseases have been looked upon as something very shameful and it has always been the women who have been accused of spreading the disease. The venereal diseases have mostly been very much related to prostitution and all action was directed towards the women. Very little thought was given to the fact that a woman, even a professional prostitute, has to be infected by an infected male before she can infect other males.

In the case of organized prostitution, there have been some attempts to introduce compulsory regular examination and, recently, compulsory penicillin treatment was introduced to cure contracted venereal disease or to keep infection away. The results have not been very promising — it is inadvisable to continue to administer penicillin once or twice a month during the time of activity of a prostitute.

In Sweden there was a system called 'reglement' which meant that the women were registered and had to be examined regularly. The result from the health point of view was very poor, as some of these women went to other doctors to be 'cleaned up' before the official examination. Through the activity of female pressure groups, it was advocated that this system of registration of prostitutes was against the rights of women. It was questioned: why should the women be registered and not the men infecting her?

LEGISLATION CONCERNING VENEREAL DISEASE

In Sweden, as in several other countries, around 1910, laws were introduced trying to supervise the venereal diseases. Every infected person was supposed to report his or her source of infection, and this source compelled to examination and treatment. These laws also gave the police some authority to assist in making people undergo treatment. These laws had a limited effect. The main impact in Sweden was that it requested the health services to provide treatment and drugs free of charge.

After serious considerations in many countries, this type of law has been looked upon as unrealistic and discriminating. In Sweden, for example, there now exists one law on protection against infectious diseases. This law consists of three parts, one for the earlier so-called epidemic diseases — cholera, smallpox, etc. — one for tuberculosis, and one for venereal diseases. This has meant that the overall regulations for each are the same and it is hoped that in future the law will see that the same responsibility is accepted from the community towards the patients with this type of diseases as by the patient himself in his responsibility of not giving chance to infect anybody else, whether he be a carrier of the germs of salmonella, tuberculosis, or gonorrhoea.

On the other hand, some discussion is going on as to whether even this type of law has any effect on the spreading of the diseases. Responsible people are not affected by the regulations: they fulfil the requirements themselves. People who cause problems will do so with or without every law. But, from the epidemiological point of view, the public health authorities should have some authority to act against persons with infectious diseases putting other persons in risk situations — be it tuberculosis or gonorrhoea.

MORBIDITY

If we look at the frequency figures all over the world, there was an increase after World War II followed by a decrease in some countries. Recently, however, it has been reported from very many countries that syphilis as well as gonorrhoea has increased in a number of cases. In Sweden, for example, with a population of 8 million, more than 38 000 cases were reported in 1970 (*Public Health in Sweden 1973* 1976): 4·5 cases per 1000 inhabitants. On the other hand, syphilis cases numbered no more than around 300. In some other countries, the figures were also rather high. In Poland, with 32 million people, the number of cases of gonorrhoea were around 50 000 and there were around 17 000 cases of syphilis. In other countries in Eastern Europe, the number of gonorrhoea cases was also very high. In Western Europe and in the United States, the figures are also increasing and from the public health point of view this is a great problem. In the U.S.S.R., according to a paper in *Community Medicine* (Hyde and Ryan 1972), the venereal diseases are going down in number but there are still many cases, in spite of the fact that every case seems to be hospitalized and treated up to complete cure. Blood tests for syphilis are made in the anti-natal clinics, and these show a decrease in frequency. According to the authors, the rate of gonorrhoea is around 0·8 cases per 1000 inhabitants, which is considerably lower than in Western European countries.

If we study a paper from China (Ma Hei-Teh 1966), we see that through an intensive struggle against venereal diseases, acting according to the political approach of that country, there has been an intensive mass-screening programme, partly through tests and partly through questionnaires. With the results of this programme, and with the co-operation of the people, the author claims that venereal diseases are social in origin and have been wiped out in China.

SOCIETAL ATTITUDES

What is the attitude of the society towards venereal diseases today? For many years, venereal disease services have been hampered by the society's outlook upon the problem as something rather distasteful associated with the lower classes. There are still many venereal disease hospitals and services all over the world that are quite 'underdeveloped' in comparison with other medical installations in the same country. In some areas, the attitude of the staff does not encourage rehabilitation of the patient.

It is astonishing that, with the trends in the modern society towards openness and frankness in discussion, intensified education and information in the schools, and in mass media, the venereal disease frequency is still so very high. Even in countries with fully developed health services, available free of charge to everybody, the venereal disease rate is far too high. At the same time, the figures show that although previously there were 5 infected men to 1 infected woman, the figures, at least in some countries, are now approaching the ratio 1:1 (*Public Health in Sweden 1973* 1976). Health education may have completely taken away fear of the disease: treatment is very effective. On the other hand, there still exists some lack of willingness to seek assistance. Also there is still the fact that too many people do not suspect that their bedmate might be infected. People tend to think that if they contract venereal disease the doctor will give them one shot and the thing is cured. The new preventive contraceptives, the pill and the intrauterine device, have diminished the possibility and/or risk of conception and therefore of congenital syphilis. But these methods have to some extent diminished the use of the rubber sheath, which is a reasonably good protection against venereal disease if properly used.

HIGH-RISK GROUPS

Statistical studies have shown that the venereal disease patient does not differ greatly from the population as a whole in many countries. However, a number of cases occur in groups which for many reasons have problems with the establishment, the police, the child-welfare authorities and, in later life, proportionally more venereal disease patients than other people are involved with alcohol and narcotic problems. In Sweden, it has been witnessed that the number of cases among very young girls has increased rapidly. In 1969 100 cases were reported among the age group 10–14 years of age and in 1971, two years later, the number of cases was 157. In 1973, however, only 69 cases were reported (*Public Health in Sweden 1973* 1976).

The situation from the public health point of view is a challenge, and there is a great deal of discussion going on about how to meet it. Information is only one part of the possible activity. In many countries, immigrants — maybe from rural areas to big cities, or immigrants from other countries — are very often reported as venereal disease cases. Lack of personal contact, increased movement of the population within countries, and migration of workers between different countries have, no doubt, contributed to the situation today.

The venereal disease situation is really challenging. We know the causes of the disease, we have a 100 per cent effective treatment method at hand — and still we cannot stop its development.

REFERENCES

HYDE, G. and RYAN, M. (1972). Control of venereal diseases in the Soviet Union. *Comm. Med.*, 7 January 1972, pp. 3–5.

MA HAI-TEH (HATEM, G.). With Mao Tse-Tung's thought as the compass for action in the control of venereal diseases in China. *China's Med.*, **85**, 52–68.

PUBLIC HEALTH IN SWEDEN 1973 (1976). Pp. 86–8. Official Statistics of Sweden. National Board of Health and Welfare. Stockholm, Sweden.

25. DIFFERENCES BETWEEN MALE AND FEMALE REACTIONS TO PSYCHOSOCIAL AND PHYSICAL STRESSORS: A REVIEW

WALTER D. FENZ and BARRY R. FOGLE

> It is likely that many studies in the literature or in a file drawer would have led the investigators to draw different conclusions if separate analyses had been made for males and females. [Kagan and Moss 1962]

We group our studies into five categories: (1) animal studies; (2) psychophysiological studies, i.e., behavioural observations, phenomenological self-reports, psychological coping processes in response to physical and psychosocial stressors, (3) psychological studies, (4) stress reactions under conditions of sensory deprivation, isolation, confinement; (5) clinical investigations.

ANIMAL STUDIES

A prominent colleague of ours, in a pessimistic mood about the state of our science, one day made the comment that, if one were to summarize all research with animals which has any bearing on human behaviour, one could easily do it on one page — double spaced. Part of the problem might be that most of these animal researchers, a few notable ones excepted, fail to point out the relevance of their work to research with humans, so that the relatively naïve human psychologist may think that his poor fellow scientist has lost his mind in his 'glass bead game' with the *Rattus norvegicus*. Therefore we approach the problem of sex differences in stress reactions in the sub-human species somewhat cautiously, and sceptically.

The British psychologist P. L. Broadhurst (1957) made the comment that 'work on individual differences in emotionality in rats should employ different criteria for each sex'. He based this recommendation on his own findings: in response to noxiously loud noise, which he found to be an excellent source of stress for rats, females defaecated less and ambulated more than males (Broadhurst 1957, 1958). This finding may not seem overly exciting, except for the fact that Munn (1950) in his scholarly *Handbook of psychological research in the rat* points out that 'urinating and defecating ... has long been used as a measure of emotionality in the rat.' In the same way ambulatory behaviour has frequently been associated with activation, or arousal, leading to problem solving. If we may draw an inference, then, males seem to respond more passively to stress, females more actively, i.e., they try to find a way out of it, rather than just sit there and soil their grill.

The stress induced to Broadhurst's rats was relatively mild; what if more intensely noxious situations are studied? Robert E. Schell and Rogers Elliot (1967) found males to be 'more emotional to relatively mild stress, but more resistant than females to more stressful experience'. The stress in their study was 'a 5 sec shock at an intensity which kept subjects jumping and squealing for its duration'.

The Schell and Elliott (1967) conclusion has only partly stood the test of time, and later research. Valle (1970), using the now famous *Rattus norvegicus*, found that in response to a mild stressor, females locomoted more and reared more, but showed the same degree of thigmotaxis, which in English means 'wall hugging' and is a sign of timidity. Thus, female subjects were more active than males, as Broadhurst (1957, 1958) suggested, but there was no difference in urinating or defaecating. And this is where science stands to-day. Conclude Schell and colleague: '... for the moment, the point is clear that sex does make a difference in response to stress. The direction and degree of difference varies with the stress and probably with the strain of the animal employed, though this latter point requires and deserves systematic exploration.' We do not really concur that it does.

Next we would like to mention two studies which deal with sex differences in mortality rate due to stress. La Barba *et al.* (1970) examined physiological reaction systems of mice regarding carcinogenesis (Ehrlich carcinoma) and mortality. Subjects were given cold temperature treatments as stressors. Males survived longer than females. Probably the most relevant comment of this paper is that 'the authors would like to caution against generalization of results'. They may apply only to the strain of mice that they studied.

Stupfel and Roussel (1968) confined male and female rats under conditions of oxygen deprivation: the mortality rate of males was consistently higher than that of females, in spite of the fact that haematological examinations and the biochemistry of the blood showed no differences between the sexes.

Another set of studies deal with differences between male and female rats in response to food deprivation.

Studies in this area seem to concur: food deprivation increases exploratory behaviour in males more so than in females. Hughes (1968) found that 48 hours of food deprivation produced a higher frequency of exploratory activity in male than in female rats; under no deprivation, males engaged in less exploratory behaviour than females. This confirmed work by Montgomery (1953), De Lorge and Bolles (1961), and Thompson (1955).

A study by Sines (1959) seems very relevant to our topic, especially in its medical, pathological implications to stress reactions. If one could generalize from this study on humans, it would be very relevant indeed but the author does not make that inference. Rats that developed stomach lesions following the stress of 48 hours of immobilization were selectively bred. Selective mating through the second filial generation was accompanied by a significant increase in the incidence of stomach lesions following the same stress conditions. These findings give additional evidence for hereditary factors controlling the development of stomach lesions under stress. Of relevance to the present review is the fact that female rats took their confinement less well than male rats: '... the females squealed and struggled more than the males and were in general more difficult to manage.' There also was a higher incidence of stomach lesions in females than in males. This had earlier been observed in work with guinea-pigs, where there also was a relationship between sex, resistance to experimental procedure, and development of stomach lesions — in the same direction (Sawrey et al. 1956). The same sex difference in resistance to stress had also been noted by Noble and Collip (1942). It would, of course, be of some interest to know what the determining variables of these observed differences are. A number of the authors cited above indicate that this is the direction of their present research, i.e. '... behavioural studies are now being conducted to determine the validity of the observed differences in activity level and "emotionality" between animals which show stomach lesions following stress and those which do not.'

Finally, another clinical investigation: Meier et al. (1963) studied sex differences in the serum cholesterol response to stress in monkeys. The decrease in serum cholesterol of the female monkeys under stress was not as great as in the males (a drop of 35·5 per cent from a control period for males, versus a drop of 19·0 per cent for females). The authors point out that it is difficult as yet to delineate the intermediary mechanisms responsible for sex differences in the relative changes in the serum cholesterol fractions. While aware that in future research such factors as altered rate of synthesis, utilization, excretion, or deposition into body tissues must be identified, the authors also lay considerable weight on possible psychological variables responsible for triggering the metabolic factors which led to the alterations in the cholesterol levels.

In the search for the intervening variables, the clinical investigations concur. Differences, by themselves, are not necessarily very meaningful findings, unless they represent a first step towards a scientific explanation as to why the differences have occurred. Unfortunately, all too often researchers have given only lip service to this fact. Research with animals, allowing for a much wider range in techniques than research with humans, should direct itself to such questions.

PSYCHOPHYSIOLOGICAL REACTIONS TO PHYSICAL AND PSYCHOSOCIAL STRESSORS

The law of initial value states that 'an autonomic nervous system (ANS) response to stimulation is a function of the pre-stimulus level' (Sternbach 1966). In the study of individual differences, especially in psychological or psychophysiological reactions to environmental change, a recognition of this fact is most relevant. Ferreira (1965) investigated a sex factor in basal palmar sweating, and found that females sweat more than males, at all age levels. Why so? It is not really known, but it does not seem to be related to differences in the known sexual hormones, since the pattern remains the same whether during pre-puberty, sexually active, or post-menopausal individuals. Physiologists would point out a number of other base differences in physiological activities between the sexes. In psychology it is even a truism to say that females score differently than males on a wide variety of psychological scales; these are basal, or as we call them in psychology, 'trait' differences between the sexes. Generally speaking, women score higher than men in 'trait' anxiety (Fenz 1967). Thus, when measuring psychophysiological stress reactions we cannot ignore possible basal differences.

In an observational study on 'factors in human endurance' in mountain climbers, deep-sea divers, long-distance swimmers, etc., Johnson (1968) refers to sex as a factor affecting responses. In relation to long-distance swimmers he points out that '... among other factors which determine performance under sress are sex differences, which include different physique and thickness of distribution of subcutaneous fat and hence isolation'.

One of John Lacey's first studies dealt with 'sex differences in somatic reactions to stress' (Lacey 1947). He used boys and girls ranging in age from 78 to 210 months and recorded cardiovascular, respiratory, and palmar conductance measures during relaxation, during reaction to a tilt-table stress, and during recovery from stress. At the time of the above mentioned publication, only palmar conductance measures had received analysis. Young girls exhibited significantly more relaxation, were more reactive, and adapted less to stress than boys. Thus, females were not only more reactive to stress, but also exhibited more physiological relaxation during rest. Lacey suggested a factor of autonomic nervous system lability, a concept he had developed over the years, If so, it represents a basal difference between the sexes, and not a reactivity difference *per se*. (It may here be noted that it is generally believed that the female also has a wider zone of cardio-vascular regulation than the male (cf. Morimoto *et al.* 1967, Dubois *et al.* 1952).)

An early study by Berry and Martin (1957) points out another important factor which has to be considered in psychophysiological studies: the factor making for individual differences may well be due to a differential psychological impact of the same stimulus on males and females. It is a well-controlled study: he selected 30 high-anxious males and 30 high-anxious females, and 30 low-anxious males and 30 low-anxious females. Each group of 30 was again divided into 3 groups, one receiving apprehension-arousing instructions, the other neutral, and the third group reassuring instructions. The study involved classical conditions of the Galvanic skin response, the unconditional stimulus being shock. Resuls indicated that the instructions had opposite effects on the conditionability of males and females. Males showed less conditioning when given reassuring instructions; females showed less conditioning with the apprehension-arousing instructions, and most with the reassuring instructions. Further, females showed greater galvanic skin response reactivity than males in all phases of the experiment: adaptation, conditioning, and extinction.

Sternbach's book on pain (1968) suggests that women are more responsive to pain than men. In the section *Stress reactions under conditions of sensory deprivation, isolation, and confinement* (p. 171) of this review we are making similar observations, and are suggesting that this may well be part of the stereotyped female role, which is, nevertheless, not at all unchangeable.

Some studies in this area are so well controlled: Legg (1965) found the opposite from Berry and Martin, i.e. that women were less reactive than men in all responses to the conditional stimulus (he did not measure responses to the unconditional stimulus). But since subjects were able to select their own shock level, females chose lower levels than males. That may well account for the differences, but for the author 'the differences remain largely unexplainable.'

The study by Bauman *et al.* (1966) leaves also a good deal to be desired. The authors point to a study by E. Katkin (1965) as a rationale for using basal skin conductance as a measure of stress, or anxiety. Katkin found that *non specific galvanic skin reactivities*, not basal skin conductance level, were a good measure of anxiety. Bauman found that females were, overall, higher in basal resistance (lower in basal conductance) than males. Basal skin resistance, as a 'between-subjects' measure, has not been found to be a reliable indicant of anxiety, but changes in basal resistance within a given subject, are useful. In the Bauman study there were no differences between males and females in amount of basal resistance change due to the imposed stress condition, nor was there a relationship between Cattell's Anxiety Scale Questionnaire (1951) and basal resistance. The finding in the overall male and female

difference may well be due to skin texture, distribution of sweat glands ... and have nothing to do with anxiety *per se*. A number of studies point to just such a basic physiological difference in sweat gland activities between the sexes (Morimoto *et al.* 1967; Brouha *et al.* 1960; Wyndham *et al.* 1964; Weinman *et al.* 1967).

Finally, a number of studies suggested that psycho-physiological differences between males and females are due to a different cognitive style, or coping process. Two studies, reviewed in the section *Stress reactions ...*, are most appropriate: Biase *et al.* (1967) found that males responded more strongly, autonomically, than females, during 3 hours of sensory deprivation; this was indicated by their sharper drop in basal skin resistance throughout the experiment. Zuckerman *et al.* (1968) determined two groups of hormone metabolites. 17-ketogenic steroids and 17-ketosteroids on a series of urine samples taken throughout an 8-hour deprivation period: females were significantly lower than males on both endocrine measures. Both psychophysiological and endocrine indicants of stress were in sharp contrast to self-report of stress and discomfort. It was suggested that free expression of discomfort adaptively reduces the impact of the stressor.

Differences in basal levels; differences in overall reactivity levels, i.e., lability levels, differences in set, or interpretation of the instructions; differentially perceived demand characteristics; psychological stereotypes determining response styles; differences in cognitive styles, or defensive operations ... these are but some of the variables relevant to psychophysiological studies of male/female differences in stress reactions.

PSYCHOLOGICAL STUDIES

One of the well-documented findings in psychological literature is the difference in scores on anxiety scales between male and female subjects: the scores of females are consistently higher than those of males. This difference is especially reliable in tests of 'trait' anxiety. This seems to be not merely an American phenomenon, but one which applied world-wide; it even applied to Greece: Vassiliou and Vassiliou (1967) found that on a Greek form of the Taylor Manifest Anxiety Scale (1953) Greek women gave a significantly higher score than Greek men. The immediate question which comes to mind is: Why are women taking life harder than men?

A study by Zohner (1970) related conformity, i.e. susceptibility to social influence, to stress, and found a differential pattern between male and female subjects: under conditions of low and high stress, males were more highly suggestible than females. The study used a task of size estimation, and instructions at three levels of assumed suggestiveness. This finding does not conform to expectations. We really do not know whether the experimenter was male or female; if the experimenter was a woman it is quite possible that her male subjects may have perceived indirect rewards for aquiescing. Anyway, we would like the study to be repeated by a male experimenter, and we seriously doubt that it is replicable under those conditions; in other words, we cannot help but feel that Martin Orne's (1961) emphasis on 'demand characteristics' was not ill founded.

Philips (1966) found that the women in his sample were not only more anxious, but also more 'acquiescent', i.e. women had a greater tendency to acquiesce, or agree with statements: if asked if they were anxious, they would be more ready to say 'yes' than 'no'. The plausibility of the acquiescence hypothesis is further supported by sex differences in role stereotypes, and in predominantly female stereotypes of dependency, passivity, and conformity (Kagan and Moss 1960). Vaughan (1966) also found that males were less conforming than women, and their scores on the Taylor Manifest Anxiety were lower.

A number of studies deal with differential defensive, or coping processes between males and females under stress. A dissertation by R. A. Rodenhiser (1967) is to the point: 'The defensive use of identification'. Identification was defined in terms of the subjects' acquisition of characteristics of the therapist in a disturbing, i.e. stress-eliciting film on psychotherapy with mute patients. He found a positive relationship between anxiety and identification and identification increasing with stress, but for male subjects only. The results suggest that stress facilitates change in self-evaluation in males but inhibits, or restricts similar change in females.

A slightly esoteric study comes to mind at this point: 'Anxiety and escapist attitudes', published in the *Indian Psychological Review*, by N. K. Dutt (1966). The author constructed a scale of 'other worldliness and self-surrender', and related its scores on an anxiety scale: the variables were highly related, and females scored significantly higher than males. This is good to know: women are not only more anxious than men, but more 'other worldly' and 'self-surrendering'.

It might at this point be appropriate to introduce three studies on sex differences in affiliation needs in response to stress. Carrigan (1966) placed both men and women under conditions of potential sociometric rejection; under those conditions, females scored significantly higher for conformity. These results confirmed results of a study by Gerald (1961): under physical threat conditions, affiliation and emotional arousal, as measured by the Galvanic skin response, were related significantly for women, but not for men. The third study is by MacDonald (1970); its main interest is in birth order differences, but it also focuses on sex differences. It is a complex study, which, in a nutshell, concluded that the desire to affiliate is more a function of anxiety in first-born males and later-born females than it is for first-born females and later-born males. The author tries hard to give an explanation for these findings.

Anxiety over parental acceptance and peer acceptance was related to shifts in moral judgment in a psychoanalytically oriented study by Birnbaum (1968). When children are made anxious about parental acceptance, they tend to regress to an earlier, more rigid stage, apparently clinging more tenaciously to parental rules in an attempt to assure themselves of acceptance; on the other hand, when made anxious about peer acceptance the shift is in the opposite, more flexible, direction. Birnbaum also found sex differences, in that girls were generally more rigid in adhering to adult rules; that is, they were less 'morally autonomous', except when a more abstract principle of justice (e.g. retribution) was at stake, in which case the boys became more rigid than the girls. These results are of interest because of the support they lend to both psychoanalytical and social learning theories of sex differences in moral development.

If one can draw an inference from the Birnbaum (1968) study with pre-adolescent children to results obtained by Crandall (1965) with adults, there appears to be a reversal shift in sex differences from childhood to adulthood; Crandall found that high-anxious men were more conservative than low-anxious men, while high-anxious women were less conservative than low-anxious women. Thus, anxiety produces increased intolerance of ambiguity in women, and a tendency in men to avoid making errors from rash judgments.

One last study on differential defensive processes between men and women in response to stress: Paris and Goodstein 1966. The authors used Byrne's (1964) 'repression/sensitization' scale, and selected equal samples of men and women repressors and sensitizors. The experimental manipulation required them to read (a) erotic literature, (b) material dealing with death, and (c) neutral material. Following these readings, they were asked to rate their anxiety, boredom, anger, sexual arousal, disgust, and 'being upset'. The investigators found no differences due to scores on Byrne's scale, but women, in general, responded more strongly to death material, in the 'emotional upset', 'anger', and strangely enough, 'sexual arousal' categories.

We have observed, then, that there are sex differences in anxiety scores; these were interpreted as reflecting greater need of acquiescence in women, in differential sex stereotypes, and in differential cognitive styles. Developmental inferences suggest that these differences are consolidated over time.

A series of studies from our own laboratory (Fenz and Epstein 1965; Fenz 1967; Brandt and Fenz 1969; and Horvath and Fenz 1971) focuses on the specificity of somatic symptoms, presumably as stress reactions, and also emphasize sex differences. Males are more prone to present symptoms related to muscle tension, females autonomic symptoms; these differences ocur in subjective report and are validated in physiological recordings under stress conditions, are found in 'normal' undergraduates and become accentuated in a psychoneurotic population. Robert Stern (1969) asked

TABLE 25.1

*Physiological changes reported to occur
before an important event*

	Males (per cent)	Significance levels	Females (per cent)
Face feels hot and flushed	19	<0·05	32
Nervous stomach	55	<0·05	66
Sweating (palms)	48	<0·05	41
Lump in throat	23		21
Cold hands and feet	14	<0·05	32
General restlessness	60		58
General body sweating	26		25
Increased heart rate	51		50
Frequent urge to urinate	16	<0·05	24
Awareness of heartbeat	43	<0·05	53

a large population of male and female students 'what physiological changes in your body usually take place immediately prior to some important event, such as a big exam, an important date, a job interview ...'. His results were shown in Table 25.1.

What the results indicate is that women generally were more prone to admit symptoms of anxiety than men; there was one discrepancy: women were less ready to report symptoms of perspiration than men.

To complement the above we like to cite a psychoanalytical study by Bradford (1968) which also focuses upon the relationship between sex differences and specificity in anxiety reactions. From the psychoanalytic model one would predict that (a) males exceed females in anxieties concerning physical threat, vulnerability, or 'castration' anxieties; (b) females exceed males in anxieties centering around social fears of rejection, embarassment, or loss of love. The study lends partial support to the psychoanalytical model: (a) there was a great overlap between men and women on fears of physical vulnerability; this is probably the result of the ambiguity in psychoanalytical theory on the incidence and importance of 'castration' anxiety in women; (b) there was a consistent and powerful sex difference in anxiety over loss of love, in the expected direction; this is congruent with a psychoanalytical interpretation of feminine psychology but can also be viewed from a social-learning theory model.

STRESS REACTIONS UNDER CONDITIONS OF SENSORY DEPRIVATION, ISOLATION, AND CONFINEMENT

Most studies on sensory deprivation used male subjects; the first study coming to our attention which used both male and female subjects was a clinical investigation by Smith and Lewty (1959). The authors had been concerned with the lack of uniformity in experimental techniques, and present the layout of a 'silent room' of their design. The study included 11 women and 9 men. The instructions were to stay in the silent room 'as long as they could stand it'. Women, in general, lasted longer than men (48·70 hours over 29·24 hours). Anecdotal information is also provided on thinking and affect, but there was no consistent pattern of sex differences.

A study by Davis *et al.* (1961) reminds us that sensory deprivation is composed not only of sensory deprivation, *per se*, but concomitant social isolation. These researchers placed two people in adjacent tank-type respirators: one set of 10 dyads was made up of males, who did not know each other; the other parallel set of dyads was made up of married couples. The married couples fared less well than the male dyads. They had been asked to stay 10·5 hours, but 9 of the male dyads stayed for the whole duration, while only 2 of the married couple dyads did. When the married couples started to talk about leaving, one partner would reinforce the other in that direction, and they would decide to leave. The authors comment that 'male and female subjects showed about the same symptoms ... but there is evidence that problems in thinking were not as severe as in experiments allowing to social contact'; this was nevertheless, more of a clinical than an experimental study.

A set of studies investigates differences during periods of deprivation of isolation, and assumes them to be related to Witkin's (1954) notions of 'field dependency' and 'body orientation'. Differences are expected on the basis of 'perceptual mode', since females are reported to be more field dependent, and males more field independent, or body oriented.

Digressing slightly for a moment, I would like to cite a study by Cohen *et al.* (1962), who compared field-dependent to field-independent males: field-dependent subjects showed higher levels of activation in terms of spontaneous Galvanic skin response activities; in comparing EEG frequencies, using three frequency bands, above 12 Hz, 8–12 Hz, and below 8 Hz, field-dependent subjects showed a proportionately greater frequency of beta waves (above 12 Hz) than field-independent subjects. Field-dependent subjects also showed greater psychological discomfort under the conditions of sensory deprivation, a higher incidence of disorganization of thought. It should be noted that this study is relevant by inference only, and also because it provided a rationale for a number of studies in the area.

Walters *et al.* (1962) based their hypotheses of sex differences under conditions of sensory deprivation on Witkin's findings of sex differences in perceptual mode. They used medical students as subjects. Contrary to prediction they found that their female subjects gave a significantly higher proportion of non-stimulus bound responses than males, i.e. they were more body oriented, or field independent in their response during sensory deprivation than males. The same researchers replicated the findings with non-medical students (Walters *et al.* 1964), under the assumption that medical students, especially female medical students, might well belong to a class of their own. Not so. Females were again more internally oriented, less field dependent than males. The findings by Walters and colleagues are opposite to expectations from Witkin's work, and by inference, from Cohen's findings.

Reed and Kenna (1964) found no sex differences among 14 male and 14 female subjects undergoing 20 minutes of sensory deprivation; his primary measures

TABLE 25.2

Studies on sensory deprivation

Authors	Type	Duration	Measures	Findings on sex differences
Smith *et al.* (1954)	Perceptual isolation	Open	Clinical observation of length of stay	No consistent differences; females > males
David *et al.* (1961)	Social isolation	10·5 hours	Clinical observation	No consistent difference
Walters *et al.* (1962)	Sensory deprivation	Open	Field dependence vs. individual psychological interview	Females more field independent; no consistent differences
Walters *et al.* (1964)	Sensory deprivation	3 hours	Field dependence vs. individual mood	Females more field independent Females select more pleasant adjectives; show no difference in selection of unpleasant adjectives
			Anxiety	Females more difficulty in breathing
			Hunger	Males > females
			Time estimation	No differences
Reed *et al.* (1964)	Sensory deprivation	20 minutes	Body image	No differences
Arnhoff *et al.* (1963)	Sensory deprivation	2 hours	Isolation disturbance	No differences
			Time disturbance	No differences
			Imagery disturbance	No differences
Biase *et al.* (1969)	Sensory deprivation	3 hours	Non-specific Galvanic skin resistance	No differences
			Basal resistance	Greater drop in males than females
			Self-reported distress	Females > males
			Somatic symptoms	No differences
Leiderman (1962)	Isolation	Open	Self-reported distress	No differences
Zuckerman *et al.* (1963)	Sensory deprivation	8 hours	Somatic symptoms	Females > males
			Other reports of distress	Females > males
			Sexual thoughts	Males > females
	Social isolation	8 hours	Need: sex, hunger	Males > females
	Confinement	8 hours	Somatic symptoms	Females > males
			Other reports of distress	
			Endocrine measures: 17-KGS; 17-KS	Males > females
Pollard *et al.* (1963)	Sensory deprivation	Open	Length of stay	Males > females

was degree of disturbance in body image. Arnhoff *et al.* (1963) similarly concluded that 'insofar as short term isolation is concerned, the ... results do not support the hypothesis that systematic differences exist between the sexes to tolerate isolation and confinement. Individual differences are greater than those attributed to sex.'

Working from a psychoanalytical point of view, Holt and Goldberger (1961) postulated that normal, but passive males should adapt more readily to stimulus deprivation, than more aggressive, masculine males, and by implication, women should adapt more readily than men. This hypothesis is opposite to the one predicted from Witkin's formulation, but in accordance with Walters' (1962, 1964) findings.

A psychophysiological study by Biase *et al.* (1967) represents a transition between studies based on the Witkins hypothesis and Holt and Goldberger's postulate and studies based on implications derived from Martin Orne's (1961) notion of 'demand characteristics'.

Biase *et al.* (1967) evaluated both physiological activity (non-specific Galvanic skin response and basal resistance) and verbal report and found that men showed greater autonomic activity than women, but women scored significantly higher on a measure of verbalized stress derived from ratings of a post-stimulus deprivation interview. These results are not consistent with the findings of Walters (1962, 1964) who reports greater indicants of discomfort in men. Perhaps this difference is related to the fact that Walters used a water-immersion technique, and the Biase study used bed confinement. The study did not support the hypothesis of a positive relationship between 'passivity' or field dependence in males and adaptive responses to isolation, i.e. the Holt-Goldberger postulate. Biase suggests as an interpretation of his findings the fact that women may feel less constrained in admitting their discomfort. This point is carried further in the following two studies.

One of the best-designed and best-documented studies in the area of sex differences in sensory deprivation is by Zuckerman *et al.* (1968), and develops further the interpretation of differences in demand characteristics, or set, suggested in his early study with Biase *et al.* (1967); the hypotheses is that females will more readily admit discomfort in sensory deprivation, when males will tend more to deny discomfort, but will show more physiological arousal. This hypothesis is based on Martin Orne's notion of the relevance of demand characteristics of the experiment in this situation linked to sex stereotypy. Our table (Table 25.2) summarized the findings; the hypothesis was essentially confirmed. An earlier, more clinical study by Pollard *et al.* (1963) came to the same conclusions. His was an open-ended study, and he found that women terminated sessions earlier than men, and more frequently: men stayed an average of 7 hours and 19 minutes. And there were also differences in verbal reports. He comments

... it would be easy to suggest that women simply were more anxious, but the subjects' own comments and their changing pattern of reported affect indicate, rather, differences in their approach to the experimental situation: to the men this was a challenge; giving up appears to have been equated with weakness, an unacceptable, unmasculine attribute.... The women, not sharing these personal implications of withstanding or not withstanding the experimental situation, did not feel obliged to stay. It is quite feasible, possibly expected for them to be weak....

Smith and Lewty (1959), whose study was the first we quoted in this review, made the comment that studies on sensory deprivation are difficult to compare because of the great variability in conditions. The same comment applies 13 years later. But some conclusions may be drawn.

1. Of all rigorous studies done in the area, only the studies by Walters *et al.* (1962, 1964) found women responding with less stress than men. The reason is probably due to the conditions of sensory deprivation which he employed, namely water immersion.

2. A number of studies found no sex differences, notably the study by Arnoff and Leon (1963) and the study by Reed and Kenna (1964). Both of them had relatively short deprivation periods.

3. The link between field dependency and greater tolerance under conditions of sensory deprivation, was not supported.

4. Under stress, as induced by sensory deprivation, men responded more physiologically (or biochemically), women more in self-report. It is quite likely that the complaining of women is an adaptive coping, or release mechanism, with the resulting benefit of less physiological arousal.

5. Differences in expected responding between males and females, namely differences in perceived demand characteristics linked to sex stereotypes are an important component in the observed differences.

A comment by Witkins *et al.* (1954) relative to their findings on differences in perceptual mode may be appropriate at this point '... women, when necessary, can respond like men ...' — when demand characteristics are equal, it is very likely that most, or all of the sex differences would disappear.

See Table 25.2 for a summary of the findings of this section.

CLINICAL INVESTIGATIONS

Reference is here made only to psychological studies based on clinical, human populations; there are only very few.

Henrichs and MacKenzie (1969) studied psychological adjustment in patients undergoing open heart surgery. Pre-operative symptoms of severe psychiatric disorder were directly related to mortality, conversively, the authors feel that attention to stress symptoms would reduce mortality rate: symptoms of pronounced anxiety in males and symptoms of emotional overcontrol in females. The efficient use of coping mechanisms thus appears to be the important factor in optimally dealing with a source of intense stress.

A number of studies deal with the 'social breakdown syndrome', i.e. the reaction of an individual to a crisis in relation to his life situation which leads to severe psychiatric disturbance and hospitalization. Beisser and Glasser (1968) report that in the sample they studied, marital stress was a significantly more frequent precipitating source of stress for women, while the stress category 'job-vocation' was a significantly more frequent precipitating source of stress for males; this could have been predicted. Between them, marital and occupational stress accounted for approximately 75 per cent of first admissions to mental hospitals.

Thomae and Simons (1967) studied what psychiatric problems are encountered by men and women in later life. Their findings on sex differences concur with findings by Beisser and Glasser (1968). Another contribution to gerontology comes from a study by Kral *et al.* (1968); these researchers studied stress reactions resulting from the relocation of an aged population. Findings showed that aged women were able to withstand the stress of relocation better than aged men.

Comparing a psychiatric population to a matched population of non-psychiatric hospital patients, Morrison *et al.* (1968) asked essentially the same question: what are the life events which lead to mental illness? But this questioning went further: do psychiatric patients differ in their life history from non-psychiatric, medical patients? Very few differences were found between the two groups. 'This report will not surprise those investigators who suggest that in susceptible individuals, life stress may precipitate the onset and exacerbation of medical as well as psychiatric disorder.' The data did not support the notion that 'psychiatric illness' is a unitary phenomenon distinguished from 'non-psychiatric illness' on the basis of the factors studied. In that, it made a substantial contribution.

As a more general comment, which is very relevant to our topic, it must be said that it is rare to find satisfactory studies of a possible relationship between psychiatric illness and life events of sociological or psychological import. The chief deficiencies of most such studies have been the lack of suitable controls, imprecision about diagnostic categories, failure to ascertain time of onset and failure to distinguish clearly between events preceding the illness and events following onset, which may have been consequences of the illness.

This is a wide open area for research.

REFERENCES

ARNHOFF, F. and LEON, H. V. (1963). Sex differences in response to short-term sensory deprivation and isolation. *Percept. Motor Skills*, **17**, 81–2.

BAUMAN, M. S. and STRAUGHAM, J. H. (1969). BSR as a function of anxiety, stress, and sex. *Psychol. Rec.*, **19**, 339–44.

BEISSER, A. R. and GLASSER, N. (1968). The precipitating stress leading to psychiatric hospitalization. *Comp. Psychiat.*, **9**, 50–61.

BERRY, J. and MARTIN, B. (1957). GSR reactivity as a function of anxiety, instructions and sex. *J. abnorm. soc. Psychol.*, **54**, 9–13.

BIASE, D. V. and ZUCKERMAN, M. (1967). Sex differences in stress responses to total and partial sensory deprivation. *Psychosom. Med.*, **19**, 380–90.

BIRNBAUM, M. P. (1968). Anxiety and moral judgment in early adolescence. *Dissertation Abstracts*, **29**, 1183.

BRADFORD, J. L. (1968). Sex differences in anxiety. *Dissertation Abstracts*, **29**, 1167.

BRANDT, K. and FENZ, W. D. (1969). Specificity in verbal and physiological indicants of anxiety. *Percept. Motor Skills*, **29**, 663–75.

BROADHURST, P. L. (1957). Determinants of emotionality in the rat: I. Situational factors. *Brit. J. Psychol.*, **48**, 1–12.

—— (1958). Determinants of emotionality in the rat: II. Antecendent factors. *Brit. J. Psychol.*, **49**, 12–20.

BROUHA, L., SMITH, P. E., DELANNE, R., and MAXFIELD, M. E. (1960). Physiological reactions of men and women during muscular activity and recovery in various environments. *J. appl. Physiol.*, **16**, 133–140.

BYRNE, D. (1964). Repression-sensitization as a dimension of personality. In *Progress in Experimental Personality Research* (ed. B. A. Maher), pp. 169–220. New York.

CARRIGAN, W. C. (1966). Sex and birth-order differences in conformity as a function of need affiliation arousal. *J. person.*
soc. Psychol., **3**, 479–83.

CATTELL, R. B. and SCHEIER, I. H. (1951). *The meaning and measurement of neuroticism and anxiety*. New York.

COHEN, S. I., SILVERMAN, A. S., and SHMAVONIAN, B. M. (1962). Psychophysiological studies in altered sensory environments. *J. psychosom. Res.*, **6**, 259.

CRANDALL, J. E. (1965). Some relationships among sex, anxiety, and conservatism of judgment. *J. Person.*, **33**, 99–107.

DAVIS, J. M., McCOURT, W. F., COURTNEY, J., and SOLOMON, P. (1961). Sensory deprivation, the role of social isolation. *Arch. gen. Psychiat.*, **5**, 84.

DeLORGE, J. and BOLLES, R. C. (1961). Effects of food deprivation on exploratory behaviour in a novel situation. *Psychol. Rep.*, **9**, 599–606.

DuBOIS, E. F., EBOUCH, F. O., and HARDY, J. D. (1952). Basal heat production and eliminatio of 13 normal women at temperatures from 22 °C to 35 °C. *J. Nutrit.*, **48**, 257–93.

DUTT, N. K. (1966). Anxiety and escapist attitudes. *Ind. psychol. Rev.*, **3**, 13–201.

FENZ, W. D. (1967). Specificity in somatic responses to anxiety. *Percept. Motor Skills*, **24**, 1183–90.

—— and EPSTEIN, S. (1965). Manifest anxiety: Unifactorial or multifactorial composition? *Percept. Motor Skills*, **20**, 773–80.

FERREIRA, A. J. (1965). Age and sex differences in the palmar sweat print. *Psychosom. Med.*, **27**, 207–11.

GERALD, H. B. and RABBIE, J. M. (1961). Fear and social comparison. *J. abnorm. soc. Psychol.*, **62**, 586–92.

HENRICHS, T. F. and MacKENZIE, J. W. (1969). Psychological adjustment and acute response to open heart surgery. *J. nerv. ment. Dis.*, **148**, 158–64.

HOLT, R. R. and GOLDBERGER, L. (1961). Assessment of individual resistance to sensory alteration. In *Psychophysiological aspects of space flight* (ed. B. E. Flaherty). New York.

HORVATH, S. and FENZ, W. D. (1971). Specificity in somatic indicants of anxiety in psychoneurotic patients. *Percept. Motor Skills*, **33**, 147–62.

HUGHES, R. N. (1968). Effects of food deprivation, deprivation experience, and sex on exploration in rats. *Brit. J. Psychol.*, **59**, 47–53.

JOHNSON, R. H. (1968). Factors in human endurance. *Brit. med. J.*, 697–700.

KAGAN, J. and MOSS, H. J. (1960). The stability of passive and dependent behaviour from childhood through adulthood. *Child Develop.*, **31**, 577–91.

—— and —— (1962). *Birth to maturity: a study in psychological development*. New York.

KATKIN, E. S. (1965). Relationship between manifest anxiety and indices of autonomic responses to stress. *J. person. soc. Psychol.*, **2**, 324–33.

KRAL, V. A., GRAD, B., and BERENSON, J. (1968). Stress reactions resulting from the relocation of an aged population. *Canad. psychiat. Ass. J.*, **13**, 201–9.

LABARBA, R. C., KLEIN, M. L., WHITE, J. L., and LAZAR, J. (1970). Effects of early cold stress and handling on the growth of Ehrlich carcinoma in BALB/c mice. *Develop. Psychol.*, **2**, 312–13.

LACEY, J. I. (1947). Sex differences in somatic reactions to stress. *Amer. Psychol.*, **2**, 343.

LEIDERMAN, P. H. (1962). Imagery and sensory deprivation, and experimental study. Aerospace Medical Division Report No. MRL-TDR-62-28.

LEGG, J. F. (1965). Differential GSR conditioning as a function of social tension and emotionality. *Dissertation Abstracts*, **25**, 2051.

MACDONALD, A. P. Jr (1970). Anxiety, affiliation and social isolation. *Develop. Psychol.*, **3**, 242–54.

MEIER, R. M., GREENHOTT, J. H., SHONLEY, I., GOODMAN, J. R., and PORTER, R. W. (1963). Sex differences in the serum cholesterol response to stress in monkeys. *Nature (Lond.)*, **199**, 812–13.

MONTGOMERY, K. C. (1953). The effect of hunger and thirst drives upon exploratory behaviour. *J. comp. physiol. Psychol.*, **46**, 315–19.

MORIMOTO, T., SLABOCHOVA, Z., NAMAN, R. K., and SARGENT, F. (1967). Sex differences in physiological reactions to thermal stress. *J. appl. Physiol.*, **22**, 528–32.

MORRISON, J. R., HUDGENS, R. W., and BARCHHA, R. G. (1968). Life events and psychiatric illness: A study of 100 patients and 100 controls. *Brit. J. Psychol.*, **114**, 423–32.

MUNN, N. L. (1950). *Handbook of psychological research in the rat*. London.

NOBLE, R. L. and COLLIP, J. B. (1942). A quantitative method for the production of experimental traumatic shock without haemorrhage in unanesthetized animals. *Quart. J. exp. Physiol.*, **31**, 187–99.

ORNE, M. T. (1961). 'On the social psychology of the psychological experiment: With particular reference to demand characteristics and their implications? Paper presented at the American Psychological Association Meeting, 1961, in New York. (Unpublished)

PARIS, J. and GOODSTEIN, L. D. (1966). Responses to death and sex stimuli materials as a function of repression-sensitization. *Psychol. Rep.*, **19**, 1283–91.

PHILLIPS, B. N. (1966). Defensiveness as a factor in sex differences in anxiety. *J. consult. Psychol.*, **30**.

POLLARD, J. C., UHR, L., and JACKSON, C. W. (1963). Studies in sensory deprivation. *Arch. gen. Psychiat.*, **8**, 435–54.

——, ——, and —— (1963). 'Some unexpected findings in experimental sensory deprivation: Psychopharmacological interaction of placebo-potentiated suggestion.' Read before the American Psychiatric Association, St. Louis, 1963. (Unpublished)

REED, G. F. and KENNA, J. C. (1964). Sex differences in body imagery and orientation under sensory deprivation of brief duration. *Percept. Motor Skills*, **18**, 117.

RODENHISER, R. A. (1967). The defensive use of identification. *Dissertation Abstracts*, **28**, 1208.

SAWREY, W. L., CONGER, J. J., and TURRELL, E. S. (1956). An experimental investigation of the role of psychological factors in the production of gastric ulcers in rats. *J. comp. physiol. Psychol.*, **49**, 457–61.

SCHELL, R. E. and ELLIOTT, R. (1967). Note on sex differences in response to stress in rats. *Psychol. Rep.*, **20**, 1201–2.

SHURLEY, J. (1962). Mental imagery in profound experimental sensory isolation. In *Hallucinations* (ed. L. S. West). New York.

SINES, J. O. (1959). Selective breeding for development of stomach lesions following stress in the rat. *J. comp. physiol. Psychol.*, **52**, 615–17.

SMITH, S. and LEWTY, W. (1969). Perceptual isolation using a silent room. *Lancet*, **ii**, 342–5.

STERN, R. M. (1969). Perceived somatic reactions to stress: sex, age, and familial occurrences. *J. psychosom. Res.*, **13**, 77–82.

STERNBACH, R. A. (1966). *Principles of psychophysiology*. New York.

STERNBACH, R. H. (1968). *Pain: a psychophysiological analysis*. New York.

STUPFEL, M. and ROUSSEL, A. (1968). Influence of sex on the resistance of rats and mice to confinement and hypoxia. *J. Physiol. (Paris)*, **60**, 379.

TAYLOR, J. A. (1953). A personality scale of manifest anxiety. *J. abnor. soc. Psychol.*, **48**, 285–90.

THOMPSON, W. R. (1955). Exploratory behaviour as a function of hunger in 'bright' and 'dull' rats. *J. comp. physiol. Psychol.*, **46**, 323–6.

THOMAE, H. and SIMONS, H. (1967). Reaction forms to stress situations: A contribution to gerontology. *Z. exp. angew. Psychol.*, **14**, 290–312.

VALLE, F. P. (1970). Effects of strain, sex, and illumination on open-field behaviour of rats. *Amer. J. Psychol.*, **83**, 103–11.

VASSILIOU, V., GEORGAS, J. C., and VASSILIOU, G. (1967). Variations in manifest anxiety due to sex, age and education. *J. Person. soc. Psychol.*, **6**, 195–7.

VAUGHAM, G. M. and TAYLOR, A. J. (1966). Clinical anxiety and conformity. *Percept. Motor Skills*, **22**, 719–22.

WALTERS, C., SHURLEY, J. T., and PARSONS, O. A. (1962). Differences in male and female responses to underwater sensory deprivation: An exploratory study. *J. nerv. ment. Dis.*, **135**, 302.

——, PARSONS, O. A., and SHURLEY, J. T. (1964). Male-female differences in underwater sensory isolation. *Brit. J. Psychiat.*, **110**, 290–5.

WEINMAN, K. P., SLABOCHOVA, Z., BERNAUER, E. M., MORIMOTO, T., and SARGENT, F. (1967). Reactions of men and women to repeated exposure to humid heat. *J. appl. Physiol.*, **22**, 533–8.

WITKIN, H. A., LEWIS, H. B., HERTZMAN, M., MACHOVER, K., MEISSNER, P. B., and WAPNER, S. (1954). *Personality through perception*. New York.

WYNDHAM, C. H., MORRISON, J. F., and WILLIAMS, C. G. (1964). Heat reactions of male and female caucasions. *J. appl. Physiol.*, **20**, 351–64.

ZOHNER, D. (1970). Environmental discontinuity, stress, and sex effects upon susceptibility to social influence. *J. genet. Psychol.*, **116**, 211–17.

ZUBER, S., PYSHKAR, D., SANSOM, W., and GOWING, J. (1961). Perceptual changes after prolonged sensory isolation. *Canad. J. Psychol.*, **15**, 83–100.

ZUCKERMAN, M., PERSKY, H., LINK, K., and BASU, G. (1968). Experimental and subject factors determining responses to sensory deprivation, social isolation, and confinement. *J. abnorm. Psychol.*, **73**, 183–94.

26. DEMOGRAPHIC AND PSYCHOSOCIAL CHARACTERISTICS OF MEN IN THE UNITED STATES NAVY AS PREDICTORS OF THOSE MEN WHO DEVELOP VENEREAL DISEASE

RICHARD H. RAHE

INTRODUCTION

A chief value of the epidemiological method in medicine is the possibility of identifying susceptible individuals to the development of particular disease entities. In this book, for example, Dr. Tottie has mentioned several identifying characteristics of persons in Sweden currently reporting to medical authorities with gonorrhea. Statistically speaking, these persons tend to be in their second and third decades of life, often they are emigrants to urban centres, they seem to be without close attachments to friends or family, and they tend to have had recent troubles with authority (school, police, etc.). These demographic and psychosocial characteristics of persons reporting to medical attention with gonorrhea are in marked contrast to such characteristics of persons reporting to medical centres with diseases such as tuberculosis. Thus, by exploring more fully, the demographic and psychosocial characteristics of persons contracting venereal disease, the better are the eventual chances of being able to identify subjects at 'high risk' to develop this disease.

Venereal disease, the most common venereal disease of today being gonorrhea, represents one of the few diseases of man that he 'brings on himself'. He does so in his sexual relations with members of the opposite sex. In the case of males, the chances of development of venereal disease can be minimized by using a condom during sexual intercourse when the health of the partner is in doubt. Failure to do so may result from lack of education in this method of prevention of the disease, or unwillingness on the part of the individual to follow this health-protective procedure. Hence, demographic and psychosocial characteristics of persons with this disease might well include subjects' level of education as well as their past behaviour in regard to non-compliance with various regulations.

In dealing with young men in the United States Navy (U.S.N.), the following demographic and psychososical factors were selected to attempt to differentiate subjects who developed venereal disease over a six-month follow-up period: age, race, occupation, education, documented recent troubles with authorities, job satisfaction, subjects' recent life-changes information, and subjects' perception of their current body symptoms. It was hoped that such dimensions of our subjects might help to assess, among other possibilities, whether it was chiefly their lack of formal education or their rebellion against authority which lead to their contracting the disease.

MATERIALS AND METHODS

Subjects were 4507 U.S.N. enlisted men aboard six large ships during 6 to 8-month cruises in the Mediterranean Sea and in the western Pacific Ocean. Approximately 7 per cent of the subjects were Negro. Extremely small numbers of American Indians and Filipinos were on board, and because of their few numbers were excluded from the following analyses. The average age of subjects was 22 years. Average education was 12 years, or high-school graduation. Fuller descriptions of the men aboard the six ships, as well as other data regarding the missions of the ships, the men's jobs, and their complete illness histories while at sea has been previously reported (Rahe *et al.* 1970*a, b*; Gunderson *et al.* 1970; Rubin *et al.* 1976).

Demographic dimensions

Age. Subjects were grouped into four categories: men 17–20 years old; men 21–22 years old; men 23–25 years old; and subjects 26 or more years old.

Marital status. Subjects were grouped as to whether they were single (never married) or currently married. Divorced and widowed subjects were excluded due to their small numbers.

Education. Subjects were grouped into four categories: those men with only a grade school education (8 years of schooling); those with 1–3 years of high-school education (9–11 years of school); subjects who completed high school (12 years of school); and those men who had taken post-high-school formal education (13 or more years of schooling).

Occupation. The various occupational divisions aboard ship were classified into 'blue-collar' and 'white-collar' jobs, with the cooks and the cooks' helpers treated as a third group. Blue-collar jobs aboard ship included working on the decks, with the ship's gunnery, and in the engine rooms. White-collar jobs included personnel jobs, supply corps, medical and dental technicians, electronics specialists, and radio-men. Cooks' helpers were men who were trained to work elsewhere aboard ship but due to their lack of opportunity or aptitude for their chosen work, or sometimes due to administrative error, they were assigned to this rather unglamorous duty.

Disciplinary actions. Subjects' recent troubles with authority leading to disciplinary actions was scored (from 0 to 3 or more) encompassing the 2 years before follow-up. This information was gathered from the men's own reports of their past disciplinary actions rather than questioning their superiors.

Race. Preliminary analyses of the data indicated that Negro sailors in our sample were slightly older (mean age of 23 years) and that they reported nearly twice the number of illness, per 1000 men per day, as did Caucasians. Thus, in the analyses to follow, Negro and Caucasian sailors were treated separately.

Psychosocial measurements

Job satisfaction. Estimations of subjects' job satisfaction was achieved through the summation of their responses to three questions regarding their work. The first question asked: 'How satisfied are you with your present job?' Subjects could answer: very much (4 points), satisfied (3 points), slightly dissatisfied (2 points), or very dissatisfied (1 point). Secondly, 'Do your present duties employ your abilities in the best possible way?' This question could be answered: very much (3 points), partly (2 points), or not at all (1 point). Thirdly, 'Are you often bored?' This question was answered either 'yes' (1 point) or 'no' (2 points). The higher a subject's total score for these three questions the higher was his adjudged job satisfaction.

The Schedule of Recent Experience (SRE) life-changes questionnaire

This questionnaire was originally intended systematically to document recently experienced life events, over the few years prior to the onset of tuberculosis (Hawkins *et al.* 1957). The design of the SRE has always been such as to include a broad spectrum of subjects' recent life-changes, including personal, social, occupational, and family areas of life adjustment.

For many years no allowances were made for the relative degrees of life change inherent in the various life-change events included in the SRE. A life change such as death of a spouse was counted the same as life change such as a residential move. In 1964, a scaling experiment for the various degrees of life-change inherent in the various SRE life-change events was carried out (Holmes and Rahe 1967).

The 42 life-change questions contained in the SRE were scaled according to the proportionate scaling method of Stevens (1966). A group of nearly 400 subjects, of both sexes, and of differing ages, race, religion, education, social class, marital status, and generation Americans were selected. They were instructed that one of the life-change events, marriage, had been arbitrarily assigned a life-change unit (LCU) value of 500. The subjects then were instructed to assign LCU values for all of the remaining life-change events in the SRE, using marriage as their module. These other LCU values were each to be in proportion with the 500 LCU arbitrarily assigned to marriage. For example, when a subject evaluated a life-change event, such as change in residence, he was to ask himself: 'Is a change in residence more, or less, or perhaps equal to the amount and duration of life change and readjustment inherent in marriage?' If he decided it was more, he was to indicate how much more by choosing a proportionately larger LCU value than the 500 assigned to marriage. If he decided it was less, he was to indicate how much less by choosing a proportionately smaller number than 500. If he decided it was equal, he was to assign 500 LCU. This process was repeated for each of the remaining life-change events in the SRE questionnaire (Rahe 1969*a*).

TABLE 26.1

Life-change events

	LCU values
Family	
Death of spouse	1000
Divorce	730
Marital separation	650
Death of close family member	630
Marriage	500
Marital reconciliation	450
Major change in health of family	440
Pregnancy	400
Addition of new family member	390
Major change in arguments with wife	350
Son or daughter leaving home	290
In-law troubles	290
Wife starting or ending work	260
Major change in family get-togethers	150
Personal	
Detention in jail	630
Major personal injury or illness	530
Sexual difficulties	390
Death of a close friend	370
Outstanding personal achievement	280
Start or end of formal schooling	260
Major change in living conditions	250
Major revision of personal habits	240
Changing to a new school	200
Change in residence	200
Major change in recreation	190
Major change in church activities	190
Major change in sleeping habits	160
Major change in eating habits	150
Vacation	130
Christmas	120
Minor violations of the law	110
Work	
Being fired from work	470
Retirement from work	450
Major business adjustment	390
Changing to different line of work	360
Major change in work responsibilities	290
Trouble with boss	230
Major change in working conditions	200
Financial	
Major change in financial state	380
Mortgage or loan over $10 000	310
Mortgage foreclosure	300
Mortgage or loan less than $10 000	170

Since this original scaling experiment, life-changes scaling studies have been performed in other locations in the United States and in several other countries. Results from all of these life-changes scaling experiments have been strikingly similar (Rahe 1969*b*). Most divergent results have been found between a small sample of Mexican-Americans versus white, middle-class Americans, and between a sample of Swedish subjects living in Stockholm versus comparable Seattlites (Kameroff *et al.* 1968; Rahe *et al.* 1971). Table 26.1 presents the list of 42 life-change events and their originally determined (Seattle) LCU values.

The practical results of these LCU weightings has been that subjects' recent life-changes information can now be given quantitative estimates in terms of the average degree or intensity of change inherent in the life-change events. In order to give incidence rates, and to find the most appropriate time interval for illness prediction, the arbitrary time intervals over which subjects' life-changes (LCU) have been summed have varied from 2 years, 1 year, 6 months, 3 months, 1 week, to 1 day.

The Health Opinion Survey (HOS) questionnaire: a measure of subjects' current perceptions of body symptoms
The Health Opinion Survey (HOS) questionnaire was originally devised by McMillan as a shortened version of the Cornell Medical Index/Health Questionnaire

(McMillan 1957). McMillan's HOS is compared of 20 brief questions dealing with subjects' perception of their psychophysiology — for example. 'Do your hands ever tremble enough to bother you?' Questions are scored on a 1- to 3-point scale. The total HOS score ranges from 20 to 60 and the higher a subject's score, the greater is his current perceptions of his body symptoms. Table 26.2 presents the list of HOS questions along with their scoring format.

It has been previously shown that Navy subjects with high intensities of recent life-changes plus high concern over their body symptoms report high near-future illness rates. Conversely, subjects scoring low on both questionnaires were seen to report relatively few near-future illnesses (Gunderson *et al.* 1972; Rahe *et al.* 1972). Whether or not these relationships would hold for a single illness (e.g. gonorrhea) was a focus of this investigation.

RESULTS

Men with venereal disease, other illnesses, or no illness reports
No cases of active syphilis were reported by any of the men. In approximately half of the cases of suspected venereal infection laboratory confirmation of infection by Neisserian Diplococci was obtained. The other half of subjects with suspected venereal disease received a diagnosis of non-specific urethritis. For comparison

TABLE 26.2

Health Opinion Survey (HOS) questionnaire

	3 points	2 points	1 point
1. Do you have any physical or health problems at present?	( ) Yes		( ) No
2. Do your hands ever tremble enough to bother you?	( ) Often	( ) Sometimes	( ) Never
3. Are you ever troubled by your hands or feet sweating so that they feel damp and clammy?	( ) Often	( ) Sometimes	( ) Never
4. Have you ever been bothered by your heart beating hard?	( ) Often	( ) Sometimes	( ) Never
5. Do you tend to feel tired in the mornings?	( ) Often	( ) Sometimes	( ) Never
6. Do you have any trouble getting to sleep and staying asleep?	( ) Often	( ) Sometimes	( ) Never
7. How often are you bothered by having an upset stomach?	( ) Often	( ) Sometimes	( ) Never
8. Are you ever bothered by nightmares (dreams which frighten you)?	( ) Often	( ) Sometimes	( ) Never
9. Have you ever been troubled by 'cold sweats'?	( ) Often	( ) Sometimes	( ) Never
10. Do you feel that you are bothered by all kinds of ailments in different parts of your body?	( ) Often	( ) Sometimes	( ) Never
11. Do you smoke?	( ) Yes		( ) No
12. Do you ever have loss of appetite?	( ) Often	( ) Sometimes	( ) Never
13. Has any ill health affected the amount of work you do?	( ) Often	( ) Sometimes	( ) Never
14. Do you ever feel weak all over?	( ) Often	( ) Sometimes	( ) Never
15. Do you ever have spells of dizziness?	( ) Often	( ) Sometimes	( ) Never
16. Do you tend to lose weight when you worry?	( ) Often	( ) Sometimes	( ) Never
17. Have you ever been bothered by shortness of breath when you were not exerting yourself?	( ) Often	( ) Sometimes	( ) Never
18. For the most part, do you feel healthy enough to carry out the things that you would like to do?	( ) Often	( ) Sometimes	( ) Never
19. Do you feel in good spirits?	( ) Never	( ) Sometimes	( ) Most of the time
20. Do you sometimes wonder if anything is worthwhile any more?	( ) Often	( ) Sometimes	( ) Never

purposes, men who reported illnesses other than venereal disease during the cruise formed a second subgroup. A third subgroup of men were all those remaining men aboard ship who reported no illnesses throughout the follow-up cruise period. These last two subgroups of men were referred to as the 'other illness' and the 'no illness' subgroups.

Out of 4197 Caucasian sailors, 297 (7 per cent) developed confirmed gonorrheal infections; 304 (7 per cent) subjects were diagnosed as having non-specific urethritis; 2407 (58 per cent) subjects reported an illness other than confirmed or suspected venereal disease; and 1189 subjects made no illness reports throughout the cruise. For 310 Negro sailors, 79 were diagnosed as having contracted gonorrhea; 36 subjects were diagnosed with non-specific urethritis; 131 subjects reported an illness other than cofirmed or suspected venereal disease; and 64 subjects reported no illnesses throughout the cruise period.

Age and marital status as predictors of subjects contracting venereal disease
Percentage distributions of Caucasian and Negro subjects for age and marital status, according to the four subgroupings defined above, are presented in Table 26.3. It was seen that Caucasians who developed

gonorrhea tended to be young — with a relatively high percentage of subjects 17–20 years of age. Caucasians with non-specific urethritis also showed a similarly young age distribution except for a higher percentage of subjects over 26 years of age than seen for the gonorrhea subgroup. If the age distributions for Caucasians with no illness reports is compared to the age distribution data for Caucasians with gonorrhea, a 2×4 chi-square analysis was found to show these age distributions significantly different at the 0·01 level.

Percentage distributions for age for the four subgroups of Negroes showed no concentration of young subjects in the venereal disease or suspected venereal disease subgroups (Table 26.3). A relatively low percentage of Negro subjects over 26 years of age was seen in the gonorrhea subgroup, however.

Perhaps due to the Caucasian subjects' younger mean age compared to Negro sailors, an overall higher percentage of Caucasians were of single marital status than were Negro subjects. For Caucasians, the highest proportions of single subjects were seen in the gonorrhea and non-specific urethritis subgroups. A 2×2 chi-square analysis of single to married percentages for Caucasians with gonorrhea to Caucasians with no illness reports was statistically significant at the 0·01 level. No similar trend was seen for Negro subjects (Table 26.3).

TABLE 26.3

Percentage distribution of age and marital status for persons contracting gonorrhea and non-specific urethritis compared to those men reporting other illness and those men with no-illness reports

(a) *Age*

	Gonorrhea	Non-specific urethritis	Other illnesses	No illness
Caucasians				
17–20 y	55	48	47	40
21–22 y	33	34	30	31
23–25 y	7	12	11	12
26+ y	5	6	12	17
Negroes				
17–20 y	36	34	42	40
21–22 y	36	31	25	27
23–25 y	22	17	9	11
26+ y	7	17	25	27

(b) *Marital status*

	Gonorrhea	Non-specific urethritis	Other illnesses	No illness
Caucasians				
Single	78	77	69	63
Married	22	23	31	37
Negroes				
Single	62	69	63	59
Married	38	31	31	41

TABLE 26.4

Percentage distribution of years of schooling and occupation for persons who contracted gonorrhea and non-specific urethritis compared to those with other illness and those with no reported illness

(a) *Education*

	Gonorrhea	Non-specific urethritis	Other illnesses	No illness
Caucasians				
8 years	5	7	4	4
9–11 years	32	26	29	29
12 years	55	60	57	57
13+ years	8	7	9	9
Negroes				
8 years	0	6	6	3
9–11 years	34	24	36	38
12 years	61	59	52	57
13+ years	5	12	6	2

(b) *Occupation*

	Gonorrhea	Non-specific urethritis	Other illnesses	No illness
Caucasians				
Blue collar	71	74	66	55
White collar	19	19	25	37
Cooks and helpers	10	7	10	9
Negroes				
Blue collar	61	69	57	54
White collar	29	19	31	27
Cooks and helpers	10	12	13	19

Education and occupation as predictors of subjects' contracting VD

The percentage distribution of subjects based upon their education and occupation is shown in Table 26.4. There were no concentrations of either Caucasian or Negro subjects with confirmed or suspected venereal disease in the lower educational categories. A similar analysis was performed for subjects' intelligence test results (standard intelligence test taken by the men upon their entrance into the U.S.N.) and again no evidence was seen for the gonorrhea or non-specific urethritis subgroups to have lower intelligence test scores than sailors in the other two subgroups.

For both Caucasians and Negroes, men with confirmed or suspected venereal disease tended to perform blue-collar jobs aboard ship, compared to subjects in the other illness and no illness subgroups. For example, 37 per cent of Caucasian subjects in the no illness subgroup had white-collar jobs compared to 19 per cent in both the gonorrhea and non-specific urethritis subgroups. A 2×2 chi-square analysis of white collar to non-white collar workers for gonorrhea plus non-specific urethritis subjects compared to the no illness subgroup showed this difference to be significant at the 0·01 level. Occupational data for Negroes showed similar but weaker trends to what was seen for Caucasian sailors (Table 26.4).

Job satisfaction and recent disciplinary action as predictors of subjects contracting veneral disease

The percentage distributions of subjects according to their job satisfaction scores and according to their numbers of recent disciplinary actions is presented in Table 26.5. For both Caucasians and Negro subjects, only a slight trend was seen for subjects with gonorrhea and non-specific urethritis to have registered lower job satisfaction scores compared to men in the other illness and the no illness subgroups.

Caucasians with gonorrhea tended to have had more recent disciplinary actions than members of the other three subgroups. A 2×4 chi-square analysis of the percentage distribution of gonorrhea subjects compared to no illness subjects for recent number of disciplinary actions showed these differences to be significant at the 0·01 level. No such trend was seen for Negro subjects (see Table 26.5).

Subjects' recent life-changes and perceptions of body symptoms as predictors of venereal disease contractants

Previous work with other U.S.N. subjects had shown that the combination of subjects' recent life-changes information (SRE questionnaire) with their perceptions of their current body symptoms (HOS questionnaire) predicted their near-future illnesses better than did either questionnaire separately (Gunderson et al. 1972;

TABLE 26.5

Percentage distribution of job satisfaction and disciplinary actions for persons who contracted gonorrhea and non-specific urethritis compared to those with other illness and those with no reported illness

(a) *Job satisfaction*

	Gonorrhea	Non-specific urethritis	Other illness	No illness
Caucasians				
3–4 (low)	21	17	22	17
5–7 (medium)	54	56	52	50
8–9 (high)	25	27	26	33
Negroes				
3–4 (low)	15	17	23	19
5–7 (medium)	57	63	48	49
8–9 (high)	28	20	29	32

(b) *Disciplinary actions*

	Gonorrhea	Non-specific urethritis	Other illness	No illness
Caucasians				
0	63	68	67	70
1	16	17	17	17
2	8	8	8	6
3+	13	7	8	7
Negroes				
0	62	69	64	57
1	19	17	18	24
2	6	14	9	10
3+	12	0	9	12

TABLE 26.6

*Percentage distribution differences for life-changes and HOS scores
for Caucasians with other illnesses versus those with no
reported illnesses*

| | | Life-changes magnitude (deciles) | | | |
		Low (1–3)	Medium (4, 5)	Medium–high (6, 7)	High (8–10)
HOS scores	Low (20–25)	−4	1	−1	−1
	Medium (26–30)	−2	−1	0	+1
	High (31+)	0	+1	+1	+5

Rahe *et al.* 1972). Therefore, for the data to follow, subjects' responses to both psychosocial questionnaires was handled jointly.

Caucasian and Negro sailors' recent life-changes scores, along with their HOS questionnaire scores, are presented in the following tables as percentage *differences* between two subgroups. In other words, the percentage distributions of scores of one subgroup are subtracted from the percentage distribution of scores of another subgroup.

In Table 26.6 the distributions for the life-changes scores and the HOS scores for the Caucasian subgroup with no illness reports were subtracted from the percentage distributions for the life-changes and HOS scores for Caucasians with other illnesses. Thus, the numbers in the Table illustrate the percentage differences between the other-illness subgroup and the no-illness subgroup for each cell in the Table. These results bear out the findings of previous studies in that the other-illness subgroup showed between 1 per cent and 4 per cent few subjects in the low ranges of scores for both questionnaires than did the no-illness subgroup. Conversely, the other-illness subgroup had between 1 per cent and 5 per cent more subjects in the cells depicting high scores for both questionnaires than did the no-illness subgroup.

When the percentage distributions for recent life-changes and HOS scores for Caucasians with gonorrhea were compared to the percentage distribution of scores for the no illness subgroup (Table 26.7). Caucasians with gonorrhea had between 2 per cent more and 4 per cent fewer subjects in the low-scoring cells for both questionnaires than did the no-illness subgroup. The gonorrhea subgroup also showed between 1 per cent fewer to 5 per cent more subjects scoring in the high cells for both questionnaires than what was seen for subjects who reported no illnesses. Although these results were in the predicted direction, the HOS questionnaire appeared to be a stronger predictor of Caucasian subjects who developed gonorrhea than did their recent life-changes questionnaire results.

When the results of the SRE and HOS questionnaires were examined for Negro subjects, divergent results from those hypothesized were seen. The Negro gonorrhea subgroup's percentage distribution of scores was compared to the percentage distribution of scores for the Negro other illness plus the Negro no-illness subgroups. (Because of the small number in the no-illness group, both comparison groups were combined.) Negroes with gonorrhea had between 2 per cent fewer to 5 per cent more subjects in the low-scoring cells for recent life-changes and HOS score than did the combined group of Negro subjects with other-illness and with no-illness reports, as well as between 5 per cent fewer to 10 per cent more subjects scoring in the high life changes and HOS categories than did the combined

TABLE 26.7

*Percentage distribution differences for life-changes and HOS scores
for Caucasians with gonorrhea versus those with no reported illness*

| | | Life-changes magnitude (deciles) | | | |
		Low (1–3)	Medium (4, 5)	Medium–high (6, 7)	High (8–10)
HOS scores	Low (20–25)	−4	−2	−1	−2
	Medium (26–30)	−1	+2	+1	+3
	High (31+)	+3	+1	+5	−1

TABLE 26.8

Percentage distribution differences for life-changes and HOS scores
for Negroes with gonorrhea versus those with other illnesses plus
those with no-illness reports

		Life-changes magnitude (deciles)			
		Low (1–3)	Medium (4–5)	Medium–high (6, 7)	High (8–10)
HOS scores	Low (20–25)	+2	−2	+1	−4
	Medium (26–30)	+2	+5	−4	+10
	High (31+)	+1	−6	−5	+2

comparison group (see Table 26.8). Here, in contrast to what was seen for Caucasian subjects, the recent life-changes questionnaire appeared to be a better predictor of Negro subjects who went on to develop gonorrhea than did the HOS questionnaire.

COMMENT

This prospective study of U.S.N. men who developed venereal disease over a 6- to 8-month cruise period utilized both demographic and psychosocial characteristics of the men which had been of value in previous illness prediction studies. The utility of these predictors in determining subjects at high risk to develop venereal disease was assessed. Results suggested that the predictors studied were only modestly successful in determining subjects contracting venereal disease — and better in the case of Caucasian than for Negro sailors.

The greater percentage of Negro sailors contracting venereal disease, compared to Caucasian men, is difficult to explain. One would have to know more about the sexual exposures of the men. For example, Negroes may have been exposed to sexual partners different (and perhaps more diseased) from those of Caucasian men.

Caucasian men who contracted confirmed or suspected venereal disease were generally young, single, employed in blue-collar positions aboard ship, and tended to have had recent disciplinary actions. They also registered slightly elevated recent life-changes as well as elevated concern about body symptoms. There appeared to be no single predictor, or combination of predictors, which strongly identified subjects who contracted venereal disease.

For Negro sailors, only two of the predictors were of value. Occupational analyses showed a disproportionate number of Negro sailors showed increased numbers of subjects developing venereal disease who worked in blue-collar versus white-collar positions, and a trend was seen for Negro subjects with elevated recent life-changes to go on to develop venereal disease.

The fact that subjects' education, and intelligence test scores, did not identify those who developed gonorrhea casts doubt upon lack of (general) education as a cause of persons contracting venereal disease. All men aboard ship were exposed to periodic written and spoken warnings regarding venereal disease, and how to avoid it, before their on-shore leave periods throughout the cruise. Despite these specific educational programmes the brighter and/or more educated sailors fared no better with this disease than did his less intellectually or educationally endowed shipmate.

The lack of strongly positive results for the demographic and psychosocial predictors used in this study suggests that new predictors should be explored. Perhaps other indicators of subjects' impulsivity or measures of subjects' inability to delay gratification would be stronger correlates of their contracting venereal disease. Defiance of authority, as measured by the men's recent disciplinary actions, was a significant predictor for Caucasian subjects who contracted venereal disease; other measurements of subjects' anti-authority feelings and actions may also be valid predictors.

In keeping with the theme of this book, a final word might be directed toward the possibility of exploring dimensions of these men's relationships with women as possible predictors of men likely to develop venereal disease. It might be postulated that men who see women in a servile role of low social importance are more likely to choose sexual partners indiscriminately, with little concern over possible venereal disease. On the other hand, it may be the case that subjects who see women as having a positive and important social role may exert care to avoid his, or her, infection by Neisserian organisms.

REFERENCES

GUNDERSON, E. K. E., RAHE, R. H., and ARTHUR, R. J. (1970). The epidemiology of illness in naval environments. II. Demographic, social background, and occupational factors. *Milit. Med.*, **135**, 453–8.

GUNDERSON, E. K. E., RAHE, R. H., and ARTHUR, R. J. (1972). Prediction of performance in stressful underwater demolition training. *J. appl. Psychol.*, **56**, 430–2.

HAWKINS, N. G., DAVIES, R., and HOLMES, T. H. (1957). Evidence of psychosocial factors in the development of pulmonary tuberculosis. *Amer. Rev. tuberc. pulmon. Dis.*, **75**, 5.

HOLMES, T. H. and RAHE, R. H. (1967). The social readjustment rating scale. *J. psychosom. Res.*, **11**, 213–18.

KAMAROFF, A. L., MASUDA, M., and HOLMES, T. H. (1968). The social readjustment rating scale. A comparative study of Negro, Mexican, and White Americans. *J. psychosom. Res.*, **12**, 21.

MCMILLAN, A. M. (1957). The health opinion survey: technique for estimating prevalence of psychoneurotic and related types of disorder in communities. *Psychol. Rep.*, **2**, 325.

RAHE, R. H. (1969*a*). Life crisis and health change. In *Psychotropic drug response: advances in prediction* (ed. R. A. P. May and J. R. Wittenborn), pp. 92–125. Springfield, Illinois.

—— (1969*b*). Multi-cultural correlations of life change scaling: America, Japan, Denmark, and Sweden. *J. psycho-som. Res.*, **13**, 191–5.

——, GUNDERSON, E. K. E., and ARTHUR, R. J. (1970*a*). Demographic and psychosocial factors in acute illness reporting. *J. chron. Dis.*, **23**, 245–55.

——, MAHAN, J., ARTHUR, R. J., and GUNDERSON, E. K. E. (1970*b*). The epidemiology of illness in Naval environments. I. Illness types distribution, severities, and relationships to life change. *Milit. Med.*, **135**, 443–52.

——, LUNDBERG, U., BENNETT, L., and THEORELL, T. (1971). The social readjustment rating scale: A comparative study of Swedes and Americans. *J. psychosom. Res.*, **15**, 241–9.

——, BIERSNER, R. J., RYMAN, D. H., and ARTHUR, R. J. (1972). Psychosocial predictors of illness behavior and failure in stressful training. *J. Hlth soc. Behav.*, **13**, 393–7.

RUBIN, R. T., GUNDERSON, E. K. E., and ARTHUR, R. J. (1976). Life stress and illness patterns in the U.S. Navy. VI. Environmental, demograhic, and prior life change variables in relation to illness onset in naval aviators during a combat cruise. *Psychosom. Med.* (In press)

STEVENS, S. S. (1966). A metric for the social concensus. *Science* (*N.Y.*), **151**, 530.

27. DISEASES POSSIBLY ASSOCIATED WITH MALE/FEMALE ROLES AND RELATIONSHIPS

J. P. HENRY

A previous chapter has presented the use of complex habitats as a means of studying the sexual role differentiation of mice. Their coping processes have been deliberately disrupted by appropriate habitat design and social deprivation of the young. Under these circumstances normal male and female behaviour is disturbed. Persistent fighting leads to a sustained arousal of the defence and alarm response. An increase in catecholamine synthesizing enzymes, high blood-pressure, and arteriosclerosis are observed. Human coronary heart disease, high blood-pressure, mammary and prostatic cancer, and anorexia nervosa are considered from this viewpoint.

INTRODUCTION

There appear to be three major subdivisions of the brain from the viewpoint of its control function. There are the two huge hemispherical association areas which constitute the huge neocortical 'social brain' (Washburn and Hamburg 1968) and physically overshadow the entire human organ. They are necessary for the prodigous, recently evolved, capacity for memory, foresight, planning, and inhibition of inappropriate action: for the speech, for the synthetic cognitive functions, and for the complex technical activity that characterizes man. A second region is the brainstem including the hypothalamus, a mechanism which harbours the physical basis of consummatory responses like eating and drinking and integrates and co-ordinates endocrine and autonomic nervous activity as well as the cardiovascular and other systems. The hypothalamus is the centre of origin of the defence and alarm responses (Mason (1968). Between these two major subdivisions and serving as a buffer and junction between them is a third zone — the limbic brain. This appears to be responsible for emotionally toned behavioural responses to the external environment. It is critical for the environmentally stable patterns of behaviour exhibited by the species in connection with the activities of feeding, drinking, courtship and mating, and the care of the young (MacLean, 1970) (Fig. 27.1).

It appears that the limbic zone interacts with the neocortical association areas (Nauta 1971) to provide coping processes (Lazarus 1966) in the course of which stimuli may be referred to previously stored memories and to inherited environmentally stable collective patterns, permitting a determination of socially acceptable and effective behaviour. One effect of isolation may be to impair development of these control processes.

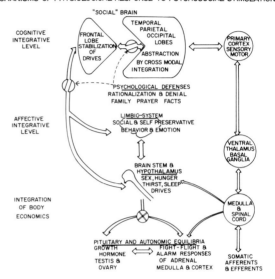

MECHANISMS OF PHYSIOLOGICAL RESPONSE TO PSYCHOSOCIAL STIMULATION

FIG. 27.1. The main current of information from the peripheral sense organs courses through the midbrain and thalamus to the primary sensory cortical projection areas. Massive neocortical cross-modal association regions provide the symbol-handling capacity needed for his culture and technology. The frontal pole connects this 'social' brain with the amygdala hippocampus, septum, and cingulate gyrus. These 'limbic' structures subserve emotion and are closely integrated with the hypothalamus which effects consummation of the basic drives. The hypothalamus together with the nonspecific reticular activating system modulates varied pituitary, vagal, and sympathetic reactions which eventually can lead to pathophysiological changes.

Under these circumstances the unbuffered stimulation will produce violent autonomic and endocrine responses as the defence (Folkow and Neil 1971) and alarm mechanisms are activated (Mason 1968). Persistence of these responses will result in the so-called diseases of psychosomatic origin (Hill 1970) (Fig. 27.1).

PATHOPHYSIOLOGICAL CONSEQUENCES OF AROUSAL OF THE DEFENCE AND ALARM RESPONSES

The previous chapter outlined the pattern of normal male and female role differentiation in the mouse. By

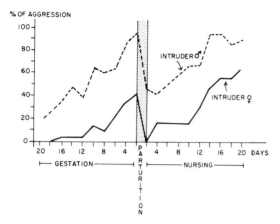

FIG. 27.2. The male mouse not only defends territory in which food is to be obtained, patrolling the box system, but he will assist in the defence of the nest from both male and female intruders. This aggressivity shows a rising sensitivity up to the time of parturition, then falls off to rise again as the nurslings mature. Modified from Beniest-Noirot: Le comportement dit 'maternel' de la souris, *Un. int. Sci. biol.*, Octobre 1956/Août 1957, p. 144, Graphique 2.

storing food well within the confines of the group's territory the male animal helps to support the female during late pregnancy and lactation. Depredations by other mice not belonging to the colony are foiled by the vigorous defensive activity displayed to intruders by the males (Crowcroft 1966) (Fig. 27.2). Mutual recognition by the various members of the group is learned and some aspects may depend on the neocortex, even in the mouse. In order to disturb this process we have employed the technique of social isolation used by Harlow (Harlow *et al.* 1971) and by Fuller and Clark (1966) with monkeys and dogs, respectively. Loss of the opportunity for social interaction with mother and peers results in extreme timidity and emotional lability when placed in a socially interacting environment. There is a dramatic failure of formerly isolated young monkeys to make adequate social discriminations. Inappropriate attacks made by them upon fully adult males and upon infants—events that never occur in a normally socialized colony — are examples of a gross social inadequacy that shows up in any demanding situation. The mating and courtship and the parental care patterns exhibited by these formerly isolated animals are all defective. This contrasts with the skilled male/female teamwork shown in groups of wild primates (Washburn and Hamburg 1968; Hamburg 1969).

Our technique for the social deprivation of mice is to raise them in 1-l glass jars from an early weaning at 12–14 days until fully mature at 4 months (Henry *et al.* 1967) (Fig. 27.3(a)). Unlike normally socialized groups, complex population cages stocked with such socially inexperienced animals appear to lack the capacity for fine role discrimination (Fig. 27.3(b)). There are fewer

pregnancies where, after delivery, the young die from neglect and as a result of constant disturbance by other females. This failure of male/female role differentiation can be demonstrated by the use of magnetic tagging and detectors at appropriate points in the habitat (see Chapter 5).

Accompanying the social disorder, there are frequent fights among the males (Fig. 27.3(b)) and the ensuing psychosocial stimulation has effects that can be demonstrated by assays of the catecholamine-synthesizing

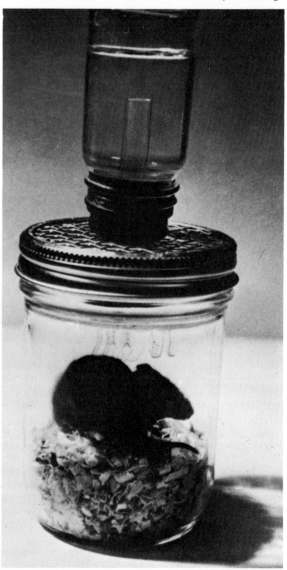

FIG. 27.3. (a) By raising a mouse in isolation in a glass jar from early weaning at 2 weeks until 4 months old the process of social adjustment can be impaired. Such animals will not form stable colonies with hierarchies of a dominant, rivals, and subordinates, but will confront each other in repeated fights for territory (see (b)).

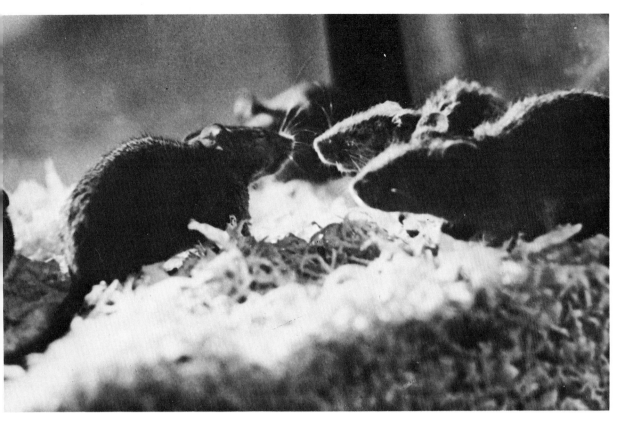

FIG. 27.3. (b) Confrontation.

enzyme content of the adrenal medulla. This shows a doubling or tripling of the levels of tyrosine hydroxylase and phenylethanolamine *N*-methyltransferase (Fig. 27.4). The former is the rate-limiting first step in the synthesis of adrenalin from tyrosine. The second is responsible for the production of adrenalin from noradrenalin (Axelrod *et al.* 1970).

There is a difference between the male and female response to a socially disordered murine community. If systolic blood-pressure is followed by measuring it in the tail once every 2 weeks, it is seen that while that of both sexes becomes elevated, in the males the increase is some 15–20 mm Hg more than in the females (Henry *et al.* 1967). This increase is sustained for as long as the violent social interaction persists (Fig. 28.4). Furthermore, in animals that have been exposed to the condition for many months, the pressure elevation persists in spite of removal from the social situation and isolation.

Histological study of the hearts, kidneys, and aortas of colonies of mice that have been in social conflict for 6 months or more shows that the sustained defence response is associated with extensive vascular damage. There is fibrosis in the heart walls and mesangial thickening in the glomeruli; there are areas of lympho-

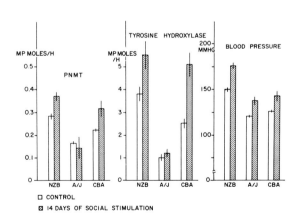

□ CONTROL
▨ 14 DAYS OF SOCIAL STIMULATION

FIG. 27.4. In strains that will fight readily, such as the NZB and CBA, even brief periods of social interaction result in elevation of phenylethanolamine *N*-methyltransferase and tyrosine hydroxylase. The blood-pressure is also elevated, rising in excess of 150 mm Hg as social stimulation is maintained over the weeks. In the AJ strain, which is more peaceable the enzymes appear to take longer to increase.

cytic infiltration in the kidneys; and there are arterio-sclerotic changes in the aorta (Fig. 27.5 (a, b, & c)). The extent of these changes varies from minor to severe; and some sexual differentiation exists on this score, for the incidence of very severe lesions is greater in the males than in the females (Henry *et al.* 1971).

The foregoing indicates that certain disorders result from sustained activation of the defence response. The animals in these socially disordered colonies suffer from hypertension and arteriosclerosis, the incidence being more severe in the males than in the females. In addition other pathological changes occur. Preliminary observations indicate that on being placed in an ongoing

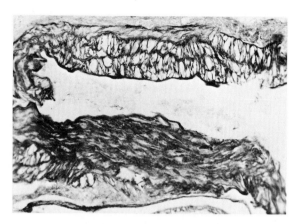

Fig. 27.5. (c) In this severely damaged aorta there is an area of invasion of spindle-shaped muscle cells which have replaced the fibrous tissue rings. On the opposite side, there is vacuolation with severe palisading.

colony as a strange intruder, the development of mammary tumours is grossly accelerated in the female CBA. The provocative stimulus appears to be a situation with which the mouse cannot effectively cope.

On the other hand, Newberry (Newberry *et al.* 1976) has demonstrated that either electric shock or repeated immobilization inhibit the development of dibenzanthracene-induced tumours in rats. There is evidence that the neuroendocrine changes involved may differ in the two cases (Henry *et al.* 1975). In Newberry's cases, the rat learns with daily repetition that aversive experiences are self-limiting. As it comes to develop reliable expectations, the animal may shift from a predominance of pituitary adrenal/cortical responses to a flight/flight sympathetic adrenal medullary pattern. The emotions involved would change from fear and depression to irritation and aggression. Similarly, in aggressive groups composed of animals socially deprived from the time of weaning; that fight chronically and suffer from high blood-pressure, the incidence of mammary tumours is not greatly increased (Henry *et al.*, unpublished observations). It is only the socialized, formerly smoothly breeding females whose social system has been disrupted that develop a sustained pituitary/adrenocortical response. We have suggested that the reason for their sustained depression would be their continued failure to return to the deeply entrenched expectations deriving from their previous life in a stable, integrated social system with an ongoing communal nursery and compatible males.

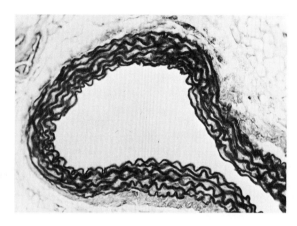

Fig. 27.5. (a) Persistent fighting between members of a socially disordered colony is associated with generalized arterio-sclerotic change in the kidneys, heart, and aorta. The three aortas shown (see also (b) and (c)) are from animals of the same age. The one shown above comes from a normal animal; the elastic rings are clearly delineated.

HUMAN DISEASE RELATED TO MALE/FEMALE RELATIONSHIPS

The preceding section cited detailed evidence that a sustained disturbance of the social system in mice that leads to severe fighting and sustained disruption of normal male/female relationships will result in cardio-

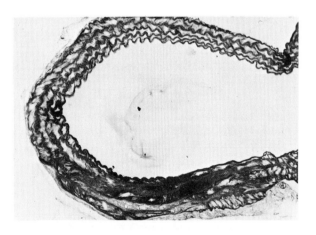

Fig. 27.5. (b) On one side of this aorta there is moderate deterioration as the elastic fibres become separated, and on the other, large 'pool' staining with Alcian Blue. The structure of the elastic rings is lost in this region.

vascular pathology. The question arises whether there is any evidence that disease in men and women may be similarly connected with sustained arousal and failure of sex-role relationships.

In 1955 there were 8 times as many cases of coronary occlusion in white males in the United States as in white females (Furman 1969) (Fig. 27.6). On the other hand, in coloured females in the Virgin Islands in 1942, the mean blood-pressure of the 50- to 55-year-olds was 168/98 mm Hg as opposed to 150/91 mm Hg for the males of the same age group (Saunders and Bancroft 1942) (Fig. 27.7). Work (Friedman and Rosenman 1974) pioneered by Freidman (1969) has thrown light on the personality of a type of man in our society who is susceptible to coronary disease. The so-called Type A is a 'work addict', who, despite great expenditure of time and effort of his job, remains dissatisfied with the progress he has made. He suffers from a sense of time urgency, he is highly competitive, he cannot relax, and his family relationships are often poor. Liljefors and Rahe (1970) in their study of Swedish twins showed

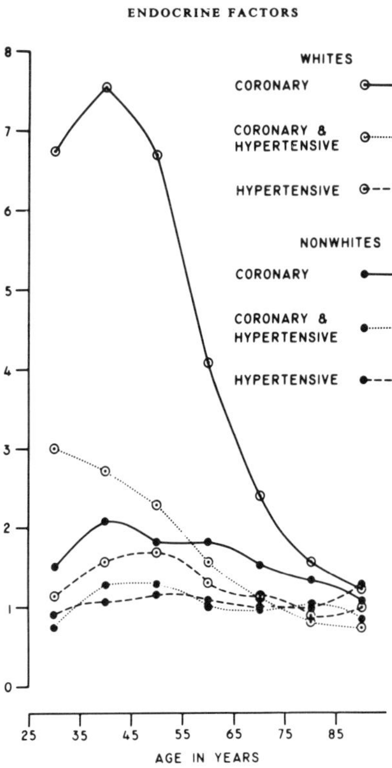

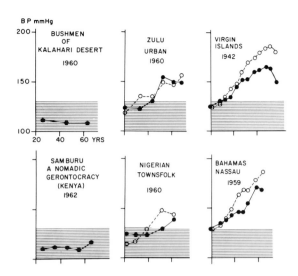

FIG. 27.7. Aging members of primitive tribes living in their ancient patterns show remarkably low systolic pressures. Recently urbanized Negroes living in Durban and near Ibadan, Nigeria in 1960 had a significant elevation of pressure as they aged. The residents of the Virgin Islands in 1942 and of Nassau in the Bahamas in 1959 had severe elevations which were significantly higher in the aging females.

ENDOCRINE FACTORS

FIG. 27.6. Curves depicting the values for the ratios of male: female age-specific death-rates in white and non-white individuals dying of coronary heart disease and hypertension in the United States in 1955. The high male/female ratio of deaths is largely limited to the white population dying of coronary or coronary plus hypertensive disease. From Furman (1969), Endocrine factors in atherogenesis. In *Atherosclerosis* (ed. F. G. Schettler and G. S. Boyd). Amsterdam.

that the twin with the most severe disease is often suffering from a sense of defeat and from sustained anxiety. In the situation described by Friedman and Rosenman (1974) it is more commonly the male who is affected and who perceives his life situation as threatening and demanding.

On the other hand, in the Virgin Islands in the 1940s, most women at age 50 had raised their families alone (U.S. Women's Bureau 1935; Weinstein 1962). Forced into the role of matriarchs in a severely impoverished subsistence economy, they had received little help from their mates. The male Virgin Islanders of the 1940s had little motivation to work and traditionally had little to do with the children. It is possible that this group of Negro women had the same high hostility to others that Harris and Singer have noted in other women with high blood-pressure (Harris and Singer 1968). Aging and unsupported by the males, left to play both roles in a struggling economy, they may well experience arousal of the defence reaction and sustained activation of the catecholamine system. Having reached the 50s, their mood may not be so much one of anxiety lest they be defeated as of indignation and suppressed anger at the ingratitude of others and lack of support from the system (Henry and Cassel 1969).

Fig. 27.7 includes 5 other cases which show the varying relationship between blood-pressure and age in social groups of Negroes. Reading from left to right, the first set represents Bushmen of the Kalahari Desert, above (Kaminer and Lutz 1960) and the Samburu of Northern Kenya, below (Shaper 1962). Both show that

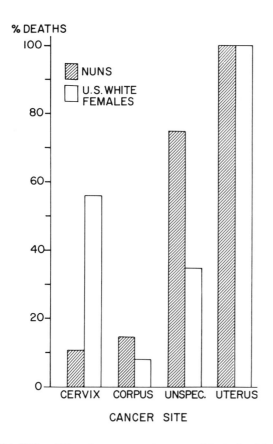

% DEATHS

NUNS
U.S. WHITE FEMALES

CANCER SITE

Fig. 27.8. Although more prone to cancer of the body of the uterus than the general population, nuns are singularly exempt from cancer of the cervix. Modified from Fraumeni, William Lloyd, Smith, and Wagoner (1969). Cancer mortality among nuns: Role of marital status in etiology of neoplastic disease in women. *J. natl. Cancer Inst.* **42**; 462, 1969.

in some groups blood-pressure does not increase with age. At the time that they were studied, the Bushmen were living in an extended family group and appeared well adjusted to their environment. The same held true for the Samburu who still occupied their ancestral lands and were a well integrated and traditional group relatively undisturbed by the ongoing social and technological revolution.

The second set of pressure tables derives from a group of Zulu living in an apartheid community outside of Durban (Scotch 1960). The old people found their tribal traditions distorted and engulfed in the new demands of the urban environment. There is a significant rise in the pressure of both men and women. The same holds for those living in a town near the city of Ibadan in Nigeria (Abrahams *et al.* 1960). These are rural people who, while adapting to cultural change, still have strong traditions from the past. In both cases there is a significant elevation of pressure in the older groups.

The third set of pressures has been discussed already for the case of the women of the Virgin Islands in 1942. Conditions in the Bahamas in the late 1950s would appear to have been similar (Moser *et al.* 1959). Taken as a whole, the data from these six surveys are typical and find support in a large number of similar observations which have been reviewed recently by Henry and Cassel (1969). They are compatible with the thesis that psychosocial factors are important in determining the level of blood-pressure in human communities.

In the case of the contemporary white male, it may be relevant that Medalie states that in Israel men who perceive their wives as insufficiently loving and supportive have a significantly higher risk of coronary disease (Medalie, personal communication). On the other hand, Nuckolls *et al.* (1972) have reported that the chances of a complication in a woman having her first baby are higher if she has had recent social readjustments in addition to the pregnancy and experiences little warm social support from husband and family. There was a significant reduction in the complication rate if they perceived themselves as well loved. In both of these cases there appears to be a connection between disease and the failure to achieve an effective male/ female role relationship.

In a recent study of sexual factors in the epidemiology of cancer of the prostate Steele *et al.* (1971) have noted that their cases gave evidence of having had a higher sexual drive than a control group. Those with this condition had more extramarital partners and also expressed frustration more often than the controls at not having enough coitus. The authors regard the data as compatible with failure 'to relieve the prostate of hormonal and other pressures related to sexual inclination'. Quisenberry noted that in Hawaii cancer of the prostate is at least six times more frequent in Caucasian men than in those of Oriental origin. He links frustration and chronic engorgement due to insufficient intercourse with the differences in lovemaking and mating habits of the two groups (Quisenberry 1960). Certainly in Western society the condition arises in elderly males in a monogamous social structure in which the accepted patterns of coitus are restricted and the sole sexual partner has a diminished oestrogen level as a result of the climacteric (Gebhard 1971). The data of Luttge (1971) indicates the importance of this latter hormone in determining unconstrained sexual activity in the human female (see Fig. 5.1, p. 43). It may be that with increasing age, in a certain percentage of sexual partnerships, the Caucasian male is not provided with adequate hormonal and autonomic nervous stimulation to maintain normal prostatic function.

The incidence of cancer of the cervix uteri in nuns is very low compared with the national average. This is a condition which is suspected of being linked to extrinsic factors of coital origin (Fig. 27.8) (Coppleson and Reid 1968). On the other hand, cancer of the breast in nuns is actually more common than in the general population (Fig. 27.9) (Fraumeni *et al.* 1969). It may

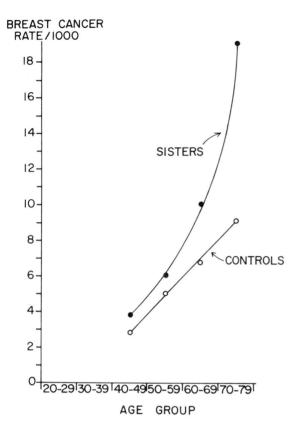

BREAST CANCER RATE/1000

AGE GROUP

FIG. 27.9. The incidence of breast cancer among nuns is actually higher than that of the general population despite their relative freedom from cancer of the cervix uteri. Modified from Fraumeni, William Lloyd, Smith, and Wagoner (1969). Cancer mortality among nuns: Role of marital status in etiology of neoplastic disease in women. *J. natl. Cancer Inst.* **42**; 461.

be suspected that breast cancer in the celibate aging female and prostatic cancer in the monogamous, aging male may both be in part attributable to a failure to achieve social psychophysiologically optimal patterns of human male/female interaction. The data of Greer and Morris (1974) would suggest this, for they find a significant association between the diagnosis of breast cancer and a lifelong pattern of suppression of feelings.

Finally the case of anorexia nervosa may be cited; this almost exclusively affects adolescent females. They often start with a dislike of being fat and restrict their diet in the desire to become attractively slim. Losing weight drastically, they become amenorrheic and lack normal expression of adolescent heterosexual needs. Occasionally starvation alternates with bouts of over-eating. Sometimes there is deliberate vomiting and purgation. The raised plasma cortisol and androgens suggest that the alarm responses are chronically acti-vated. The parents often present psychosocial and male/female relationship problems themselves. The

patients appear to be avoiding or being grossly ambiva-lent about taking the plunge from parental dependence and childhood into sexual maturity and womanhood (Crisp 1970). The features of this disease point to a failure in establishing a normal male/female relation-ship and to the dangerous physiological disturbances that can follow a blocked development of the sexual drive.

THE ROLE OF THE COPING PROCESS IN CONTROLLING THE LEVEL OF THE DEFENCE ALARM RESPONSES

Lazarus has contributed greatly to understanding of the relationship of stress to the psychological mechanisms known as the coping processes (Lazarus 1966). It is clear that they are of the greatest importance in deter-mining the extent to which the defence and alarm responses will be aroused in any particular social situation. It was hazarded in the introduction that these processes may be dependent on the interaction of the limbic system with the neocortical association mechan-ism. Their effect is to determine the level of arousal induced by an emotionally stimulating event and the evidence shows they will inhibit adrenocortical arousal in potentially highly stimulating situations.

Thus the pioneer studies of Friedman *et al.* (1963) with the parents of leukaemic children showed the role of such psychological coping mechanisms in preventing arousal as expressed by an increase in 17-OHCS excretion, and the current studies of Katz *et al.* (1970) with women awaiting biopsy of a threatening lump in the breast point to the same direction. In work showing a significant correlation between the 24-hour level of adrenocortical hormone excretion in the urine and effectiveness of defences as independently evaluated by psychiatric interview, they note the role of denial and displacement, but also comment on more positive mechanisms. Indeed they find an association between active prayer and faith and stoicism/fatalism and the lower levels of adrenocortical arousal.

In an elegant related study of responses to the threats of the war in Vietnam, Bourne (1971) has described how by the coping process of 'ignoring the dangers surrounding him and transforming himself from a sensitive man into an insensitive technician of war with illusions of invulnerability and immortality the professional Special Forces soldier loses his identity in his military unit and gives himself entirely to the job at hand'.

Bourne used two groups, i.e. helicopter ambulance men and seasoned troops awaiting attack in a Special Forces camp. In both he observed an actual decrease in adrenal cortical activity during the period of acute danger as measured by the daily output of 17-OHCS in the urine. On the other hand, the officer and radio operator at the camp who were under considerable strain in dealing with headquarters had increased levels. Similar observations have been made with astronauts while circling in earth orbit. Quite unexpectedly they were shown to have lower levels of 17-OHCS excretion than during control periods (Lutwak *et al.* 1969).

PHYSIOLOGICAL MECHANISMS UNDERLYING THE COPING PROCESSES

Nemiah has recently presented evidence in support of the French psychiatrist Marty's observation of the peculiarly 'operational thought' that is commonly found in patients with psychosomatic disorders (Marty and M'Uzan 1963). They appear to be unable to make a verbal discrimination between various feelings and they have a paucity of drive-related fantasies. In fact, their thought content seems to be rigidly focused on external environmental events. Nemiah speculates that their lack of mental association and fantasy represents a deficiency in connections between the limbic system and the neocortical 'sociocultural' brain (Nemiah and Sifneos 1970). According to this theory, this type of personality has cut himself off from effective participation in the behaviour required for effective cosummation of the various limbic-system-based patterns including those for male/female relationship, i.e. for **mating and for parent/child attachment. For the symbols** representing these drives are projected by the mammals onto their mates and their young. It presumably requires interoceptive attention towards emotional and fantasy activity to sustain an active relationship with these symbol carriers. This Nemiah and Sifneos (1970) point out is just what a person with an 'operational

thinking' attitude is not equipped or motivated to accomplish. It is relevant that Nauta (1971) suggests that frontal lobe deficiency may lead to interoceptive agnosia which he defines as an impairment of the ability to integrate certain information from the internal milieu with the environmental reports provided by the neocortical processing mechanisms. The result of such deficiency may be a loss of efficiency of the coping processes.

Galin (1974) proposed that the mental events in the right hemisphere that are associated with affective responses may not be transferred to the left because of functional suppression of traffic across the corpus callosum. This would help to explain the lack of fantasy in operational thinking and would change the location of the block postulated by Nemiah from the limbic neocortical interconnections to the process of inter-hemispheric transfer. Future studies may show whether either or both hypotheses are correct.

The socially deprived animal fails to respond effectively in a social context to the so-called environmentally stable patterns or instincts. There is a failure to behave in such a way as to cushion the impact of external stimuli. As a result there is a more intense arousal of the hypothalamic and midbrain consummatory areas. The consequent arousal of the defence and/or the alarm responses can then result in the initiation of physiological events whose cumulative effect can be a serious and sustained disturbance of the basic physio-**logical control mechanisms. The ensuing repeated acute** and chronic disturbances of respiratory, cardiovascular, gastrointestinal, and other vital functions will eventually progress to the pathological changes of active disease processes.

REFERENCES

ABRAHAMS, D. C., ABLE, C. A., and BARNARD, B. G. (1960). Systemic blood pressure in a rural West Africa community. *West Afr. med. J.*, **9**, 45–58.

AXELROD, J., MUELLER, R. A., HENRY, J. P., and STEPHENS, P. M. (1970). Changes in enzymes involved in the biosynthesis and metabolism of noradrenaline and adrenaline after psychosocial stimulation. *Nature (Lond.)*, **225**, 1059–60.

BOURNE, P. G. (1971). Altered adrenal function in two combat situations in Vietnam. In *The Physiology of Aggression and Defeat* (ed. B. E. Eleftheriou and J. P. Scott), pp. 265–90. New York.

COPPLESON, M. and REID, B. (1968). The etiology of squamous carcinoma of the cervix. *Obstet. Gynecol.*, **32**, 432–6.

CRISP, A. H. (1970). Psychological aspects of some disorders of weight. In *Modern Trends in Psychosomatic Medicine*, Vol. II (ed. O. W. Hill), pp. 124–46. New York.

CROWCROFT, P. (1966). *Mice all over*. London.

FOLKOW, B. and NEIL, E. (1971). *Circulation*, pp. 560–83. London.

FRAUMENI, J. F., LLOYD, J. W., SMITH, E. M., and WAGONER, J. K. (1969). Cancer mortality among nuns: role of marital status in etiology of neoplastic disease in women. *J. Natl.*

Cancer Inst., **42**, 455–68.

FRIEDMAN, M. (1969). *Pathogenesis of coronary artery disease*, pp. 75–135. New York.

—— and ROSENMAN, R. H. (1974). *Type A behavior and your heart*. New York.

FRIEDMAN, S. B., MASON, J. W., and HAMBURG, D. A. (1963). Urinary 17 hydroxycorticosteroid levels in parents of children with neoplastic disease. *Psychosom. Med.*, **25**, 364–76.

FULLER, J. L. and CLARK, L. D. (1966). Genetic and treatment factors modifying the post isolation syndrome in dogs. *J. comp. Physiol. Psychol.*, **61**, 251–7.

FURMAN, R. H. (1969). Endocrine factors in atherogenesis. In *Atherosclerosis* (ed. F. G. Schettler and G. S. Boyd), p. 376. Amsterdam.

GALIN, D. (1974). Implications for psychiatry of left and right cerebral specialization. *Arch. gen. Psychiat.*, **31**, 572–82.

GEBHARD, P. H. (1971). Human sexual behavior: a summary statement. In *Human sexual behavior* (ed. D. S. Marshall and R. C. Suggs), pp. 201–17. New York.

GREER, S. and MORRIS, T. (1975). Psychological attributes of women who develop breast cancer: a controlled study. *J. psychosom. Res.*, **19**, 147–53.

HAMBURG, D. (1969). Observations of mother-infant interactions in primate field studies. In *Determinants of infant behavior*, Vol. IV (ed. B. Foss), pp. 271–95. London.

HARLOW, H. F., McGAUGH, J. L., and THOMPSON, R. F. (1971). *Psychology*. San Fransisco.

HARRIS, R. E. and SINGER, M. T. (1968). Interaction of personality and stress in the pathogenesis of essential hypertension. In *Hypertension: neural control of arterial pressure*, Vol. 16 (Proc. Council for High Blood Pressure Research, Am. Heart. Assoc.), pp. 104–13. New York.

HENRY, J. P. and CASSEL, J. C. (1969). Psychosocial factors in essential hypertension: recent epidemiologic and animal experimental evidence. *Amer. J. Epidemiol.*, **90**, 171–200.

———, MEEHAN, J. P., and STEPHENS, P. M. (1967). The use of psychosocial stimuli to induce prolonged systolic hypertension in mice. *Psychosom. Med.*, **29**, 408–32.

———, ELY, D. L., STEPHENS, P. M., RATCLIFFE, H. L., SANTISTEBAN, G. A., and SHAPIRO, A. P. (1971). The role of psychosocial factors in the development of arteriosclerosis in CBA mice: observations on the heart, kidney and aorta. *Atherosclerosis*, **14**, 203–18.

———, STEPHENS, P. M., and WATSON, F. M. (1975). Force breeding, social disorder and mammary tumor formation in CBA/USC mouse colonies: a pilot study. *Psychosom. Med.*, **37**, 277–83.

HILL, O. W. (1970). *Modern trends in psychosomatic medicine*, Vol. II. New York.

KAMINER, B. and LUTZ, W. P. W. (1960). Blood pressure in Bushmen of the Kalahari Desert. *Circulation*, **22**, 289–95.

KATZ, J. L., WEINER, H., GALLAGHER, T. S., and HELLMAN, L. (1970). Stress distress and ego defenses: psychoendocrine response to impending tumor biopsy. *Arch. gen. Psychiat.*, **23**, 131–42.

LAZARUS, R. S. (1966). *Psychological stress and the coping process*. New York.

LILJEFORS, I. and RAHE, R. H. (1970). An identical twins study of psychosocial factors in coronary heart disease in Sweden. *Psychosom. Med.*, **32**, 554.

LUTTGE, W. G. (1971). The role of gonadal hormones in the sexual behavior of the Rhesus monkey and human. *Arch. sexual Behav.*, **1**. 61–88.

LUTWAK, L., WHEDON, G. D., LaCHANCE, P. A., REID, J. M., and LIPSCOMB, H. S. (1969). Mineral electrolyte and nitrogen balance studies of the Gemini VII fourteen day orbital space flight. *J. clin. endocrinol. Metab.*, **29**, 1138–40.

MacLEAN, P. D. (1970). The limbic brain in relation to the psychoses. In *Physiological correlates of emotion* (ed. P. Black), pp. 130–44. New York.

MARTY, P. and DE M'UZAN, M. (1963). La pensśee opératoire. *Rev. Fr. Psychanal.*, **27**, 345–56.

MASON, J. W. (1968). "Overall" hormonal balance as a key to endocrine organization. *Psychosom. Med.*, **30**, 791–808.

MOSER, M., MORGAN, R., HALE, M., HOOBLER, S., REMINGTON, R., DODGE, H., MACAULAY, A. (1959). Epidemiology of hypertension with particular reference to the Bahamas. *Amer. J. Cardiol.*, **4**, 727–33.

NAUTA, W. J. H. (1971). The problem of the frontal lobe: a reinterpretation. *J. psychiat. Res.*, **8**, 167–87.

NEMIAH, J. C. and SIFNEOS, P. E. (1970). Affect and fantasy in patients with psychosomatic disease. In *Modern trends in psychosomatic medicine*, Vol. II (ed. O. W. Hill), pp. 26–34. New York.

NEWBERRY, B. H., GILDOW, J., WOGAN, J., and REESE, R. L. (1976). Inhibition of Huggins Tumors by Forced Restraint. *Psychosom. Med.*, **35**, 155–62.

NUCKOLLS, K. B., CASSEL, J., and KAPLAN, B. H. (1972). Psychosocial Assets, Life Crisis and the Prognosis of Pregnancy. *Amer. J. Epidemiol.*, **95**, 431–41.

QUISENBERRY, W. B. (1960). Sociocultural factors in cancer in Hawaii. *Ann. N.Y. Acad. Sci.*, **84**, 795–806.

SAUNDERS, G. E. and BANCROFT, H. (1942). Blood pressure studies on Negro and white men and women living in the Virgin Islands of the United States. *Amer. Heart J.*, **23**, 410.

SCOTCH, N. A. (1960). Preliminary report on the relation of sociocultural factors of hypertension among the Zulu. *Ann. N.Y. Acad. Sci.*, **84**, 1000–9.

SHAPER, A. G. (1962). Cardiovascular studies in the Samburu Tribe of Northern Kenya. *Amer. Heart J.*, **63**, 437–42.

STEELE, R., LEES, R. E. M., KRAUS, A. S., and RAO, C. (1971). Sexual factors in the epidemiology of cancer of the prostate. *J. chronic Dis.*, **24**, 29–37.

U.S. WOMEN'S BUREAU (1935). The economic problems of the women of the Virgin Islands. *Bulletin 142 of the United States Women's Bureau*.

WASHBURN, S. L. and HAMBURG, D. A. (1968). Aggressive behavior in Old World monkeys and apes. In *Primates: studies in adaptation and variability* (ed. P. Jay), pp. 548″68.

WASHBURN, S. L. and HAMBURG, D. A. (1968). Aggressive behavior in Old World monkeys and apes. In *Primates: studies in adaptation and variability* (ed. P. Jay), pp. 548–68. New York.

WEINSTEIN, E. (1962). *Virgin Islanders: cultural aspects of behavior*. Glencoe, Illinois, U.S.A.

28. THE RELATION BETWEEN FAMILY CONSTELLATION AND PSYCHOSEXUAL DISTURBANCES

LARS LIDBERG

INTRODUCTION

The studies of Money *et al.* (1955, 1957) on psycho-sexual differentiation in children with anomalous hormonal 'setting' have shown in a convincing manner that a child acquires during rearing a behavioural pattern that is characteristic for males or females, and that psychosexual masculinity or femininity does not follow automatically from biological sex. The first-born child or the only child has different personality characteristics from other children. Galton (1974) showed that a significant majority of prominent English scientists were either an only, or the first-born, son. McArthur (1956) described the first-born as an adult-orientated, sensitive, and serious person as contrasted to the peer-orientated, easygoing, and friendly second-born, and Sampson (1965), who summarized several studies, found that although first-born or only children more often attained positions of intellectual eminence they were less likely to express overtly aggressive feelings or be an empathic and sociable, outgoing person. Palmer (1966) found that the first-born develops a harsher superego (identifying with authority, discipline, parental prohibition, and moral values) and is more inclined to choose occupations involving a parent-surrogate role.

In the light of these findings it seems probable that being the first or the only child may also have a bearing on the tendency to develop psychosexual problems. Before I started my studies, Breckenridge and Vincent (1943) were the only researchers to indicate this. They stated that men who were the only or first-born children had 5·72 times the average number of divorces while those who were the middle children had only 0·58 of the average number. In a preliminary study (Lidberg 1972) I have shown that patients with psychosexual disturbances have older parents than the population mean, and that they more often are the only or the first-born child. The psychosexual disturbances studied were impotence or premature ejaculation. Some authors consider premature ejaculation is associated with emotional immaturity (Abraham 1927) and others with neurotic personality (Simpson 1950) or that it is a kind of psychosomatic disease (Schapiro 1943). Kinsey *et al.* (1948) argue that it represents a biologically 'superior' reactivity. There are authors who do not separate impotence from premature ejaculation (Noy *et al.* 1966; Blend 1967). Some of my patients suffered both from impotence and premature ejaculation and others suffered from premature ejaculation before they became impotent. Taking this into account, together with the fact that there was no great difference in our findings between patients with impotence and premature ejaculation, I have not separated these two groups.

METHOD

Impotence was taken to mean the inability to achieve an erection *before* or *during* coitus. Premature ejaculation refers to ante-portal ejaculation, ejaculation immediately after insertion, or ejaculation which the patient can not delay despite strong conscious effort to do so. The necessary criteria to establish the diagnosis type of premature ejaculation were habitual ejaculation occurring at a time undesired by, and against the will of the male, and resultant conflicts with the sexual partner. The background data were obtained in a uniform manner, but formalized questioning did not take place. The sample was unselected. However, those patients who mainly described urological or psychiatric symptoms were referred to urological or psychiatric departments. Most of the patients were residents of Greater Stockholm.

The age of the parents of my sample was compared with figures from a special census taken in Sweden in 1935/36 (SOS 1950). From this census it is possible to calculate the median age of parents of people of roughly the same age as our patients in the whole Swedish population. Since the age distribution was positively skewed the median was used to describe the age of the parents. The sample consisted of 235 outpatients who had consulted the author for psychosexual disorders at the RFSU Clinic (The Swedish Association for Sexual Education) from October 1964 to October 1968. A few of them had been referred by general practitioners or psychiatrists. Only 34 presented disturbances other than impotence and premature ejaculation. Examples of these other disturbances are: anxiety about masturbation (8), anxiety about being homosexual (6), and anxiety about size of genitals (4). One hundred and eleven patients showed symptoms of impotence and 90 of premature ejaculation. Both symptoms were present together in 32 patients. The older patients more usually complained of impotence, in agreement with the findings of e.g. Kinsey *et al.*

RESULTS

Age of the parents

The parents of the patients are relatively older than those of the general population. The median age of the fathers of our patients at the time of birth of patients born in 'complete' homes (not illegitimate or from a broken home) was 36·1 years and of the mothers was 33·0 years. In the Swedish population the median age of the fathers of children born in wedlock was 29·8 years and of the mothers 26·4 years, according to the previously mentioned population census (SOS 1950).

Position among siblings (see Table 28.1)
Twenty-six per cent of our patients who grew up in 'complete' homes were an only child or the only son. The frequency of only-male-child differed significantly from the population average. Of those persons in Sweden born between 1900 and 1935, 10·94 per cent were the only child, according to the 1935/36 census (SOS 1939). As rather more boys than girls were born, the frequency of only-male children in the population can thus be calculated to be 6 per cent at the most. Among our patients they amounted to 11 per cent. This high frequency of only-male-child cannot be explained by the high incidence of older parents in the patients. The fact that older parents usually have more children than young ones, should, on the contrary, compensate for the over-representation of the patients who were the only son of older, and hitherto childless parents.

TABLE 28.1

Family conditions of patients with premature ejaculation and impotence

	Number of patients	Percentage
Incomplete home		
Born out of wedlock	7	4
Broken home before the age of 16	8	4
Complete home		
Only child	22	11
Only son	30	15
Oldest child, not the only son	39	24
Others	95	42
Total	201	100

Occupation of the patients
The results we obtained regarding occupation of the patients have previously been reviewed (Lidberg 1972). The proportion in technical professions was high — 32 per cent (average: 12 per cent; SOS 1973) — as was the proportion of men employed in office administrative work — 10 per cent (average: 5 per cent).

DISCUSSION

Great expectations in regard to performance from the only or the first-born boy is still very obvious cultural heritage in the occidental, patrilineal community. This tradition, with emphasis upon the right of primogeniture, has become less pronounced recently, but still prevails in the middle-class of Western culture societies and places high values on future goals, individualism, and independence.

Adler (1927), who described the psychological effects of achievement, stressed the importance of an individual's ordinal position. Expectations that may promote occupational success and promotion can also cause insecurity and the tendency to develop problems in sexual relations. Accordingly, Herell (1972) has shown that first-born boys are over-represented among military leaders but are also more inclined to develop neurotic disorders than boys who are not first-born.

Other studies have confirmed that first-born children have more independent intellectual attitudes than later-born children (Becker *et al.* 1964) and that they are more inclined to identify particularly with authority, discipline, parental prohibition, and moral values (Palmer 1966). The parents' insecurity and inexperience in child-rearing may also be of importance with respect to oldest or only sons. That first-born children are exposed to a greater measure of parental control — not only during infancy — has been shown in a Swedish study of 820 schoolchildren aged 10–14 years (Schaller 1972). This parental control leads to an accentuation of performance expectations and social success.

Milton (1958) found that mothers with sexual anxiety were characterized by a rearing behaviour that best could be described as strict and non-permissive. In his analytical study, which was made on 379 mothers whose children were at a maternity home, Milton was able to show statistically that such rearing behaviour, which is not obviously related to psychosexual behaviour (excessive demands in table manners and cleanliness, particularly concerning toilet functions) can have an influence on sexual adaptation. Kayton and Borge (1965) showed that there were significantly more only children or only sons among patients with obsessive/compulsive character disorders than in a control group of other patients, and were of the opinion that the conditions for the only son and for an oldest son were similar.

Kayton and Borge (1965) thought that the parents' insecurity when confronted with the rearing of the first-born child resulted in tendency to use intellectualized, verbal communication with the child, causing emotional isolation and lack of development as well as a premature superego development in boys. The excessive demands and restrictions made on the only child or the only son might cause insecurity and contribute to future psychosexual disturbances. Why patients with relatively old parents have psychosexual disturbances may thus also be related to a more authoritarian rearing.

In a Swedish study of conscripts Bliding (1974) found that among men who were under psychiatric consultation those who were born when their mothers were more than 30 years old or fathers more than 35 years old tended to be raised in a more authoritarian style than others. He also found that only children were more seldom married.

In England, over-representation of higher social classes has been shown in patients with psychosexual disorders compared with patients seeking advice for general psychiatric problems (Johnson 1965; Cooper 1968). The psychiatric departments in Stockholm do not report distribution of social class, but the socio-economic educational level in my sample was high. Also the proportion of my sample in technical professions was high. The proportion of men employed in office administrative work was also higher in my sample than in the town and county of Stockholm. This preponderance of technical and office administrative occupations has been found previously in an unpublished report concerning outpatients with psychosexual disturbances from the RFSU Clinic (Dahlin 1969). My sample was not large enough to permit a differential study of the profession of the oldest or the only child compared with the others. The preponderance of technical and office administrative occupations in the sample of patients may be seen as a manifestation of their tendency to avoid emotional and personal contact and to deal with problems in an intellectualized way, a tendency which can contribute to psychosexual disturbances.

REFERENCES

ABRAHAM, K. (1949). Ejaculation praecox. *The international psychoanalytical library 1927*, No. 13 (ed. E. Jones). London.

ADLER, A. (1927). *Understanding human nature*. New York.

BECKER, S. W., LERNER, M. J., and CARROLL, J. (1964). Conformity as a function of birth order, payoff and type of group pressure. *J. abnorm. soc. Psychol.*, **69**, 318–23.

BLEND, D. (1967). Sex and its problems. IV. The impotent male. *Practitioner*, **198**, 589–96.

BLIDING, Å. (1975). Psykiska insufficinesreaktioner under militär grundutbildning. Thesis, Lund.

BRECKENRIDGE, M. E. and VINCENT, E. L. (1943). *Child development*, p. 155. Philadelphia.

COOPER, A. (1968). A factual study of male potency disorders. *Brit. J. Psychiat.*, **114**, 710–31.

DAHLIN, O. (1969). Erfarenhet av sexuell rådgivning. (Manuscript)

GALTON, F. (1874). *English men of science. Their nature and nurture*. London.

HERRELL, J. M. (1972). Birth order and the military: a review from an Adlerian perspective. *J. individ. Psychol.*, **28**, 38–40.

JOHNSON, J. (1965). Prognosis of disorders of sexual potency in the male. *J. psychosom. Res.*, **9**, 195–200.

KAYTON, L. and BORGE, G. F. (1967). Birth order and the obsessive-compulsive character. *Arch. gen. Psychiat.*, **17**, 751–4, 1967.

KINSEY, A. C., POMEROY, W. B. and MARTIN, C. E. (1948). Sexual behaviour in the human male. Philadelphia.

LIDBERG, L. (1972). Social and psychiatric aspects of impotence and premature ejaculation. *Arch. sex. Behav.*, **2**, 135–46.

MILTON, G. A. (1958). A factor analytic study of child-rearing behaviors. *Child Devel.*, **29**, 381–92.

McARTHUR, C. (1956). Personalities of first and second children. *Psychiatry*, **19**, 47–54.

MONEY, J., HAMPSON, J. G., and HAMPSON, J. L. (1955). An examination of some basic sexual concepts: the evidence of human hermaphroditism. *Bull. John Hopk. Hosp.*, **97**, 301–319.

——, ——, and —— (1957). Imprinting and the establishment of gender role. *Arch. Neurol. Psychiat.*, **77**, 333–6.

NOY, P., WOLLSTEIN, S., and KAPLAN-DE-NOUR, A. (1966). Clinical observations on the psychogenesis of impotence. *Brit. J. med. Psychol.*, **39**, 43–53.

PALMER, R. D. (1966). Birth order and identification. *J. Consult. Psychol.*, **30**, 129–35.

SAMPSON, E. E. (1965). The study of ordinal position: antecedents and outcomes. In *Progress in experimental personality research* (ed. D. Maher), Vol. 2, pp. 175–228.

SCHALLER, J. (1972). *Ordinal position and parental control*, Volume 2, page 17. Psychosocial Reports. Göteborg, Sweden.

SCHAPIRO, B. (1943). Premature ejaculation. *J. Urol.*, **50**, 374–9.

SEARS, R. R., MOCCOBY, E., and LEVIN, H. (1957). *Patterns of child rearing*. Evanstone.

SIMPSON, L. S. (1950). Impotence. *Brit. Med. J.*, i, 692–7.

SOS [OFFICIAL STATISTICS OF SWEDEN] (1939). *Recensement de la population en 1935/36. Le recensement partial de la population en mars 1936: nombre d'enfants et décédés dans les marriages.* Stockholm.

—— (1950). *Mouvement de la population en 1947.* Stockholm.

—— (1973). *Population and housing census 1970.* Part 7. Stockholm.

TAINTOR, Z. (1970). Birth order and psychiatric problems in Boot Camp. *Amer. J. Psychiat.*, **126**, 80–6.

29.   CYCLICAL HORMONAL ACTIVITY

JOHN CULLEN

EQUALITY AND SAMENESS

One of the most welcome phenomena of our time is the articulate and persuasive voice of half the world's population for liberation and equal rights. I refer, of course, to the emergence of women from a situation in which they have throughout history been deprived of an effective voice in the decision making which shapes our physical and psychosocial environment. Naturally such a revolutionary movement tends to be selective or to exaggerate some claims. There is, for example, the tendency to confuse equality with sameness. This chapter will seek to identify differences between men and women, differences in very fundamental biological processes and differences in cultural determinants.

Of all the baselines against which change is measured in science, time is the most enduring. It therefore seems worth considering how men and women interact on a shared time scale. This requires us to identify sex differences in the schedule by which life is lived and to indicate some of the rhythms which interweave in very complex ways either in individual men and women or in their relationships to each other.

THE MENSTRUAL CYCLE

The most obvious of the sex-linked biological time sequences is the 'lunar cycle' of sex hormone activity in women — the menstrual cycle. Lunar biological cycles are so called because they have a periodicity similar to that of the phases of the moon, 28–30 days, although not necessarily in phase with it. Menstruation is a great time marker in women's lives. Its onset is the watershed between childhood and womanhood, celebrated in most cultures except our own with great ritual and solemnity. No one knows fully why the menarche should occur at a particular age and explanations based on climatic or ambient light differences tend to give way to genetic and racial theories. Once it has started it recurs, regularly in most women. Again no one knows why it should recur with a lunar periodicity in the human and other primates or why the oestrus cycle in the rat, for example, should recur every 4 or 5 days. Menstruation stops as inexplicably as it began but as inevitably as the ageing process itself.

Despite our lack of knowledge about the most obvious phenomena of the menstrual cycle we can speak with more certainty about other aspects of it. We know, for instance, that the menstrual cycles are activated by and are under the control of two hormones — oestrogen and progesterone. We know that production of these hormones is controlled by two other hormones, follicle stimulating hormone and luteinizing hormone which are secreted by the pituitary gland at the base of the brain. The pituitary gland is controlled by the hypothalamus, and this part of the brain is under the influence of the functions of which include perception, thinking, learning and memory. We know, further, that oestrogen and progesterone influence behaviour and mood. Indeed, progesterone or its metabolites or synthetic progesterone-like compounds may act on the brain as powerful anaesthetics in their own right. In fact more than 10 years ago I participated, at Cambridge, with Derek Russell Davis in experimentation with these compounds on their usefulness in facilitating abreactions in psychotherapy. I gather this work has been taken up again recently in the United States.

INFLUENCE ON MOOD, BEHAVIOUR, AND HEALTH

The stage is now set for an examination of the way in which these profound changes in the internal processes of a woman's body can influence her mood, behaviour, her health, and above all her relationships with her most intimate companions — almost invariably her husband and her children. Her family's health may suffer if a woman is under stress. She may suffer serious psychological disturbances, especially around the time of the menses or just before their onset. They also occur just after childbirth. Now, these are the times at which levels of progesterone in the blood-stream are dropping to very low values after previously sustained high ones. Hamburg *et al.* (1968) give a very clear account of their own studies of women who show post-partum distress or distress during the menstrual cycle. Their findings support those of Coppen and Kessel (1963) which indicate that approximately 25 per cent of all women experience moderate to severe distress in their menstrual cycles just before or during menstruation. This distress, they point out may involve pain, diminished concentration, and impoverished judgement, behavioural changes with withdrawal from social activity or lowered work performance, and mood changes such as depression, irritability, and anxiety together with a variety of symptoms related to disturbances of water balance or of the cardiovascular system. We have, therefore, a situation in which 25 per cent of women experience recurring exposure to a stress situation between 400 and 500 times in their lives. This cycle of change in a woman's psychobiological programme takes place in a complex psychosocial context with husband, children, and colleagues as the principal social contacts.

Kagan (1972) summarizes 'current and well supported speculation by the concept that "stimuli arising from psychosocial situations can promote health or cause disease". If such situations are adapted to the organism's needs or the organism can adapt to the situation, health ensues. If not disease results. ... When changes are frequent and extensive, the chances of failure of adaptation increase.' Over the past 20 years or so Katharina Dalton (e.g. 1953, 1955, 1959, 1960a,b,c, 1961, 1964, 1966, 1967, 1968) has been patiently cataloguing the coincidence of serious deviations from healthy adaptation in women in the premenstrual phase or during menstruation. All sorts of disasters seem to occur at these times. More mothers take their sick children to the doctor — twice as many. More schoolgirls fail their examinations or achieve lower grades or are punished for misdemeanours. More women commit indictable crimes or become disorderly prisoners. More women have accidents, attempt suicide, or are admitted to mental hospitals. This is an incomplete list but none-the-less it is an astonishing epidemiological phenomenon with enormous implications as a psychosocial stress stimulus. It is surprising then that we are so little aware of it as a day-to-day experience. This we may suppose is due to the rather absurd attitudes both men and women have towards this particular biological rhythm; and has incurred an almost total neglect in developing health policies to answer the problem. It is only if a woman herself seeks medical help that some relief may be offered. Meanwhile these women, their husbands, and their children must cope as best they can.

The effects on the children can be subtle and unrecognized. I have already mentioned Dalton's findings about the timing of medical referral of sick children. Recently she has found similar distributions of the admissions of children to hospital with illness or after accidents. These are obvious disasters for both child and mother, but a major coincident (to say the least of it) in their aetiology is hardly ever recognized. But the effects may be even more subtle and difficult to recognize. Help in delineating the intricacies of these influences can come from the concepts and findings of learning theorists in psychology. One of the most active apostles of this approach, Ferster (1961), has analysed the role of consistent reinforcement patterns in parents' behaviour towards their children, with special reference to autistic children. The factors he describes can be applied with equal relevance to normal children. A mother who undergoes gross changes in mood and behaviour on a lunar cycle can hardly be experienced as consistent by a child whose expectancies are diurnal. It may be that not only the formation of a child's behaviour may be influenced in this way but even his psycho-endocrine and autonomic nervous system stress responses may be set in abnormal patterns just as surely as by the regular return of an aggressive drunken father to the home. Of course I do not suggest that most women do not try to rise above their mood changes, but it takes great effort and the effort also can

show. The work of Miller and Di Cara (1967, 1968, 1969) has shown that profound changes may be brought about in visceral and glandular responses by repeated learning experiences. Just 10 years before the publication of their work I had argued (Cullen 1960) that somatic learning of this kind must be expected: 'The question of the symbolism of symptoms depends on the personality structure of the individual case. This individual personality structure, of course, depends on memory and the previous experience and learning of the patient on the basis of his inherited capacities. The whole somatic system including the skin is no less involved in this learning process than the central nervous system.' Here, then we have the outline of the model for the generation of disease and disease precursors — the learning of both behavioural and somatic responses under reinforcement schedules arising in the psychosocial stimulus situation. Filling out this outline (see Fig. 29.1) will be a continuous process as new findings are made, but there is already a vast amount of knowledge which must be incorporated and applied.

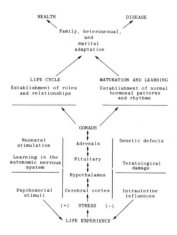

FIG. 29.1.

SECONDARY CYCLES IN FAMILY MEMBERS

We shall turn now to the men who are married to these women — and who father and relate to their children. Do they, too, have cycles — monthly cycles like women? Richter (1968) has argued that both men and women are born with a female brain with female internal clocks, and that the monthly rhythms are suppressed by the appearance of male hormones in the male child about the time of birth. He uses evidence from animal studies that female cycling of glandular activity can be restored in the male under certain conditions. Be that as it may there is undoubtedly in some men a lunar periodicity in the recurrences of episodes of certain diseases. Dalton has claimed that these are

198

found to be in synchrony with the premenstrual phase of the wife of the sufferer and are therefore to be regarded as a response to the woman's mood or behaviour change. Motoring accidents incurred by men have also been said to occur most frequently around the premenstrual phase in their wives. Whatever we may ultimately find out about rhythms in men, we must taken into account the socially and culturally determined cycles of mood, behaviour, energy, and vigilance. The work/leisure cycles, monthly pay-days, and so on can all profoundly influence change in behaviour and mood in men. Somehow or other these must coexist with similar cycles, as well as hormonal cycles, in their women, however asynchronous their patterns may be. The rhythm of family life is also determined by these cultural clocks and the woman may have to perform uniformly in relationship to this time scale, however much it may be out of phase with her own internal biological clock. Levels and expectations of sexual responsiveness may also run to different rhythms in men and women. Michael (1968) has shown the variation in sexual arousal and behaviour of primates over the menstrual cycle and Hamburg (1968) has shown that women report a similar phasic pattern in their sexual interests. It can be seen then that asynchrony in the partners periodic experience may lead to sexual problems in conflicted marriages and that this may be disasterous for both the marriage and the health of the partners. The occurrence of any of the other untoward effects described by Dalton can have an equally damaging effect on either partner.

THE EFFECT OF THE MENSTRUAL CYCLE ON ROLE AND IDENTITY

Before giving a brief illustrative overview of some of our clinical material from the Psycho-Endocrine Research Centre of the Department of Psychiatry, University College, Dublin, I would like to mention another aspect of menstrual cycling in women. This is the way in which it is seen to establish role and identity in women. Women have attitudes to their menses — often very complicated attitudes. They may consciously or unconsciously accept or reject the biological and psychological reality of the status menstrual cycling confers. Often these attitudes reflect those of the mother or stem from the experience of the menarche either as a normal milestone, an unexpected disaster, or a frustratingly delayed status achievement. This is a commonplace of the psychiatric history and is frequently found to be bound up with subsequent attitudes towards sex and marriage. Women are not always glad that they are women. Almost always, however, they regard the occurrence of menstruation as a confirmation of their femininity. At the menopause they may fear the loss of their femininity or sexual status. Both the onset and the cessation of the menses are often charged with conflict about identity in relationships with men.

ANOREXIA NERVOSA

A condition which we have investigated and treated in a fairly large number of cases now is anorexia nervosa. This condition, as is well known, occurs almost exclusively in young women and only very rarely if at all in young men. We find that most of these girls have had difficulties in identifying with their mothers and in relating appropriately to their fathers. The have difficulty in accepting their feminine role and identity and may be deeply confused about this. Indeed an explanation of naïve simplicity may be advanced that their self-imposed emaciation is designed to abolish their female bodily configuration. Whatever the merits of this type of teleological explanation we have been invariably successful in our treatment of these cases when we achieved three goals — weight gain to near normal levels, insight and acceptance of femininity, and the establishment or re-establishment of monthly cycles. We achieve the latter by giving oestrogen and progesterone in sequential form followed by low doses of clomiphene. This usually triggers off spontaneous monthly cycling but the cycles resemble those normally found around puberty, in being mainly anovulatory. They persist and hopefully will eventually settle down to a more mature pattern. As one might expect in girls in a situation of severe conflict we almost invariably find also that they show very high levels of adrenal gland activity during its diurnal cycle and that their adrenal gland responses are extremely sensitive in the Synachten Test. We have used this as a guide to their level of psychosocial adjustment and if this is progressing favourably, with a return of more normal levels of adrenal rhythms, then menstrual cycling will continue spontaneously after induction. In these cases, then, the establishment of menstruation is a touchstone of identity adaptation.

PSYCHE AND HORMONES

In the Psycho-Endocrine Research Centre we see many curious manifestations of the vulnerability of the complex rhythmic patterns I have described. There is the case of the two very attractive sisters, both happily married and who both came to seek help for their infertility. Neither, although in their early twenties, had ever menstruated. This did not seem to have raised any question about their sexual identity either for themselves, their parents, or their husbands. Both turned out to be genotypically XY male (see Fig. 29.2) and therefore will never either menstruate or have children. The implications of cases of male intersex testicular feminization syndrome like these will be discussed elsewhere in the book.

The chemical similarities and interchangeability of the sex hormones which determine the obvious bodily evidence of sex difference (see Fig. 29.3), their common source, and the interchangeability with stress hormones from the adrenals provides a matrix within which many

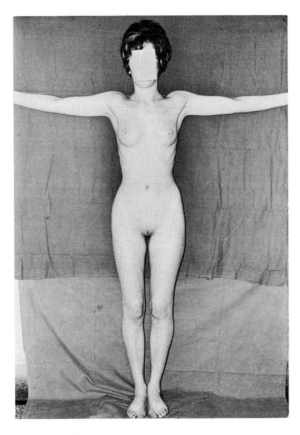

FIG. 29.2. Testicular feminization syndrome.

bizarre cases occur. One 28 year-old woman suffered much marital conflict, and had an alcoholic mother. She showed gross hyperactivity of her adrenal glands, probably accounting for her high levels of circulating androgens, and as a consequence had frustratingly increased libido to nymphomaniacal levels with hirsutism as an embarassing accompaniment. Her marriage has broken down. Then, on the other hand there was the man who had developed breasts and a failing libido. He has encouraged a *ménage à trois* with another man living in his house, to the utter confusion of his children, and his wife is suffering from stress. His blood shows unusually high levels of oestrogen. How early this hormonal anomaly was present we do not know.

We have seen many other cases where biological sex caused stress situations — cases, for example, of adrenal virilization in women, who showed hirsutism and a tendency to suppression of the menstrual cycle; cases of infertility with a vicious circle of stress, disappointment, and suppression of menstruation. And of course the endless cases of premenstrual tension, often with abnormal blood levels of oestrogen and progesterone, and with husbands reacting variously, for example by over-eating, obesity, and hypertension; alcoholism; or, in one case, by becoming a diabetic.

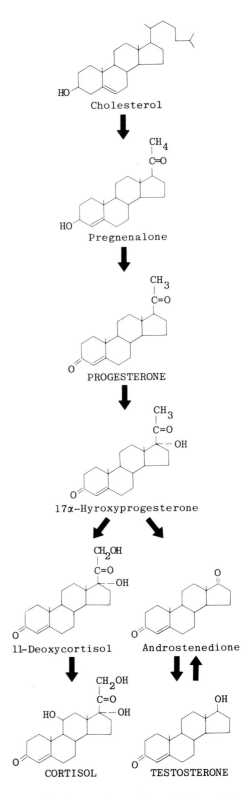

Cholesterol

Pregnenalone

PROGESTERONE

17α-Hyroxyprogesterone

11-Deoxycortisol   Androstenedione

CORTISOL   TESTOSTERONE

FIG. 29.3. Some pathways of steroid biosynthesis.

A crude model of the processes involved in such cases might read as follows:

STRESS
↓
Excessive adrenal activity
↓
Increased output of cortisol precursor
↓
Increased circulating sex steroids
↓
Suppression of gonadotrophins from the pituitary and the hypothalamus
↓
Interference with normal gonadal functions
↓
Disturbed menstrual cycles; erratic or abnormal sex drives;
↓
Aggression in marriage

This simple model gives only a glimpse of the biochemical complexities involved. However, challenge and opportunity frequently go together. We now have techniques for measuring levels of all these hormones in the blood and, within the limits of ethics and tolerance of venipuncture, we can now undertake dynamic correlation studies between hormonal status changes and variations in psychophysiological parameters. We can, with the insights from the experimental findings in the psychology of learning devise more meaningful experiments into the ways in which hormonal patterns change with time, with experience of recurring patterns of stress, and with many other variables relating to life style. There is also the opportunity for therapeutic intervention, using either natural hormones or synthetic hormones, which are available in increasing variety, to enable us to attempt restoration of normal rhythms and cycles. There are hazards in this, of course. Perhaps the most obvious are those which have been associated with the pill of which the most frequent and most disturbing are the reports of hazards of depression, and risk of suicide. Hypothetical biochemical models for this finding have involved neurochemically active substances such as tryptophan and serotonin.

Our own studies

In our laboratory we are in the early stages of long-term experimentation involving methods which incorporate the theoretical constructs which I have outlined above. The work is with human subjects, both patients and volunteers. Up to now we have been concerned:

(a) to get a clinical overview of the range of case material available and to derive hypotheses from these;

(b) to build up the necessary assay techniques, equipment, and skilled biochemistry staff;

(c) to develop tests for behavioural variables which are sufficiently reliable and sensitive and to train the appropriate staff;

(d) to encourage a broad interdisciplinary approach. This is, perhaps, the most important of all.

The joining of our team by a systems engineer, Dr. Noel Murphy, who is a lecturer in the Engineering School of the University has helped us solve many problems which could not have been resolved from within the frames of reference of the life sciences.

DIURNAL RHYTHM OF ADRENAL ACTIVITY

Before concluding I would like to mention another hormonal cycle — the diurnal rhythm of cortisol production and adrenal activity. Whether there are sex-determined differences in this cycle is not clear. This is surprising in view of the gross differences in life style and patterns of stress challenge between the sexes. We have already described how the activity in the adrenal gland may be implicated in sexual functioning. Then, there is the coincidental sleep/waking rhythm. How this relates to adrenal circadian rhythms is not clear. Within sleep itself there are cycles of different patterns of brain electrical activity which are said to be important factors in preserving mental health. What does seem to be certain is that there are people who have circadian patterns which are the reverse of what we expect normally. This may be more common than our culturally imposed work/rest rhythms suggest. The distribution of work-times selected by employees allowed to select their shift would bear this out. Also it has been found that medical students given access on a 24-hour basis to audio-visual aids in a university library distributed their work so that 25 per cent of them used the library between the hours of midnight and 7 a.m. We do not know whether marriages between spouses whose circadian rhythms are synchronous are better than those where they are asynchronous.

These diurnal cycles are relatively easy to detect, but there may be cycles which recur only once a year or less often. An interesting suggestion by Franz Halberg of the University of Minnesota, who, incidentally, invented the term circadian rhythms, is that there are possibly circannual rhythms in the excretion of 17-ketosteroids in men. The urinary secretion of 17-ketosteroids in men is at levels equalled by women only when they are pregnant. Excretion of these substances varies in different pathological and physiological conditions. So in the end it may turn out that women have to adjust to male hormonal rhythms but of a much more devious and secretive nature! Perhaps the ultimate confirmation of male chauvinism will come as the full story of the prostaglandins unfolds. These hormone-like substances which were first named by the great Swedish biochemist, Ulf S. von Euler, were found by him to be highly active substances found in human semen (amongst other places where they are found is in the menstrual fluid of women) and they are now known to have marked effects on the blood-pressure, on the contractility of the uterine muscle, and on a whole range of other physiological activity. They are probably implicated in the formation of cyclic adenosine monophosphate, which is one of the key factors in the relay of specific hormonal messages throughout the body; and both substances seem to be keyed into the communication networks of the body, especially in the cell membrane which is the ultimte interface between the living and non-living worlds. Perhaps the female can absorb male prostaglandins when the lunar cyclical changes in her genital tract allow it.

Discussion of the ways in which the cycles of change in the physical environment interact with biological cycles must be left to the fascinating studies of the 'clock-biologists'. One of the earliest of these was the Swedish Nobel Prize Winner for Chemistry in 1903, Svante Arrhenius (1898) who perhaps would not now find many supporters for his theories about the influence of atmospheric electricity on biological rhythms in health and disease. However, he was wise to speculate about the ways in which men and their environments interact. Only by such seeking will man survive in our world with its harmonies with the great cycles and rhythms of the universe.

REFERENCES

ARRHENIUS, S. (1898). Die Einwirkung kosmischer Einflüsse auf physiologische Verhältnisse. *Skand. Arch. Physiol.*, **8**, 367–416.

COPPEN, A. and KESSEL, N. (1963). Menstruation and personality. *Brit. J. Psychiat.*, **109**, 711–21.

CULLEN, J. H. (1960). Psychological mechanisms in the psychosomatic skin affections. Paper read at Cambridge University Conference for Dermatologists. In *Progress in the biological sciences in relation to dermatology* (ed. A. Rook), pp. 197–206. Cambridge.

DALTON, K. (1955). The premenstrual syndrome. *Proc. roy Soc. Med.*, **48**, 337.

—— (1959). Menstruation and acute psychiatric illnesses. *Brit. med. J.*, i, 148.

—— (1960a). Effect of menstruation on schoolgirls' weekly work. *Brit. med. J.*, i, 326.

—— (1960b). Schoolgirls' behaviour and menstruation. *Brit. med. J.*, ii, 1647.

—— (1960c). Menstruation and accidents. *Brit. med. J.*, ii, 1425.

—— (1961). Menstruation and crime. *Brit. med. J.*, ii, 1752.

—— (1964). The influence of menstruation on health and disease. *Proc. roy. Soc. Med.*, **57**, 262.

—— (1964). *The pre-menstrual syndrome*. London.

—— (1966). The influence of a mother's menstruation on her child. *Proc. roy. Soc. Med.*, **59**, 1014.

—— (1967). The influence of menstruation on glaucoma. *Brit. J. Ophthalmol.*, **51**, 692.

—— (1968). Menstruation and examinations. *Lancet*, , 1386.

—— and GREENE, R. (1953). The premenstrual syndrome. *Brit. med. J.*, i, 1007.

FERSTER, C. B. (1961). Positive reinforcement and behavioural deficits of autistic children. *Child Devel.*, **32**, 437–56.

HAMBURG, D. A., MOOS, R. H., and YALOM, I. D. (1968). Studies of distress in the menstrual cycle and the post-partum period. In *Endocrinology and Human Behaviour* (ed. R. P. Michael), pp. 94–16. Oxford.

KAGAN, A. (1972). 'Experimental evaluation of the role of psychosocial stimuli in disease as a guide to rational health action.' Paper read at the Conference on Experimental Behaviour Basis of Mental Disturbance. Ireland 24/28 April, 1972.

MICHAEL, R. P. (1968). Gonadal hormones and the control of primate behaviour. In *Endocrinology and human behaviour* (ed. R. P. Michael), pp. 69–93. Oxford.

MILLER, N. E. and DI CARA, L. V. (1967). Instrumental learning of heart rate changes in curarized rats. *J. comp. Physiol. Psychol.*, **63**, 12–19.

—— and —— (1968). Instrumental learning of vasomotor responses by rats. *Science (N.Y.)*, **159**, 1485–6.

—— (1969). Learning of visceral and glandular responses. *Science (N.Y.)*, **163**, 434–45.

RICHTER, C. P. (1968). Periodic phenomena in man and animals. In *Endocrinology and human behaviour* (ed. R. P. Michael), pp. 284–309. Oxford.

SESSION 4

Prevention of stress and disease originating from male/female roles and relationships

30. THE EPIDEMIOLOGIST'S AID TO THE EVALUATION OF PREVENTIVE HEALTH ACTION

AUBREY KAGAN

THE PROBLEM

The health planner, advisor, or decision maker is frequently faced with a dilemma. Increasing ill health, thought to be due to social change, demands that he take action. But what action *can* he suggest when:

(1) he is not sure whether it will do good or harm, but suspects both;
(2) he doesn't know who it will benefit and who it will harm, or how much;
(3) he is not sure what it will cost, but suspects a great deal.

Under these circumstances, which are all too common, the only ethical approach is to evaluate the proposed action on a small scale in terms of safety, efficacy, and cost. There are many ways in which the epidemiologist can help health action, in this chapter I will discuss his contribution to evaluation.

It is only by evaluation that the people the epidemiologist serves, and many others in a similar situation, will be protected from dangers, learn from mistakes, and find a rational effective approach to disease prevention. Although the importance of evaluation is now understood by the medical profession, it is practised only very occasionally and usually very reluctantly — but on these occasions with considerable success (Cochrane, personal communication; Mather *et al.* 1971).

THE DIFFICULTIES

The reasons given for reluctance to do what seems essential are ethical, technical difficulties, and costs. The epidemiologist can help in all these aspects of evaluation (Kagan 1971, 1972, 1974).

Ethics
The essential ethical problem is that evaluation is a form of experimentation. We do something, we are not quite sure what its effect will be, but we want to find out what happens. There is no doubt that this is an experiment, and there is equally no doubt, to my mind, that unbridled experimentation might be and has been both dangerous and harmful to the subject. However, it is not necessary to treat people like guinea-pigs in order to carry out experiments. Under certain conditions, experimentation is both reasonable and ethical. The conditions are that the subject should know what the experiment is about, what can be done, and the reasons why, and

then should be free to volunteer or refrain. The experiment must be carried out in a humane way and everything must be done to minimize dangers to a level that the ordinary person is accustomed to take during his ordinary life activities. Not only should all this be done, but, to use the words of Hailsham (in a sense that he did not intent) it 'should be seen to be done'. Preferably, the problem should be of importance to the people taking part in the experiment. Under these circumstances, experimentation is ethical and we should not hesitate to say so, nor should we disguise our intention to experiment by using words such as 'intervention' or 'controlled trial'. The obverse of the situation is that all action that is unevaluated is an experiment, but carried out in such a way that we cannot learn from the experiment. In my opinion, that is unethical.

Technical problems
The predicament. Technically, the situation is due to inherent difficulties in the problems to be tackled that are unlikely to be met without modification of traditional methods.

The usual process of discovery depends upon thought, observation, and experiment. Thought directs observation along a particular pathway; observation sends thoughts in a particular direction. These processes lead to a hypothesis which is then tested. The results of this lead either to an acceptable theory or to one that needs further testing, to a change in hypothesis, or to the realization that a further set of observations is indicated — and so on.

There is an element of chance in choosing the right observation, the right hypothesis, the right conditions for observation, and the right test situation. That is why the majority of ideas and hypothesis prove to be sterile and chance observations may be productive.

A negative result is useful only if the false hypothesis or inadequate health action is in some way related to the correct hypothesis or action, so that its disproof directs attention to the latter; or if by thus excluding one of a few possibilities attention is directed to the others. In any event, unless the first hypothesis is luckily correct, observation and experimentation have to be repeated.

This process of discovery has succeeded and is tolerable when the procession between thought, observation, experiment, and back again is fast and inexpensive. A train of thought can be followed, modified, re-tested, or cast aside, and a new idea can then be put through the same process. Under these conditions the process results in discovery sufficiently often to receive acclaim and acceptance and to have resulted in the undoubted advances of science that we now experience. When the process is slowed down, e.g. the chances of hitting upon the right idea get slighter, or a need emerges for large-scale prolonged observation and tests, the frequency of obtaining useful results is greatly diminished. The expense of procession becomes great and the expense of repetition enormous in terms of manpower, materials, and time.

This describes our predicament. The number of factors suspected, and therefore to be observed, is great. Observation of representative samples of large numbers of human beings under habitual conditions is required. The number of possible associations is great because not only are the number of suspect factors large but it is likely that combinations of factors should be examined. The number of hypotheses arising is large. Tests of hypotheses of prevention of disease seldom takes less than 2 years and often take longer. Discovery is the exception. False hypotheses leading to sterile results are the rule. Repetition of the process becomes necessary but inexpedient in terms of effort, time, and money.

INCREASING THE EFFECTIVENESS OF EPIDEMIOLOGICAL METHODS

We cannot do without the iterative process of 'thought, observation, test'. We must make it more effective. This might be achieved by:

(1) improving study designs;
(2) better forms of mathematical analysis of data;
(3) greater and known precision of observation;
(4) more efficient assessment of larger numbers of subjects;
(5) multipurpose action — several hypotheses or health actions tested simultaneously; observations made at the same time, that by suitable analysis will enlarge our understanding of the whole system.

In particular, attention should be paid to:

(a) the definition of relevant factors;
(b) the definition, testing, and modification of methods for assessing these factors and establishing their precision and bias;
(c) the problem of control groups;
(d) the achievement of high response and the maintenance of adherence to the study;
(e) follow-up;
(f) numbers and type of subjects;
(g) costs.

The definition of relevant factors
I will not deal with (a) here except to say that, usually, factors connected with safety and cost and ways in which the health action is potentially dangerous are forgotten.

Assessing these factors
Methods for measuring various factors and the ways in which these can be improved and tested for precision and bias have, in recent years, been fairly well established. At any rate, the principles are now available for doing this. So are the principles for reducing bias when it cannot be tolerated. One point can be emphasized here. It is now popular to refer to 'the process of standardization', by which is meant carrying out measurements in a uniform way with the same kinds of instrument. This is sometimes useful but does not necessarily lead to precision or lack of bias. The essential feature is 'calibration'. For this, standards are necessary and when these are available or made available, then any kind of instrument in any person's hand may be calibrated so that it is comparable with any other kind of instrument in any other person's hand. But it is not sufficient simply to stablish procedures for measuring relevant factors. It is necessary during the course of a study to exert a continuous 'quality control'. Priciples for all this have now been set out.

Controls
The kinds of controls that have been used are: randomization of individuals to the 'treated' or the 'control' groups; historical controls, and natural situations. Of these, the first, apart from exceptional circumstances, is the most reliable method. It is, however, rather difficult to arrange. Some notable examples in which this has been achieved in testing the effect of treatment on subjects and the effect of mass health screening can be mentioned. One approach, which, perhaps, could be described as the 'heroic' is where doctors are persuaded that random assignment of patients to 'case' and 'control' is reasonable. For example, this has been done in testing whether home or hospital treatment is better in the treatment of the acute coronary case (Cochrane, personal communication; Mather *et al.* 1971); whether 'outpatient' injection of varicose veins is as good as or better than 'inpatient' surgery; and is being used at the moment to evaluate the effect of clofibrate on subjects with raised serum cholesterol in primary prevention of coronary heart disease. A less heroic but very ingenious way is being used in the evaluation of mass health screening. In London, England (W. W. Holland, personal communication) and Titograd, Yugoslavia (D. Djordjevic, personal communication) random samples of individuals of a particular community have been assigned to a regime of mass health screening and the controls to a regime of the traditional medical approach. These two groups will be compared for mortality, morbidity, disability, utilization of health services, and costs of health services. This clever procedure has also been used in New York (Shapiro *et al.* 1967) to establish the value of mass health screening for cancer of the breast. Here, it is obviously unethical to screen a large group of women and assign at random those in whom a cancer has been found to a

treatment and a non-treatment group. It is quite ethical, however, to invite a random half of a large group of women to take part in a screening programme and to compare the kinds of cases that are found by the screening procedure and the usual procedures as well as the ultimate effect on the individual. There are notable difficulties in this procedure but it looks as though they can be overcome.

Analysis is greatly strengthened by precise data and adequate controls. When sufficient data is available to show interrelationship between the parts of the system, it may be possible to use systems analysis techniques to simulate the whole system and show how it works in many different conditions.

Achieving high response

Problems of response are now fairly well known and it seems that if one approaches almost any community in a manner that is in keeping with, and not against, their cultural mores and traditions, and if one treats them as human beings, something of the order of 80 per cent will respond. Of the remaining 20 per cent, if one takes care to make individual enquiries into the reasons for non-response, it is usually possible to reduce it to 10 per cent without much difficulty. After this, improvement of the response rate becomes difficult and may not be worth the effort. Little is known about adherence to prolonged regimes, especially when these are unpleasant and uncomfortable.

How are people motivated to take part in an experiment? I think that there is a large body of data that might give us an insight into this, particularly in efforts to study the effect of reduction of cigarette smoking and the taking of drugs to prevent high blood cholesterol, glucose intolerance, high blood-pressure, but this needs to be analysed.

Follow-up and number and choice of subjects

The problem of follow-up and numbers of subjects and costs are all related. If a study is to continue for 3 or 4 years, it is rather important to carry it out on a population that is not going to move very much during that time. It is necessary to investigate this point before a study starts and it is necessary to incorporate into the study design some arrangement for keeping in contact with the subjects even if they do move. Evaluation of health action often requires a very large number of man-years of study — something of the order of 50 000 to 100 000. There are several ways in which this number can be efficiently reduced. These are by improved precision, to characterize each subject for each factor studied, by studies of high-risk subjects, and by better choice of end-points. It may also be assisted by developments in application of mathematics to the analysis of the data.

A little more could be said here on the subjects of 'high risk' and choice of 'end-points'. It is very clear that if the incidence of the end-point (disease) in the 'treated' and the 'controls' is 1 per cent and a ½ per cent per annum respectively, then a very large number of man-years of study will be required. If this could be increased for example to 15 per cent and 7 per cent, the number of man-years could be reduced considerably. This can be done sometimes by choosing high-risk subjects. Of course, there is a price to pay and that is that the study does not cover all kinds of persons at risk to the disease.

Another approach is by choosing an end-point which is likely to have a very high incidence in the 'treated' and a very low incidence in the 'controls' or vice versa. This may require using one end-point as the key indicator and two or three other supporting end-points. An example could be given for the evaluation of prevention of coronary heart disease by reduction of high blood-pressure or high blood cholesterol. It is possible to conceive of a study in which the treated and untreated were compared for incidence of coronary heart disease, incidence of all disease, mortality from coronary heart disease, and mortality from all disease. The differences would be of the order of 3–5 per cent, compared with 1–3 per cent. This would be difficult to show. But supposing a third end-point were included, namely the frequency and extent of myocardial infarction in subjects who died in the treated and the untreated: the differences then would be likely to be of the order of 10 per cent and 80 per cent, and this could be shown in relatively few cases. Of course, this could only be shown by the deaths, and there would be relatively few deaths. But calculations have shown that, if one were concerned with middle-aged males aged 50 ± 5 years, and the treatment reduced the incidence and mortality of coronary heart disease by 50 per cent, then it is very likely that with as few as 6000 man-years of study it would be shown that the treated had less myocardial infarction than the untreated. With the same sample size it would be possible to say that the incidence and mortality of coronary heart disease and other disease was no greater in the treated than the untreated, and the conclusion that the treatment was effective in reducing myocardial infarction could be drawn. This sort of reasoning is somewhat speculative, but is based on information from population-related autopsy data and is quite likely to be correct. If so, a study could be reduced from the generally accepted level of 100 000 man-years to something of the order of 6000 or, to be on the safe side, 10 000 man-years — a 90 per cent saving.

Costs

One of the many reasons given for the failure to evaluate health actions is the high cost. Can this be reduced? Is it really high? One of the striking features of many health actions that need to be evaluated is that many of the expensive features for different problems overlap. For example, it should be possible to choose a dozen problems that could be carried out in the same sample frame, in the same sample of subjects, by the same observers, and in the same places. Many of the observations would be in common, but a few additional ones peculiar to each problem would have to be added. The number of subjects would have to be increased but the facilities for follow-up would be the same. I have made calculations elsewhere (Kagan 1970) which indicate that where a dozen problems tackled separately might cost something in the region of £10 million, tackled together they would cost only £4 million. Multipurpose testing is extremely likely to reduce the cost. Furthermore, by including additional observations related to the problems under study, useful information may be obtained for very little additional cost.

Is the cost of evaluation really high? The cost of not evaluating can be enormous in actual money spent, in money wasted and, above all, in harm done. Since nearly all our health measures are expensive and dangerous, we can assume that money spent on evaluation will be repaid. It is a little like our policy with regard to buying a house or anything else that is going to cost us a lot of money. Before buying it, we get an expert to decide what its weaknesses and merits are. We are prepared to spend perhaps 1 per cent of the total cost on this, and that would be a very reasonable expenditure for evaluation of health actions. One factor that has changed appreciably the cost and feasibility of multipurpose health actions is the development of technology for examining large numbers of people for large numbers of factors. To my mind, evaluation is the proper use of automated multiphasic health testing at the present time.

STRATEGY

We wish to test hypotheses and evaluate health actions. Retrospective and prospective studies, as they are often carried out, only suggest hypotheses or give support — or the contrary — for existing hypotheses. Prospective studies give clearer results and better information on the interrelation of numerous factors than restrospective studies, but are more expensive.

However, by including experimental approaches in a prospective study, hypotheses may be tested and health actions evaluated. This implies altering some of the conditions in boxes 0, 1, 3, 4, or 6 of Fig. 1.1 (p. 3) in a sub-group of subjects, and not altering them in another sub-group which is used as a control. Comparison of events in the 'altered' and 'control' sub-groups tests the effect of the alteration. This, given suitable conditions, is only a little more difficult than observation/analytical prospective studies, but the ethical and technical conditions mentioned in the previous section must be observed.

Systems analysis
A number of health workers, inspired by reports from business and industry, believe that 'systems analysis' will give a deep and broad understanding of health problems in a shorter period of time. This remains to be demonstrated for health problems (and for all but a few types of industrial problems). However, if one could develop a mathematical model of the whole system (see Fig. 1.1, p. 3) that could be used to stimulate the real situation, it might be a useful way of understanding what would happen to the various parts of the system under very many different conditions. This possibility is worth exploring. In my view, the best way of attempting this is to obtain a good idea of the interrelationships of the parts of the system (Fig. 1.1) by experiment and observation, to translate these into mathematical terms, and to relate forecasts derived from simulation to observations of real events. the observations for this can be included with little extra expenditure into a prospective experimental study.

The strategy that I therefore advocate is a prospective experimental study in which several health actions, and hypotheses of mechanism, stimulus, or interacting variables are tested, and at the same time, observations are made of the interrelationships of many other factors included in the boxes of Fig. 1.1.

Examples
Here I will give a rough outline of two studies of the type described above that are likely to be ethical, possible and useful, and, at the same time, test some elements of the general concepts that control of psychosocial stimuli and their effects prevent ill health due to male female roles or relations. The details would depend on local circumstances.

Prevention of unwanted pregnancy and gonorrhea in adolescents (15–19 years). There is a good deal of evidence that the incidence of gonorrhea is high and rising in young people and that unwanted pregnancy is frequent and harmful for mother and child. Thus a recent Franco/Swedish special study showed the incidence of gonorrhea to be about 1 per cent in boys and 1·9 per cent in girls aged 15–19 years (WHO 1970). It is difficult to know the frequency of unwanted pregnancy in girls at this age but depending on definition its incidence may be as high as 6 per cent. Evidence supporting the harmfulness of unwanted pregnancy to the child born of rather older women is available (Forsmann and Thuwe 1966). The evidence for or against harmfulness of unwanted pregnancy in younger girls is not well documented. Opinion is generally in the direction of it being more harmful than for older women. There is speculation, but not much evidence, that sex education may be harmful. There is considerable doubt about its efficacy and the relative efficacy of different approaches.

It would thus be beneficial to conduct a study to show the dangers, effectiveness, and costs of various measures to prevent gonorrhea and unwanted pregnancy in people aged 15–19 years. We shall use the following symbols:

Minimal or standard sex education: M
Special sex education: S

		T (60)	−T (60)

Peer group advice: G
Special treatment facilities: T
Selye stress: St
Precursors: P
Disease in general: D
Gonorrhea: V
Unwanted pregnancy: U
Difference between expectation and
perceived situation (satisfaction)   E

Hypotheses to be tested: †That treatments G, S, T, GS, GT, ST, or GST, in conjunction with M, are better than M alone.

We will also seek to show the relative benefits of each treatment and who is benefited and who is harmed by each.

An attempt will be made to forecast the needs and costs of application of effective treatments on a large scale.

Interactions — between treatments, effects, stimuli psychobiological programmes, mechanisms, precursors, diseases, intervening variables — will be qualified.

Social situation. We shall define two types of sex education. The minimal (M) will be of the type normally given to all schools. A special form of sex education (S) that is believed, but not known, to be effective will be designed and given to some of the children. In many communities M will have been given to all children, in which case S, G, and T will be additional.

In some schools 'leaders' amongst the children will be identified and they will be co-opted, motivated, and instructed in giving advice to the other children (G).

Special facilities (T) for making it easy for children to receive advice on sexual relationships, advice on and facilities for contraception, treatment of venereal disease, and unwanted pregnancy will be provided for some of the children through the schools, family doctors, clubs, or other arrangement, whichever is thought to be the most suitable.

Psychological stimulus. Satisfaction, or the difference between expectation and the perceived situation (E), with: work, play, home, friends, sexual relations, and male/female relations; and with sexual instruction, peer advisory group, and special treatment facilities will be determined at 3- or 6-monthly intervals.

Psycho-biological programme. At the commencement of the study each child will be assessed for home circumstances; attitudes to authority (parents, teachers), to peers and siblings, and to the opposite sex; physical and mental health; IQ; school performance; and 'Selye stress' response to a standard load.

Mechanisms. During the course of the study changes in attitude to authority, peers, and members of the opposite sex, and change in habitual 'Selye stress' response will be determined.

†Better in the sense that they reduce V, U, and D.

Precursors. During the course of the study general health, physical and mental health, work performance, promiscuity, pregnancy, use of contraceptives, and interpersonal conflict will be monitored.

Disease. Time of occurrence of gonorrhea, unwanted pregnancy or other disease, and the disability and outcome will be determined.

Intervening variables. Social class, siblings, and attitudes of parents and siblings will be determined. Life-change events in the family and in the child will be assessed.

Study design.

1. Children enter into the study at age 14–15. Follow up will continue till age 19. It would be an advantage if some kind of follow up could be arranged for a longer period.

2. About 12 000 boys and 6000 girls are needed for this study. This is because the frequency of end-point is greater in girls than boys. If they do not go to mixed schools advantage can be taken of this by studying fewer girls' schools.

3. Assuming about 100 boys and 100 girls aged 14 or 15 per school about 120 boys', or mixed schools, will be needed, and about half the number of girls schools.

4. These will first be randomized to two groups of 60 schools. One group will receive M and the other S (or S + M). Each of these two groups will be randomized to a further two groups of schools, only one of which will receive G. Each of these resulting four groups will be randomized to two more groups of schools, only one of which will receive T. Table 30.1 outlines the 'social situation' constitution of these groups. Number of schools is shown in parentheses.

TABLE 30.1

		T (60)	−T (60)
M (60)	G (30)	M,G,T (15)	M,G (15)
	−G (30)	M,T (15)	M (15)
S,(M)† (60)	G (30)	(M),S,G,T (15)	(M),S,G (15)
	−G (30)	(M),S,T (15)	(M),S (15)

†(M) signifies that in some communities all children in all groups have had a basic sex education prior to the commencement of the study. This will not disturb the study design.

5. Psychobiological programme and intervening variables will be assessed at the commencement of the study. Social situation, stimuli, mechanisms, precursors, disease, and some intervening variables will be assessed or monitored at 3- and 6-month intervals.

6. These assessments will be made independently of knowledge of the treatment group to which the subjects belong.

209

Prevention of personal and family ill health by control of conflict between husband and wife. According to Gebherd (Chapter 16 of this book) and others, a high proportion of husbands and wives suffer from conflict over sexual, domestic, or work roles. Conflict can by itself be a disability, but this is not always the case. Conflict is associated with minor and, sometimes major illness. It is not known whether the conflict is the cause or if it is reduced whether benefit or harm will result. We shall use the following symbols:

Husband:	H
Wife:	W
Children:	C
Conflict (or difference between expected and perceived situation) in sexual, domestic or work roles:	E
Selye stress:	S†
Life-change score:	L
Counselling to reduce E:	T
Substitute flight/fight activity:	R
Disease:	D

Hypotheses:
(1) T reduces E whether S^+ or $S^\pm$;
(2) R does not reduce E whether S^+ or $S^\pm$;
(3) T reduces D (in H, W, or C) only when S^+;
(4) T reduces D (in H, W, or C) when $S^\pm$;
(5) T reduces D (in H, W, or C) only when it reduces S;
(6) T reduces D (in H, W, or C) only when it reduces E.
(7) R reduces D only when it reduces S^+;
(8) R reduces D only if E is high.

Interaction between stimulus, psychobiological programme, mechanism, precursors, disease, and intervening variables will be quantified.

Stimulus. The difference between expectation and perceived situation (E) in male female sexual domestic and work roles will be assessed in H and W separately during the course of the study.

Psychobiological programme. Attitudes to male/female roles and S response to a standard load will be determined for each H and W.

Mechanism. Change in attitude and change in habital S will be assessed in each H and W during the course of the study.

Interacting variables. Counselling on male/female roles will be given to some subjects, others will be instructed to take a substitute flight/fight activity such as extra exercise (R), others will receive neither of these 'treatments'. Other interacting variables such as social class, number of children, hobbies, life-change event score will be measured in H, W, and C.

† All husbands and wives will be assessed for S in response to a standard load. The highest one third will be assigned to the S^+ group and the other 600 to the $S^\pm$ group.

Precursors. Satisfactions, attitudes, symptoms, work, play activities, heart-rate, blood-pressure, sedimentation rate, serum cholesterol, and glucose tolerance will be assessed at frequent intervals in H, W, and C, and mental and physical development of C and school activity will be recorded.

Disease. All specific disease, disability, and attendance for medical advice will be recorded.

Study design.
(1) 900 husband-and-wife pairs and the households in which they live will be studied. If the focus is on child health the pairs should be representative of the husbands and wives aged 25–34 in the community. If the focus is on the health of the husband and wife the pairs should be representative of husbands and wives aged 45–54.
(2) Each of the pairs in $S^\pm$ or S^+ group will be randomly assigned to T, R, or neither R nor T (−RT) group.
Fig. 30.1 outlines these groupings. Number of families in each group are shown in parenthesis.

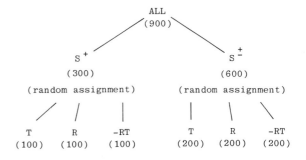

Fig. 30.1.

Studies of the kind briefly outlined above require considerable thought and care to be technologically tailored to particular circumstances in which the study will be carried out. They are only given as examples. Many other different problems might be more important. If so it would be desirable to give thought to the possibility of combining several hypotheses testing studies where there is overlap in sampling, subjects, observers, investigators, and place of investigation. In this way very considerable savings in cost and effect may be made.

SUMMARY

The health adviser or decision maker often is impelled to make decisions on health action when he does not know who will be benefited and who will be harmed, and to what extent. He may suspect that benefit may not be great and harm may be considerable. Further in modern times he will know that cost will be high. It is in such circumstances that an evaluation of the health action on a small scale — to learn if, and how, it should be applied on a large scale — is essential.

Consideration is given of how the epidemiologist can overcome ethical obstacles and technical difficulties, and minimize the costs of evaluation.

Two examples of multi-hypotheses testing studies are given which at the same time and for the same cost will give a reasonable chance to examine a systems analysis approach.

REFERENCES

FORSMANN, H. and THUWE, I. (1966). One hundred and twenty children born after application of therapeutic abortion was refused. *Acta Psychiat. scand.*, **42**, 71–88.

KAGAN, A. R. (1970). 'Automated multiphasic health testing (AMHT) in research.' WHO Internal Document ENCD/70.3.

—— (1971). Epidemiology and society, stress, and disease. In *Society, stress, and disease* (ed. L. Levi), Vol. 1, pp. 36–48. London.

—— (1972). Evaluation of mass screening for health: needs, difficulties and possibilities. *Publ. Hlth Lond.*, **86**, No. 3, 119–24.

—— (1974). A review and a suggestion for studies to test hypotheses. In *Life, stress, and illness* (ed. E. K. Gunderson), Chapter 3. Springfield, Illinois.

MATHER, H. G., PEARSON, W. G., READ, K. L. Q., SHAW, D. B., STEED, G. R., THORNE, M. G., JONES, S., GUERRIER, C. J., ERAULT, C. D., MCHUGH, P. M., CHOWDHURY, N. R., JAFARY, M. H., and WALLACE, T. T. (1971). Acute myocardial infarction: home and hospital treatment. *Brit. med. J.*, iii, 334.

SHAPIRO, S., STRAX, P., and VENET, L. (1967). Periodic breast cancer screening: the first two years of screening. *Arch. environm. Hlth*, **15**, 547–53.

WHO (1970). 'Franco-Swedish pilot project on the surveillance of communicable diseases, particularly venereal diseases'. WHO Internal Document /VDT/70.312.

31. SEX ROLES AND RELATIONSHIPS: SOCIAL POLICY AS A MEANS OF PREVENTION OF PSYCHOSOCIAL DYSFUNCTION

CAMILLA ODHNOFF

Helmer:	First of all, you are a wife and mother.
Nora:	I no longer believe that. I believe that I am first of all a human being, just as much as you are — or at least I will try to become one.
Helmer:	You are talking like a child. You don't understand the society you live in.
Nora:	No, I don't. But I shall try to learn. I must find out who is right: society or I.

[From *A doll's house*, by Henrik Ibsen (1891)]

THE OFFICIAL SEX-ROLES IDEOLOGY: EQUAL ROLES, EQUAL RESPONSIBILITY

From the beginning of the 1960s a strikingly constructive and progressive debate has been going on in Sweden concerning the roles of men and women, and equality between sexes. The Swedish Social Democratic Government has also made what are probably the world's most advanced public official declarations concerning the political objectives of full equality between men and women. The Government report on the position of women, for example, which was delivered to the United Nations in 1968, probably shocked other countries by demanding, among other things, the liberation and emancipation of men. In this declaration to the United Nations, the Government has adopted a sex-role ideology stating that boys and girls should be treated alike, and both should be brought up for the two roles they are to fulfil in working life and in the family. Men should share housework and child-care equally with women and the birth of a child should entail the same restrictions or interruptions in the gainful occupation of a man as of a woman. Women undoubtedly give birth to children and perhaps also breast-feed them but this does not always mean that a woman is better suited to care for a child. And, above all, it does not mean that for the rest of her life she is predestined to wash, dress, and feed the child, run the household, and serve her husband to any greater extent than he is supposed to serve her, the child, and the common household.

In the report to the United Nations it is stated that:

The measures to raise the status of women recommended in resolution No. 1133 as well as in certain of the suggestions included in the Secretary-General's 'Annex II' are felt to be relatively isolated from the general policy in various fields aimed at economic and social progress for the population as a whole. However, experience from both Sweden and other industrial countries suggests that the question of women's rights must be viewed as a function of the whole complex of roles and the division of labour imposed on both women and men by upbringing, tradition and practice (and to a lesser extent by legislation). A decisive and ultimately durable improvement in the status of women cannot be attained by special measures aimed at women alone; it is equally necessary to abolish the conditions which tend to assign certain privileges, obligations or rights to men. No decisive change in the distribution of functions and status as between the sexes can be achieved if the duties of the male in society are assumed *a priori* to be unaltered.

The aim of reform work in this area must be *to change the traditional division of labour* which tends to deprive women of the possibility of exercising their legal rights on equal terms. The division of functions as between the sexes must be changed in such a way that both the man and the woman in a family are afforded the same practical opportunities of participating in both active parenthood and gainful employment. If women are to attain a position in society outside the home which corresponds to their proportional membership of the citizen body, it follows that men must assume a greater share of responsibility for the upbringing of children and the care of the home. A policy which attempts to give women an equal place with men in economic life while at the same time confirming woman's traditional responsibility for the care of home and children has no prospect of fulfilling the first of these aims.

Most political parties in Sweden have declared their support for the radical view that men and women should play the same roles in all fields, and they have worked out comprehensive programmes for this. Representatives of employers' organizations and the big trade unions have in public interviews backed the radical standpoint.

SOME EFFECTS OF NON-EQUALITY

The 'fatherless society': children's 'woman-world'

Many children today grow up in surroundings where men play a minor role. At home, in the nursery school and in the lower and middle classes of the comprehensive school, as well as in their free time, they are almost entirely with women. Men in their occupationally active years have very little opportunity to be with children during the day. There is a great lack of 'father-figures' in the child's day, and particularly the boys feel the absence of any man they can identify with.

For boys this woman-world raises the problem of how to defend themselves against following the woman-role. A divergence from and refusal of 'femininity' becomes for them a condition of life. They are impelled to conform strictly to their gang and their own sex in order to assert their 'masculinity'. Because of the absence of father-figures in their daily life they lack securely built-in control over their behaviour. The over-compensatory masculinity and the violence used against others — for instance, girls, women, and old people — against handicapped persons and immigrants of various ages, or the risk of social deviations with various forms of alienation, such as alcohol and drug addition, even among younger boys, tells a clear tale of the boys' psychosocial dysfunction in the 'fatherless society'.

The price of 'manliness'

An article in a magazine for parents contained the following: 'Up until teen-age, girls feel that they have a much better life than boys, and boys agree with them; but then the situation is reversed....' We may ask, however, whether the man's role in the family, in working life and in society *is* better, and more human. Men must qualify themselves for leading and responsible positions, according to traditional sex-role ideas. They must accept hard, dirty, and dangerous work — of those involved in occupational accidents 85 per cent are men. Heavy demands, severe working pressures, responsibility, stressful shift work, and so on also reap victims. The Swedish sociologist, Rita Liljeström, writes:

In the man-society, those men who have failed in their supporter role form a sizeable bottom layer. they have never had the choice of being supported and protected, of living close to children, of finding comfort in the reality of personal relationships, of being soft and tender, of making themselves attractive and adapting to a partner who gives them security and prestige. These men have never been able to scrape together the bride-price, and in the factories there are many men who pay the monthly instalments with worn-out backs. Now that we are really discovering the disadvantages for men that are involved in our inherited conception of sex-roles. The 'price of manliness' is high; and, as I said earlier, it begins to be paid early in a man's life. The adjustment problems of boys are greater. Nervous disturbances such as bed-wetting, speech defects, motor hyperactivity and emotional outbursts are commoner among boys. In family guidance centres most of the cases are boys. Likewise in the help-classes in schools. [Liljeström 1968]

The following statistics bear Liljeström out:
   Suicides, 1969: 1242 men, 508 women;
   In alcoholic institutions, 31 March 1972: 2678 men, 125 women;

In youth welfare schools, 1 April 1972: 580 boys, 115 girls;
In youth prisons, 31 December 1970: 463 boys, 9 girls;
In prison, 31 December 1970: 4544 men, 120 women.

Mortality statistics show that men have a higher rate than women in all age-groups, except the oldest. Apart from the 'accident peak' in the 20s, male mortality is highest in upper middle age. In the early 1950s the mortality risk for male 60-year-olds was about 35 per cent greater than for women in the same age-group: now it is about 70 per cent greater! For younger men — 35-year-olds — the mortality risk is also increasing alarmingly. Stomach ulcers, coronaries, and other stress diseases are much commoner among men than women in this age-group.

However, the highest price for 'manliness' paid by many men was described in slightly different terms in a Stockholm school enquiry a few years ago, when a very high percentage of both boys and girls answered 'No' to the question: 'Can a father ever have the same emotional contact with his children as the mother?'

Myron Brenton (1967) an American sociologist, has made a special study of the males among his compatriots. He collected psychological and sociological data and interviewed sociologists, family counsellors, almoners, and psychiatrists. Without doubt, many of Brenton's observations are generally valid and apply also to the Swedish father — for instance, that it is easier to make a lot of money than to be a good father.

In another American study, over 600 married women, questioned as to their view of their husband's roles, placed the supporter role first, then the father role, and thirdly the husband role. The father is thus obliged to base his self-esteem primarily on his occupational role; his personal relations to wife and children rank lower, even in the eyes of his wife.

The same women ranked their corresponding three roles as follows: first mother, then wife, and thirdly home-maker. Consequently — in relation to what was said earlier concerning the price for manliness — it is perhaps psychologically easier for girls and women to perform low-status work, since their self-esteem has little to do with their occupational role. The roles of good mothers and wives are those which women are traditionally brought up to and those which they cultivate and rank first in the fields of education and personal relations. These facts are perhaps also generally valid and applicable to relationships and family life in Sweden.

A REPORT ON THE PRESENT SITUATION

The lack of equality

Visitors from abroad who are not particularly familiar with present conditions in Sweden may be under the impression that equality between men and women already exists here, or at any rate that Sweden has gone a very long way towards achieving equality between the sexes. The unusually open approach to sexual questions, the relatively unprejudiced attitude towards unmarried mothers, and the comparative rarity of the so-called 'double-standard' probably have helped to create such an impression.

It is true that women and men have largely the same legal rights and that all education, except military, is open to both sexes. But if we define equality between men and women in terms of equal influence and power, an equal position on the labour market, equal responsibility for home and children, and equal pay, we must admit that we still have a long way to go and we do not compare very well even with many other industrialized countries: and that, with our various social policy measures, we have made only a relatively small advance towards a real freedom for both men and women to combine their roles at work in the family, and in society.

Sex roles and schools

In our country, schools make no distinctions between girls and boys. They are no longer kept in separate classes, and expectations are the same for both sexes as regards work and study objectives.

Although the school system treats girls and boys alike, differences in their behaviour are evident: the boys get into trouble at school, they tire of school more often, they fight more, play truant, and they have worse relations with their teachers. More boys than girls have reading and writing difficulties and are assigned to special instruction. And boys tend to get lower grades.

Girls, on the other hand, adapt better to the teacher's instructions and advice. They are 'neat and orderly'. They speak and read better than boys of the same age. They hardly ever fight — and so on. By the time they get to school girls have already adapted to a 'womanly' identity, with the subordinate and relatively passive qualities predominating.

At schools equality between the sexes is practised, yet girls and boys use educational opportunities differently, so firmly are they tied to the sex-roles by old habits and values current in families, working life, and society at large. The girls generally value themselves lower than boys. They have also traditionally been influenced by their parents' failure to encourage them as much as the boys to continue their education.

The sex difference is apparent today at every point where a 'free-choice' between various possibilities is offered in the school system. The boys take one decision and the girls another. In 1970–1, in the seventh grade of a reformed comprehensive school, the boys chose technical subjects first and then German. (English is compulsory.) The girls chose German and French rather than technical subjects. Half of the boys and 77 per cent of the girls put languages first. Of the boys, 42 per cent put technical subjects first, but only 0·6 per cent of the girls! Ninety-three per cent of the boys as against 20 per cent of the girls choose wood- and metal-crafts, while 7 per cent of the boys and 80 per cent of the girls choose needlework!

The same tendency is seen in further education. In two- and three-year theoretical courses in 'continuation schools', girls choose languages, humanities, and social sciences rather than physics, mathematics, and technical subjects. The latter are chosen by the boys. In the vocational courses in continuation schools, which more accurately reflect working life, we find the sex-role pattern still more pronounced.

In the Autumn of 1970, boys constituted 85 per cent of the students in technical courses and 92 per cent at those in occupational courses for industry and crafts, but only 14 per cent of the students in courses for service occupations and — strikingly — *only 6 per cent* in social care courses. The girls who trained for industry were largely in the textile fields. Girls generally take shorter courses than boys. In universities and colleges, girls constituted almost 70 per cent of humanists in the Autumn of 1970. Among law students 31 per cent were girls and the percentage was about the same in medicine; but only 9 per cent of technical college students were girls.

The pupils' choice of occupational guidance — e.g., in comprehensive school grades 8 and 9 (at ages 14–16) gives cause for further reflection:
She gives preference to health-care and care of the sick, hygiene, and beauty care, followed by office work and teaching.
He prefers apprenticeship to engineering, construction, and metalwork occupations. Then comes electrical work. Health-care and care of the sick are at the bottom of his list.

We are therefore entitled to wonder how far the little girls of today have progressed beyond the idealistic pictures painted by poets a century ago.

INTERESTS AND OCCUPATIONAL AIMS

What else do we know about what kinds of jobs young people aim for today? Thirteen-year-old girls in Gothenburg want to be nurses, children's nurses, hairdressers, office workers, elementary school teachers, or shop assistants. Fifty-nine per cent of the girls questioned wanted one or other of these six occupations! The boys, on the other hand, wanted occupations that paid well and they viewed education as a means to get ahead.

The expectations up till now centred on girls as regards education and choice of occupation have not stimulated them to take more than short training courses, leading to an occupation of domestic, nursing, or teaching type, which they would follow while awaiting marriage and children. Boys, on the other hand, have been taught from early years that they will have to support a family and the education they get must pay off. They may have to give up interests and hobbies for these considerations. As parents we may be said to have favoured the girls in a way by allowing them to follow their job interests and desires. We have made few demands on them as regards the capacity to support themselves and perhaps their children. And we have indulged this attitude at the expense of the boys, who more often hear the words 'you must!' in their working life.

A male and a female labour market

When girls go out to work they encounter a different kind of labour market than do boys. Indeed, there still exists a labour market divided on the basis of sex.

The 'female labour market' is distinguished from the male by the fact that it covers so few occupations. A study including about 300 occupations shows that some 75 per cent of gainfully employed women are confined to only 25 occupations, while less than 14 per cent of the men are in these occupations. More than half of the 25 are connected with the feminine sex-role. Women are expected to tidy up, care for the sick, look after homes and children, see to their appearance, nurse the aged, look after animals, and handle the food requirements!

A similar division into masculine and feminine exists in other occupational areas. Only in a few areas have men and women to any considerable extent identical working assignments. These are mainly professions that require longer training, such as medicine and teaching. Commerce and catering constitute a further exception, certain jobs having been performed for a long time back by both men and women. The post office and local government traffic service are new fields where men and women have the same tasks.

The division into two separate labour markets means that the sexes have little chance to compete with each other in working life. This means it is hard to compare the wage scales. The typical 'masculine' and 'feminine' jobs are evaluated by different standards. An undisguised undervaluation of women occurs also when they are paid less than men for exactly the same work. The 1968 Education Enquiry showed, for instance, that a woman economist or engineer rarely rises to the same salary level as a man in an identical position.

The price of 'femininity'

The Low-Income Enquiry which studied the position of low-income groups in Sweden gave the following data concerning the division into 'masculine' and 'feminine' on the employment market and in other areas. Women constitute two-thirds of all those in low-income groups, although they amount to only one-third of those in full-time employment. Three-quarters of the women earn less than Skr. 20 000 a year, while 3/4 of the men earn more than that sum. Half of the men earn more than Skr 24 000, but only 1/10 of women earn more than that.

In various enquiries, the population pyramid shows that women more often leave the employment market. There is equality at the start: the 15–25 year age-group for both sexes; but subsequently women leave the employment market to play their roles in bringing up

and taking care of others. Their return to employment at a later stage in life never restores the balance in the pyramid. Moreover, there are many obstacles in the way of the woman who wants to go back to work after interruption. The fact is that the married woman who wants to go out to work or to remain at work rarely has any real choice between home and a job. The child supervision facilities available suffice for barely one quarter of the women who are already out in employment. Other forms of service are also inadequate. The ideal that the man is the breadwinner is deeply rooted in both politicians and employers — and also, indeed, in many people in employment, both women and men! Women are looked on — and they also to a large extent still look on themselves — as a reserve labour supply with the modest demands for jobs, pay, and promotion. From the very moment she comes into the employment market a woman begins to pay the price of 'femininity' by accepting what is offered to her, and she often submits to discriminatory treatment just because she is a woman.

The biggest obstacles, however, may exist within her own family. Men and children have got used to being personally looked after in a well-run home and being provided with clean clothes and good food without themselves having to devote any effort to such trivial matters.

The lack of female policy-makers

It may be noted that women only to a very small degree have taken responsibility — or indeed have had a chance in Sweden and other countries to take responsibility — for evolution in politics and professional life. It is still the men who speak on behalf of women and children. It is the men who plan, negotiate, and decide for the women. In this connection, as in so many others, the women merely provide service for the men. They fix refreshments or stay at home to look after the children.

In 1921, Swedish women were given the right to vote, and yet today, 50 years later, their voices are so little heard! We see men as almost the sole representatives of the Swedish people. Women, says the Swedish sociologist, Edmund Dahlström, seem to represent 'an off-centre interest — in common with groups like fishermen, teetotallers, and small businessmen.'

Here are a few political and occupational statistics on this point:

Parliament, 1972: 300 men, 50 women
Government, 1972: 17 men, 2 women
Local government, councillors, election 1970: of 18 327 elected only 2557 are women
Schools, 1971: 65 per cent of teachers in comprehensive schools are women, but only 4 per cent of headteachers are women.

The proportion of women in the various local political committees is also worth noting. Here too, the traditional sex-role attitudes come through: women deal with matters relating to children, they sit on child welfare boards and social welfare boards, but apparently they are not needed on building committees, where home construction and living environments are planned, to anything like the same extent!

In the trade unions, the situation is as follows (1970): *Members of LO* (Swedish Confederation of Trade Unions): 1 199 603 men and 480 532 women.
Members of the LO Board: 15 men and 0 women.
Members of TCO (white collar employees): 372 051 men and 285 674 women.
Members of the TCO Board: 8 men and 2 women.
Members of SACO (university graduates): 81 191 men and 33 800 women.
Members of the SACO Board: 13 men and 2 women.
Thus, among the active politicians — those in the inner trade union circles who make decisions — there are few women, but many men, in spite of the fact that women have an equally large share of social responsibility.

Conclusions

These facts from Sweden are, of course, valid to some extent in all the industrialized countries of the West. The pattern of women's and men's different responsibilities and possibilities and the traditional sex-roles are much the same everywhere. The difficulties created for men and women, as well as the third party — children — by these deeply engrained sex-role patterns are probably deeply felt everywhere.

However, in Sweden and other countries we are witnessing the development of another family pattern with a sex-role ideology in theory and practice — even if this is going slowly — where men and women work side by side and jointly take responsibility for the children and have a chance to develop their relationship with each other and, not least, with the children. But the problems are not less for those who choose to open new paths and try other family roles than the conventional ones.

A NEW FAMILY PATTERN

The family structure

How does the family look today? As a rule, the household is small. One third of households in Stockholm consist of one person, another third consists at the most of two persons. Young people, childless couples, and pensioners predominate; families with children constitute less than half of the households. Half of such families have only one child, a further one third have two children at the most. Fifty years ago 55 per cent of the families contained three or more children; today the figure is down to 12 per cent. The Family Policy Committee reports that in 1971 of all mothers with new-born children about 18 per cent were not married. Of the unmarried mothers about two-thirds lived together with the father of the child. There were totally about 140 000 single parents with children under 16, of which 40 000 lived together with some other person, usually the other parent.

The family pattern that emerges from current statistics in Sweden indicates that the individual passes through successive forms of living with others, which may generally be described as follows:

1. The two-generation family — that is, the nucleus family, with parents and growing children.
2. The young people's group which functions in a loose way for a year or several years and from which respective nuclear families gradually detach themselves.
3. A couple community within the group, which for most of them again becomes the two-generation family (1) in a collective framework, which in various phases of the family's life may again become clearly defined.
4. The third generation's little family with big needs for collective togetherness and for services.
5. Persons who are outside both family and other group life.

The boundaries between these categories are, naturally fluid, since one gradually evolves into the other. A big problem today is that so many people live in isolation in one- and two-person households.

New family patterns are also developing. One is the picture drawn, for instance, in *The affluent worker in the class structure* (Goldthorpe *et al.* 1969), which depicts the worker and his personal relationships. The double-career family is also emerging as a new pattern.

The worker in the affluent society

The first example concerns the well-off worker in a fast-expanding industrial district. The investigators find that the worker's obligation in his role as *pater familias* bring harder pressures on him to increase his income by means of shift — or overtime work. His role obligations hardly allow him to take part to any great extent in trade union activities or in clubs connected with his work or mixing with colleagues in his free time. The worker apparently devotes his time and efforts primarily to his family; his wife and children edge out colleagues and political interests. Gardening, looking after the house and the car and other property take up all his time and energy, at the expense of his interest in public affairs. He usually votes for the Labour Party; however, his feelings of solidarity are mainly connected with his own family. His feeling for the common good in work-places and in society at large, it seems, are thereby weakened. The wife usually works, unless she has small children. This is the picture of a 'new' working family which resembles neither the traditional working-class family nor the middle-class family.

Is this type of family represented in Sweden? We do not know. Data concerning conditions in Swedish worker families are still inadequate. However, we may be fairly sure that there has come into being a 'new family' in which the father provides both economic and emotional contributions, even though the extension of working hours, partly resulting from the longer distances between his home and his work cause his economic contribution still to predominate.

The family with double roles

The 'new' worker family where the man has more emotional involvement with wife and children may perhaps be viewed as a forerunner of the 'family with double roles' or 'double careers', where husband and wife take equal shares of work inside as well as outside the home. Interest must now be focused more on this latter type of family to see how the sex-roles and relationships work out and the consequences of double work for both partners, positive or negative, particularly as regards the effects on the children and their total living environment. Studies of women and men in 'double-career' families indicate that this kind of family so far is commoner in the well-educated upper middle class, though in Sweden it also occurs among ordinary employee groups. These families apparently do not have conventional sex-role ideas, but give their children the chance of a variety of role identifications.

All the families studied mention the following kinds of strain, which, in extreme forms, may cause psychosocial dysfunction:

1. *Overwork and over-strain*. Neither the man nor his wife has any service available in the home. They have no one who 'backs them up' and relieves them of the burdens of household chores, care of children, social obligations, and so on. All this must be neglected or else be distributed among the family members. No outside domestic help can be obtained. The free time spent in common requires planning and arranging. Vacations mean a great deal to personal relations.

2. *Exposure to external sanctions*. The women who has a job or a career is exposed to suspicion from women who follow a different family pattern. They expect her to be a poor wife and mother and perhaps even a selfish person who allows occupational interests to take precedence over the traditional sex-roles and relations. This sensitivity to criticism for not being at home with her children may sometimes be aggravated by her own uncertainty as to how she can manage the care of the children and somehow work her way onwards. The employment situation can be planned, but if there is no one to look after the children there is no margin of safety, and the family lives from hand to mouth. The children, however, gain one thing from this situation and that is the active attention of their father. That they suffer relatively little from their father's occupational role is something of a consolation for having less of the mother's attention.

3. *Doubt as to personal identity and worth*. Most spouses in double-career families say that they experience periods of doubt and role-insecurity. They were brought up on traditional sex-role lines and lack models for the unconventional patterns they are working towards. The wives go through times of uncertainty and depression when they become more sensitive to criticism. The men, in turn, give up the current masculine

privileges to back up their wives' occupational interests, and consequently have episodes of resentment and negativism, feeling that they have had to turn their back on job opportunities and other interests in order to look after their family. Most families have their 'tension-limits' within which they must try to compromise.

4. *Less time available for social life*. All families have friends who generally are colleagues of one or the other spouse. The wife's more prominent colleagues give her support and maintain her occupational identity in relation to her husband's colleagues. These friends become the couple's common friends. However, the families have less time for contact with their neighbours. They keep up only the most important family relationships, and feel some guilt that they have no time to see more of their relatives.

5. *Co-ordinating the occupational cycle and the life cycle*. The roles in family and occupational life change with time. It may be hard to co-ordinate phases of occupational life with demanding phases of family life. All the time it is a question of a continuous adaptation dynamism.

On the plus side may be reckoned the following. The families in the studies under consideration all say that a good income is a precondition for their way of life. To be able to devote themselves to their work the spouses must be able to afford some extra expenditure for their family life. The essential gain, however, is the possibility of self-realization, and the bringing out of latent qualities, getting things done, and creating and expressing the personality. All the women said that an essential part of their identity was connected with their work. The men experienced a kind of 'vicarious identification' with their wife's career. Their women were realizing in their work something that the men had a personal interest in but which they could not find a full outlet for in their own occupations. 'Once one has tried the pattern with both spouses having a career it is difficult to change over to anything else.'

SOCIAL POLICY AS A MEANS OF PREVENTING PSYCHOSOCIAL DYSFUNCTION

To deal with the problems outlined above, which accompany both the traditional sex-role pattern and family relationship and the new patterns, characterized, among other things, by 'Father's return to the fold', and to make possible a third role that is equally important, the social role for both men and women, we shall have to make efforts over a wide area. Concrete political measures are needed in all sectors of society.

Political action and involvement must proceed on two levels. In the first place, it must result from practical concrete measures aimed at preventing or arresting the psychosocial dysfunction that we observe today resulting from sex-role ideas and the relations and cooperation between people close by and in society at large. In the second place, these pragmatic measures must be complemented and supported by various legal measures which aim at promoting further development, particularly as regards taxation, marriage, social welfare, child welfare, housing, and the environment, which will meet the requirements of children and adults — as well as labour legislation, accident prevention legislation, and so on. Here it is not only politicians in the Government and Parliament, in the various political parties, and in local government who have responsibility for information, education, and political action but also the trade unions and, not least, the private individual who as a political being can force the pace of development. Nor should we forget the researchers. By means of research into the living environment of men, women and, most of all, children and the opportunities for them to express their latent capacities in the family, at work and in society, the researchers can affect developments and help the decision-makers in public life towards wider knowledge of human requirements and social imagination in planning and in decision making.

The need for information
One might think that people are well informed concerning the effects of a more or less rigid attitude in sex-role questions and the consequences of this for society, in the labour market, in social insurance, in matrimonial legislation, and so on. This, however, is not so. Young people still marry or live together without enough knowledge of the economic and legal consequences for the man and the woman.

Many employers still harbour definite prejudices about women workers and maintain that women have a higher absenteeism rate and more interest in their home and children than in their work, and that they are better suited to certain kinds of dull work, that they are content with less pay, and so on. They assume that men are readier to do overtime and attend meetings whenever and for as long as desired and that they always have 'home service' so that the lack of baby-sitters, for instance, does not affect their work in any way.

The flood of information today is almost overwhelming. However, the information that pours over us from the mass media, from newspapers, magazines, radio, TV, films, and all kinds of advertisements and brochures, is highly coloured by traditional sex-role ideas and often gives a faulty picture of reality; it exaggerates the 'manly' and the 'womanly' and helps to create ideal pictures of a real man and woman who have no connection with reality and infuses new life into the old prejudices.

At the same time the mass media create a gap between dream and reality. For many housewives the difference between words and actions is enormous. On the surface she is praised as the good wife, the source of family happiness, but within themselves many feel that, in fact, they are the family doormat. To prevent false expectations and ideas concerning family and work

roles in boys and girls, men and women, we need much information and data on the actual situation for these groups. We must also investigate the chances of changing this and of creating more equal conditions in which factors like sex and race would not be discriminatory. No one would be expected to do this or that just because they happened to be born male or female.

Naturally, attempts to provide information and to influence sex-role attitudes in schools and work-places have only a limited effect. No basic change can be produced by such means. Realities can be changed only by thoroughgoing measures. And it is, of course, reality that must be changed if any real change in attitudes is to be brought about.

The need for education
The education of children, young people, and adults — not least women — and parents — must be one of the most important factors in bringing about any real change in the present situation, in eliminating discrimination against women primarily, and in preventing psychosocial dysfunction resulting from sex-role attitudes that prevent people from constructing a personal identity in relation to others.

Nursery school. The main contributions to the prevention of psychosocial dysfunction are those made during a human being's most formative years — at the pre-school age. The really big efforts must be devoted to children in this age-group. The nursery school is, therefore, one of the principal instruments for an integrated, pedagogical, medical, social, and psychological prophylactic effort on behalf of children and parents. It is a necessary complement to the child's over-all possibility of realizing its innate potentialities and developing into a democratic person who can cooperate with others and work for improved living conditions for everyone. The nursery school is also necessary for parents as a complement to the home and a support for men and women in their roles as parents, as workers and politically active members of society.

Society's objectives for care and development of children was stated in April 1972 by the Swedish delegate to the UNICEF board meeting in New York as follows:

The purpose of society must be to promote the health of all children and ensure for every child an adequate material standard in a good social environment.

Society must, moreover, in cooperation with parents, endeavour to provide for every child the best possible conditions for the development of its emotional and intellectual potentialities.

The development of the child is enriched by having it participate at an early stage in a living culture, not just as a passive listener or spectator but as an active culture-bearer who preserves and carries onward the art of self-expression in speech, song, music, dance, colour, and design. One of the principal elements in personality development is the ability to communicate with other people through language, image, and movement and from person to person communicate thoughts, opinion, needs, and emotions.

Through positive stimulation the basis can be laid for the development of the child into an open, considerate human being who can both think for himself and cooperate with others. The child should be encouraged to seek knowledge in a creative way and employ it for the improvement of not only his own but also other people's living conditions.

The Committee on Child Centres has proposed a pedagogical programme for the nursery school from this viewpoint and has specified priorities as to which groups of children and parents with small means should be given access to the nursery schools.

The objectives of the nursery school must be based on the needs of the child and family and their changing position in society. The possibility of improving this must also be among the aims.

The child must attend nursery school from an early age if it is really to provide him with a better start in life. The equality requirement is particularly obvious as regards children in the most unfavourable starting positions — children with physical, psychic, social, or language handicaps — but it is important to provide all children, regardless of sex, with better conditions as they start their years of school and later life.

I have already indicated the differences between boys' and girls' choices of educational and occupational paths. During the pre-school years the groundwork is laid for the development of the adult personality. A child must from the very beginning be able to develop confidence in himself and his abilities as well as trust in others. The development of personality depends on the conditions present at the beginning and at that stage the people around the child constitute the principal element. If the child meets a response to his most important needs and has an emotionally warm and dynamic environment where he can make his various discoveries, he will learn to take intitiatives, cooperate, and take responsibility later in life.

The Committee on Child Centres gives a very wide interpretation to the conception of pedagogy: we are almost always in 'learning situations', and in interplay with others a dialogue goes on in which the parties influence one another. On this basis, the Committee maintains that all adults are teachers and influence the general development of the child.

As regards the matter of a proper identity and adult models, the nursery school is thus extremely important for the child's basic sex-role ideas. If children are in a nursery school where men and women work together and all have the same responsibility for teaching and there is no division of tasks along sex-role lines, then in the long run this practical example will provide a lesson in the sex-role subject.

The pre-school should, for the sake of close contact, be located near where the children live. It should not, for instance, be located near large work-places, even if this may be feasible in exceptional areas where work-places and dwellings are relatively integrated.

The child needs contact with people in different age-groups, so efforts should be made to bring places of recreation for various age-groups into contact with the pre-schools and their environment. In other words, the pre-schools should not be isolated institutions. The pre-school must be viewed as an important component of the entire dwelling — and contact-environment. It must be seen as a natural centre for human contact in any given neighbourhood and a source of support for everyone, but particularly for newcomers and for immigrant families. It must function as an important link in a network of closer and deeper relationships and contacts, involving people of different ages, occupations, and ways of life. It must be able to offer children a warm emotional environment and a range of activities that help them to develop physically, psychically, socially, emotionally, and intellectually.

The pre-school should maintain an open attitude towards society in order to show children the truth about the world around them — for instance, by means of visits to work-places, institutions, and libraries in their neighbourhood. The pre-school should also be open to visits from outside, from both adults and children. Nor should we overlook its important function of creating contact between children and old people.

In the day-homes, we are now trying to get away from the system we have hitherto had, with the children divided into narrow age classes, and instead we form them into groups in the age-range of 2½ to 7 years. It can mean a lot to a small child in the way of emotional security if it can be in the same group for all its time in the day-home. Instead of the competitive spirit that can easily develop in groups of children of the same age, we are trying to create in the children a feeling of mutual confidence, consideration, and responsibility for one another. In the new groups, there are more people around whom the younger children can turn to for help with clothes, food, and their various occupations, while the older ones get useful training in looking after others.

There is little point in trying to teach children cooperation in theory: they have to experience how it works out in practice by seeing how the staff work together and with the children and their parents. They should also be given some idea, in the course of the day's work, how people try to overcome difficulties and solve their problems in a democratic society.

The Committee emphasises that *all* pre-school staff should participate in the teaching and that the work should be divided up according to their personal inclinations and capacities rather than on the basis of formal qualifications, as happens now. We have therefore arranged an experiment in Swedish nursery schools with work-teams in which all staff members with similar or relatively similar jobs cooperate closely. These work-teams include not only pre-school teachers and children's nurses but also kitchen and cleaning staff.

In Sweden we have also experimented with so-called sex-quotas in order to get men to work in the pre-school system. This, of course, is only an emergency measure. It can open this door for the men, but cannot bring about much change in the composition of the staff.

With the help of the Board of Labour we have also organized a child-nursing course which has taken in an equal number of men and women. The men who work in day-homes after such training feel that their work there is essential and they are pleased with their new occupational role. In Gothenburg an experiment has also been made with unemployed men who work in the day-homes under so-called relief programmes, and are paid by the Board of Labour. Here, too, the men have gained valuable new experience in working with small children. We have also tried the experiment of allowing young men who do not wish to bear arms doing their compulsory military service work in the day-homes. The results of this have been favourable. I think some imagination is required to induce the men to go to work in the pre-schools, and to utilize the job offers and make this work seem a positive alternative for men who are unemployed, or doing their military service, or who need a sabbatical year off from other work, and so on. Perhaps in this way we can get the men to remain in these schools and train for work with small children.

For the sake of both men and children we must try to break up the traditional sex-role pattern in pre-schools and not allow yet another generation of children to lose their freedom to function as human beings without inhibitions resulting from inherited sex-role ideas.

The new comprehensive schools and continuation schools. In the new comprehensive schools and continuation schools in Sweden, our children and adolescents are brought up to think critically and independently and are encouraged to improve not only their own but also other people's living conditions in a democratic society. An essential part of the education of children and young people is education in sex-role questions in both theoretical and practical — that is, creative — subjects. Regardless of their sex, and their preferences, girls and boys are instructed together in wood and metal handicrafts and in textile crafts in the lower and middle school forms. In the higher forms, unfortunately, they must choose one or the other, although regardless of sex. There ends, for the time being, their all-round training and there, where the pupils still are allowed to make a 'free choice', the sex-role attitudes break through. Instruction in home- and child-care is given to both girls and boys in the last two grades of the comprehensive school. Moreover, it is the duty of student advisors in comprehensive and the continuation schools to provide guidance and facts and try to stimulate girls and boys to adopt a less traditional sex-role attitude in their choice of educational and occupational paths. Good sexual education is also essential in preventing psychosocial dysfunction.

It is perhaps too early, for the results are still inadequate, for a general evaluation of the new schools' sex-role education. So there is all the more reason to devote time and energy to school instruction and policy on this subject. The compulsory comprehensive school has a unique opportunity to reach all children between the ages of 7 and 16. After this, as many as 90–95 per cent of children aged 16–18 go on to various kinds of education in the higher school forms. If schools take their opportunity to show the way towards alternative possibilities and solutions to the problems of sex roles, identities, and relations, we shall probably soon get a generation with the knowledge and courage to realize the aim of equality between man and woman and to find unconventional ways for people to find both occupational and social engagement in their roles as parents and partners.

Certain subjects, I feel, are particularly important when it comes to changing current attitudes, and these are civics, psychology, and languages, particularly the mother-tongue. Civics gives children insight into our modern society and its development and all its positive and negative features as revealed in politics, social planning, working life, social security arrangements, economic problems and so on. Sound knowledge of conditions around them, as well as in society at large, is absolutely necessary for both men and women.

Psychology gives children insight into their own personality development and can help them to strengthen their identity and better understand the interplay of forces around them; it can help them to cooperate with others and find solutions to those conflicts and aggressions that so spoil things today for people whose perspectives are distorted by negative instincts and impulses. For this reason it is of fundamental importance for them to have a right conception of themselves and confidence in their sex roles.

Language training, particularly in the mother-tongue, is essential for everyone. There is much talk today about 'political poverty' — i.e. the poverty of men and women who have no command of language, who are unable to express their needs, desires, and opinions and do not know how to influence the course of their own lives and the situations they find themselves in. Poverty of speech, in combination with low self-esteem, creates psychosocial dysfunction. Decision-makers, social workers, physicians, psychologists, and others are not always attentive to people's relative inability to express their needs or to the poverty in words and other means of self-expression that many still suffer from. This applies particularly to women, who have low self-esteem, poor education, and little insight into political or 'masculine' language.

By making available knowledge and instruction in the three areas mentioned, schools can help to produce in the not-too-distant future a generation of people with a better understanding of personality development in themselves and others, whose ability to express themselves and influence social policy in all fields will put them in a better position to bring about changes in living conditions.

Adult education. Adult education is an area where the Government will have to make much greater efforts during the coming decades. In Sweden today, about 80 per cent of the people have no more than an elementary school education. In the near future, just as many of the young people will have some form of continuation school education as their basic education.

It is important that the older men and women be compensated for the lack of education in their early years. Rapid changes in society, the restructuring of economic life, new living patterns, and our democratic form of government all entail a demand for better-educated citizens. Adult education is an important means of attaining objectives of family policy such as equality between women and men, as well as greater physical and psychic security for people in their family role.

There must be more adult education available to enable women to go out on the labour market and follow occupations corresponding to their interests and capacities. There must also be more adult education for other groups who are in a weak position and are threatened by unemployment. This applies particularly to older and handicapped persons and to single parents, both women and men. Men need more education if they are to fulfil satisfactorily their role in looking after the home and family. The men of today are often handicapped in this area. We must also work out an adult education organization that will counteract the economic, social, geographical, and sex-role obstacles which prevent adults from getting an education and that will provide equal conditions for women and men.

In Sweden we have three main possibilities for facilitating retraining for the labour market, particular as regards people with little basic education:

1. We have adult education provided by the government in the daytime and evening. In all the larger government districts this education is given free in the form of further general education corresponding to that available in comprehensive and continuation schools. In the Spring of 1971, these courses were taken by 85 000 people, including 50 000 women.
2. We have the education provided by the Board of Labour, the so-called preparatory courses intended to improve the general qualifications of students in subjects such as mathematics, Swedish, physics, and chemistry.
3. We have the occupational training given in the Board of Labour courses.

Housewives with little basic education are regarded as 'unemployed' and are therefore given educational allowances during occupational training. In 1970, the Labour Board courses were taken by 118 000 persons, of whom half were women.

However, women often follow sex-role patterns in selecting these courses and they take shorter courses than the men, this in spite of the fact that the Board devotes considerable resources to information and occupational guidance and aptitude tests, in order to encourage both women and men to make a less conventional choice of education and occupation. The trade unions are deeply involved in these questions and participate in the Labour Board's activities.

Adult education resources must also be channelled to a larger extent towards supporting the weaker members of society: older workers, both women and men, handicapped persons, and single parents. The last-named group consists mainly of women who are generally poorly educated and have low self-esteem. They are doubly handicapped by their small chance of obtaining decently paid work which would enable them to support themselves and their children, and by the difficulty of finding a job near their home and child-supervision.

To prevent psychosocial dysfunction it is most important that these women should be given the chance of a reasonable standard of living. Great efforts will have to be made to go out to them and provide advice and aid, particularly as regards occupational guidance. To give encouragement, particularly to the poorly-educated groups who have not yet taken any initiative to obtain adult education, the Swedish Confederation of Trade Unions (LO) has begun a programme to locate and pinpoint such groups in their work-places.

The social problems connected with adult education are very complicated and in the near future we must find ways to make adult education effective as a means to prevent psychosocial dysfunction and to remedy existent dysfunction.

Parent education. Efforts must also be made to provide children, young people, and adults with a good training for parenthood. Very recently the 1968 Government Committee on Child Centres published its preliminary report entitled 'Pre-school'. The Committee proposes training for parenthood. This, it says, should be provided by institutions which we all have to do with at some stage of our lives — namely, the school, antenatal clinic, and child welfare centre.

The Committee emphasizes the importance of education for parenthood in the comprehensive and continuation schools, in connection with pregnancy and after birth:

Education for parenthood should probably be given in three phases, corresponding to the periods of their lives when people need support and new knowledge. It is essential that the parent regard his (or her) upbringing of the child as something meaningful for both persons concerned. Such education must therefore focus partly on the parents as educators and partly on general principles of development for the sake of the child. [Barnstuge-utredningen, 1971.]

The obligations of employers
A better balance must be achieved in the distribution of parent's tasks in and outside the home. This means that the present lopsided arrangements must be corrected, and that the parents of small children must be relieved of the very heavy work-load they now carry.

It is not enough merely to build day-care centres and provide housing allowances. It must also be recognized by parties on the employment market that children are valuable members of society and that the parents of small children — both fathers and mothers — may have obligations towards their family that take precedence over their job. Such obligations may justify a shortening of working hours and taking days off the job in case of sickness or other problems at home. In this context it would be advisable to study how reductions in working hours could best be distributed over the working week with view to making it easier for husbands to do their share of work in the home.

Planning of housing areas

Public planning must also take human beings into account. If people are to function, the planning of workplaces, dwellings, and service facilities must be co-ordinated. These things are important for everybody but they are vital for single parents. It is the needs of these people that we must keep primarily in mind when formulating our requirements for the future living environment, and it is their situation that must provide the driving force towards economic solutions that make good dwellings in good environments available to everyone.

A governmental committee in Sweden, the Service Committee, was appointed in 1967 to study the different aspects of service facilities in residential areas. Among environmental requirements listed by the Committee are:

1. Nurseries for all children whose parents cannot look after them at home because of employment or for other reasons, but also as an environmental requirement warranted by the child's own needs.
2. Playing and recreation areas for young and old.
3. Community services for cleaning, laundry, catering for the old, the sick, and the handicapped.
4. Commercial services for those who wish to exchange housework for work outside the home, and to buy instead the services the worker at home would otherwise have provided.
5. Opportunities to buy daily necessities also for those with normal daytime working hours.
6. Facilities for stimulating and contact-creating activities both during the day for all children, youngsters, housewives, shift-workers, and pensioners who stay at home, and also in the evening for all day workers who, thanks to expanded services, have time and energy over for activity that everyone can experience as meaningful and pleasant.
7. Safe, reliable, and comfortable means of transport.

The Committee has declared as its opinion that the role of service for residents in the community development process is to lighten the burden of wearisome household tasks, increase the scope for development of personality and pursuit of healthy activities, and to help establish increased security, equality, and fraternity. The Committee also considers discussion and priority of urgent importance, the main purpose here being to establish the nature and extent of the community's responsibility and its contributions to the provision of service.

One way out of many to reach these goals mentioned above is to integrate the different service activities. The main purpose of integration of this kind is to form better contact between people and the groups in residential areas but also to increase social safety for different groups, e.g. the elderly, the sick, and the disabled. Another important purpose for integration of service facilities is to save money. Integrated solutions will normally decrease costs for erecting and running the buildings and activities.

The main purpose of integrating different service activities in service facility complexes in residential areas is to increase the security and the fraternity between people in the neighbourhood units. One way to reach this goal is to use primary and comprehensive schools as bases for different activities and to use the different premises and work-shops for all groups and individuals in the residential areas.

Brickebacken. The Service centre of Brickebacken, the latest neighbourhood unit just outside the town of Örebro, some 200 kilometers west of Stockholm, is the first integrated service facility complex erected in Sweden. The area contains 1900 dwellings for c. 5000 inhabitants and the centre was inaugurated in September 1971. The centre at Brickebacken, which is located in immediate contact to the dwelling area, comprises premises covering a total area of some 11 000 m² grouped around a central covered and heated street for pedestrians. The core of the centre is a resident service bureau, a comprehensive school, a recreational centre and a supermarket. The purpose of the resident service bureau is to act as an agency for other resident services. The supermarket contains a small shop which is open in the evenings. The school's kitchen and the dining room have been enlarged so that they can be used not only by the pupils but also as a dining room for the staff and the public. The dining room can be rented for private parties and the kitchen serves meals to take home. Premises for hobbies and so on, which automatically belong to the recreational centre, have been amalgamated with recreational premises belonging to other institutions and the same has been done with the church and library premises. The centre also includes premises for medical care, dentist, and an indoor swimming-pool (see Fig. 31.1).

The social and economic situation of families with children are matters which are largely connected with living service facilities. If we provide the parents with services that enable both of them to go out to work we are also improving the family's economic situation and perhaps also its social and emotional situation. If we

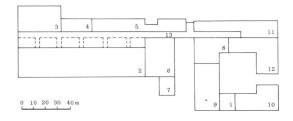

FIG. 31.1. Plan of integrated service facility complex in Brickebacken, Örebro, Sweden.

1. Resident service bureau
2. Comprehensive school
3. Recreational and sports centre
4. Club
5. Workshops and hobby
6. Library
7. Church
8. Restaurant and cafeteria
9. Supermarket
10. Post office, bank, and other shops
11. Medical and health centre
12. Local offices of the housing concerns
13. Indoor pedestrian street

provide a dwelling large enough to allow people to be apart or together, as they wish, we are thereby lessening psychic and social dysfunction. If we create a good environment where children can go out and play and where adults can be with them and provide them with stimulation in an atmosphere of security, then we are also lessening the strains that particularly mothers at home with small children are exposed to in the insecure environments that exist today in our new dwelling-areas.

Family service centres/health centres
We should also develop centres that provide a more open kind of play activity for children of all ages, where adults of all ages also can participate. This would be an important complement to the pre-school and for a long time ahead it would help to meet the need for teaching supervision of young children.

The Committee on Child Centres considers that health- and family service centres must also be provided in connection with the pre-school in the dwelling-area. These would provide an integrated service with prophylactic child care and social care as well as child and adult health services; and a co-ordinated team of physicians, social workers, psychologists, family counsellors, children's nurses, and others would be able to give each child and adult the support and assistance they need.

A first modest step towards all this can be taken by co-ordinating the existent neighbourhood facilities — for example, the child welfare and central social welfare board functions; the child welfare centres, maternity centres, the children's and young people's psychic care services, and possibly the family counselling offices. By means of simple and direct cooperation with people from the various services mentioned doing their particular job in a wider framework, we can also

achieve a kind of teamwork in this area that will be rewarding for both the parents and children who use the social services and those who provide such services.

The most important thing, therefore, is to create a good total environment for the child. If we do this we shall have succeeded in putting into effect a sizeable sector of prophylactic social policy. Big investments in little people, I think, will show a good profit in the future. As head of the approved schools in this country I can testify, at any rate, that the neglect and mistreatment of young children cost a great deal of time, energy, and money to rectify later in their lives.

The aim must therefore be to meet the needs of all children and parents for pre-schools and recreational homes of various kinds in the districts where they live — both old and new districts; and to give all children a year, or several years preferably, in some type of pre-school before they enter comprehensive school. This, as I said, is the essential practical measure of social policy that should be put into effect over the whole field. This is the measure with widespread and deep-reaching effects that will do much to remove present difficulties and prevent new problems from arising.

LEGISLATION

Political action also takes the form of legislation and various public measures to guarantee everyone, regardless of sex, a certain minimum security in various directions. It takes the form of legislation concerning marriage, taxation, social welfare, child welfare, housing, environment, conditions of work, accident prevention, and so on.

Marriage, fiscal, and social welfare legislation
Marriage, fiscal, and social welfare legislation are closely related. If, here in Sweden, we exalt the principle of equality between women and men, we must also recognize the consequences of this.

Marriage legislation
We have an educational policy that makes no distinction between girls and boys and we have no sex-segregated school classes. Our children and young people have already begun to follow the consequences and the lessons of equality they learned at school. Both girls and boys get themselves a kind of occupational training that enables them to choose patterns of living and living together in accordance with their own interests and values, instead of wanting merely to be supported or looked after.

The new freer kinds of family relationship also must be given due recognition by the legal system. This can help to prevent the psychosocial dysfunction that still occurs today as the result of efforts to follow an unconventional mode of living. This, of course, does not mean that the conventional kind of matrimony must be broken down and destroyed as a cohabitation and family pattern, but it does mean that in future we must try to give the other patterns that people may choose for living together a large degree of legal equality with matrimony, as regards the social and economic consequences. Present family law will probably become part of a wider system covering people living together, of which the basic principle will be that the family is a voluntary form for economically independent free individuals living together.

Community between people is a vital necessity in our society, but a close emotional contact is best developed and deepened if based on economic independence. It cannot be strengthened by means of laws and regulations that demand more of one than of the other partner. In August 1969 the Minister of Justice appointed a Governmental Committee with the responsibility of carrying out an investigation concerning present legislation on family law.

An important part of the terms of reference runs as follows: 'Marriage should be a form for voluntary cohabitation by independent persons. The function of legislation in this connection is to solve practical problems not to privilege one form of living together above others.' Thus the terms of reference of the Committee are based on an entirely changed idea of marriage which is seen as a form of voluntary living together by two independent persons. In a few years we can expect people to enter into marriage with a simple and neutral registration procedure which later on can be supplemented, for those who want to, with a religious or civil wedding ceremony.

Consequently the Committee will simplify the forms for entry into marriage but it will also simplify the forms for dissolution of marriage. If the spouses mutually agree on dissolution of their marriage they should be able to get an immediate divorce without a separation period. The Committee is giving considerate attention to the rules for maintenance. The obligation for alimony between spouses will be reduced to a minimum.

This Committee is carrying out an extremely important and comprehensive investigation aiming at, in the field of family law, equal treatment of people by society, irrespective of sex, irrespective of they are living alone or in some form of co-habitation.

Tax reform
An important *tax reform*, implying a change over from joint taxation to individual taxation was entered into force in 1971. Hitherto we had double tables, which hit unmarried persons rather heavily and which was less severe for married persons. The married man had double privileges compared with his unmarried colleague. For one thing he was taxed at lower rates and secondly he was able to make a tax reduction for his wife. The principle behind the new proposal is that all people shall be regarded as economically independent individuals and that society shall adopt a neutral attitude to the form of cohabitation which people choose. The support of the society shall be given where

there is a need, to children, to the aged, to the sick and to the handicapped.

Now, one cannot carry out such a radical reform without transitional regulations. We have a large group of families in which the woman has no possibility of entering into gainful employment even if she wanted to. She may be too old to receive training, or is living in a place where there are no job opportunities, etc. For this reason a tax support for these families will remain during a transitional period. But it will be given in the form of a reduction of the final tax instead of, as earlier, the income on which tax is paid. Tax reduction by progressive taxation is of greater value to those who have a high income than to those who have a low income. We have that effect now eliminated.

Social legislation
Another area which is usually directly dependent on sex-role ideas is that of *social legislation*.

Social security must be made available to men and women on equal conditions in all areas. Special treatment for either sex causes disturbances and imposes improper demands — for example, the man's efforts to provide the maximum amount of security for the woman, or vice versa. In general, what is needed is a social insurance system that gives people security, regardless of their sex, in situations such as the following: in sickness, unemployment, old age, childbirth, and during child care.

Let me take just one example of inequality in this area: when she has a baby, a woman is entitled to a fairly long period off work, for physical and psychic reasons. Should not a new father also be given the chance to participate from the start in his child's development and at the same time support his family in the altered situation brought about by the arrival of the child? We now have a fruitful discussion going on in this country concerning men's equal rights to 'paternity leave'. The trade unions and other groups have supported this proposal in their family policy programmes.

As regards other areas of legislation, I would mention working environment and accident prevention legislation, which have a great effect on human relations. The psychosocial dysfunction that accompanies shift work and heavy industrial work, for instance, has not been sufficiently studied as regards its impact on men's and women's ability to function in their sex roles and family relationships; and the effect of these factors on the children has not been studied — at least not in this country. Reasonable hours of work and good working conditions in which no sex discrimination occurs are a necessary requirement for the future.

Building legislation and housing legislation that takes into account what the individual needs in the way of a good dwelling and a good external environment are also preconditions for the prevention of psychosocial dysfunction. In this country the Building Law Enquiry is now considering such matters.

NEED FOR RESEARCH

There is much research going on about men's and women's sex roles. The effects of the traditional sex-patterns are also being studied. However, it may be noted that there is much less research about the unconventional family patterns and relations that are now developing. We need purposeful research concerning the possibilities for men, women, and children, as human beings, of finding expression for their latent potentialities in the family, in working life and in society at large. We know very little, for instance, about children's environment and the chances of improving it. What do sex roles mean to children? When all children get a chance to go to pre-school, what will this mean for them and for society? What changes and improvements can be made in the short and in the long run? Research in several areas is required. Through their studies the researchers can promote development and give politicians the tools necessary for their decisions. To a large extent it is towards children and their 'alien land' that researchers must devote their efforts.

CONCLUSION

The question of sex roles is merely a part of the apparently confused pattern of modern society. The pattern is a mixture of will, reality, need, and resources. A plurality of values is characteristic of the present time. A gap between old and new is found in all areas. Therefore, we must find the least common denominator in order to push the pace of development and eliminate the obstacles that rise in our way. To concentrate on neutralizing the negative consequences of, for instance, sex-role prejudices is one such denominator. In this connection I am naturally looking towards the younger generation. They are building the new society and we must clear the way for them. Children and their living environment must therefore be given priority. For their benefit we must take prophylactic measures and at the same time try to repair the damage done to the older generation and to those who are still young.

What does it mean for the evolution of society that men and women are so isolated from each other in their roles at work and in the home? What has it meant for the development of the world that the so-called masculine attributes of activity, extroversion, hardness, aggression, and coldness have largely characterized the decision-makers while the passive, introverted, soft, yielding, and tender women have merely accepted the decisions?

Theories, technology, and the capacity to destroy have run away out of all reasonable relation to human needs, says the Swedish writer, Eva Moberg; while wisdom and the ability of people to live together have remained at a mediaeval level. This could not have happened if the men's role had included more participation in the world of child and home and if the women's role had included more participation in public affairs. It is simply impossible to achieve a greater degree of maturity without more all-round human development. We cannot divide up the sexes into one which is warlike and one which is life-preserving without bringing deadly consequences for humanity. Both sexes must become both life-preserving and responsible members of society.

REFERENCES

BARNSTUGEUTREDNINGEN (1971). *Innehåll och metoder i förskoleverksamheten*. Diskussions-PM från 1968 års barnstugeutredning. Stockholm: Allmänna Förlaget, 1971.

BRENTON, M. (1967). *The American male*. London.

DAHLSTRÖM, E. (ed.) (1967). *The changing roles of men and women*. London.

FACKFÖRENINGSRÖRELSEN OCH FAMILJEPOLITIKEN, LO:s familjepolitiska rapport, 1969.

FAMILJ OCH SAMHÄLLE, TCO:s familjepolitiska rapport, TCO-Prisma, 1970.

FREDRIKSSON, I. (1970). *Die Stellung der Frau in Schweden, Modellfall Skandinavien?* Hamburg.

FRIEDAN, B. (1968). *Den feminina mystiken*.

GOLDTHORPE, J., LOCKWOOD, D., BECHHOFER, F., and PLATT, J. (1969). *The affluent worker in the class structure*. Cambridge.

GRØNSETH, E. *The dysfunctionallity of the husband provider role in industrialized societies*. Oslo.

HOLMBERG, R. (ed.) (1966). *Kynne eller kön? Rabén och Sjögren*.

HOLTER, H. (1970). *Sex roles and social structure*. Oslo.

JOHANSSON, S. (1970). *Om levnadsnivåundersökningen, Låginkomstutredningen*. Stockholm.

KORPI, W. (1971). *Fattigdom i välfärden, Tidens samhällsstudier*.

KVINNORNA OCH ARBETSMARKNADEN. FÖRDOMAR, FAKTA,

FRAMTID (1971). Arbetsmarknadsstyrelsen, Stockholm.

LÄROPLAN FÖR GRUNDSKOLAN (1962). Skolöverstyrelsen. Kungl, Stockholm.

LGR 69. LÄROPLAN FÖR GRUNDSKOLAN (1969). Utbildningsförlaget Liber AB, Stockholm, Sweden.

LILJESTRÖM, R. (1968). *Jämställdhetens villkor. Män och kvinnor i dagnes värld*. Stockholm, Sweden.

NASH, J. (1965). 'The father in contemporary culture and current psychological literature.' In *Child development*. Society for Research and Child Development, Chicago.

NATIONAL CENTRAL BUREAU OF STATISTICS (1975). Stockholm, Sweden.

PEDAGOGISKA MEDDELANDEN nr 5/1970, The Royal Board of Education, Stockholm, Sweden.

RAPOPORT, R. and RAPOPORT, R. (1971). *Dual-career families*. Harmondsworth, England.

SELLERBERG, A.-M. (1971). *Sociologiska aspekter på barntillsynen*. Lund, Sweden.

SOU (1970). Boendeservice 2, **68**, report 2 presented by the Service Committee.

SOU (1971). Boendeservice 6, **28**, report 6 presented by the Service Committee.

SWEDNER, H. (ed.) (1970). *Socialvård och Samhällsförändring*, artikeln Fattiga barnfamiljer i Malmö av Kurt Sjöström. Stockholm.

SVENSSON, A. (1971). *Relative achievement: school performance in relation to intelligence, sex and home environment.* Göteborg Studies in Educational Sciences 6. Stockholm, Sweden.

THE SWEDISH INSTITUTE (1968). *The status of women in Sweden.* Report to the United Nations, Stockholm.

THIBERG, S. (1968). Samhällsplanering för service. *Hertha,* **3**.

32. SEX EDUCATION IN SCHOOLS IN DENMARK

PREBEN HERTOFT

INTRODUCTION

Experience acquired in one country on the subject of sex education cannot be applied as a matter of course to another, because the way this subject is taught, and the way it is understood, must be related to a number of basic factors inherent in each society. Examples of such factors are traditions, religious beliefs, the general level of education, women's rights and their place in society, the type of social and sexual legislation, the extent of family planning, etc. Even when these factors *are* taken into account sex education may not necessarily be accepted: it generally meets with a varying amount of opposition. It is usually necessary to challenge a number of conventions if sex education is to be successful, though the means of doing so will vary from country to country.

In fact hardly any country today has at its disposal a pattern for sex guidance in its schools. The Scandinavian countries are puritanical in this respect, contrary to popular belief. These countries are in the middle of a development which is, as yet, far from complete. I would like to review this development, as it has occurred in Denmark. Those interested in a more detailed account of its background — including the contents of a number of reports of commissions and the results of certain Danish sexological investigations — should consult the paper by the Danish psychiatrist Henrik Hoffmeyer (1970).

In the following I shall briefly discuss the meaning of the term 'sex guidance', then describe the rules governing sex guidance in schools in Denmark. Finally, I shall consider the results which may be expected from this guidance, and how far such guidance can go. I wanted to stress that I do not see myself in the guise of a missionary, that I recognize the subjectivity of much of what I am about to say, and that I am quite prepared to change my present attitude as and when the problems are further elucidated.

THE MEANING OF THE TERM 'SEX GUIDANCE'

The Swedish psychiatrist Torsten Sjövall (1963) divides the concept of sex guidance into two parts which he calls 'sexual information' and 'sexual education'. He describes sexual information as the 'imparting of exclusively factual knowledge on sexuality as a biological function', whereas the purpose of 'sexual education' goes much deeper and is defined as 'an instruction in the best way

to integrate these facts in the prevailing psychosocial situation.' If I underline this differentiation it is not really because I find the expressions particularly well chosen, or the definitions really adequate, but because it seems right to differentiate between the purely informative aspect of sex guidance, which is an account of straight facts (not necessarily biological facts only, but also the importance of the psychological and the social factors), and that aspect of sex guidance which goes deeper, where the educator is not content merely to inform, but attempts to promote certain patterns of behaviour and attitude, and to warn against others — to put it bluntly: where he moves from straight information to subjective propaganda.

It is characteristic of Sjövall's classification that sexual guidance is referred to as a purely theoretical matter, and that the possibilities of practical instruction are not even mentioned. Sjövall is not to blame for this as it is characteristic of the entire Western tradition, but it is nonetheless thought-provoking. In the case of many other areas of education we would consider it absurd to be content with theoretical training. Let us take a simple example such as swimming. It is not only by telling them how to swim, and describing the pleasure and the dangers pertaining to it, that children are taught to swim. We train them in a swimming pool. As far as sex life is concerned, however, we expect that a little theoretical guidance is enough, and that the rest will follow. In the Western world there is no tradition for practical training in the so-called art of love, as it is known in both the Near and the Far East, and the rule is that adult sex life is hidden from the children. It is only in recent years that some opposition has developed against this attitude. The observation of primates, for example, points to the need for a certain apprenticeship in the sexual field to enable apes to find out about mating at the age of puberty.

Man, however, is no ape, and sex guidance is a much more radical subject than swimming lessons. Let us therefore set aside the practical and experimental aspects of sex guidance, despite their importance, and restrict ourselves to its theoretical aspects. Whether sex guidance in the future should on the whole remain theoretical and the pros and cons of really practical information and training on the subject of sex, can be discussed elsewhere. Going back to our starting-point, we must ask ourselves: is the school to restrict itself to providing *sexual information*, or is it to deal with so-called *sexual education* too? Let us consider the rules governing sex guidance in Danish primary schools, which children attend from age seven.

RULES GOVERNING SEX GUIDANCE IN DANISH PRIMARY SCHOOLS

At the turn of the century the view that schoolchildren ought to receive sex guidance was already a matter for discussion in Denmark. Thus, at a school meeting in Copenhagen in 1907, it was accepted that 'the act of procreation is not indecent in itself'. Thus pacified, public opinion decided that school children should at least be taught human reproductive biology. It took a long time, however, to integrate the subject into the school curriculum. It was not until the 1930s and the 1940s that some progress was made on sex guidance in the schools, particularly in the larger towns — in rural areas the children have, up to this day, had next to no sex guidance at school.

Research undertaken in the beginning of the 1960s (Report of the Committee on Sexual Education 1968; Hertoft 1968) revealed that approximately 50 per cent of Danish schoolchildren received some sex guidance during their years at school — seldom more than one or two hours, and often in the form of a speech made to a large group of 14-year-old schoolchildren. It is not surprising that this teaching method was very unsatisfactory. Sweden, on the other hand, has had compulsory school sex guidance since 1956. Influential opinion in Denmark was still of the opinion, however, that schools were not to concern themselves unduly with sex guidance.

This opposition was clearly substantiated when the first two television broadcasts on sex guidance for schools were at the planning stage. One of the most trustworthy psychiatrists in the country had been invited to produce the broadcasts, but even before they were shown more than 80 000 protests were registered. The broadcasts were not particularly controversial, and tempers simmered down quite rapidly. Subsequent schools television broadcasts did not give rise to any commotion. Through the 1960s a government commission (The Committee on Sexual Education) worked on the problems relative to sex guidance for schoolchildren of all ages. One of the commission's two final reports (1968) recommends the introduction of compulsory sex guidance for all Danish schoolchildren; and from 1971 onwards, sex guidance has been a compulsory subject in Danish primary schools. The new rules were accepted by majority vote, but met with strong opposition from small groups from ultra-right and ultra-left parties. Prior to the new legislation in this field, detailed 'Directives regarding sex guidance in primary schools' (Folkeskolens laeseplansudvalg 1971) were published. The introduction sets out the following aims for sex guidance in the schools:

Frankness: The school must endeavour to promote frankness regarding the sexual aspects of human life.
Confidence: The school must endeavour to propagate this frankness by its own confidence-inspiring attitude towards the children.
Knowledge: The school must endeavour to impart a knowledge which:

(a) may help to avoid a feeling of insecurity and fear from which problems might otherwise develop (freedom from fear);
(b) may contribute to the development of understanding of the connections between sex life, love life, and social life (understanding the connections);
(c) may enable each child to discover for himself the points which are most in harmony with his own personality (liberty of choosing standpoints); and
(d) may stress the importance of a sense of responsibility and courtesy in the field of sexuality (comprehension of responsibilities).

The directives indicate that instruction must adhere to three main principles:
(1) the so-called '*concentric*' teaching principle (see below);
(2) the teaching must be *integrated* into the general curriculum of the school; and
(3) the teaching must be in the form of *conversations and discussions* with the children.

The concentric principle
This means that teaching about sex begins while the children are small — during their first year at school. It becomes progressively more detailed, in step with the children's development. The directives state, *inter alia*, 'Any subject may, in principle, be treated at any time. The teaching programme deals with the whole question, and is limited only by the consideration of the children's stage of development and maturity.'

The principle of integration
The directives indicate that 'the topics dealt with in sex guidance must be integrated into the school's general curriculum. Efforts should be made to avoid sex guidance being dealt with primarily or exclusively in special talks or under specific conditions.'

The aim of the integration is to stress that human sexuality should not be presented as an isolated facet, but as part and parcel of human life. The directives also state:

It [human sexuality] is not exclusively a physical question (concerning, for instance, anatomical or physiological phenomena), nor is it exclusively a technical question (such as birth control), but neither is it so emotionally accentuated that it cannot be treated impartially and objectively. The problem must be evaluated, and then shown as one of the many facets of life. It is not sufficient merely to evaluate straight sexual satisfaction, or the begetting of children. Sexual life must be presented as something of value to all aspects of human life, be it from the personal, the family, or the community angle. This is why the subject must be integrated into the school's general curriculum. Sexual questions must be dealt with when the opportunity arises in connection with the topics being discussed by the class at a given time. Almost any topic can serve as starting-point.'

Conversation and discussion
The principle that tuition should be in the form of conversation and discussion serves to guarantee, *inter*

alia, that the children understand what is being said, become involved, and have the chance of talking themselves; moreover, 'education through talk and discussion will very likely provide each child with a greater chance of discovering the conceptions which harmonize with his own personality.'

If guidance along these lines is to succeed, it *must be made compulsory*. It is not possible, just because a topic provides the opportunity of drawing in the sexual aspects of the question, to send one or several of the children out of the classroom for half the lesson and most of the next. The official directives emphasize that co-operation with the homes is a must in this, as in all other essential respects, but that the school does not propose 'to take anything away from the homes'. It is pointed out in the directives that the school's sex guidance must be comprehensive and objective; it says, for example, that 'all parents must rest fully assured that their children will not be influenced in a prejudiced way, which may differ from the home's views. Parents must be confident that the basic ethical views are presented factually and objectively.' Just as it is compulsory for the children, sex guidance is mandatory for the schools.

It has been made possible for a school in a transitional period to supplement integrated sex guidance with what is called a 'comprehensive representation of the main topics concerning sex guidance', and to give these lessons to the sixth and the ninth forms, 13 years and 16 years old respectively. However, the long-term aim is to integrate sex guidance completely into the school curriculum. Certain restrictions regarding the preparation of the lessons have been imposed upon the teachers:

(a) the use of so-called 'vulgar terminology' is prohibited;
(b) sex guidance which could be construed as personal advice must not be given to any individual child;
(c) information about the technique of sexual intercourse is prohibited, nor must any other technique aimed at achieving an orgasm be elaborated upon;
(d) the use of photographic material is prohibited at all stages of sex guidance activities, whether it represents masturbation, sexual intercourse, or other erotic situations.

The justification of these restrictions states that: 'the restrictions are imposed partly to safeguard the teacher, so that his teaching cannot give rise to unjustified criticism, partly to avoid the real possibility of overstepping the line into the field of medicine, and lastly for the sake of those children who come from homes where the overstepping of these boundaries is found particularly offensive.'

A large majority of parents and of teachers consider the new directives on sex guidance as a step forward compared with the past; they think that matter-of-fact guidance in this important field is necessary in a community whose members are exposed to innumerable sexual stimuli through press, books, advertising, etc. It has been pointed out that the task is beyond many parents' abilities; it is reassuring, therefore, to know that the schools are endeavouring to make up for this parental failing.

A number of small groups have criticized the present arrangement. Some, more particularly, have deplored its mandatory character and assert that an attempt is being made to impose opinions and to take the responsibility for their children away from the parents.

Others criticize the arrangement for not being radical enough. They regret that the school authorities do not leave it to the teachers to choose their own terminology; this counteracts the wish for 'integration', as everyday language differs from official, clinical-sounding terminology. Many are dissatisfied with the prohibition of photographic illustrations — they refer to the peculiar attitude of the country that authorizes pornography and yet prohibits the use of factual photographic material of sexual situations. And all this in spite of the directives which state that some of the children are bound to have pornographic literature and pictures which they bring to school, 'whereby the opportunity might arise to a general discussion on pornography'. Again on the subject of pornography, it is mentioned that 'a broader view of sexuality may be expected to de-dramatize the interest in pornography'. So although pornographic picture material may be drawn into sex education, at least theoretically so if the pupils bring it themselves, it is forbidden to use non-pornographic representations of sexual situations, although these could serve particularly well to demonstrate the difference between pornography and normal sexuality.

The prohibition of *technical* sex guidance has also met with opposition and it has been stressed that this is a subject which many older children are curious about. It has been mentioned that some of the most widely read books on sex guidance, Bent Claësson's (1971) *Boy and girl; man and woman* for example, contains four-letter words, photographs of masturbation and of sexual intercourse as well as technical advice, and that it is to be regretted that these books, which find favour with the young, are not to be used in teaching.

All in all, however, it must be said that the new system seems in many ways to aim at being a compromise between many divergent views — from the most conservative to the most radical. However, it is characteristic that nobody today has dared state officially his opposition to sex guidance *per se* — only its form is discussed.

COMMENTS ON THE OBJECTIVES OF THE DANISH RULES

A review of the aims of sex guidance in Danish schools shows that they are defined by the terms: *frankness*, *confidence*, and *knowledge*. Special emphasis is laid on knowledge, as this keyword is particularly carefully elaborated. This 'knowledge' is to contribute to (a) freedom from fear, (b) understanding of the link-up of facts, (c) liberty to make one's own decisions, and (d) understanding of one's responsibilities. One might say: 'beautiful words'. One might add: 'a certain lack of stringency'. And in the end, one might well be very doubtful about the school's ability to shoulder the task thrust upon it. It is clear that the aim is to delve deeper than what is encompassed by the term sexual information and reaches beyond so-called sexual education. As theory is one thing and practice another, the factual result is likely to be that the teaching of knowledge will be more successful than the imparting of attitudes.

Consider the following two questions:

(1) what can, and what cannot be obtained by means of information — information being taken in the broadest sense of the word?
(2) is the school's sex guidance programme to be merely informative, or is it to be more than that, and different?

It is, as often happens, easier to pose the questions than to find the answers. But all those who work with sex guidance must consider them, and try to come to their own conclusions.

THE MEANING OF KNOWLEDGE

In Scandinavia in the 1930s and 1940s, the situation was quite simple. At that time sex guidance was considered as a doubtful business and met with fierce resistance from most people. At the same time ignorance was enormous, and its consequences numerous and absurd. Perfectly normal behaviour such as, for instance, masturbation, gave rise to unnecessary anxiety and alarm because people did not know any better; unwanted pregnancies, with all their sequels, occurred simply out of ignorance of contraceptive remedies, poor distributional facilities, and doctors' reluctance to provide birth control guidance. At that time sex education was realized to be necessary but the idea was simply to impart the necessary guidance to as many as possible, and the value of this aim could not be disputed. Many hoped probably, in the heat of the battle, that most sex problems would be solved provided people were sufficiently well-informed. Others were well aware that although sex guidance would solve some problems, it certainly would not solve them all — but they did not find it timely to say this too loudly, for fear of harming the cause. It was important not to provide the opposition with more ammunition, as there was already enough to fight about.

Things have changed today, fortunately — and a less stark appraisal of the possibilities of sex guidance can do no harm. Even today, many people think that provided enough is known — not only about contraceptives, but about how man and woman satisfy one another sexually, most of the problems are solved, particularly if the rules of the community became somewhat broader.

It would be nice to think that provided man knew what was right, he would act accordingly. But man is more than an intelligent being who follows logical rules, and this has wide implications on our behaviour and attitudes in nearly all important spheres, including that of sex. Man is largely guided by impulses other than his intellect, and knowledge acquired exclusively through the intellect must be of restricted (but by no means unessential) value. Such knowledge is often a necessary criterion for making the 'right' decision, the most sensible and rewarding in a given situation — but it is not the only one. Occasionally knowledge acquired by intellect conflicts with other aspects of our personality, and quite often that sort of knowledge fails us and we act, looking at it rationally, in an incomprehensible fashion.

A realistic appraisal of the possibilities of sex guidance would presuppose due consideration of these irrational facets of human nature. Opponents of sex guidance, who attach all sorts of harmful effects to it, have one thing in common with some of its supporters who have an exaggerated faith in what it can achieve: they perceive man as an uncomplicated entity. Sjövall (1967) says, very aptly: 'traditions and myths are more powerful determinants of human behaviour than are factual knowledge and logical reasoning.' He bases his contention on Freud, who often dealt with this subject in his works and perhaps most vividly in a paper dated 1937 (Freud 1964), where he examines the importance of giving children factual knowledge in the sexual field:

I am far from maintaining that this is a harmful or unnecessary thing to do, but it is clear that the prophylactic effect of this liberal measure has been greatly over-estimated. After such enlightenment, children know something they did not know before, but they make no use of the new knowledge that has been presented to them. We come to see that they are not even in so great hurry to sacrifice for this new knowledge the sexual theories which might be described as a natural growth and which they have constructed in harmony with, and dependence on, their imperfect libidinal organization — theories about the part played by the stork, about the nature of sexual intercourse and about the way in which babies are made. For a long time after they have been given sexual enlightenment they behave like primitive races who have had Christianity thrust upon them and who continue to worship their old idols in secret.

I think that, particularly where sex guidance for children is considered (how to teach it, and how early in life), people tend to forget what qualifications children have for accepting and understanding what is explained to them; many are inclined to think that they are just miniature adults. We should make use of investigations into children's comprehension of sex guidance at different age levels and we must learn to avoid bringing them into conflict with their own concepts. The Danish psychologist Ruth Iversen (1968) seeks 'a more comprehensive attitude to the irrational and emotional factors in small and older children which represents their faithfulness to early childhood'.

There is no doubt that too many well-meaning educators in the sexual field have offended this 'faithfulness to early childhood' with clumsy attempts at guidance. All who have dealt with small children, watched them at play and listened to their talking, have had the opportunity to confirm Freud's experiences; we know also how inconstant children's interest is in detailed explanations on sexual questions, and that the same thing has to be explained time and again before they 'understand' it the way adults do. There are many examples to show that this 'faithfulness to early childhood' may mark an individual for many years after puberty — even if the true link-up of facts has been intellectually grasped. One, rather droll, example will serve to show this.

During some research work undertaken by myself (Hertoft 1968), 400 young men, 18–19 years old, had to account for their sexual behaviour, knowledge, and attitude. One of the questions they were asked was: at what age did you realize 'how children are made'? One of them smiled diffidently and replied: 'It took me an awful long time to understand that even the king and queen do it the same way', and he was no doubt thinking of his own parents. If endeavours had been made very early to teach him 'how it is really done', it might have confused him, at best done him no good, and at worst harmed him and interfered with the development of his understanding of himself.

It is a fact that children cannot be told the whole truth, and by saying this I am not attempting to reintroduce stork into the nursery. But one must not remain blind to the fact that the myth was not fortuitous, and that in some ways it was connected with 'reality', because there are many kinds of reality, for both children and adults, whether we like it or not.

What is valid for small children is also valid for older ones, as well as for adults. Sex guidance acts on only one personality level, at which sexual adjustment and behaviour are related to all parts of the mind, some difficult to reach and difficult to influence, in particular by ready-made statements, soothing assurances, and good advice. If this is true, it is even more so when giving guidance on sex problems. Sjövall (1963) remarks sarcastically that 'many educators stubbornly indulge in wishful thinking when they state that sex guidance is the only means of combating difficulties caused by psychological problems.' From much of the advice given today — and this is reflected in a number of books on sex guidance — one may get the impression that all the problems can be solved to everybody's satisfaction provided a few physical difficulties are removed. What counts, they say, is some insight and some knowledge of the right mechanics. If only it were that simple — though I wonder then if it would be as exciting as it is! Let us take another practical example.

In the course of the above-mentioned examination of 400 young men's sexual behaviour, knowledge, and attitude (Hertoft 1968), they were, *inter alia*, questioned about their knowledge of birth control and the use of contraceptives. It appeared that the majority of them knew of the most common contraceptives, but that only about 50 per cent of the sexually experienced used them regularly. Among those who had made a girl pregnant — nearly all pregnancies were primarily unintentional — a lesser number of boys, approximately one quarter, had used contraceptive devices regularly. They could give many more-or-less plausible explanations for this, but not one of them said that ignorance was the main reason.

This is a phenomenon well known from numerous other investigations: people *know* about contraceptives: women have a pessary in a drawer, but they don't use it in the end even if their common sense tells them that they must on no account become pregnant at this particular moment. Factors other than common sense intervene, some of them very complicated. This is all very well-known and understood; but it must also be clear that plain sex guidance will serve no purpose if in practice it is not simply a question of knowledge.

Different results are obtained with the more recent contraceptive methods — the IUD and the pill — these appear to be very much more effective than the pessary or sheath. The whole explanation can lie in the fact that the new methods are more acceptable than the old ones. A contributive factor is undoubtedly that whereas the use of the older contraceptive methods depended entirely on the individual's attitude *at the actual moment of sexual intercourse*, a time-dependent factor has been introduced with the new methods: they act independently of sudden wishes and impulses and do not allow the same latitude as the old methods in respect of the factors which defy ordinary logical thinking and so-called common sense. The failure of the old methods was not due to ignorance, it was due to something imponderable which makes even the best kind of sex guidance yield only limited results.

I think it best neither to overrate nor to underestimate sex guidance, but to recognize both that it does have an intrinsic value, and that it serves no useful purpose to attribute to it an importance which it can hardly claim in an otherwise well-informed community. The aim is, first and foremost, to provide each individual person with a certain fund of knowledge which he may use to the extent which he himself finds correct and can manage. Just as we find it quite natural that every person in this country should have the opportunity of learning to read and write, without expecting that such knowledge will increase his capacity of leading a harmonious life and of understanding himself and others (even though it may have some influence), we must accept that, primarily, sex guidance represents only the fulfilment of a requirement which has remained unsatisfied for far too long, but such a fulfilment will not necessarily bring about a solution to difficulties which may be the result of man's sexual drive and actions.

ETHICS AND SEX GUIDANCE

It was laid down in an early Danish directive (1961) that sex guidance 'must aim at forming the children's character and contribute to their harmonious development'. Considering that only 50 per cent of the children benefit from sex guidance at that time, and that those who did seldom received more than a total of 2 hours' instruction, there is an ironical side to this statement. But, regardless of the number of lessons schools devote to sex guidance, they will not find it easy to gain that much of an influence. If we do accept — and there is much supporting evidence — that the basic attitude and character of a human being are formed at a tender age, that they are a result of hereditary and environmental factors, that they follow nonverbal, alogical paths, then it becomes clear that factors quite different from the school have the decisive influence in this connection. It follows that even if parents never intentionally say one word of sex guidance to their children, their influence is more crucial in 'forming the children's character' than the school's will ever be, and that parents cannot, as a matter of course, disclaim all responsibility for their children's education and leave it all to the school. They do indeed influence their children in the sexual sphere, whether they wish to or not.

In the present educational directives (Folkeskolens laeseplansudvalg 1971), the words 'character-forming' are wisely left out, but it is stipulated that, in the field of sex guidance, the school must impart to the children a knowledge which helps, *inter alia*, to strengthen their sense of responsibility and consideration for their partners. This sounds most attractive, though one may well ask whether these are not just pretty phrases. Could this paragraph on the aims of sex guidance not just as well have been left out? It is really so absurd to imagine a form of sex guidance which does not aim at influencing the children, but leaves it to them to decide on their personal attitude according to their own lights? One could equally well ask: should not sex life, each individual's sexual development, bear the stamp of an ethical attitude? If not, where will we end? I do not wish to be misunderstood or accused of harbouring views which are alien to me, so I must reply that sex life and sexual development must naturally bear the stamp of ethics; but that this is an altogether different problem, not necessarily connected with sex guidance. Further, ethics in sexual questions are closely related to the individual's attitude to human problems in general, from which it is difficult to isolate them; sexuality is but one manifestation among others: man is an entity, albeit not always a harmonious one.

It cannot be denied that schools endeavour to influence children ethically in all spheres of education: it can hardly be otherwise, although the views held up as right may be open to discussion. However, in my opinion, it is misguided to aim at a particular ethical goal either in general education or sex guidance. It is, in addition, probably fairly useless to try to encourage any particular ethical attitude, for the attempt is doomed even before it starts. Henrik Hoffmeyer (1962) sheds light on this when he says:

It is every home's privilege and duty to bring up its children according to ethics which are considered right. On the other hand, when we touch upon the information and education given by schools, doctors, etc., the problem is a different one. We come across children with widely differing biological [constitutional] backgrounds, and coming from different social, cultural and religious surroundings. Even if we wanted to, we would be unable to dress this motley flock in ethical conformity. Nor would we be able to motivate them, through school or other educational activities, to an ethical behaviour which is more or less at variance with their earlier acquired attitude, which long ago served as the foundation of their individual behaviour.

But Hoffmeyer adds:

We can try, conversely, to find out whether there exists a common ethical denominator, some basic principles, acceptable to the majority of the children. Is not such a principle to be found in the question of responsibility?

This may be true. But, just as we can look for a common denominator, is it not possible to refrain from looking for anything? Is anything to be gained from the exercise, except more words? Do we have to magnify this hitherto so neglected subject to such proportions? Are we unable to treat sex guidance in the same matter-offact way as other subjects? Could we not try to give a comprehensive orientation without ethical furbelows; stress how widely differing behaviour and attitude can be; and explain which biological, social, and psychological factors affect behaviour? Although most sex guidance has hitherto been given to 14-year-olds or thereabout, it need not be rose-tinted like confirmation speeches (who, anyway, believes in the usefulness of such well-meant wishes and advice?) which, if they make any impression at all, seldom influence the confirmation candidate.

Despite my belief that schools must not claim a fundamental attitude to what is right and wrong where sex life is concerned, I do not wish to recommend — as some have — that the teacher should adopt a 'neutral' attitude to his subject; this makes teaching impersonal and boring. Jakobsen (1965) is right, I think, when he says that 'the teacher must be realistic and objective, yet this subjective attitude is the sounding board of his audience's attention and reaction. This is why the 'standard lecture', which schools and doctors regularly endeavour to find, is of little value. Only the teacher's interest gives life to the subject.' I believe it right that the teacher should express his personal opinion, provided it is made quite clear that it is his opinion and that it may be of no value to others. As far as possible it should be left to the teacher to choose his own vocabulary — provided it is understandable; if he has to use words that do not come naturally to him, for instance to 'latinize' what could just as well be said in the mother tongue, or to employ more common expressions that he is wont to use, something forced and alien appears in his teaching — instead of being normal, it becomes special. Simplicity, straight-forwardness, and frankness are part of what should characterize sex guidance, as they do other subjects. Sex guidance is not different. It is perhaps more difficult for some teachers to be simple, straightforward, and frank when they teach this subject, and if it is so, they should either decline from teaching it, or at least be aware of their handicap and not make a virtue of it. Sex guidance should not be strained or awkward or, worse, intimidating, nor should children feel outraged or morally affected.

CONCLUSIONS

The foregoing should make it clear that it is, in my opinion, the unquestionable duty of the school to give sex guidance as effectively as possible; that it should deal with the psychological and social as well as the biological aspects of sex life; moreover, that it will fare much better if, in the main, it restricts itself to informing, and refrains from futile attempts at influencing the children's sexual attitude. The school should give them a foundation upon which they can build in accordance with their own attitude.

In the past schools could have been reproached for neglecting this duty. It is praiseworthy that they are now beginning to make up for lost time. But there is a new danger attached to this: first, that schools may overrate their importance in this field, and set themselves unattainable goals; and secondly, that by approaching the subject in too conservative and rational a fashion they might succeed, instead of helping the children and the young, in intimidating them by not giving due respect to their individual ideas and fantasies.

Sex guidance must be a discipline on a par with other school subjects, yet it must not be forgotten that it is not quite like them. Not because sexual questions are specially taboo, but because man's sexuality is so complex and so vast, contains so much which is irrational and obscure that both teacher and pupils are involved in it to a far greater extent than they are in subjects which can be taken up or dropped at leisure. Whether we like it or not, sexuality is part and parcel of our daily life; it presents a challenge to schools, and should be the object of its particular attention.

SUMMARY

What is one to understand by the term 'sex guidance'? The valid rules for it in Danish schools are reviewed and commented upon. It is emphasized that sex guidance should be compulsory in all schools, but that the discipline differs from other school subjects and should therefore be the object of special care and attention.

REFERENCES

CLAËSSON, B. (1971). *Dreng og pige, mand og kvinde* [Boy and girl, man and woman]. Copenhagen, Denmark.

FOLKESKOLENS LAESEPLANSUDVALG (1971). *Vejledning om seksualoplysning i folkeskolen* [Directives regarding sexual guidance in primary schools]. Copenhagen, Denmark.

FREUD, S. (1964). *Analysis, terminable and interminable*. Standard Edition of the Complete Psychological Works, Vol. 23, pp. 233–34. London.

HERTOFT, P. (1968). *Undersøgelser over unge maends seksuelle adfaerd, viden og holdning* (with an English summary) [Investigation into the sexual behaviour of young men].

Copenhagen, Denmark.

HOFFMEYER, H. (1962). *Sexuel Opdragelse* [Sexual education]: *Festskrift til Karl Evang*, pp. 70–84. Oslo, Norway.

——— (1970). 'Development of sexual education in Denmark.' Paper presented at the 3rd FONEME International Convention, Milan.

IVERSEN, R. (1968). Discussion comments. Nordic Summer University, Sexology Group, Copenhagen.

JAKOBSEN, L. (1965). Den profylaktiske undersøgelse af børn efter 6 års alderen [The prophylactic investigation of children after the age of sex]. *Ugeskr. Laeg.*, **127**, 1559.

33. PREVENTION OF SEXUAL INADEQUACY BY SEX EDUCATION AND MARRIAGE COUNSELLING

JOSEF HYNIE

SEX EDUCATION

Childhood

A person's future sex life is affected by events right from the beginning of his life and so a child's upbringing can have an effect on his relationships with other people later in life. Too much fondling in childhood can make a person into a selfish pleasure-seeker in sexual relationships, but an upbringing without tenderness can have equally disastrous effects. Children model their ideas on the male and female role in life on the behaviour of their father and the mother, and the absence of one parent often results in problems in later life.

Children should learn to help others, to help round the house, and to share with other people. I think that coeducation is also very important to teach children to relate well with other children of both sexes.

It is important that children are given comprehensible and frank answers to their questions about sex. Naturally children are not capable of a full understanding of sexual matters, and it may be difficult to interpret their questions correctly. Parents should guard as much as possible against their child witnessing disturbing episodes. Often an isolated event, such as witnessing or experiencing rape, can have a long-lasting psychological effect on a child, with the result that he can never form stable sexual relationships in adult life.

Parents are often very worried if they see children playing with their genitals, but there is no cause to be; and it is better to distract the child's attention than to punish him, as the latter course may cause deep-seated neuroses. Sometimes children masturbate for a particular reason, for example they are suffering from phimosis or intertrigo. These conditions should be treated promptly, and problems of insufficient sexual differentiation — hermaphroditism or hypospadias — should be corrected. For example, if boys can only urinate in the female manner problems will arise at school and they may suffer stress and doubts about their sex. The full operation in these cases cannot be done until puberty, but in severe cases we have introduced an early operation to elongate the urethra so that a penoscrotal angle that enables the boy to urinate standing is attained.

PUBERTY

Puberty has traditionally been a time when young people are given warnings about the possible results of 'wrong-doing' — venereal diseases, the possibility of an unwanted pregnancy, etc. The way in which some parents impart this information to sensitive young people could make them develop neuroses. The necessary information on menstruation, nocturnal emissions, masturbation, etc. can be given in an objective and factual manner, and in addition young people can be introduced to the concept of adult love for another person. At puberty I think young people should also be prepared so that they are able to cope sensibly if they find themselves faced with problems such as venereal disease, an unwanted pregnancy, or abandonment.

THE INTERVAL BEFORE SEXUAL LIFE BEGINS

The divorce rate is known to be highest in couples who marry very young, and in Czechoslovakia we are thinking of introducing a minimum marriage age of 20 for young men, as has been done in Poland, where the early results seem encouraging. However, problems arise here, as sexual maturity occurs about 5 years before this.

Many years ago sexual continence was recommended in this interval. Some people still choose this course, although they are acting contrary to the popular trend and their voice is not often heard. Sexual continence is possibly not so difficult for girls. Professor Galla (1968), Dean of the Faculty of Philosophy, interviewed girls of 18–19 who were in their first year at Charles University, Czechoslovakia. It emerged that what they felt was most lacking from their relationships with young men was romance. Intellectuals and artists were more felt to be less lacking in this regard than sportsmen. Again, these are feelings that do not run with the present tide of public opinion. One factor that may make it easier for girls to practise abstinence is that according to Kinsey *et al.* (1953, pp. 144–6, 353, 714–24), the peak of a woman's sexual desire and capacity to have orgasms occurs after the age of 30. But in young men that culmination occurs at about 20 and slowly decreases thereafter. But continence is possible for young men and can be made easier if they channel their energies into other activities and realize that nocturnal emissions or masturbation are quite natural when sexual tension is high. An interesting job and varied leisure activities are important.

Many young people do experience a full sex life in the interval between puberty and marriage and do not desire to have children. They should therefore have some knowledge of contraception. Very often they practise coitus interruptus, which has disadvantages for both partners, as does use of the condom. The pill and the IUD have different disadvantages. Gedda (1970), in Stockholm, demonstrated changes to chromosomes, chiefly polyploidy, after the use of hormonal contraception, and warned against this method with regard to the possibility of genetic changes. IUDs can cause inflammation and other complications, even, in some cases, sterility. Sterility can also follow an abortion, although the risk of this is decreasing in countries where abortions are performed only in hospital under good conditions. Criminal abortions are naturally much more dangerous. Young people should be told about the potential problems and left to make their own decisions and to take responsibility for them. Full sexual life brings obligations and duties to each partner.

Good use can be made of the interval between puberty and marriage to prepare young people for marriage. They can be instructed on such matters as the economic problems of running a house and the care of babies and their nutrition. A good preparation for marriage is the best way to prevent stress situations later.

MARRIAGE COUNSELLING

I discussed some of the stress factors that can arise in marriage in Chapter 22. There are three major stress areas that most often bring couples to crisis point and divorce. The wrong choice of marriage partner, problems with sexual life, or other problems, such as a clash of personalities.

The choice of partner

Naturally one chooses a marriage partner whom one instinctively likes, and feels attracted to. In some countries material assets are also considered important. The situation is I think simplified in countries such as Czechoslovakia where nobody owns property to any great extent. One should also feel that one's partner will be a good father or mother. Sometimes people attach too much importance to physical attraction and find later that their partner's character is not as appealing as their appearance.

I think it is important for an engaged couple to visit each other's homes and become acquainted with the life-style of the parents and the way they organize their marriage, which will have been a model for their children. A man who has a dominant father may have problems if he marries a woman whose mother was the dominant partner. A woman may grow more like her mother over the years in her opinions, and also her attitude to sex. If the backgrounds of the boy and girl are very different this may cause lifelong problems. Finally the couple should spend sufficient time alone to get to know one another.

Sexual disharmony

Young people sometimes want advice about whether they should have sexual relations before marriage to test whether or not they will be compatible. First trials are not always reliable indicators of future compatibility. Often the couple are too inexperienced; but it should be possible for the couple at least to ensure that they are both physically capable of sexual relations and attracted to one another.

Nevertheless about a quarter of the people who come to our consulting rooms are young men having problems with their sexual life at the beginning of marriage. In many cases treatment brings good results. Self-confidence is very important; and sexual activity should not be forced: it is better to wait until it awakens naturally, or the lack of success will create a new stress and a vicious circle is started. The partner's behaviour is also important. She does not help her husband if she is not interested, or frigid, but if she is too passionate she may also hinder the development of the sexual relationship. Understanding and tolerance will help her husband more than reproaches or taunts for his lack of success. And she should not expect sexual life to be perfect right from the beginning, and refuse her husband's attentions if it is not. Practice makes perfect!

Some men blame their lack of success on their wife and test their potency with other women. But his can lead to feelings of guilt, and fear of being found out by their wife, and add further stress to the situation.

Couples sometimes cannot initiate sexual relations because they are both inexperienced. In these cases instruction and guidance are necessary. The couple are also examined to ensure that the failure is not due to a physical defect in either partner.

Like eating, sex is not only for practical purposes but also for enjoyment. So there are many variations that can be practised; and there is no problem if when there is love between the partners they mutually enjoy unusual sexual practices. But if one demands such a practice which the other finds repugnant, as I discussed in Chapter 22 (e.g. masochism or fetichism), the marriage is greatly stressed and may end in divorce.

Sexual life is sometimes possible until 70–80 years of age, if the partners are in good health. It is more often stopped by prejudices than by necessity. It is natural that after 50 sexual desire is not as strong as in a young person. The initial reactions in both the male and the female are slowed down and prolonged; and orgasm does not accompany every copulation. The number and intensity of contractions in orgasm are reduced. Before a couple reach the age of 50 they should know that such a 'slowing-down' process takes place in both sexes but that sexual relations can still be successful. Naturally understanding and lesser expectations from both sides and the continuation of desire for the other partner are necessary conditions.

Other problems

Often economic problems can cause stress. In Czechoslovakia we try to minimize these by instructing older schoolchildren on the problems that can arise in running a household. Usually both man and wife are employed; and the man should be willing to take on his share of running the household. Often the necessary understanding between husband and wife is missing.

Another frequent cause of stress in a marriage is differing views on the upbringing of children. Each may insist on his own system, often taken from the tradition in his own family, and is not ready to accept the system the other partner believes in. Marriage counselling can sometimes alleviate such situations by giving objective advice.

Where there is disharmony we use Leary's (Mellan 1970) method to evalute the personality of each partner. Where hostility and dominance are high in both partners it is hard to reconcile the couple (see Chapter 22).

SUMMARY

Doctors know the stress factors that can arise during sexual development and can help to prevent sexual inadequacy in adults by advising schools on sex education. This chapter deals with the problems of sex education in childhood, puberty, and in the interval before marriage. Doctors sometimes participate directly in marriage counselling by advising on matters such as how to choose a partner, and the problems that can arise in marriage.

REFERENCES

BIBBY, C. (1946). *Sex education*. London.

BOARD OF EDUCATION (1964). *Handbook on sex instruction in Swedish schools*. Stockholm, Sweden.

DOLBERG, G. and GRISSLER, A. (1966). Zum Aufbau der ärtzlichpsychologischen Ehe- und Sexualberatung als Bestandteil der Ehe- und Familienberatung. *Dte Gesundh Wes.*, **21**, 1768–75.

GALLA, J. (1968). Personal communication. Prague.

GEDDA, A. (1970). Symposium of IFA on Hormonal Contraception, in Stockholm, Sweden.

GRASSEL, H. (1967). *Jugend–Sexualität–Erziehung*. Berlin, Germany.

HERTOFT, P. (1969). Sexual behaviour of young men. *Symposium Sexuologicum Pragense*, pp. 50–4. Prague, Czechoslovakia.

HYNIE, J. (1970). *Lekárska sexuológie* [Medical Sexology]. Martin, Czechoslovakia.

KINSEY, A. C., POMMEROY, W. B., MARTIN, C. E., and GEBHARD, P. H. (1953). *Sexual behavior in the human female*. Philadelphia.

LEMAIRE, J. G. (1967). *Les conflits conjugaux*. Les Editions Sociales Françaises. Paris, France.

LINNÉR, B. (1965). Society and Sex in Sweden. Stockholm, Sweden.

——— (1967). *Sex and society in Sweden*. New York.

PŘÍHODA, V. (1963). *Ontogenese lidské psychiky*. Stát. pedag. naklad, Prague, Czechoslovakia.

34. MARRIAGE COUNSELLING AND SEX ROLES IN SWEDEN

BIRGITTA LINNÉR

INTRODUCTION

Psychosocial welfare does not mean only economic welfare and milieu welfare. It also includes emotional welfare. Counselling, therapy, and education should be regarded in the context of the whole social/political and preventive mental health programme. I would like to present a brief review of marriage counselling; family-planning counselling; and the most recent areas of education, especially with regard to the new male/female roles and relationships, in Sweden.

MARRIAGE COUNSELLING

In Sweden child and youth counselling centres were started in the 1930s, sometimes in close connection with the psychiatric clinics at the hospitals or with the Board of Child Welfare. In the 1940s counselling bureaux for sexual problems and family planning and abortion problems were started. And in the 1950s family counselling agencies were formed for marital crises as well as family crises. Now, in the 1970s there is a broadening concern for counselling and educational programme in the social welfare and family welfare services.

Therapeutic counselling is either governmentally-supported, municipally organized, or private. Some counselling is also performed by the various churches. There is also the RFSU, The Swedish Association of Sex Education, which is part of the International Planned Parenthood Federation, which organizes counselling in sexual problems and family planning, and training and educational programmes (Sjövall 1971; Swedish Council for Sex Education 1970). The therapeutic counselling and treatment available in Sweden are mainly based on psychodynamic theories and principles.

An interesting development has taken place since the 1930s, when the emphasis of counselling was on the problem of the child, to the 1950s when the focus was on husband/wife problems, and to now, when there is more emphasis on the interaction and the interrrelations of the family as a whole, with the possibilities of family treatment and family therapy. Indeed, interest is centred not only on the family but on improving the psychosocial health of society in general (Linnér 1972; Svala 1972).

The Municipal Family Counselling Bureau in Stockholm
Parliament decided to support family counselling work in 1960, but as early as 1951 the Municipal administra-tors of Stockholm had started an experimental counselling bureau. The Municipal Family Counselling Bureau is an independent section of the Child Welfare Board. The Bureau offers professional help with interpersonal problems in marriage and family life. It was mainly conceived for crises situations in male/female relationships — interpersonal counselling. This service also includes divorce counselling. All residents of Stockholm can apply for consultation, which is free. The clients come voluntarily, and both women and men seek help in emotional crises. Young people seek help more often than middle aged or old people, often therefore before the crisis has frozen their relationship into a noncreative partnership. This was confirmed by recent research work (Statens Immigrationsverk 1972; Högström and Karlsson 1972). Young couples also come to discuss the pros and cons of legal marriage. They are given all the available information to enable them to make up their own minds.

The work of the counselling bureaux is based on the pluralistic ethical views prevalent in Sweden. 'Marriage' and 'family' are interpreted in a broad sense to include legal as well as informal marriages and families. Divorce and remarriage are accepted on equal terms for men and women.

There are three bureaux, in different parts of the city, staffed with social case-workers as family counsellors. Each team also consists of a psychiatrist, gynaecologist, child psychologist, and lawyer. Each bureau also has a psychoanalyst as a consultant for the staff.

Interviews are held individually or jointly with a couple or a family. Group therapy with couples is a part of the work. The length of time for which clients have contact with the bureau depends on the needs of the clients. Besides the group work mentioned above the staff has 'young-couple courses' with informal discussions about psychological relationships; emotional crises and their solutions; and sexual relations, including information about contraceptive techniques, what it means to be a parent, etc. (Linnér 1972).

Since 1969 one counsellor has been nominated as family life consultant.

There is a growing demand for the bureaux to help with giving information in schools.

FAMILY-PLANNING COUNSELLING: SOME CONCRETE EXAMPLES

I would like to give some concrete examples of family-planning counselling, as the availability of this is important in improving male/female relationships.

The National General Post Office in Stockholm employs gynaecologists on its staff health department. These people give information and advice on contraceptive techniques to the women employed, and give lectures to newcomers and young people in the in-service training programme. In the beginning this work had to be done against some resistance because the administrators and doctors, mostly men, did not see this counselling as a matter really necessary for or relevant to health care. Dr. Kajsa Sundström, most senior of the gynaecologists employed at the Post Office, said to me: 'If the employers can give so much attention and money for a cancer-detection drive, I consider it equally important that contraceptive advice is provided as a health service. It will comfort many women who secretly fear pregnancy in exactly the same way as a negative smear relieves those who have imagined that they have cancer.'

When we started the municipal marriage and family counselling bureau in 1951, it seemed quite self-evident that we should have a gynaecologist in the team and provide services for family planning. I think this was the first bureau of its kind in the world to give advice on modern contraceptive techniques, as this was still very controversial in most countries (Linnér 1968; Swedish Institute for Cultural Relations 1971).

In Stockholm an experimental 'sex bureau' has been started for students from comprehensive schools and, as head of the medical and health programme for the Stockholm schools, Dr. Sven-Ivar Rollof said in an interview: 'The bureau wants to prevent rash sexual debuts, abortions, and unwanted pregnancies. The bureau gives individual counselling and is planned primarily to function as a counselling bureau for both boys and girls, and secondly to help the students with contraceptive techniques of different kinds.' When I talked with Dr. Rollof, he stressed the importance of young boys having a chance to come to the bureau and discussing such problems as premature ejaculation. Boys are often a neglected group in this area. Dr. Rollof emphasized that this centre for sex counselling services for schoolchildren was the first of its kind in the world.

The gynaecologist Dr. Bengt Persson, from the University Hospital in Uppsala said, in a sex-education programme for secondary-school pupils in which both of us participated: 'Don't hesitate to come to the clinic for consultation on family planning. We will not talk to your parents: this is a matter between you and your doctor. You don't have to borrow your mother's pills, or to buy pills on the black market in Sweden; you can talk confidentially with the gynaecologist at the clinic or maternity health centre.' The students in public schools in Uppsala have requested improved sexual counselling, including family planning. At university level family-planning advice is a part of the student health programme.

In Borlänge, an industrial city with a high proportion of young people, the municipal administrators have started a youth centre with various activities, where personal counselling and advice in the sexual area and family-planning advice are available. In recent years similar youth clinics have been set up in various places in Sweden, especially in the metropolitan areas (Sundström 1976).

Public institutions and family planning

At public institutions such as homes for mentally retarded and physically handicapped persons, youth institutions, hospitals, prisons, etc. there is a certain acceptance of the reality of sex life (Katz 1972; Nordquist 1976). For example, at the home for the mentally handicapped in Uppsala men and women are allowed to have a double room and the woman can obtain the pill. As the Administrator said to me: 'It is self-evident that our inmates should have the necessary sex education and contraceptive services.'

At the home for physically handicapped in Stockholm young people have had the same facilities available for some years. There are still many problems for the handicapped. This was confirmed by Inger Nordquist, social worker and leader of a working group dealing with psychosexual questions of the handicapped, when she said at the World Congress of Rehabilitation International in Sydney, Australia (Nordquist 1972):

the capacity to reach a harmonious sexual life does not entirely depend on the handicapped person himself, but still more on his environment. There need not be more psychological problems in the existing sexual life of the handicapped than in the sexual life of the non-handicapped. The problems are instead problems of communication — both in transport and contacts, and also, for some people, technical problems. But the greatest problem existing is the lack of knowledge in the personal environment of the handicapped individual.

This open attitude is so far quite exceptional in the world today, but there is a tendency towards more open tolerance and acceptance. However, certain radical groups feel that this whole area is very neglected and that insufficient advances have been made. And indeed much remains to be done.

SEX ROLE EDUCATION

Sex role education has to be seen in the context of a general movement, beyond the legal emancipation of women, towards complete equality between the sexes — equality extending over the entire range of rights and responsibilities open to human beings. I will discuss here sex role education in schools, mainly, and focus on the new balance between men and women in the marital and family area.

Elementary education

The first prerequisite of educational parity is that boys and girls be given the same elementary education free of charge. Pupils ought not to be hived off according to sex into different classes or schools. Another prerequisite is that children should not in the course of their education be given the idea that certain jobs and professions are suitable for men and others for women. On the contrary, schools should aim at making it clear to pupils that the differences between individuals of the same sex are greater than any average differences between the sexes as a whole. Textbooks and other teaching aids ought not further to entrench traditional ideas concerning the separate roles of the sexes but on the contrary provide information designed actively to combat them.

The new curriculum

A basic change in attitudes and in indoctrination in the area of sex roles was introduced in the comprehensive-school system when the new curriculum was taken in 1969. In practice the sex roles education is integrated in different subjects as modern languages, vocational orientation, psychology, and religion and is not taught as a separate subject *per se*. Sex role education has particular relevance in subjects such as social science, family life and sex education, and child-care education.

It is not only in the theoretical subjects that the new sex roles are debated and taught but also in the practical subjects such as home economics, the use of textiles, and manual handicrafts. As an example, manual handicrafts were once entirely monopolized by males, but now both sexes learn side by side in modern manual handicraft workshops. Home economics is now obligatory for everyone. Child-care education is also obligatory for both boys and girls in order to give both sexes the same responsibility in the traditional woman's role.

In 1970, The National Board of Education initiated a sex roles project in order to study possible ways of helping the schools perform their task of 'working towards equality between men and women — in the family, on the labour market, and elsewhere in society (*Current Sweden* 1975). Since 1975 all 6-year-old children have the legal right to 3 hours a day of pre-school, and children who for special reasons require special support or stimulation can have a place in pre-schools at an earlier age. This is in conjunction with the programme of child care, which affects all families.

These are attempts at changing the traditional patterns. So far no clear effects have been visible, however. To quote one of the leading office-holders in the National Board of Health, Annika Baude, at the International Conference on Social Welfare in San Juan, Puerto Rico, July 1976: 'girls as well as young people as a whole have considerably raised their educational level, but their concentration on those professions traditionally dominated by women has not changed despite the fact that all instruction during the basic school period is identical for boys and girls' (Baude 1976).

Teacher training. In the teacher-training programmes sex role education is integrated as a 'sex role theme' for all groups of teachers, ranging from religion to science. In the various summer-workshops of 1970

discussion focused for the first time on the evolving responsibilities for men and women — and how to deal with those responsibilities.

School textbooks. Another aspect of sex role education is what is presented in school textbooks about modern sex roles, both in the text and the illustrations. Many textbooks still keep to the traditional sex roles and that continuous revisions have to be made in order to minimize the gap between the new objectives and the material used in the actual teaching. I quote from an article in *Hertha* (Westman Berg 1969):

The traditional roles of the sexes are hammered into the minds of infant schoolchildren on virtually every page of every textbook they use, as has been pointed out by both Swedish, Norwegian, and Finnish reviewers. The mothers work about the house, dressed in aprons; the girls too wear aprons, bake little cakes, put their dolls to bed, help their mothers, and so on. Fathers — and sons — on the other hand are depicted in more varied situations. In addition to this, boys and girls are attributed different characteristics. Girls are invariably described as conscientious, dutiful, tidy, and helpful, but at the same time passive and timorous. Boys are sometimes described aggressive towards each other, disdainful to girls, untidy and forgetful, but without any suggestion of reproach being made for these failings. Boyish pranks are acceptable, but one never comes across girls blithely contravening the rules laid down for them.

A recent textbook (Linnér and Westholm 1972) on family life and sex education offers a good example of the new approach of sex roles. The quotation is taken from a chapter on equality between woman and man:

In the double standard system, women have frequently been 'seduced', 'slipped', or 'been driven by passion' into sexual relations, just as the attitude of men has often been to 'see how far one can go'. The double standard long had the support of the law, which, until as late as 1920, spoke of man's *right* but women's *duty*, regarding marital intercourse. On the psychological plane, people believed the dogmas concerning man's *activity* and woman's *passivity* — about man as the active *subject* and woman as the *object*. With the new tendency toward equal expectations of both men and women, equal norms and demands — in the sexual area of life also — we see a new type of involvement and psychosexual mutuality.

With a better balance in the relationship between man and women, there are possibilities for increased tenderness and satisfaction — the 'give-and-take' principle. What is more, foundations arise for mutual respect and acceptance of responsibility, for oneself, and one's partner. The tendency toward a more positive and equal sexual experience is counteracted by the commercial exploitation of our sexual interest. In advertising and sex industry, for example, women continue to be used as erotic symbols, as objects of pleasure for men.

Family life. Family life education is already on the curricula, but there is an interest in having the programme broadened. Among others the parent/teacher association has proposed an all-inclusive 'subject' covering family laws; psychosocial relations, including intra-relationship crises and their solution; and sexual relations, including family planning and information on contraceptive techniques, etc. The Government Committee on Child Care and Child Welfare, working since 1973, has recently proposed a new type of parent education based on the dialogue pedagogical method used in study circles and other small-group work.

Sex education has been compulsory in Swedish schools since 1956, and is integrated in the whole school system (Karlsson 1974; Linnér and Westholm 1972). Boys and girls have the lessons and discussions together. The basic philosophy is one of acceptance of the dual role of sex life, meaning both for pleasure and for procreation, on equal terms for men and women. The guideline should be as in a recent proposal by the Governmental Sex Education Commission: 'The moral implications of the sexual behaviour of men and women should be judged equally. The argument that women are not equal to men should be totally dismissed' (Nordquist 1976).

The Government Sex Education Commission presented their final report in 1974. The report has two main parts, 'Analysis and considerations' and 'A proposal for a teachers' handbook'. The Commission has based its proposals for the comprehensive-school sex education and human relationship programme on empirical research with a rational regard for the realities of life (Swedish Department of Education 1974; *Current Sweden* 1974).

We have now become an immigrant country, and more than 120 different nationalities are represented in Sweden. It is estimated that about 20 per cent of all marriages and stable relationships are with one or both partners from another country, and in many cases with an alien cultural background. In 1971, the National Immigration and Naturalization Board issued a pamphlet for the information of immigrants to Sweden, called *Women and men. Sex — things you ought to know* (Statens Immigrationsverk 1972), which was published in several languages. The intention was not to impose on the readers what might be called the Swedish attitude towards sex, family planning, and abortion, but solely to give non-Swedish speaking people acess to information on a subject area where ignorance can lead to personal tragedies. The pamphlet was written in consultation with the National Board of Health and Welfare and the Swedish Association for Sex Education. The official authorities therefore had stepped into a field which they avoid in most other countries.

The pamphlet was not successful. It had been written without consulting immigrant groups and without paying enough attention to the 'cultural shock' of the immigrants and other complexities. Later a research project was started, supported by the Elise-Ottesen-Jensen Fund, in which immigrant organizations, institutions, and clergymen were involved (Blomquist and Schwarz 1975).

Some years ago the National Board of Education initiated summer workshops for teachers of immigrant students, focusing on subjects such as: 'Should the school sex education programme be regarded as an undue interference of the immigrant groups?' 'Family law and the immigrant groups'; 'Sex and psychological relations in various cultural patterns — representatives from different cultures present their background'; 'Sex and personal relationships in different religious traditions'. The growing interest in cross-cultural research (Kellogg *et al.* 1975; Kozakiewicz and Rea 1975) in sex education came to the fore at a symposium for doctors, school nurses, and other health personnel, arranged by the International Union of School and University Health and Medicine in Stockholm in June 1974. For the first time in the history of the Union sex education at school was on the programme and a whole day was dedicted to the subject (Linnér 1975).

THE BROADENING INTEREST IN PERSONAL COUNSELLING AND EDUCATION

There is an increasing interest in psychosocial counselling and education as a part of the whole mental health programme in Sweden. In the recent proposals by the Governmental Family Law Commission the need for extended family and divorce counselling was taken into consideration. And the Secretary of State, Department of Health and Social Security, underlined in spring 1970 the needs of improved and extended counselling possibilities in the problem areas of living together: 'Through a continuous extending of the services, I consider it important to improve possibilities for counselling and help in questions of psychosocial interrelations.' In order to cover the recognized need of qualified counselling and therapy, the Swedish National Board of Universities and Colleges of Further Education (1975) are at present studying a programme of training in psychotherapy and psychosocial case-work as part of the academic curriculum.

In summer 1972 the Government appointed a working Commitee to suggest improved counselling and educational possibilities in the area of family-planning services.

When Parliament passed the new Abortion Act in 1974, permitting a woman to decide herself at an early stage of the pregnancy about abortion, it also authorized improved and expanded contraception counselling as well as improved family-planning education. This in the spirit of the principle that it is better to prevent than to cure. A Committee on Health Education at the National Board of Health and Welfare was commissioned to work on a long-term programme for information on family planning in Sweden. An essential part of the information given is aimed at young people. The intention is not simply to provide information on contraceptives, but above all to motivate young people to use them. Information of this kind, which is designed to influence attitudes, will necessarily also deal with questions relating to the sex roles and to human relationships in the wider sense (Liljeström 1974; Sundström 1976).

Finally, it should be mentioned that the programmes do not work so well as they are intended to. In spite of our basic philosophy of equality a lot of problems remain. But is not that what one should expect in a transitional period like this, both nationally and internationally?

REFERENCES

BAUDE, A. (1976). *Education as a tool for promoting equality*. National Board of Health and Welfare, Stockholm, Sweden.

BLOMQUIST, B. and SCHWARZ, D. (1975). *Sweden — relationship problems of immigrants*. IPPF (Europe) Regional Information Bulletin, Vol. 4, No. 2. London.

CURRENT SWEDEN (1974). The State Commission on Aspects of Sex and Personal Relationships in Teaching and Public Information. No. 43.

—— (1975). Free choice — theory and reality. Summary of a report from the sex roles project, Swedish National Board of Education. No. 95.

HÖGSTRÖM, A.-S. and KARLSSON, B. (1972). *Den kommunala familje-rådgivningen i Stockholm*. Stockholm, Sweden.

KARLSSON, H.-J. (1974). *Sex education in Swedish schools*. The National Board of Education, Stockholm, Sweden.

KATZ, G. (1972). *Sexuality and subnormality. A Swedish view*. National Society for Mentally Handicapped Children, London.

KELLOGG, E., KLINE, D., and STEPAN, J. (1975). *The world's laws and practices on population and sexuality education*. Medford, Massachusetts.

KOZAKIEWICZ, M. and REA, N. (1975). *A survey on the status of sex education in European member countries*. IPPF (Europe). London.

LILJESTRÖM, R. (1974). *A study of abortion in Sweden. A contribution to the United Nations World Population Conference*. Stockholm, Sweden.

LINNÉR, B. (1968). The sexual revolution in Sweden. *Impact Sci. Soc.*, **18**.

—— (1972). *Sex and society in Sweden*. New York.

—— (1975). *Sex education and family planning — a world dilemma*. The VIIIth Symposium of the International Union of School and University Health and Medicine, Stockholm, 1974.

—— and WESTHOLM, B. (1972). [Sex education package for 'Gymnasieskolan' (age 16 and older)]. Stockholm. Student's pamphlet and Teachers' Guide available only in Swedish. Transparencies: 'Sexualliv and Samlevnad' by Berg, Linnér, Westholm, and Wallin. 48 transparencies, illustrated subjects are: anatomy and hormonal interaction, sexual activity, pregnancy and childbirth, family planning, venereal diseases, social welfare and counselling. Commentary booklet (English translation available): *Sex and personal relationships. Outlines for lessons and commentaries for the transparencies*.

NORDQUIST, I. (1972). *Sex, handicapped individuals and their environment*. The Swedish Central Committee for Rehabilitation (SVCA), Stockholm.

—— (1976). *Education of professionals and staff-members about sex questions of disabled persons*. The International Clearing-House on Social and Sexual Questions for Disabled Persons. Stockholm, Sweden.

SJÖVALL, T. (1971). *Responsible parenthood and sex education*. Background paper on Sweden. IPPF (Europe). London.

STATENS IMMIGRATIONSVERK (1972). *Women and men. Sex — things you ought to know*. Stockholm, Sweden.

SUNDSTRÖM, K. (1976). Young people's sexual habits in today's Swedish society. *Current Sweden*, No. 125.

SVALA, G. (1972). *Sweden*. Country profiles. New York.

SWEDISH ASSOCIATION FOR SEX EDUCATION (1970). *What Swedes teach about sex*. New York.

SWEDISH DEPARTMENT OF EDUCATION, SEX EDUCATION COMMISSION (1969). *Om sexuallivet i Sverige* [on sex life in Sweden]. Official Reports, SOU, **2**.

—— (1974). *Sexual-och samlevnadsundervisning* [Sex and Personal Relationships in Teaching and Public Information]. Official Reports, SOU, **59**.

SWEDISH INSTITUTE FOR CULTURAL RELATIONS (1971). *Society and sex in Sweden*. Stockholm, Sweden.

SWEDISH NATIONAL BOARD OF UNIVERSITIES AND COLLEGES OF HIGHER EDUCATION (1975). *Utbildning i psykoterapi och psykosocialt arbete* [Education and training in psychotherapy and psycho-social case-work]. UKÄ 1975, **24**.

WESTMAN BERG, K. (1969). School books and roles of the sexes. *Hertha*, **5**.

35. FEMALE AND MALE ROLES — SCHOOL AND EDUCATION

MARGARETA VESTIN

THE TASK

Listening to speeches and reading the papers before and during this conference concerning male/female relationships and problems, the *educationalist* must ask: What do all these conflicting facts tell *us*? We are responsible for the upbringing of children and the education of youth, we have to prepare young people for adult life. Can we benefit from all this material, these visions?

My task, as a member of the central school authorities in Sweden, is to get informed and, when informed, to distribute information, making it well structured for students on several levels, teachers or potential teachers, parents, and other concerned with education and training, as well as to stimulate debate and activities.

The official goals and guidelines for comprehensive and the upper secondary schools (the gymnasium) in Sweden stipulate that: 'The school should try to promote equality between men and women — in the family, on the labour market, and in the life of the community at large. It should provide orientation on the question of sex roles, stimulating pupils to discuss and question the present state of affairs' (Läroplan för grundskolan 1969). This task is stressed in many ways throughout the general recommendations for school activities and in the various syllabuses.

In the case of sex roles there is a separate chapter in the general recommendations for the comprehensive (9-year basic) school. Here are some extracts (Läroplan för grundskolan 1969):

By the terms of the aims and guidelines of the curriculum, the school is to promote equality between the sexes — in the family, on the labour market, and in the community at large. This should be achieved partly by treating boys and girls equally, partly by the school counteracting in its work the traditional attitudes to sex roles, and stimulating the pupils to debate and question the differences between men and women in respect of influence, working duties and wages that exist in many sectors of society.

Swedish schools are completely co-educational, with the same syllabuses, timetables, and courses for boys and girls. Equal treatment, however, does not involve simply boys and girls being given the same teaching and being stimulated to interest themselves in the same type of tasks in different subjects; it means also that the school must have the same social expectations of both sexes. The school must assume that men and women will in the future have the same roles, that preparation for the role of parent is as important for boys as for girls, and that girls have reason to be as interested in their careers as boys.

Children starting school (in Sweden at 7)† often have many stereotyped ideas about what a boy/man and a girl/woman should and should not do. They are often subjected to pressure from their surroundings to adapt to the traditional sexual roles, by the attitudes of many adults, by the approaches adopted in the mass media etc. It is the task of the school to make the pupils aware of this influence, and to stimulate them to analyse it and discuss it critically.

'Sex role education' is to be given in conjunction with all school activities. At the lower levels, teaching on the question of sexual roles should be designed above all to offset stereotyped ideas by giving a more differentiated picture of reality. In the higher classes, the question of sexual roles should be set in its psychological, social and economic context. The reasons for and consequences of differences in the status of men and women on the labour market, in the family, and in public life should be discussed in a manner that will make pupils experience the question of sexual roles as one that is exciting and can engage them, by virtue of its importance both for the individual and society at large. Pupils should be stimulated to collect their own information and bases for discussion from the cinema, radio, television, books for young people, newspapers and magazines, political debates, etc.

The curriculum underlines especially the importance of dealing with the responsibility for and within the family as a prerequisite for equality on the labour market and community life as a whole. Within the subject known as 'family questions' the following is said concerning young people as future home-makers:

They must be aware that a necessary condition for equality between the sexes on the labour market and in society in general is that the responsibility for care of the children and domestic work be divided equally between men and women within the family. At this age level, pupils should also be in a better position to see the importance of life both in the home and in the community being based on cooperation between independent and equal people, a cooperation characterized by loyalty and respect for each person's individuality.

The manifestation of existing sex roles should of course be dealt with and discussed in connection with educational and vocational orientation and guidance (known as 'syo')‡ theoretically and practically. The guidance work should be active:

†Age 7–9: lower level, 10–12: middle level, 13–15/16: upper level, 16/17–18/19: upper secondary (gymnasieskolan), 7–16: education compulsary, 16–18/19 optional education and training.

‡Syo stands for study (Studie-) and vocational (Yrkes-) orientation (Orientering). In Sweden the term 'Orientation' includes guidance.

If the 'syo' specialist (the guidance officer, counsellor) merely acts as intermediary of information that has been sought after, then syo does not become a strong counterweight to the influence of home environment, companions, mass media, etc. 'Syo' should counteract any such limitations in the choice of vocation as, for instance, are due to social background, sex, want of motivation to analyse his situation, etc., even if this leads to questioning a decision made by the pupil and to rendering the choice more difficult in that the alternatives experienced only tend to increase.

THE SITUATION TODAY

Against this background, the school authorities found that in reality the sexes were by no means equal. Even if the school as such undeniably affords an example of the fact that boys and girls need not be treated differently — they have the same timetables and syllabuses, the same rights and obligations, and they are taught together, enjoy the same qualifications, and have the same right to further education — it is the traditional attitudes and behaviour relating to careers and adult roles which dominate the picture (see Fig. 35.1).

When asked who ought to do the following tasks, groups of boys and girls aged 13 answered as follows (Dahlgren and Wallin 1971).

Task	Boys	Girls
Needlework, knitting	only for girls	only for girls
Cooking, baking	only for girls	only for girls
Care of small brothers and sisters	only for girls	only for girls
Wash the dishes	only for girls	for both sexes
Look at war-films	only for boys	only for boys
Mending things at home	only for boys	only for boys
Washing the car	only for boys	only for boys
Competitive sports	for both sexes	for both sexes
Run errands	for both sexes	for both sexes
Make one's bed	for both sexes	for both sexes
Smoke	for both sexes	for both sexes

There were many other questions which did not differentiate boys from girls. But it is significant that, although *some* changes have no doubt occurred, young

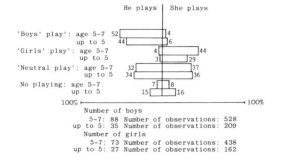

FIG. 35.1. How boys and girls take part in 'boys' play', 'girls' play', and 'neutral play' during observations in nursery school (Englund *et al.* 1974).

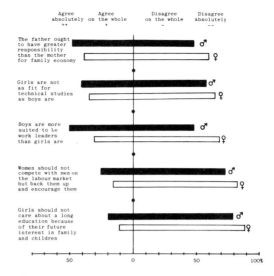

FIG. 35.2. How 1217 boys and 1142 girls aged 12–13 responded to statements on sex roles in 1969–1970 (boys: filled bars), (Vestin 1974).

people in these ages are still very traditional in their attitudes despite a good deal of discussion in families and in school.

Boys and girls in grade 6 (about 12–13 years old) answered some questions concerning sex roles as shown in Fig. 35.2. And when the students were asked the same questions a few years later (about 18–19 years old) — what had they to say? Figure 35.3 gives some

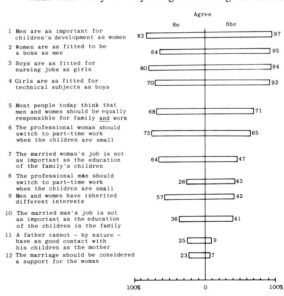

FIG. 35.3. How 328 boys and 286 girls aged about 18 in upper secondary school answered statements concerning sex roles (a selection from 38 items). The answer 'agree' stands for 'agree absolutely' and 'agree on the whole'. The other alternatives, not presented here, were 'don't agree at all', 'don't agree on the whole', and 'don't know' (Bronstrom and Gustafsson 1973).

243

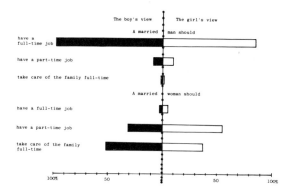

FIG. 35.4. Attitudes in 16-year-old boys and girls about division of labour between family and working life.

examples from a large questionnaire. Attitudes of boys and girls aged 16 to division of labour between family and working life are given in 35.4.

In 1976 the final, third investigation was made in schools: the results have yet to be analysed. It could be that young people are developing a more open attitude. Combining the answers in Fig. 35.3, items 6 and 8, with the corresponding answers in Fig. 35.4, it seems as if *either* the 16-year-olds are more traditional than the 18-year-olds *or* that attitudes have changed in recent years. But popular literature, popular music, advertisements, etc. present a picture of manhood and womanhood which theoretically *could* be biologically determined and which in any case seems to be quite natural for today's adolescents. Their romantic atmosphere contradicts more trivial values and dreams at school and in workplaces.

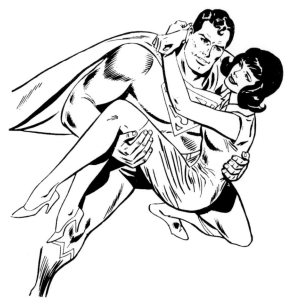

FIG. 35.5. The real man and the real woman.... Or just a dream?

Even if one understands young people, how are we to cope with both the visions *and* the realities? We want both boys and girls to stand on their own feet, be self-confident, and fitted to cope with all sorts of matters in the family and on the labour market.

The Swedish labour market† has practically no obstacles to a completely free choice for boys/men and girls/women. Even the last preserve of men — the armed forces — will in all probability be open to women in a few years. Yet in many respects there is still one labour market for men and another for women, besides — of course — a lot more men than women at the top.

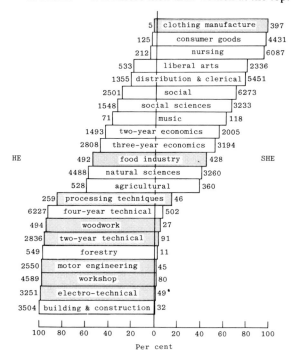

FIG. 35.6. The general pattern for choice of stream in upper secondary school (figures in percentages) (Statistical Central Bureau 1976).

The different ways in which boys and girls make use of their capabilities clearly starts before school and does not change very much during school either. The curricula for education and training are highly indicative — as seen above — helping teachers, vocational counsellors, and others to pin down the lack of concern for equality. But there are so many obstacles to consider, not just the real ones but imaginary ones, too. Certain questions have to be elucidated so that they can be tackled properly in education and teacher training.

Which are the sex differences which are amenable to change and which are not? What are the facts, the values, the prejudices? Which relationships between the sexes seem us to be good/bad? Will some of the

†The Swedish people = 8·2 million. In labour force = 2·3 million males and 1·8 million females. Adults not in the labour force = 0·6 million males and 1·2 million females.

244

conceivable changes generate stress — and if so, how can we prepare for this? I do not consider that the question of stress — when altering sex roles — is a crucial problem but it is still serious enough to merit the attention of educationalists. The strategies for a programme of change ought to be discussed among the many authorities and organizations concerned with education and training, social welfare, family politics, labour market policy, and so on.

SEX ROLES — A PROGRAMME OF CHANGE

In November 1970 the National Swedish Board of Education informed the Ministry of Education of a programme to strengthen the work of the Board concerning sex roles. A project in the form of a commission representing all sections within the Board as well as National Labour Market Board and the Joint Female Labour Council should consider ideological and practical problems from many aspects and present suggestions and proposals for their solution.

Briefly, the aims of the project were:
to collect, structure, and distribute material of an experimental, scientific, statistical, etc. nature, from experience and from literature and the like, which could clarify and advance the work concerned;
to serve the schools — administration, planning, instruction, guidance, etc. — with this data bank; as well as
to serve the institutions for training and further training of teachers and other persons inside and outside school who take part in education and guidance;
to assist with the corresponding information in the developmental work concerning curricula, syllabi, teaching aids, etc.;
to encourage responsible persons and institutions inside and outside school to further scientific or other forms of developmental work in the field, thereby assisting the representatives for schools and education to realize the intentions in the curricula;
to find forms for combining the efforts of school authorities with the corresponding labour of other responsible authorities and/or groups and organizations.
The project was intended to work with documentation, observation schools (pilot studies), teaching experiments, etc., and more specialized studies such as studies of which factors induce girls to be less interested, or have less aptitude, than boys in physics and technology, or which factors are taken into account when boys and girls choose a practical vocation.

A team worked on the documentation and development of curricula. Summer courses of a pilot character were to have been held. Study material for parental meetings had to be edited, etc. When collecting data for all this work it was necessary to consider such fields as human biology and medicine, anthropology and cross-cultural studies, psychology, pedagogics, sociology, economy, literature, arts, technology, etc.

In the summer of 1975 the 'sex role project' published 'A freer choice — equality-programme for schools' (Vestin 1975). The proposals are now being considered by school authorities, teacher training colleges, and many other institutions and organizations. During autumn/winter 1976–7 the opinions and proposals from the field as well as from the Board of Education (and other official organizations) has to be summarized and considered. The Government will then decide their standpoint and ask Parliament, if necessary, for changes in laws, curricula, etc.

Part One of the report describes the development and socialization of the distinctions made between the sexes, as seen by different specialists. One chapter is devoted to the reasons why sex roles appeared in the first place — the old chestnut of heredity and environment. A brief description is given of the physical and mental manifestations of sex roles and of their reflection in different forms of human behaviour. The programme chapters also include factual summaries on certain points.

The project was deliberately focused on facts and viewpoints capable of shedding light on current conditions and interpretations of facts and values — for instance, aspects of sexual differences and role patterns as evidenced by research and by personal observation. As the work proceeded, it became more and more obvious that people's ideas as to what forms of behaviour are genetically determined and what forms constitute variations between members of the same sex are not always very well founded. People (including school representatives) invariably state a series of entirely superfluous categorizations into masculine and feminine, often through sloppiness of speech and with reference to trivialities which, taken together, can have a certain effect.

Our ideas concerning what suits men and women respectively are not incomprehensible: they are reflections of a past age and outdated patterns of life. Often they are based on an understandable confusion of male and female with masculine and feminine. The report opens with an introductory section on terminology. Throughout the report we tried to maintain a distinction between features and characteristics which exist for biological reasons, those which are acquired (learned), those which have been allotted us through the structure of society and those which are solely concerned with predominance (a majority of men or a majority of women) in courses of training or study, in occupations, and in different positions.

Clearly we must distinguish between sexual identity, which is a fairly stable ingredient of the personality of a boy or girl, and the sex role, which is more changeable and ductile. This partly has to do with the tact and care with which we must meet newcomers (and their parents) to our education in this field.

In the second part of the report the need for change is stressed. This need is discussed together with related issues. The background view is geared to the programme section. An outline is given of the pros and cons of existing roles and of the view of humanity and society on which curricular proposals and alterations need to be based. But there are limits to the action we can take, which in turn restricts the scope available for change. The exact location of the boundaries is very much a matter of values and priorities.

Misunderstandings often arise concerning the implications of changes in sex roles. In particular it must be emphasized that there is no question of denying the existence of male and female qualities. Nor is there any question of denying the happiness that can be derived from conjugal life, the family, and children — on the contrary, the needs and wellbeing of children are among the principal motives for altering sex roles.

But the role of the father needs to be emphasized more, while that of the mother needs to be correspondingly deglorified. It should also be added that the object of the exercise is not to 'drive all women out of the home, put all their children in public nurseries and force everybody to get a job'. The aim is to give both men and women the opportunity and the right to go out to work *and* still have time and energy left over for their families and children.

The fact remains, however, that both men and women need to be emancipated from a great deal of the compulsion implied by the labels of masculine and feminine. Women are subjected to a more palpable discrimination, and our very economy is partly based on the existence of sex roles. In so far as society must be prepared for a perpetuation of sex roles, it will be up to future generations to work for changes in this respect, for instance through the medium of politics and the trade union movement. It is the task of schools to equip students in such a way that they will be both willing and able to work to this end. The curriculum requires school work to be conducted accordingly.

A large part of the report is devoted to proposals and suggestions concerning different ways and means to start or support changes in sex roles and social, psychological, and economic conditions in and out of school. Although it is not easy, one must definately try to avoid stressing approaches and actions. In this section the report deals with all kinds of teaching questions. Some special consideration is devoted to the use of language, the question of natural sciences and technology, handicraft, and physical education (which are sexually segregated after the middle level of comprehensive school), the problems of making technology and nursing compulsory subjects for both boys and girls, ways to make practical classes instruct both boys and girls to cope with daily practical skills, and to give a grounding for all manual skills. Consideration is also paid to the school as model of society in terms of occupations and functions dominated by men and women respectively, and also to the pedagogical structure and physical environment of school. The members of the project maintain that it should be a source of strength to schools to be able to alter patterns in their own sphere — as a

reflection on current sex roles in society at large. Pupils need good examples in their daily school life.

Attention is paid to study and vocational guidance. This can be made more effective if it is started as early as junior level, with more frequent study visits, discussions concerning occupations for boys and girls, and so forth. Increased vocational guidance in comprehensive school can be partly of a steered nature, and proposals to this effect are also made regarding upper secondary school. On the other hand, study and vocational guidance cannot be expected to have much effect as long as a host of other influences drive girls in one direction and boys in another, for instance as regards the main responsibility for the domestic role and for leadership functions. Great attention will have to be paid to this point in school work.

One important item on the programme concerns the basic and in-service training of school personnel as well as parents and adults in general. Partnership in various forms and in various sectors is also proposed with institutions and groups outside school. This is absolutely essential if the initiatives taken by schools are to have any effect, one of the main themes of the report being that spot measures are unlikely to have more than a temporary or superficial effect. Thoroughgoing consultation and agreement are needed between different parties, not least as regards the priorities given by authorities and other pressure groups to their resources of personnel, time, and finance.

Curricula and syllabuses are usually accompanied by supplements which go into greater detail concerning methods, progression, etc. in the light of the goals and main teaching items for the subject or subject area concerned. The project has compiled a description of goals containing proposed amendments to the Education Act, 'Goals and guidelines' and other documents. These proposals concern the duty of the school management to promote equality of status between men and women, as well as the inclusion in the curriculum of the question of school as a total environment with a bearing on sex roles among students. Various detailed proposals in this 'supplement chapter' concern the comprehensive school and upper secondary school curricula, teaching materials and a documentation term. Goal definitions, a check list for educational publishers and teachers, and a rough outline of progression are presented in appendix form. Consideration is also given to the question of objectiveness in textbooks. A new series of textbooks (for the three levels in basic schools and useful also for nursery and upper secondary schools) is being produced with financial and editorial help from the sex role project. It is also intended that the report itself, with its appendixes and supplements (including those from the 'model schools'), should provide a more versatile aid to teaching and in-service training pending the completion of the manual. The plan is to keep the latter up to date by issuing periodical supplements. It is also necessary to have a *policy* for *actions* for realizing a programme as a whole and in detail.

PROPOSALS RELATED TO DIFFERENT LEVELS OF DECISION-MAKING

The report and programme chapters are rounded off with a survey of desirable measures (addressed to the Government and Riksdag [The Parliament], SÖ [The National Board of Education], the individual Local Education Authority, or the individual teacher). The proposals according relate to three levels of decision making. It is important to realize that a number of proposals concern measures which are decided on by individuals, who can therefore accept or reject them according to their personal situation. This is very much the case with matters concerning teaching content, contacts with colleagues and parents, one's own in-service training, etc. Some of the administrative or organizational proposals may be easier to put into effect if two other sets of proposals are carried through, namely those of the 'SIA' Commission (SIA = 'the internal organization of schools) on the internal organization of schools and those of the 'SSK' Commission (SSK = the schools, the State, and the municipalities).

A programme as wide-ranging as that presented here is bound to combine the visionary approach with minor adjustments and changes of principle with highly practical, specific alterations. This is in the nature of the subject. Sex roles are acted out in broad social contexts, in private life and by the individual. Unlike other, more limited problem areas, they concern everybody, and to a great extent they also concern children who are not yet born. Care and consideration must be combined with a certain boldness. The members of the project do not consider this balancing trick to be entirely beyond the bounds of possibility.

In conclusion, in more specific terms, the essentials of some of the goals can be outlined as follows:

Proposals at immediate level — basic demands

1. It can be made a basic requirement of teaching and guidance for schools to ensure that *every boy* and *every girl* is in some context or other given information about, an opportunity to discuss and — preferably — arrive at a personal opinion concerning sexual identity, sex roles, and the social conditions by which sex roles are reflected. A sex role which may constrict the individual personality admittedly derived from biological reality but is perhaps above all a product of learning and social expectations. Students must have the chance of discussing possible remedies for the lack of equality between men and women.

2. In response to a second fundamental requirement, schools can arrange instruction and contacts with working life (theoretical and practical introduction to working life) in such a way as to enable *every boy* and *every girl* at some point during their school career to try occupations that are dominated by the *opposite sex*. Practical experience of this kind will impart greater substance to discussions concerning sex roles.

3. Schools can stipulate that their own educational, physical, and personal structure — at present displaying much the same patterns as the community at large — must be revised so that they are more conducive to the equalization of sex roles. There are many school sectors which are dominated by boys or girls, men or women, and which are therefore unsuitable models for the adult roles of young people at school. This applies to alternative subjects, teacher and school management recruitment, the structure of other school personnel, school buildings etc.

4. Schools should be able to assume that all their staff members, school management included, have acquired (in their basic training) or will acquire (by means of in-service training) a knowledge of pedagogics in general and their own subject area/school level in particular, as well as a knowledge of the implications of sex roles for the individual, the family, and society. One extremely important factor in this context is an awareness of one's own attitudes and values in this sector and of the importance of one's own role for the pupil's process of identification.

5. Schools can and should take the initiative in establishing cooperation with others. An equality programme in school cannot be put into effect without consultation and collaboration with many parties outside the school. If students can also be induced to help establish and maintain outward contact of this kind on a formal or informal basis, so much the better. Among other things it is important to avoid a predominance of either sex in all organizations concerned with discussion and decision making, e.g. joint committees, the organization of relationships between school and working life, and school management committees.

Some measures requiring central/ministerial decisions:

6. Additions and amendments to the Education Act and to the 'goals and guidelines' for school work. A clearer statement of the equality programme is needed, for instance with regard to school as a total environment.

7. Certain alterations to the structure of senior level and upper secondary school, possibly entailing alterations to time schedules, the aim being to make it easier for boys and girls to choose more independently of sex role conventions and to gain more varied experience.

8. Wider practical vocational guidance, facilitating both completely free choices and a controlled period in which boys try their hand at 'girls' jobs' and vice versa. If possible, more practical elements in the work of upper secondary schools as well.

9. Experiments involving certain sex quotas. Proposals concerning experimental activities. Various means should be tried of improving the admission prospects of the 'minority sex'.

10. Information and training measures for school personnel, parents, etc. (These have already started.)

11. The establishment of documentation services in association with other authorities and organizations,

including Nordic bodies and (to a certain extent) on an international basis.

12. Financial and personnel resources to facilitate a second stage, comprising research and development, evaluation planning, special experimental measures, etc.

SOME CONCLUSIONS

One of the main themes of the report and draft programme from the project is that each boy and girl must be given instruction and insight concerning his/her role in working life and society as well as his/her role in family life. Besides being a matter of equality and justice, this is very much a question of the wellbeing of children and individuals — and therefore of society as a whole.

When trying to change attitudes and behaviour with a view to equality (not similarity!) one must not confuse identity and role. Even if the 'core gender identity' is intertwined with sex role stereotypes one must try — when small boys and girls start school — not to disturb their security as a boy or a girl. As a teacher one has to observe and diagnose their stereotypes and very cautiously begin to question them. The same applies in contacts with parents: respect for the individual and a careful approach.

The role of education is partly to give young people sufficient security and self-esteem to act against the traditional expectations of how boys and girls ought to be and behave. One has to teach them to differentiate biological and acquired traits (and that is not at all easy), and to understand and cope with roles which may not fit their personal disposition. As a teacher you also have to provide information about and debate different forms of discrimination — material and mental. But this is where the trouble starts — who is discriminated against, from which aspects, and by whose values? By and large, it is women throughout the world who are discriminated against most. Her 'value' is lower than the man's.

Which is the sex that is discriminated against? Could it not be the sex which has (and perhaps finds it satisfying) to make money, to make a career, to take difficult decisions, to take part in or perhaps stimulate war and violence, to be instrumentally strong and brave ... if not, he is not a 'real man'. He misses out on the closeness of children, and warm, soft personal relationships that may not be 'useful' or result in him making more money. When the female situation is discussed, the observer often starts with male values: the male way of

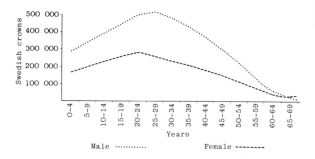

FIG. 35.7.   How the periodical *Bankvarlden* (Banking World) esteemed men and women in 'lifetime cost' Valines in 1970 (*Bankvarlden* 1970).

life is the ideal, the criteria of how the role should be formed. Today one has to try to combine the best in the male and the female role in a proportion to fit *the individual*. The sex identification (the feeling 'I am a man', 'I am a woman') should be strong enough to admit the individual to take whatever role he/she lives.

School authorities, as well as other responsible authorities and organizations, must in my opinion debate just these basic values of masculinity and femininity at all levels in society, and try to initiate this debate in their own fields. It is not sufficient just to provide instruction *about* sex roles, but they must also *alter* the sex-role pattern among students *and personnel*, train young people in the tasks of the opposite sex, and arrive at a balanced distribution in all sorts of studies, jobs, interests, and status among younger and older members of school society.

We must help young people to get rid of *our* prejudices.

POSTSCRIPT

This conference — and especially Dr. Lazarus — discussed the stress which could result from altering the sex roles. I can today underline the fact: it is stressing to alter the personal situation in favour of a new, even if you understand the importance of a change. The debate in Sweden is by and large in favour of taking also rather radical steps to create equality between the sexes. But to avoid serious stress effects it is necessary to be tactful, careful, understanding, to take your time.... School and education must work — in my opinion — with softness where other groups can afford to be more tough.

REFERENCES

BANKVÄRLDEN (1970). **5**.

BROSTRÖM, L. and GUSTAFSSON, B. (1973). *Vilken inställning har gymnasieskolelever könsrollsfrågan?* [Attitudes among students in high-school to sex roles]. Mjölby, Sweden.

DAHLGREN, H. and WALLIN, E. (1971). *Attityder till manligt och kvinnligt bland elever på grundskolans högstadium* [Attitudes to masculinity and femininity among students in the upper level in the compulsory school]. Göteborg, Sweden.

ENGLUND, K., MATTIESEN, E., and ÅNEVALL, K. (1974). *Könsrollsuppfattningar på dagis* [Attitudes to sex roles in the nursery school]. Örebro, Sweden.

────── (1969). *Läroplan för grundskolan 1969* [Common recommendations] (Decided by the National Board of Education).

RIKSDAG (1969, 1970). *Läroplan för grndskolan 1969; Läroplan för gymnasieskolan 1970* [Goal and Directions for schools] (Decided by Parliament).

SANDBERG, E. (ed.) (1975). 'The goal is equality.' Paper presented at the FN Conference, Mexico City.

────── (1975). Skolöverstyrelsens könsrollsprojekt: Ett friare val — jämställdhetsprogram för skolan [A freer choice — programme for equality within education]. Stockholm. (Short summary also available.)

STATISTICAL CENTRAL BUREAU (1976).

VESTIN, M. (1974). *Könsroller, studie- och yrkesval.* Stockholm, Sweden.

────── (1975).

──────, HÖRNQUIST, and SALMSON (1976). Some information concerning sex role questions and programs for development of equality between men and women, particularly within the field of education. Report to UNESCO, Geneva.

────── (1971). U 68. Rapport 2. Val av utbildning och yrke. Stockholm.

36. THE REPRODUCTIVE RELATIONSHIP: A MENTAL HEALTH VIEW

FERDINAND R. HASSLER and NORMAN SARTORIUS

Valid and reliable data about mental health aspects of human reproduction are very scarce. A number of studies have been done but there are very few which have been well documented and from which definite consequences can be drawn.

Why is this so? It is difficult to imagine that this very important field has escaped the interest of experts working in human reproduction and in behavioural sciences. Psychiatrists and behavioural scientists have done research into most aspects of human functioning; the experts in the field of human reproduction are people with wide visions and deep concerns about the populations with whom they work.

One of the most likely explanations for this situation is the sharp delineation which exists between experts working in these two fields. They each pursue their own main interests and traditionally links between them are weak. Sexologists are working between the fields but their number is small and the number of experts in the other fields who accept them even smaller.

The regrettable lack of information in this field could perhaps partially be explained by the practical methodological obstacles that any research in this field has to face. The complexity of both human reproduction and mental health are such that work on definitions of concepts and development of methods of quantitative measurement progress very slowly.

Even simple demographic data lose their meaning when they are mentioned in discussions about this field. Marital status tells us little, either about reproductive behaviour or about psychosexual functioning. The problems become greater when one moves to complex terms such as motivation, attitudes, the process of decision making or mental wellbeing.

Sociocultural and economic factors play an enormously important role in definitions of concepts in this field and consequently in any research which is undertaken. The term 'adolescence' for example, is used very often but its definition is poor. In most instances adolescence is defined by chronological age and it is usually said that a person between the ages of 15 and 19 is an adolescent. But is this really so? A girl of 8 or 9 in India who takes full care of her 2-year-old sister cannot be compared with a girl of the same age who goes to school in Europe. A young man of 16 who is employed and father of a child in Indonesia has a different life pattern from a boy in high-school in Holland. In Teheran, for example, a few years ago, 8 per cent of all divorced and not re-married women were aged 15–19, and in this age group there were almost 30 times more women than men (Sartorius 1971). It is easy to see that there are at least three definitions of adolescence: the biological,

the psychological, and the sociocultural definition. All three of them vary considerably from country to country or even within the same country.

In addition to the difficulties of definition of terms there is the difficulty of disentangling the components of the reproductive relationship and defining factors influencing it. The economic and sociocultural development of different countries has a considerable influence on the patterns of human relationships in the community. These relationships in turn are the decisive factors in the structure of the reproductive relationship. The impact of assuming responsibility for a family differs according to age when such responsibility is assumed and so does the stress which this responsibility may represent for the individual. Sociocultural factors have a considerable influence on the stability of the formalized union. It is very difficult to identify and measure the different factors hidden in the vague term 'culture' and this complexity is another reason for the absence of data obtained by controlled and prospective studies.

The cultural diversity of sexuality and reproduction is strikingly contrasted by two anthropological studies recently reported in *Psychology Today*. In this article, Marshall and Messenger (1971) report the practices of the inhabitants of two islands — one a small island off the coast of Ireland and the other a spot of land called Mangaia, the southernmost of the Cook Islands in the South Pacific.

The sexual culture of the Irish island is described as follows: sex is never discussed in the home when children are about; almost no mothers advise their daughters. Boys are better advised than girls, but the former learn about sex informally from older boys and men, as well as from what they see animals do. Adults rarely give sexual instruction to youth, believing that after marriage nature takes its course. The average marriage age is 36 for men and 25 for women, and 29 per cent never marry. The men share the belief that sexual intercourse is debilitating. They will desist from sex the night before they are to do a job that takes great energy. Sex is seen as a duty by women, that must be endured and there is much evidence that the female orgasm is unknown or at least considered a deviant response. Men do not approach women sexually during menstruation or for 4 months after childbirth; a woman is considered dangerous to the male at these times. Secrecy surrounds elimination. There is a lack of a 'dirty-joke' tradition. Dancing allows little body contact. Clothing is always changed in private, sometimes under the bedcovers, and islanders ordinarily sleep in their underclothes. They continue to wear them during coitus, which is practised only in the male superior position and is invariably initiated by the man.

At the other end of the spectrum, on Mangaia in the Cook Islands, sex for pleasure and for procreation is reported as a principal concern of the population. The islanders demonstrate that concern in the startling number of children born to unmarried parents, and in the statistics on frequency of orgasm and the numbers of sexual partners. A flick of the eye, a raised eyebrow in a crowd, can lead to intercourse without a word. Coitus is the usual outcome of heterosexual contact and frequently precedes personal affection. There is sensuousness and open provocation in the local dance. The folk tales feature explicitly detailed accounts of sexual acts and organs. Girls learn about sex and develop the appetite for it at 12 or 14 years, about the time of the beginning of menses. Most boys do not commence their sexual life until they are 13 or 14 and have undergone a superincision. A male 'expert' performs the superincision and then imparts sexual knowledge and training to the neophyte — later locating an 'experienced' woman who practises various acts and positions on him. Particularly stressed is the ability to bring a partner to climax several times before he reaches his own, and to achieve mutual orgasm. Mangaian men generally agree that the really important thing in copulation is to give pleasure to his partner — so that it is the woman's orgasm which gives the man a special thrill, separate from his own orgasm. It is believed that women must 'learn orgasm' and that a man who teaches a woman to have it is a 'good man'. Parents encourage their daughter to have sexual experience with several men. They want her to find the man who is the most congenial — among those whose other social and material assets make them eligible as potential husbands. Illegitimacy does not carry the social stigma in Mangaia that it does in the Western world. Two areas of widespread extramarital activity are openly acknowledged. One is the woman's inclination to return to the man with whom she first enjoyed intercourse. The other is the belief that a normal human being must have a regular outlet, so that for example, men who are away travelling are not condemned for selecting other women.

PSYCHIATRIC PERSPECTIVE

In psychiatry much has been written — particularly by psychodynamically oriented writers — about the pathogenic role of sexual functioning in the genesis of psychosis, psychoneurosis, personality disorder, and the psychophysiologic disorders. Harper's review (Harper 1959), for example, describes 36 theories of psychology and psychiatry; most of these schools of thought place considerable emphasis on aspects of sexuality.

Much information is becoming available also regarding the biological aspects of sexuality. Data is being accumulated and theories developed regarding the control of behaviour by the brain through such mechanisms as the limbic system. However, at this stage it is difficult to state practical implications and much work remains to be done regarding the neurophysiology, neurochemistry, and genetic aspects of sexuality.

It is probably true, as noted in a study by Pinderhughes (1972), that most patients and most psychiatrists believe there are significant interrelationships between many psychiatric disorders and sexual functions. Pinderhughes also states that there is the general feeling that psychiatrists should, and indeed frequently do, discuss these relationships and problems with their patients. However, he noted that there was no general agreement on the nature, content, or usefulness of these discussions; nor is there a reliable, organized body of knowledge that indicates the degree or the circumstances in which sexual functioning may contribute to the development of psychiatric disorders or may be affected by the psychiatric conditions. Many of the beliefs held by psychiatrists and patients and encountered in the psychiatric literature have not been substantiated and many of the beliefs are in sharp conflict with one another. All too often professional beliefs seem to be based more upon an indoctrination process rather than upon data obtained by sound research.

PSYCHOLOGICAL ASPECTS OF PARENTHOOD AND PREGNANCY

The problem of the unwanted child has received some attention in psychiatric literature in the past. In recent times attention is switching to the problem of the unwanted parent. The generation gap and the struggle between generations are the topic of a number of studies but little definite information has come out of these. There is general agreement that the structure of families has changed. (There is also agreement that the change has been faster in the last few decades than ever before, although there is little evidence supporting such contentions). In the United States, for example, the proportion of women married at a given age has increased over the years. In 1940, 61 per cent of women over 15 were married; in 1968 the proportion was higher (68 per cent). Almost 90 per cent of women in their late 20s were married in 1968; in 1940 this figure was significantly lower (74 per cent vs 84 per cent). As Rossi (1972) points out, people are not against the institution of marriage: if they divorce they will most probably get married again. However, the tendency to divorce has certainly increased, even in families with children.

It seems that the happiness of both partners and a harmonious marriage has a higher value than before: on the other hand consideration of views and interests of other people (including children) and social norms, including e.g. religion, seem to have lost some of their importance. It is very difficult to judge whether such a trend is beneficial or socially dangerous.

The same applies to the importance of another, once obligatory criterion of a successful marriage — that of having children. A number of surveys of the families questioned said that they wanted to have children; yet the same surveys showed that families now resort rather more freely to abortion, contraception, and permanent sterilization. In a number of countries the need to have children has been modified and although most couples express the desire to have children this is with the proviso that they can control the number of children and the time when they are born.

The problem of motivation for or against pregnancy is of crucial importance. Sociocultural pressures, personality characteristics, and previous experience play an important role in the decision-making process, but the number of studies about factors influencing the decision-making process is small and the studies rarely withstand rigorous scientific testing. The motivation for contraception and acceptance of family-planning measures has received some attention: the motivation for or against pregnancy much less. This motivation undoubtedly varies according to the level of socio-economic development; the availability, the cost, and safety of contraceptive measures; and the personality of the user and their perception of the factors of importance for decisions.

The situation is equally unclear in the field of choice of birth-control methods. In a number of countries, the predominant measure to space and limit the number of children is abortion. The decision to select this 'post-conception' family planning is influenced by a variety of factors, none of which is simple and easily measurable. A number of studies on the psychological and physiological consequences of abortion have been carried out, but the results of such studies are frequently contradictory. In all cases, abortion is a physical stress and even if a termination of an unwanted pregnancy may be a relief for the unwilling mother and father, physical complications may occur. The role of the psychiatrist in the field of abortion has been mainly one of providing a sanction for an otherwise prohibited measure. Surveys have shown that many of the 'medical' indications for abortion have been psychiatric, although it is more than likely that most of the people who have received a psychiatric diagnosis to justify a legal abortion were no more mentally abnormal than the rest of the population. It has been reported that the frequency of severe mental disorder following abortion is low; however, it may be dangerous to draw conclusions about the mental health of the women who had abortions from data provided by reports which are available for legal abortions because of the large number of illegal abortions about which we know very little.

Various psychological states in the mother have been described to influence the course of pregnancy, labour, and delivery but results of the investigations in this field are not conclusive. Extramarital pregnancy, for example, has frequently been suggested as a cause of premature delivery, i.e. the rejection of the foetus. Unfortunately a similar aetiology has been advanced for postmature delivery.

A number of psychological symptoms have been described as appearing in pregnant women. The frequency of such symptoms varies from survey to survey and ranges from 0 per cent to 80 per cent of all pregnant women. The variation probably reflects the characteristics of the observer and the culture and definition rather than the true differences between populations. The type of symptoms described in pregnancy varies considerably: from hypersensitivity of taste and smell to emotional ability and irritability and preference for certain kinds of food. It has been claimed that many women report a positive improvement of health in the second half of pregnancy but it is difficult to state whether this feeling of wellbeing results from the disappearance of discomfort experienced in early pregnancy, from the anticipation of a wanted child, or from psychophysiological changes. More severe cases of psychological disorder have been described under the blunderbuss term 'post-partum psychosis'. The frequency of this condition varies from report to report — with recent studies showing up to 7 cases per 1000 live births. Older studies have shown lower numbers. Different types of psychopathological syndromes have been described: schizophrenia-like conditions, affective disorders, exogenous reaction-type syndromes, and, in some cases, a neurotic or psychopthic-type reaction. Obstetric complications seem to play a minor role in the occurrence, but occurrence of mental disorder in the family or previous mental disease seem to be of importance. It seems that the condition is more likely to be found in women over 30, in unmarried women, and in women who have their first child.

Studies of possible psychological complications that occur when a contraceptive method is applied appear to be of great importance. This is particularly true for methods which result in permanent sterilization such as vasectomy and tubectomy. Practically nothing is known about the later psychological wellbeing of people who have the operations. Some reports seem to indicate that as many as one-quarter of men who have been vasectomized experience psychological disorder varying in kind from mild neurosthenic syndromes, impotence, and marital discord to serious disorders such as psychosis (N. N. Wig personal communication). The results of studies directed to this problem are often of doubtful value because of methodological shortcomings and restrictions inherent in the study of phenomena in this field. These include cultural taboos, questions of the right to personal privacy, shame, and shyness as well as the lack of personnel who could adequately assess the situation.

Another problem which has received relatively little attention is the relationship between the type of personality and type of contraception chosen. It may well be that volunteers for vasectomy already have psychological difficulties. Alternatively the opposite could be true. We have no data which would direct us in either direction.

The recent years have witnessed a considerable increase in publications concerned with mental health aspects of human reproduction. A review of these reveals that:

(1) although a large number of studies have been carried out few have resulted in reliable data;
(2) the number of studies done by teams composed of mental health specialists and family-planning specialists is very small;
(3) the definitions of phenomena which are being studied in this field vary from study to study and from researcher to researcher;
(4) there do not seem to exist comparative cross-cultural studies in which the researchers utilized a uniform methodology;
(5) although there is some data concerning serious mental disorders influencing the human reproductive relationship there is little information about the role that 'mild disorders' play in this respect;
(6) the number of longitudinal studies with clearly defined aims and long-term follow-ups of cohorts of users of family-planning methods is growing but there are few concerning mental health.

GUIDELINES FOR INTERVENTION

The following guidelines† for members of the health professions, educators, legislators, and administrative persons reflect the general thinking of many mental health workers in the Western societies, who have written most proliferously. These 'guidelines' should not be perceived as definitive knowledge, but merely as an attempt to express a 'nodal point' reflecting current thinking and serving as a basis for discussion.

1. Sexual behaviour is most productively viewed as a function of interpersonal relationships and reflecting the total life pattern and experience of an individual. In this regard, it is helpful to view sexual and reproductive behaviour as representing a merging of many different dimensions, with great variations in the experience of each person. Thus, when working with or thinking about individuals, it is not helpful to classify a particular activity or sexual act as normal or abnormal, as positive or negative, or as masculine or feminine.

2. Each individual has a right to choose those manifestations of sexuality that he prefers. However, since culture vary widely in the behaviour they accept, each individual must be prepared to pay the price for choices which are unacceptable to the social group in which he lives.

†Suggested in part by the report, 'Marriage, the family, and human sexuality in medical education' (1966) (Bowman Gray School of Medicine, Winston-Salem, North Carolina) and the report, 'Sex and the college student' (1965) (Group for the Advancement of Psychiatry, New York).

3. People usually have the capacity to fulfil the biological needs of sexuality and reproduction with a minimum of outside intervention. However, assistance in the psychological and emotional spheres seems to be fairly frequently needed in many societies, and should be made available in the framework of general health — and other community services.

4. Professionals coming into a therapeutic relationship with others have the responsibility of helping their clients to understand the alternatives among which they may choose and to point out the implications of their choices in terms of the social and personal values of their habitat. Therapists have neither a right nor a responsibility to make the choice for any individual — other than their own selves of course — except where self-injury or exploitation of one individual or a group by another is concerned.

5. The capacity for discretion constitutes an element of mature judgement. Sexual activity that is not private is likely to be disturbing to others, so that a person's failure to insure the privacy of a sexual act places it outside the private domain and into the realm of public concern. On the other hand, a person's privacy requires respect and activities privately practised with apropriate attention to the sensitivities of others, need not be of direct concern to society.

6. People who become involved in a very bizarre behaviour or repeated sexual transgressions may be suffering from an underlying mental or emotional disorder. Referral to appropriate sources of treatment or counselling should not, of course, be limited to situations of extreme behaviour, but should occur also during times of temporary stress, as a means of promoting normal development, and hopefully, mental health.

7. Health services and other 'helping' agencies should provide as a regular part of their programme ready access for their clients to confidential consultation regarding problems related to human sexuality. Immediate medical assistance should be available to people concerning areas such as family planning, questions related to actual or possible pregnancy, venereal diseases, and sexual inadequacies.

8. In most instances consultation by a well-trained person will be helpful in distinguishing between persons with mild or transient manifestations who are likely to be helped by brief therapy and persons with conditions based on serious impairment. Although treatment can often be exceedingly helpful in various sexual problems of a psychological nature, it can achieve little result without the motivated participation of the individual. Additionally, it should not be assumed that therapy or counselling can be relied upon to prevent or even to alleviate future deviant behaviour, thus periods of repeated assistance may be necessary.

9. Staff members of units providing assistance can often receive substantial help in their usual daily work with their patients or clients through consultations and in-service training programmes that provide technically

sound information and open discussion of conscious and unconscious factors influencing behaviour and value systems.

10. Sex education is increasingly seen by many as an important preventive measure. Since countries have widely differing attitudes about instruction in sexual matters, no specific formulation of subject matter will fit the variety of moral, ethical, and religious positions that various societies reflect. However, where courses are taught, it is suggested that they should (a) clarify for participants their personal set of values, society's position, and expectation, and the individual's integration of these two; (b) identify and correct misconceptions by providing an opportunity for open and objective discussion on any and all sexual issues; and (c) provide factual information regarding areas such as human sexual physiology, contraceptive methods and techniques, development of interpersonal relationships, and means of acquiring social-coping skills.

AREAS FOR FUTURE RESEARCH

The survey of literature and contacts with people and agencies working in the field indicated that there is a number of topics which could be of great interest and considerable scientific importance if they were studied with proper methodology and by qualified researchers. These topics include:

(1) the meaning and perception of stressful events in pregnancy;

(2) the 'positive' effect of pregnancy on mental health;

(3) the association between hormonal and psychiatric changes during pregnancy;

(4) studies of factors contributing to infertility and reaction to infertility;

(5) the change of roles of both partners in the reproductive relationship in the course of adolescence, parenthood, and old age;

(6) personality characteristics contributing to the choice of contraceptive method and personality characteristics contributing to good and poor effect of the contraceptive.

At least initially, future research should concentrate on:

(a) the development of valid and reliable instruments and procedures acceptable and applicable in the context of the particular culture in which the studies have been carried out;

(b) studies directed towards the assessment of prevalence and incidence of psychiatric complications connected with family-planning procedures;

(c) study of factors that play a role in the major decisions in human reproductive relationship (e.g. marriage, abortion, etc.);

(d) long-term prospective controlled comparative studies aiming at the assessment of the role of sociocultural factors on the reproductive relationship.

REFERENCES

EYSENCK, H. J. (1971). Introverts, extroverts and sex. *Psychol. Today*, **4**, (8).

HARPER, R. A. (1959). *Psychoanalysis and psychotherapy: 36 systems*. Englewood Cliffs, New Jersey.

KINSEY, A. C., POMEROY, W. B., and MARTIN, C. E. (1948). *Sexual behaviour in the human male*. Philadelphia, Pennsylvania.

MARSHALL, D. S. (1971). Sexuality — two anthropological studies, too much in Mangaia. *Psychol. Today*, **4**, (9).

MASTERS, W. H. and JOHNSON, V. E. (1966). *Human sexual response*. Boston, Massachusetts.

MESSENGER, J. C. (1971). Sexuality — two anthropological studies, the lack of the Irish. *Psychol. Today*, **4**, (9).

PINDERHUGHES, C. A., GRACE, E. B., and REYNA, L. J. (1972). Psychiatric disorders and sexual functioning. *Amer. J. Psychiat.*, **128**, 1276–82.

ROSSI, A. S. (1972). Family development in a changing world. *Amer. J. Psychiat.*, **128**, 1057.

SARTORIUS, N. (1971). Psychosomatische Störungen des Adoleszenz: Epidemiologische Erforschung. *Psychosomat. Med.*, **3**, 93–102.

37. TOPICS FOR FUTURE RESEARCH ON SEX ROLES AND RELATIONSHIPS

JOHN MONEY

1. Diagnostic observation of coitus to gain improved understanding of the relationship of the partners, especially partners who are dissatisfied.

2. Classification of human sexual/erotic types, for more precise description and for improved matching and guidance of partners.

3. Detailed documentation of the relationship between erotic imagery and erotic practice, with special attention to the biographical origin of erotic imagery.

4. A study of the lives of people engaging in unconventional sexual activities, e.g. promiscuity, consensual adultery, polygamy, communal sex and family life, group sex, and bisexualism, in order to ascertain the long-term effects.

5. Biographical long-term, sexual/erotic studies of individuals of known special history, e.g. prenatal excess androgenization or deandrogenization, or early childhood sexual trauma.

6. Long-term prospective studies of the outcome, in adolescence and adulthood, of childhood gender anomalies and/or unusual erotic experiences.

7. A more honest and frank documentation of the sexuality of childhood.

8. Experimental studies in childhood of, for example, the response to, and long-term effects of seeing erotic representations as part of a programme of sex education.

9. The long-term effects of removing traditional taboos on childhood sex play in relation to the sex education of childhood — for example in special experimental communities, such as the kibutzim of Israel.

10. More complete ethnographic documentation than has so far usually been recorded of the relationship between childhood sexual mores and adult erotic and sexual partnerships — domestic ethnography included.

11. Psychosocial and biographical field studies of changing sexual mores, including a study of women's and men's liberation.

12. Psychosocial and biographical field studies of the use and/or neglect of contraception prior to or after marriage, with special attention to the long-term effect.

13. Psychophysiological studies of hormonal contraceptive effects.

14. Studies of the sexual partnership and family life when one of the pair has an atypical sexual status or injury, e.g. intersexuality, transsexualism, paraplegia, irreversible impotence, traumatic genital loss, and so on.

15. Development of prosthetic devices and procedures for the genitally handicapped of all ages.

16. Use of hormones, e.g. anti-androgens, and other pharmacologic products as adjunctive to the treatment of severe and disabling paraphilias.

17. To parallel animal research, the development of research procedures adjunctive to open-brain surgery for identifying sexual pathways and nuclei in the human brain in psychosexual health and disease.

18. Drug-induced enhancement versus diminution of erotic sensation and orgasm.

SYNOPSIS OF GENERAL DISCUSSION

AUBREY R. KAGAN

Plenary discussion on the highlights of the papers in the previous chapters, discussion in six subgroups each day on special aspects, discussion after plenary presentation of summaries of subgroup deliberations by their respective chairmen, and post-symposium thoughts sent to the editor amounted to about 50 per cent more words than the rest of the book. Much of the argument was repetitive and scattered. The editor therefore asked me to bring together in summary form the discussion on selected topics from all the symposium sources. In doing so I have tried to give some of the flavour of forward, backward, and lateral thinking that interdisciplinary occasions of this sort inspire.

It has not always been possible to ascribe each statement to a particular person. Sometimes they did not identify themselves. Collective statements, e.g. summary reports of subgroup discussions to plenary session are often referred to without assigning origins. I apologize to those whose remarks are not acknowledged and also for any errors that may have resulted from my mis-interpretation in the course of summarizing some of the recorded statements. Some topics have had to be left out altogether. There has been no attempt to summarize all that was said.

The main headings and topics of the synopsis are:-

The Concept of Normality
Psychosocial Stressors
Mechanisms
Precursors and Disease
Sex Education
Action Now
Research Priorities

THE CONCEPT OF NORMALITY

It was considered essential to discuss this from several points of view. All agreed that *statistical* norms, such as the observed average, plus or minus one or two standard deviations, were useful. Such information is needed to know the existing state of affairs in a particular situation. Mead, Money, and Gebhard cautioned that much of the data available at the conference, were derived from 'developed' countries of the West.

Social norms

Norms of behaviour differ so greatly between societies — in some societies, Mead told us, the women do the heavy work and the musculature of men is relatively undeveloped — that it is necessary to describe social norms for each. But it is one thing to describe these for scientific purposes and another to regard them as 'established'. Bancroft warned: 'Whenever a social norm is established, particularly in relation to male/female roles, and sexual behaviour, this is likely to cause stress to some who would regard themselves as abnormal, and to provide support for others. It is therefore of importance to recognize the social implications of establishing norms and to realize that these implications are extremely complex. There has been a tendency in the past for norms to be established for scientific reasons and incorporated into a set of social norms.

The dangers of this are particularly great when society is changing its views. At such times *ideals* are often put forward in the guise of 'norms'. These new aims might result in a better life but their consequences are complex and impossible to forecast. Bancroft, Kagan, and Mead agreed that new ideals should not be accepted without prior evaluation of the consequences. Mead, reporting a subgroup discussion, said with respect to the concept of normality of sex roles and relationships:

All human societies have concepts of what constitutes an appropriate type of sexual behaviour. Here we more or less confined ourselves to the question of types of sexual behaviour and not to the whole question of roles and statuses, i.e. to such questions as deviant types of behaviour, homosexuality and so forth. It is characteristic of our own tradition to stigmatize the disapproved as abnormal.

Mead thought this was a very important point and said that every society disapproved of such behaviour in a different way.

We have invented this notion of abnormality which we apply. Almost all cultures reject male homosexuality, or insist upon it being heavily institutionalized. This may be regarded as related more to the establishment of viable hierarchies than to the question of the society's fertility rate. However, at the present time, when fertility is being devalued, homosexuality is being more tolerated than it has in the past. In very primitive societies the unmarried female state is usually not tolerated.

Mead continued to say that the question of norms for a given society needed careful definition and clarification. She said this was difficult but first her subgroup had tried to do what Dr. Money and Dr. Gebhard suggested, by considering the statistically validated means and ranges for a given population. These needed to be distinguished from the biological adequacy of that behaviour for the survival of that society. This was, Mead thought, a slightly different slant than that used by the others, because here biological function in the individual was not being discussed, but rather the possibility that the social norms of a society may violate the survival possibilities of that society, e.g. the very long periods of socially approved celibacy — the lives of monks — that are found in some societies. Next, there was a notion of the norm as the construct of social desirability. The subgroup got into major difficulties here, with, for example, the extent to which social desirability should be confused with statistical normality. Male and female relationships functioned in all societies to regulate reproductivity, childcare, mutual care, and sexual competitiveness and envy. In most stable societies, these processes were relatively self-regulated, but at times of rapid social change like the present, attempts to change particular expectations of male/female relationships could result in great individual hardship and distress.

Human response to sexual stimuli. Research in this field throws light on the establishment of sexual preference and choice of partner as a basis of individual variation; gives a background against which sexual variation can be assessed, and also upon some of the bases of individual sexual inadequacy. The sub-group reached a consensus that the enormous richness and range of variety of primate and human behaviour made it desirable to avoid in our current stage of knowledge the imposition of narrow educational objectives and male and female role relationships. It was felt very strongly that the attempt to eradicate previous inequalities in our own society over time by imposing new fixed positions, was undesirable.

Sex roles
Socially determined norms. Gebhard saw sex roles as primarily socially determined phenomena, depending mainly on physical strength on the one hand and reproductive function on the other.

Sex roles in our society are marked by rather simplistic dichotomous thinking. We think in terms of males being big, females small; males strong, females weak; males aggressive, females passive; etc. This has lead to the idea that the female who is large or strong is somehow less feminine; and that a small or a weak male is somehow less masculine. In brief, we arbitrarily assign certain attributes to each gender and then define gender according to these attributes, really circular reasoning. Obviously, these ideal traits do not suit the personalities or physiques of many people, and consequently stress is caused.

In addition, our mass media have assigned women numerous other roles and role obligations. The wife must be a companion, a business-woman, a cook and a nurse, a mother, a lover, an interior decorator, and so forth. Inability to meet all of these unattainable ideals produces in some women feelings of inadequacy, guilt, and resentment. Anthropological data show that one major determinant of sex role is age. Children are often treated much alike, but with the advent of reproductive capacity, the two genders are sharply differentiated to establishing different ideals of behaviour and dress. Many societies have puberty rites which signal diffusion of sex roles. Once, however, the reproductive years are over, there is less emphasis on the sex roles and the two genders become often much more similar in behaviour and even appearance.

'Good and bad' women. Gebhard explained that in Judeo-Christian tradition there was the concept that there were two classes of females, essentially the good female and the bad female. The Old Testament extolled the virtuous woman and condemned the harlot. This polarity of thought has led males to categorize women into (a) good women, who tend to be rather sexless mothers, whose world centres on the home and the children, the good girls whom one marries and converts into mothers; and (b) the bad women, who tend to be the sexual ones, who are enjoyed but not married. This sharp distinction still existed, particularly in Latin America and also in the Mediterranean world.

How did this division into good and bad come about in Judeo-Christian tradition? Gebhard suspected that it was borne from the ambivalence that men had towards woman in the Near East and Europe. On the one side women were viewed as mothers and the givers of food and life, and, of course, as irresistible attractions. In early agricultural societies the major deities were often female, the earth goddess, the great mother, and some of these female deities were specifically sexual, as, for example, Isis, Astorite, and Aphrodite.

On the negative side, there were four items. First of all, men resented the power of female attraction. For the sake of a female a man would risk his wealth, social position, his friendships, and even his life. Secondly, women were seen as the enemy of spirituality and religion, because, according to men, they personified sexuality and the carnal side of life. Thirdly, because women could not compete with men in terms of physical strength, they were forced to pursue their goals through persuasion, through subterfuge, deceit, and intrigue.

Males always react very negatively to such indirect, feminine, let us say, techniques. Thus the average male thinks intrigue is somehow worse than a good, clean battle, and that poison is far more evil than the sword. Fourthly, men have always been concerned about the magical qualities of females, these inexplicable creatures that give birth and who bleed and exhibit erratic behaviour during some cycle that corresponds to a lunar cycle, plus the universal fear, of course, of menstrual blood. Obviously, females are dangerous creatures. So we have this ambivalence. On the one hand there are things that are desirable and loved, and on the other hand things to worry about and dread. This, of course, reinforces that simple dichotomy of good women and bad women, and is the fallacious reasoning that impedes female/male relationships to this day.

'Romantic fallacies'. Gebhard pointed out that society continues to promote various romantic fallacies which engender stress. Some of these represent unattainable ideals, which therefore give rise to feelings of guilt and inadequacy. Others are so contrary to human inclination that subscribing to such ideas guarantees trouble. He gave a few examples. One was, that for each person there is only one true love in the world waiting to be discovered, and that it is a mistake to marry anyone else. This was obviously ridiculous. Another romantic fallacy was that you can love only one individual at a time. Two simultaneous loves must detract from one another, since a person has a limited amount of love to give. Kagan wondered how many marriages that romantic fallacy had broken. Another was that only

love justifies sexual activity, which is otherwise construed as coarse or animalistic, and so on.

Most of we males have argued against that particular fallacy. We know now, from recent research that males and females are basically alike, and that their intellectual and emotional capacities are equal. The idea that females are inherently less sexually responsive is being seriously questioned. Most of the alleged male/female differences appear to be culturally produced. While some of these culturally produced, artificial distinctions may have been socially useful back in a hunting society or an early agrarian society, many of the distinctions are now useless or injurious in an urban, technological civilization.

Money said:

I have recently come to think not so much of the Judeo-Christian tradition but one which is bigger still, and that dates from possible þre-history around the Mediterranean littoral and all around the Golden Crescent, or the Great Crescent, I mean the area in which one had the greatest manifestation of the double standard. I have a sort of hypothesis that I want you to comment on. I wondered whether this may have some relationship to the fact that this is the part of the world where cities grew first, and it is also the part of the world where slavery was very important in the development of cities, and also the part of the world where women were held in harems, so that they were really the equivalent of slaves. So there were two kinds of women.... You could only build cities in those times if you had slaves to do all the labour and I wonder if there may not be a broader, sociological connection with the sexual behaviour that we are heirs to now. And by contrast I can see a completely different tradition which Preben Hertoft has told us about in the Scandinavian countries. I found out last year when I was in Finland, to my surprise, that this tradition of 'night-courting' which the Finns translate from their language in the delightful terminology 'taking your nightlegs for a walk', actually can also be found down through Hungary and in through the French Alps in remnant form, or at least up to the nineteenth century. It seems to represent a totally different tradition of the north as compared with the Mediterranean and Near East area. Perhaps one can indeed see the great areas of the world, where still there are remnants of very ancient traditions of how the sexes meet together. I see another great difference along the Papuan/Melanesian belt, with a totally different set of customs.

Gebhard replied:

Well, you are certainly right about the Fertile Crescent area. I recall in the code of Hittite laws which must go back to about 1700 B.C. at least, they very carefully distinguished between, you might say, respectable women on one hand, and on the other hand, female slaves, who were lumped together as a group, which would bolster your argument.

Mead said that surveys being made of the distribution of song and music and language were beginning to get the very early areas of civilization well defined, certainly the northern area that came down into Korea, where the civilization was different from that in fertile countries such as North Africa in early times and the Mediterranean.

But Mead considered the confusion between shedding blood and fertility was a more important point.

When you begin to get human sacrifice, and the idea that the blood will advance and water the fields and advance the well-being of society, you begin to get very contrasting attitudes towards blood that are rather different from ones you get in these northern societies. So I think that we have to go way back, to the ambivalent attitudes towards bloodshed, and the bloodshed that is connected with defloration, and with menstruation.... We have to go back to the beginnings of incest to the idea whether you do or do not shed the blood of your own, and that this underlies the later dichotomy.

In very simple societies like New-Guinea the ambivalence could still be found. Menstrual blood was thought to be terribly dangerous, but you could also use it to cure somebody. There was a connection with female magic. You could cool it by pouring hot water on it. There was an endless series of such ambivalences connected with blood and they went way back before the cities were built.

Mead also discussed more specific ambivalences. She said that although we had discussed alternative life-styles that had recently been invented, nobody had mentioned a nun: a perfectly good alternative lifestyle within the Judeo-Christian religions. A woman could choose chastity and celibacy and have a life of her own, or be a family member, and neither one of those were evil. They were alternatives. The point was that one could not have both a family and an individual life. That dichotomy, Mead considered, had been at least as important as the dichotomy between the 'good' and the 'bad' women, and between the prostitute and the virtuous woman.

Odhnoff referred to a recent German survey on matrimony as seen from the male and female angle. The great majority of men considered marriage, kitchen, and nursery to be the highlights of happiness for the women, and a great satisfaction to themselves. While 92 per cent of the men claimed that their marriage was happy, only 19 per cent of women joined this song of praise. The rest of them complained bitterly.

Attitudes to sex. Gebhard from his surveys in the United States presented data indicating that abstinence from sexual activity was more difficult for the male than the female. Bancroft challenged the data and both agreed with Linnér that there was 'considerable individual variation'. Mead, discussing this point and the notion of 'orgasm' referred to the importance of cultural factors. She thought it was important to realize that the American conception of sex was very close to that of defaecation, and that this was the total notion of male sex in the United States. Everybody in the United States knew it was bad to be constipated: one was in very bad health, and in great distress; and sexual frustration was seen in the same way. She then considered the Chinese and Indian view of male sex, which was that it was depleting, that one was losing a vital substance.

If you can keep the vital substance in, it will nourish you and especially nourish your spiritual life, which will bloom under this cultivation. You get a totally different picture. We have a lot of material on Chinese abstinence from sex for very long

258

periods, and there is an enormous fear on the part of young men of what will happen to the essence of their nature if they loose too much of this stuff.

Mead also commented on another point that Mrs. Linnér made about the difference between some women and some men with respect to experience of orgasm. She said she had worked in societies where there was no recognition of a female orgasm whatsoever, and found few women wo knew what it was. These women knew it only individually and subjectively. Mead considered this was confirmation that orgasm was a potentiality of the female, but it did not need to be realized in a particular society at all. She told us that in 1928 the ideal of the Manus, a very compulsive anal group of people, was that a daughter slept with her father and a son slept with his mother, so that the parents never had to sleep with each other. But the men went out and captured prostitutes occasionally. Although they claimed they took no pleasure in sex, the women tried to kill the prostitutes. They were jealous of their husbands having sexual relations with anyone else. After the social revolution which like all revolutions tried to change the family and sexual life, the men were permitted to have love affairs. This was regulated. The men were expected to fall in love with a girl before they married them. After marriage they were expected to have love affairs. If a man became interested in a woman, it was her duty to sleep with him at once, to 'unfix his thought', which otherwise became 'constipated' on this woman. Mead added that, at present, the Manus were specializing in long-term adulteries. Their attitude was: It is wonderful to have a mistress. You don't have to sleep with her: wives you have to sleep with, but a mistress you can talk to.

Linnér emphasized the importance of orgasm and the recent awareness of women to the right to enjoy this but Money counselled against setting orgasm (especially simultaneous orgasm in both partners) as the objective of all sexual intercourse with the corollary that if it was not achieved sexual intercourse was inadequate.

Michael summarized the opinion of himself and others in indicating the difficulty of deciding whether orgasm occurred in female animals.

There is a problem about female orgasm, it seems to me. You know, men can't lie. Women can lie, or tell stories. I was just thinking of the whole problem of assessing the motivational state of the female, both in lower animals and in humans. We really have very little data on what there is in it for the woman in sex.

Michael added that it was relatively easy in the case of the male animal, because most of the behaviour initiative was with him and the consummatory thing was obvious. He ejaculated.

This can be looked at and scored in a behavioural situation. But there are very few situations where you can see what the consummatory thing is for the female. There are, perhaps, two species of animals, where there is something that is analogous to orgasm. The female cat, as many of you know,

has a so-called after-reaction which is a very rigorous rolling and rubbing behaviour, that is supposed by some authorities to be an external sign of orgasm. And in the rhesus monkey, we have described a condition called the clutching reaction. At the moment of the male's ejaculation the female rhesus monkey turns around and clutches at the male ... and at the same time she looks into the face of the male and lipsmacks. At other times it is very important for female rhesus monkeys not to look at male rhesus monkeys, because the direct look between the animals is a threat. One can show that this reaction, this clutching reaction, which can be quite violent, is under hormonal control. The incidence of it would increase with estrogen treatment and can be inhibited by progesterone treatment.

Hormones and social factors in relation to sexual intercourse. Michael illustrated from his studies of primates that copulation frequency was related to oestrogen level in the female. Different pairs of monkeys behaved differently at the same hormonal levels. Some appeared to be 'ill-assorted', showing low sexuality throughout the oestrous cycle. There was a great variation in the pattern of behaviour, reminiscent of the human situation. He referred to data on humans from North Carolina which suggested a similar relationship between frequency of sexual intercourse and oestrogen in the female. Cullen commented that he had come to a similar view on the effect of endocrine factors in the menstrual cycle and the interpersonal relationships between husband and wife. The husband needed a real understanding of the mood changes in his wife in order to avoid conflict and stress. Engström confirmed that oestrogen therapy caused sexual arousal in the female. Cullberg thought that the studies relating hormone status and sexual arousal in women were not as conclusive as animal studies. In his view the easiest way of explaining the heightening of human sexuality during the first two weeks after menstruation was that many couples have a period of abstinence during menstruation.

Referring to female interest in sex after the menopause Gebhard said that, from his data, in the absence of vaginal atrophy, interest continued certainly for a decade beyond the menopause — till about 60 years of age. 'Beyond that we don't have enough cases.' Mead thought that 'if the culture believes that sex gets better as you get older, it gets better. If it believes it gets worse, it gets worse.' And she thought people's ideas on this could probably be changed.

Child-rearing. Linnér and Odhnoff felt that men and women had equal rights and equal duties in domestic care including the washing, feeding, and generally handling the young child. Legislation with regard to maternity leave, employment hours and times, and social benefits could and did make this possible. Money reported from a subgroup discussion about parentalism being an example of sex-related behaviour which was not genuinely sexually dimorphic. But there was a sex difference, however, in the threshold of its arousability. In rats, in which parentalism was supposed to be sexually dimorphic, in that male rats did not show it, personal history could make a difference in the behaviour of the animals. He described an experiment in which a new litter of pups were put with an ordinary male rat every day.

Persistence was rewarded because after two weeks the male started behaving like a mother. Possibly something happened to the pituitary/adrenal system, but that has not yet been discovered. What the animal did do was to make a nest, to retrieve the young, put them in the nest and hover over them, but, of course, he could not lactate.

Now that child-rearing could be independent of the power to lactate in humans they could overcome the problem of the male rat. But we were not at all certain that this would be a good thing in the sense that breast-feeding though not essential was still to be encouraged. Nor was it at all clear what the consequences of 'father-feeding' *per se* would be for the baby. There was considerable evidence (*Society, stress, and disease,* Vol. 2) that the early baby-handling period enabled a special relationship to be established between mother and child which was of importance to the child's subsequent development. Would baby care shared by the father (a) weaken this relationship; (b) provide an alternative (particularly when the mother/baby 'fit' was poor); (c) generally strengthen the 'baby/mother/father fit'; or (d) have little effect?

Biological norms. Although many of the differences between societies are due to geographic, economic, and cultural factors, customs, mores, and laws, there are underlying biological characteristics of men and women common to all societies. Can such biological norms relevant to male/female roles and relationships be defined? Do social norms of these relationships sometimes conflict with biological norms? The evidence that social and cultural factors can profoundly influence fundamental physiological reactions as well as behaviour related to sex roles made it difficult to answer the first question. Discussion centred around phyletic considerations of human behaviour, biological differences in men and women, and animal studies relevant to both.

Phyletic considerations: sexuality, pair bonding, and male dominance. Kagan suggested that a somewhat speculative approach to

what most people might have in common in relation to male/female roles is to consider the anatomy, physiology, and cultural characteristics of people and in particular to consider those characteristics that seem most common for most people, and then to see if these characteristics may have had survival value in the times when our genes were being affected, namely, the tribal-hunter half-million years. I have made a naive attempt at this and it becomes rather clear that anatomically and physically men and women are designed to be highly sexual.

At the social level it is not so easy to look at things because they are so overlaid by culture. It seems there is a prevailing, but by no means unique form of behaviour characterized by a tendency to a prolonged trial period with one or more successive persons to form a pair bond, a tendency to a prolonged pre-copulatory phase, and a tendency to form a long-standing pair bond of mutual care and child-raising. Although people vary in this, the tendency seems to me to be there. We have celibate, polyandrous, and polygamous groups and communal intercourse and child-rearing, but they are extraordinarily uncommon.

Male/female pair bonds are probably strengthened by intense sexuality. The strength of this pair bonding is rather clear, because even in the most permissive or polygamous societies there is a tendency to form them for mutual care and child-rearing. Very speculatively, these things could have been of survival value in a hunter/food-gathering era and could therefore have become part of the human gene pool, the high sexuality contributing to reproduction and strong pair bonding which itself makes possible the prolonged child-rearing which is so necessary for the human young. But this could also have been produced by communal care. On the other hand, an argument that is used in favour of pair bonding is that it would support co-operation amongst the males whilst they were hunting. And certainly, this co-operation was essential for survival, but would communal mating, for instance, have done the same thing? These are wild speculations and I think we shall never know the answer. On the whole, I have, for emotional reasons, a preference for the pair bonding technique. I think it has the edge on communal mating and communal care.

I think the pair bond has had some advantage in present society for the health of the people so bonded. This is an observation that has been made over a very long period of time and which is applicable wherever you can make the observation: i.e. the married are healthier than the divorced or widowed. This may be because the relatively healthy marry or stay married, but even if that were the case, pair bonding would still be important for genetic survival.

It is very likely that some of the roles that in the hunter-tribe were sex-related at an early stage remained so. Women had to look after children most of the time. Their role would include maintenance of the cave, and food-gathering near the home. As a result they may well have been given or taken over as well the role of caring for the sick, injured, or exhausted males. And this combined domestic function may have given rise to what I think, certainly exists in the majority of societies today, however egalitarian, namely, an overt or apparent male dominance. I say apparent, because often the hand that rocks the cradle rules the world.

Mead preferred the word 'achievement' to 'dominant' because

dominance and submission take so many different forms in different societies. But achievement is male and public life is male and has been throughout. Now public life may be chasing elephants or making speeches or dressing dolls. And I have studied societies in which the most public and noble thing a man does is to dress a doll. But if he does it, it is achievement and it is public. If women do it, it is private and non-achievement. Whereas having children is the female correlate of achievement. And the other point is that action closer to home has been female right through history as far as we know: walking about with a baby on your hip is not easy and it is not something you do chasing elephants.

She added that as a result of this female food-gathering activities were close to home, for shellfish, berries, and so on; and large-scale activities requiring a great deal of muscle tended to involve males even if it took 20 men to do something that could be done by 30 women. Nevertheless the tendency was to use 20 men to pull a heavy log, rather than 30 women, and in the case of one log, one human being, Mead said you would be pretty sure the human being was a male. There was a heavy emphasis on the greater physical strength of males.

Michael illustrated how a change in male/female dominance can take place. He reported how a single pair of male and female rhesus monkeys were studied throughout the course of the pregnancy of the female. The story started before day 0 of gestation. The pair were well assorted, they showed rhythms of sexual activity in relation to the cycle, the male was responsive and sensitive to the female's endocrine state, and the female was allowed to conceive at a controlled mating, so it was known exactly when she became pregnant. Michael picked up the story at about day 80 of gestation. As pregnancy proceeded from day 80 to about day 130, the male responded to the female with mounting behaviour and increasing sexual interest in her. He clearly expected that the relationship was going to go on. As pregnancy proceeded, a very astonishing thing happened, namely, the gradual introduction of aggressive behaviour, mainly originating from the female of the pair. The male continued to show sexual interest, and she increasingly rebutted and refused his mounting attempts — the development of female dominance. And this was a female — half the size of the male, and with no canine teeth — who started to hit and bite him with increasing frequency. The male would attempt to mount, and then leap away from the female: he was scared stiff of her. Michael stressed some important observations in this study. One was the expectancy of the male that the sexual relationship would continue as previously, which it did not. Another was the developing female dominance. And yet a third was the amazing male tolerance towards the female when she was pregnant.

Lazarus asked whether the male was unable to deal with feminine aggression in mammalian species because of the inhibition against attacking females, so that the female who braved it out with the males would usually be tolerated. But Michael said that this was not the case in primates. Under usual conditions the 'female who showed any aggression towards the male would be likely to get very severely beaten up'.

'Group co-operation'. There was according to Mead much bias in the literature on the ability of women to work in groups.

The ability of either males or females to get on with each other in co-operative ways is totally a function of social organization. If you have the kind of society, for instance, in which men have to move into their wives' community, the men never form as cohesive a group as the women in that community. We are accustomed to the situation where the woman moves into her husband's community, and never makes the kind of friendships that are made in adolescence, and it is usually regarded as disloyal to her husband if she talks to the wives of his business associates, or a fellow employee, or members of his family.

Mead said that Lionel Tiger assumed that pre-*Homo sapiens* there was a kind of male pair bonding, for which there was no proof. He assumed that it occurred early, and was promoted by elephant hunting and so on. Mead considered that it took just as much bonding and co-operation to stay home as it does to leave, maybe more. She said that in cases in which females — or males — were allowed continuous association right through life the influence of social organization could be seen. Males tended to be organized around public activities, and females around the home and the care of children, and very often female co-operation was a function of kinship, because it was domestic and localized. But Mead saw no evidence whatsoever that there was more capacity for co-operation in males or females as such.

Aggression/submission in animals. Muscular strength. Michael showed, by reference to Barrier Reef fish, that first encounters between conspecifics were aggressive. The males and females were identical in appearance but the latter would reduce the aggressive atmosphere by assuming a submissive, tail-down posture.

When we move up the evolutionary scale to the primate, studies in our own laboratory have shown that the same mechanisms are operative, that there is also the approach/escape conflict, and that behaviour has to become ritualized in order to turn the aggression, which I am hypothesizing was built-in — in evolutionary terms — right from way back. The interacting primates, and, I suggest, the interacting humans, have somehow to redirect their aggression from the pair that are brought together and have to interact for mating purposes, in some way on to the environment.

In a wide range of mammalian species 'there is marked physical dimorphism, the male being heavier, stronger, and equipped for aggression. There are very few specific exceptions, e.g. the female hamster'.

Biological similarities and differences between men and women

Imperative differences. Money and colleagues came to the conclusion that there were only four 'imperatives around which sexually dimorphic behaviour manifested itself in human beings — women menstruate, gestate, and lactate, and men impregnate'. Science and technology had already made inroads into these 'four immutable mountains' e.g. with regard to the need for lactation, and might change the needs for some of the other roles. Other differences were of degree, or could at certain critical stages of development be optional and physiologically or socially determined.

Gender identity. This last contention was illustrated by Money in relation to the way people identify themselves, or are identified by others, as male or female and the consequences of this.

261

The determinants of gender identity range all the way from genetic factors to psychosocial. I like to emphasize this, because we still are heirs of the nineteenth century in these matters and therefore with perilous ease fall into the trap of dichotomizing the biological versus the social and psychological determinants, or the cultural ones. It has much greater scientific productivity in the long run if one sees a sequential pattern. I like to make the analogy with a relay race in which each one of the determinants is a runner in the race and he carries the program to the next determinant, so to speak. One of the things that has in some ways been astonishing to me from the study of intersexual or hermaphrodite people is that the genetic determinant *per se* has a very brief moment of influence.

The genetic determinant was not a long-term influence continuing into adult life in any direct sense. Its moment of influence was in writing the programme for the differentiation of the undifferentiated gonadal tissue in the foetus, so that these gonads once having differentiated would continue the programme to dictate the prenatal foetal hormones, which then in turn carried the programme on to the differentiation of the external genital morphology.

The fetal hormonal influence has its say on the genital dimorphism of anatomy of sex organs. And also, as has become evident in the last 8–10 years in a burst of new experimental activity … it has its influence on certain dimorphic pathways in the brain, particularly, it would appear, in the region of the hypothalamus in the limbic system. The study of human intersex people is the only way that it is possible at the present time to make comparisons with animal studies, and there one does indeed find that there is a close parallelism with the primates and also with the lower animals.

By inference one can assume that there are some aspects of human gender-identity differentiation which have their beginnings in these dimorphically different pathways in the brain. I do not propose to deal specifically with this in any further detail, except to say that one sees this manifestation quite clearly in the case of girls who have been masculinized before birth by an excess of male sex hormone.

These girls were tomboys. Money explained that he used this word because they were not transformed into boys or transsexuals or lesbians, but had differentiated the female gender-identity with a tomboyish flavour. He said that some of these individuals, because they were born with the external genitalia differentiated as a penis and an empty scrotum, had been raised as boys. These individuals then had their tomboyish traits very easily incorporated into their masculine differentiation of the gender-identity, and were not recognized as different from boys who were genetically male.

The brain dimorphism feeds its influences to the formation of juvenile gender-identity and carries on its influence to the ultimate formation of adult gender-identity, so that a genetic female may be regarded as a male.

Because of the appearance of the sex organs at birth, those mighty little words 'it's a boy; it's a girl', news that spreads fast soon after delivery, influenced other people's behaviour and in a very literal way they determined millions, billions of transactions from the time of birth until the time of death.

And so the sex of assignment, in rearing, is not just simply a one-shot type of thing, but it is continually re-emphasized and repeated throughout life.

When it was joined with the influence of the sex organs in the development of the child's own body image, one saw the extraordinary and in a way unbelievable influence of culture for those of us who have been mostly inclined to think in terms of instinct. It is really truly remarkable how much remains to be differentiated after birth with regard to gender-identity. I think one may say fairly safely that gender-identity, even its deformities that may be manifested later on, e.g. in the paraphilias, is completely differentiated in childhood in the prepubertal years and what happens with the onset of pubertal hormones at puberty is rather that there is a change in the threshold for the illicitation of sexual arousal and sexual response, rather than the building in of anything new with regard to the content of the imagery which will have arousal value. And so one finally sees all the pathways feeding together into the formation of adult gender-identity, which maintains itself with remarkable stability and continuity, except there may be in some cases a change after the intervening influences of brain damage or brain deterioration, and sometimes one sees in senility changes in adult gender-identity, that would have been quite unthinkable when one knew the person at the height of adulthood.

I would like now to emphasize the extraordinary importance of the postnatal period differentiation and to do that I want to show you slides of some patients.

The first one seems to be completely unremarkable; a simple play picture of two children; except that if you have a look at the next slide now you will see that the little girl actually began her life and spent seven months of her life as a little boy and then had an accident which completely obliterated the penis. It was a long story as you may well imagine and it had its solution in having the little child reassigned as a girl, and this reassignment was finally accomplished at the age of 17 months.

The next slide which summarizes most of what I could say in two hours, is a picture of this little girl at 5½ years in my office, quite unrehearsedly hamming up for her picture in a way that her brother would never have done.

The next picture showed a man and a woman who had the same diagnosis of gender and prenatal history. They were both genetic male hermaphrodites born with two imperfectly formed testes, imperfect in the sense that they were highly unlikely to be fertile. But they were assigned a different sex and had completely different gender-identities. Money told us that the boy was a college boy who had fallen in love with a girl and would not be particularly remarkable if one came across him in the course of either one's social or professional life. One would accept him as a college boy. And likewise one would accept the girl as a secretary, which is her job; one might employ her and never realize that she was in fact a genetic male who had been born with an enlarged clitoris and two undescended testes.

262

This picture also is a testament to the extraordinary power of sex hormones given at puberty, since you see a perfectly normal female body there, the result of oestrogens administered after castration at the age of 11.

In the next slide, you have a very nice and ordinary looking family picture. But the special feature here is that the father is a genetic female, who grew up as an extremely unhappy transsexual lesbian girl and finally underwent sex reassignment.

The special point Money made was not that the man was accepted as a man by all of his work-mates, who had no conception whatsoever of the medical history, but that he was also accepted as the father by the girl, who was the illegitimate daughter of the woman.

She reacts to her 'father' in exactly the same way your daughter, I trust, would react to you. She has no concept that both her parents are genetic females and she is a very seductive, flirtatious little girl with her father in the way that little girls of eight years old are supposed to be.

The next slide shows two people who both have the adrenogenital syndrome. They both wanted to change their sex, but the one on the left had been ostensibly assigned as a boy and could not accept the confusion in differentiating his gender-identity, and differentiated an ambiguous one instead of a unitary one, and then decided that the best way to solve the problem would be to change to be a girl.

The young person on the other side had exactly an opposite story. Money continued:

I am particularly interested in one fact with regard to the one on the left, who is just beginning to grow her breasts from cortisone therapy. About nine years after the change the girl was able to talk with total freedom. Just last year she told me that the one single factor that had helped her finalize her decision was that at age 12, mark you, when she was living as a boy, she had tried to have a love affair with a girl who was interested in her down the street. She found it was not rewarding, but very perfunctory, if I may use my own word. At the same time she had found herself spontaneously to be attracted to a young man that visited the house, a family friend who was five or six years older, and she knew that for him she had the true feelings of love, and she did in fact marry him eventually. and that feeling of being able to fall in love was for her the final conviction that she should not live as a boy any longer, but should change over. The other young person has not a similar story to tell, but he now does have romantic feelings toward girls.

Money said he had specially chosen these slides to emphasize that in these cases the discordance in gender was postnatal, and the genetic and prenatal genders were concordant. This special sort of ambiguity had to be resolved, and was resolved in opposite ways by each person.

Endocrine secretion. Persky found a relation in young men and women between 'aggression' and plasma testosterone levels. Young men had a much higher level of plasma testosterone than young women. But the levels in men fell with age whilst those in women did not. In sexually aroused male monkeys plasma testosterone rose several-fold. In men sexually stimulated by self-masturbation there was no such change. Henry referred to Rose's work which associated a rise in testosterone level with increased social status and vice versa. He pointed out that probably 'masturbation is not associated with any great change in status' and Mead pointed out that it was not an interpersonal response.

Male/female differences in *reaction time to sex hormones*: Michael said that in many mammals, including primates, withdrawal of sex hormones by castration and administration of sex hormones from exogenous sources was followed by rapid onset of behavioural changes in the female, but only after a delay of several weeks or months in males. This was not an effect specific to the hormone because treating female monkeys with androgens was also followed by abrupt changes. Michael added that women were exposed to considerable and rapid changes in oestrogen and progesterone level during the menstrual cycle.

We know these hormones produce effects on mood and on behaviour, on irritability, on whether you are looking outward or looking inward, on the psychologic orientation. This is something that the male simply does not have to contend with, he is not subjected to these changes in his internal chemistry in the same way that the female is. Now whether or not this change in blood chemistry constitutes what you might call a biological constraint on the female is an open question, and it is a hot one too, but one might speculate that there are certain professions, certain occupations, certain social roles to which the female might be more suited than the male, and some to which she might be correspondingly less suited.

Lazarus was of the opinion

that while these large fluctuations are taking place, and possibly some mood changes — although I have not seen evidence of this — the woman is taking care of her children and maintaining her home, working in an office, doing her professional job, teaching, writing her research papers, or whatever it is she is doing, throughout all this, in other words transcending or perhaps coping with or habituating with these kinds of surges of hormonal activity, because her primary motives, if you like, or goals, seem to be the main factors that control her behaviour. So while I think it is important to show what she has to contend with, if indeed she has to contend with these surges, nonetheless what she does shows very little disruption of her normal activities. One last word on this. We have been talking about how men and women differ biologically or physiologically. One of the things we have not talked about are the needs that men and women share in common when they build a life together. For example: needs for belonging and love, perhaps, for identity or individuality, for a stable frame of reference about the world and values, for transcendence of one's animal nature, and what Fromm talks about as human nature.... Presumably, if these can be regarded as needs, biologically speaking, they are by and large needs shared in common between men and women, and they undoubtedly have much greater power and importance in governing the way in which we live and the problems that we have, and the stresses that we have to deal with, and the sources of gratification that we have, than the kinds of hormonal differences that have been discussed so far in the symposium.

Catecholamines: Frankenhaeuser's data (Chapter 21) showed that girls and women at rest had similar adrenalin excretion levels to boys and men respectively. But during the performance of mental tasks the male adrenalin levels increased considerably but the female levels did not. This was speculatively interpreted by Henry as showing that the 'males pushed harder'. Mead felt that 'culture can overlay this sort of thing', giving as an example the effect of culturally determined physical activity on development of musculature in women and the lack of it in men, and women's ability to 'put on a spurt' when they are commonly called upon to do so. Frankenhaeuser thought it was not so simple to interpret her data. The men and women had performed equally well and there was no evidence that men had tried harder or the women less hard. It might just be that men were hyper-reactive or women hypo-reactive. Perhaps the latter had a more economical way of responding and this fitted in (very speculatively) with the longer life-span of women.

Frankenhaeuser concluded:

What is important to me is that we have those hormonal differences, differences in hormonal functioning between sexes, not only of sex hormones, but also in hormones like adrenalin, which we know influences emotional balance, and therefore also presumably it is very important to the whole question of social roles, and social adjustment in general. So I want to agree with all these previous speakers who have said that we lack hard data on this subject, and I want to emphasize that here is an area where indeed we could very easily get more hard data, because all these problems are problems that can easily be studied, both in laboratory studies and in field studies. It is strange to me that so little attention has been paid to this whole area which, it seems to me, is a way to get at the whole problem of biological constraints, if there are any, and which they are in the case of male/female social roles.

Levi referred to studies he had done which showed that women responded to pornographic films with less sexual arousal and less increase in catecholamine excretion than men. This was comparable to Frankenhaeuser's findings in response to mental exertion. He wondered if hypo-reactivity in women was a general or a specific response. Bancroft's results were different. He had found that women had less sexual arousal than men to pictures of the opposite sex but nearly the same response to pictures of sexual activity.

Biological/social conflict. There was no doubt that biological constraints could and did give rise to social constraints, but Money stated: 'One has to respect biology, but one can't expect it to tell us our norms' — and Lazarus said that it was useless to talk in general terms about this. One had to give specific instances on which action could be based. Arne Engström emphasized the need for this in reminding the conference that in the political/administrative/adviser triangle often the first and last changed frequently and with the change there was a change in views. The administration, which remained steady was therefore in a powerful position for maintaining its point of view. The need for rational specific advice was therefore great.

Specific instances were mentioned where the female or the unborn child were at special risk to environmental hazard (e.g. lead poisoning, radiation, German measles) and when society, therefore, was expected to take special action. Kagan gave as an example the problems of family planning in a rural Turkish village:

It is the custom in these villages to have large families, and this probably arises from the biological need to have enough people to cultivate the land and produce the food for the community at a time when the children did not survive very often. The custom is still there, and I understand from some of my colleagues that this works particularly through two channels. The mother, mother-in-law, auntie, and other ladies of the village think that a married girl who is not pregnant is abnormal. The husband takes the same view for a rather different reason. He tends to think that unless he has four sons, his old age will not be cared for, and so he produces, according to his subjective social pressure, a large family until he has got four sons. Now we introduce here a social change which results in survival of the children, and this produces a biological pressure and not enough food. If that is seen by the community, aren't they going to change their social attitude? Aren't they going to reduce their family-size? If they did not, of course, and nothing else was done, they would fail biologically.

Mead raised the question:

Is it good for women to have children? I mean, good for individual women to have a child. We have just had a decision in the Supreme Court in one of our American states — in a case prosecuting a midwife, a male midwife, I might add — that childbearing is a disease and therefore belongs to the medical profession. Now I would like to keep clearly before us as we plan for women as human beings: that child-bearing is what they were designed for, anatomically, and physiologically, so that not having a child is in a sense a physical deprivation or an attack or an affront to the organism. On the other hand, is this merely in the psychosexual realm? Some of the psychiatric evidence would suggest that women who can have children and don't would be psychologically maimed. But that a woman who had no husband, for instance, would not be psychologically maimed, or a woman who had a hysterectomy would not be psychologically maimed.

Mead thought that all available data (e.g. numbers of cases of cancer in women who have and who have not had children) should be used to plan for the future. Society could either be planned to let every woman have at least one child, if she was physically capable; or so that women who were good at having children had, say, seven, and other women did not have any. These were both very important alternatives, and very relevant to bringing up children, to social legislation, and so on.

Engström considered that child-bearing was not a physiological necessity in the sense that the life-expectancy of women without children was not decreased. Excess mortality due to parity increased only with the fourth child. Cancer of the uterine cervix, which was low in nuns was associated more with sexual experience than childbirth. Reduced mortality from cancer of breast in women who had born children seemed to be one of the few clear advantages in physical health.

Henry confirmed that in female mice longevity was not related to child-bearing. Cullberg, speaking as a psychiatrist, noted shock reactions occurring

when a woman is deprived of the possibilities of having children, as during sterilization investigations and after hysterectomy and after the menopause. These shock reactions are sometimes very strong, but it is difficult to say if they are stronger than could be expected from the cultural expectancies toward the woman to have children, or that there is some kind of deeper lying hereditary determinant.

Mead thought we should consider the large collection of clinical cases of women who become creative after they were told they would not have children, or any more children, either because of an early hysterectomy, or being widowed with several children, or because of the menopause. Women who showed no creativity or very little creativity before this became painters, poets, scientists, and so on. The question of *creativity and its relationship to having children* was important from the point of view of social planning. If there was a difference in the impulse towards creativity in women who do or do not expect to have children, then society's arrangements for the role of males and females, say in the area of contributions to society, would be different. It was conceivable that major discoveries in mathematics were more likely to be made by the one millionth man than by the one millionth woman. On the other hand, Mead thought, there might be forms of creativity which were just as significant for culture which had never been tried out, because women had never been given the opportunity. Mead emphasized that not one single public, or cultural field was known in which women made an equal or greater contribution than men. We could decide to give this advantage to men, because it was correlated with the fact they did not have children, and had other areas of achievement. Or we could give an equal chance to men and women for different kinds of creativity, both of them however being rooted in their biological capacity to have or not have children. This would affect social roles, and affect them at the very apex of importance. Therefore, in other words, we decide that either

if you let women be physicists you would have some more physics, of a very different sort; or you decide if you clutter up the classes of physics with women you won't get as many great physicists. You see, it makes a great deal of difference, and this affects education, affects the logistics of whether the wives should go where their husbands are, or if a man is married to a woman who is a potential great physicist, should he move?

The relationship between childbirth and creativity was open to doubt but if it were correct there would be a very definite relationship between what was known about possible biological constraints and social roles.

Lazarus was still unconvinced that anyone had shown a specific biological constraint arising from male/female relationships influencing specific societal factors. The only thing that had offered a glimmer of this relationship had been Mead's observation, which Lazarus thought was very clever, about prostitution. It had never occurred to him before 'that males would not be satisfactory for prostitution because of the nature of their sexual apparatus.... I don't know how important this is for the issues that are of great interest in the formation of society and social change.'

Mead went on to clarify her point:

I am not talking about prostitution in the market place, you know. I am talking about the fact that women, in order to keep the family going, will tolerate almost anything, and can, because all they have to do is lie still. Now there is data that was presented about the German study, where 19 per cent of the women were satisfied and 92 per cent of the men. This is an example of what I am talking about. But whenever you get a demand in society for male potency, that is beyond the males' willingness to give, you get problems, and I see this all the time in primitive societies: societies in which the men spend their lives complaining that the women want more copulation than they are prepared to give, and they are not going to give it.... It was this that I was talking about, when I said prostitution. It is in the broadest sense; i.e. you will accord sex satisfactorily to the other partner in return for other non-sexual benefits; food, shelter, a quiet house, children getting on well, your husband doing well next day, when he gives a lecture. These are the things that I mean by prostitution.

Masculinity/femininity: a continuum. The participants were agreed that although social arrangements still often polarized attitudes to men and women in anatomical, physiological and behavioural terms it was, with few exceptions, better to characterize men and women according to their measurements on the same two continua. Gebhard and Money found this concept most practical and the former referred to Beech, who had recently told him that for many years he had been troubled because he thought of masculinity and femininity as opposite ends of one scale. The less masculine you were, the more feminine you would be by definition; or the more masculine you were, the less feminine and so on. This concept, however, did not fit with a lot of the research work he was doing with animals. Finally he developed another concept that was much more sensible. It fitted with his experimental data and made good sense to everyone he had told about it. That is, masculinity and femininity should not be conceived of as being on one scale. Each should be conceived as a separate scale and a person's position should be rated in terms of both scales. Beech said that the average person, if he is a male, rates high on the male scale, and somewhat lower on the female scale. But some individuals can rate low on both scales or high on both scales. Gebhard considered that this concept of two separate scales made a lot of sense, and cleared up many problems that had plagued us before.

PSYCHOSOCIAL STRESSORS

General concept

A stressor situation due to psychosocial factors arose if there was perceived threat to perceived needs, whether or not these were real. Under such circumstances the individual or group was called upon to adapt and if this was impossible or inadequate the situation was likely to be pathogenic. Important 'needs' were likely to be those defined by Maslow, i.e. related to safety of the individual, species or community; sense of belonging and love; self esteem and status; sense of self-realization. Kagan thought the symposium should be concerned with such situations in relation to male/female sexuality, pair bonding, and aparent male dominance.

Some features of male/female roles and relationships

The interpersonal relationship. Cullen saw the relation between male and female, with regard to sexuality, pair bonding, marriage, mutual care, and child-rearing, as the closest interpersonal relationship that commonly exists in human experience. He considered that through it there had developed 'a very big repertoire of coping mechanisms for instance for handling aggression, and stressful situations in work and in play'.

Mead pointed out that this special domestic relationship between men and women spilt over to work relationships, often with ill results. For example in many countries it was still many times more stressful for a woman to be a doctor than for a man.

Aggression. Michael and Henry showed that aggressive reactions are an integral part of the interaction between conspecifics (in fish, mice, primates) that come together when they need to mate. Normally the aggressive responses were quickly modified and redirected. The initial signal for this redirection was a 'submission' response on the part of the female. The agonistic quality of these encounters was dampened down during parturition and was associated with hormonal changes.

Michael speculated that much stress in human courtship and the marital state might occur as a result of failure to reduce and redirect the agonistic interaction. Cullen postulated that hormonal changes in a woman's menstrual cycle might, by causing mood and behaviour changes including sexual responses, which, being inexplicable to the male partner, become a source of stress. There were cyclic social and cultural factors in the male (e.g. weekend availability) and possibly male hormone cycles as well, which might cause conflict. Following on a thought arising from Frankenhaeuser's identification of 'day' or 'night' catecholamine secretors Cullen wondered if 'night' people might not be the wrong companions or mates for 'day' people.

Biological and social maturation. Hynie pointed out that the time gap between biological readiness to have sexual intercourse and reproduce, and social readiness to bear the responsibility, had been in the past, and was still to some extent, accompanied in many countries by societies' opposition to sexual relationships at an early age. The stressors from such a situation had in many countries been reduced by social permissiveness and the availability, not always accompanied by the successful use of, contraception. In many countries legislation had made it easier for young people to study, work, or be out of work, and still be able to afford the necessities of family life. Nevertheless, according to Liljeström, the conflict between biological and social maturation was rising again because 'the reproductive age coincides with the age at which the young adult is trying to establish his or her place in the world of production. The situation becomes even more precarious, when, as is the case today, the differentiation of roles is questioned.'

Liljeström thought that traditional role differentiation and more modern role sharing (at home and at work) both had their good points and their sources of stress. The former made it difficult for the man and woman to replace each other as providers, reduced the contact between the father and children, and made it difficult for the mother to take an equal share in self-expression and community activities and responsibilities. Role sharing was liable to end up with poorer services in the home for all and was associated, in today's society, with the stressors of uncertainty due to role confusion. Linnér and Odhnoff felt that society had made it to some extent, and could make it to a much greater extent, economically, morally, and ethically possible for a role-sharing system to work; and even for one-parent families, where the one parent exercised his or her profession, to be viable and healthy. Bancroft, Kagan, Mead, and Money considered that before venturing into the unknown by applying such methods on a grand scale society should assure itself that by doing so it was not creating severer stressors on, for example, the children.

Gender-identity. Bancroft noted a reciprocal relationship between gender-identity, the choice of sexual object, and method of relating to one's sexual partner. In particular he referred to data which supported the notion that disturbances of maternal and paternal relationships undermined 'the masculinity of the developing male'. Money gave many clinical instances which supported the view that upbringing influenced strongly and adversely male/female relationships in later life. More hopefully he showed how such difficulties could be prevented or, if they had already occurred, could be ameliorated. Both these sets of data underlined the importance of their warning that new and untried approaches to child-rearing arising from male/female role sharing should be approached with caution.

Social expectations. Mead pointed out that every society had different expectations for men and women in terms of anatomy, physiology, temperament, and capacity. If the individual boy or girl, man or woman, differed from society's expectations a stressful situation arose.

Many socially assigned traits were not 'intimately connected at all with the primary sex characteristics or the primary reproductive tasks of each sex'. The less the connection the more likely is there to be stress.

The little girl who matures too early, or the little girl who matures too late according to the expectation of the society; the boy who matures too late; the very short man; and the very tall woman are almost uniformly disadvantaged, (although occasionally, if height is applied to the aristocracy, a very tall aristocratic woman may have a reasonably better time than the tall plebeian woman might have). And in general, I think we can say that the less related the traits that are imputed the more likely there is to be stress. If you simply impute to women that they have breasts, most of them do, and although there will be some disadvantages in having either too long breasts in a country like Bali, or too slight ones in some African tribes, nevertheless the fact that most females have breasts, makes it fairly easy to be a female. If, however, you begin imputing some elaborate form of temperament or skill or beauty, that is not intimately related, you get the same sort of difficulties you get with race, when you tie in with skin colour all sorts of other characteristics that are utterly irrelevant to skin colour. In our rapidly changing society at present you can see shifts in stress-related conditions, e.g. in the United States the shift in incidence in ulcers from women to men from 1900 to 1940, and the present vulnerability of middle-aged males.'

Conflict between social expectancy and possibilities for achievement were instanced. Lazarus spoke of the tendency to make it a moral imperative for women to take an achievement role in society when the number of positions that could be gratifying were very small. Goodman mentioned the discrepancy between the philosophy of equal rights for men and women and the absence of equal rewards. Mead, referring to the United States spoke of girls who were socialized to be human, and then married and put in the suburbs, and told that they could only perform a series of routine domestic tasks. You can start with humanity and end up with a restricted sex role. This was equally true for boys who thought they had an interesting career ahead of them and then ended up working all their lives in a dull job in an accountant's office. 'In both these cases you have a wide, generous, variegated socialization, and the narrow realization'.

Lazarus, referring to the 'paradox of social policy', and Mead both pointed out the dangers of jumping from philosophy to social action without prior evaluation in a complex field.

'We can very easily overemphasize the controversies amongst ourselves about sexual degree of aggression then project it out on the world as if it were really the causative factor.'

Specific problems

Marriage. Difference between expectancy and reality was thought to be the cause of much trouble in married life. Much that was essentially socio-economic and needed to be treated from that point of view was wrongly regarded as essentially medical or psycho-logical e.g. lack of money, space, and privacy. In many countries there was a great deal of commercialization of sex via mass-media and pornography which portrayed unattainable ideals of romantic marriage on the one hand and the desirability of acrobatic and marathon sexual activity on the other. Functions of marriage such as to protect women and children and ensure inheritance were fast being taken over by social agencies, or the need for such functions as disappearing. In spite of this marriage was still popular in such societies probably as an index of commitment. Nevertheless divorce was becoming more common and the mutual care between husband and wife was probably diminishing in quality and quantity. This might account in such countries for the increased mortality rate in the middle-aged males, who were more vulnerable to lack of care than middle-aged women. It was thought that this state of affairs was due to ambiguity about roles and disappointment in the gap between what was expected and what was perceived as reality — for example a recent survey in the Federal Republic of Germany showed that only 19 per cent of married women were content with their married life.

Hertoft and Trost reported that unmarried cohabitation was common in Scandinavian countries and becoming commoner. Trost had found that such liaisons were less stable than married ones even when the age of the couples was taken into account. He thought that this indicated that the cohabitations were to some extent 'trial marriages'. Linnér pointed out that in Sweden social services were equally available to all whereas the civil laws were still more advantageous to the married.

Contraception. Linnér referred to the stress in women to whom family planning was denied and who had to resort to illegal abortion if they wished pregnancy to be terminated. Others pointed out that contraception was not an unmixed blessing. Psychosocial stressors could arise when contraception, e.g. the pill, was freely available. Cullberg classified these stressors as: hormonal effects on mood, e.g. depression during the first few weeks of adapting to the pill; intra-psychological effects on the woman taking the pill, e.g. a feeling that she was chemically sterilized; interpersonal psychological effects, e.g. causing or revealing fear of sexual inadequacy by removing physical excuses for withholding sexual intercourse.

Engström pointed out that the pill was often effective in reducing premenstrual pain and Cullen thought that by matching the pill to the woman it was already possible to reduce premenstrual emotional disturbance in many cases.

The full psychological implications of oral and other types of contraception were not yet understood. The condom, a male-controlled device, was unpopular with men. The intrauterine device, which had a number of practical advantages, including perhaps in some respects a prolonged menstruation, was certainly not without physical as well as psychological disadvantages. Vasectomy had been shown to be both efficient and popular with married couples in an English survey several months after the treatment had been made freely available *to those who wanted it*. The data from India was, according to Hassler not so reassuring. In some surveys 25 per cent of vasectomized men complained of impotence. But controls were not available for comparison.

Cullberg thought it was necessary to know of the stressors arising from perceived sociological 'threats' in situations where contraception was freely available but not yet freely accepted.

Critical events. Pregnancy, the post-partum period, spontaneous abortion, perinatal death, elective abortion, and divorce were all cited as life-change events connected with male/female roles and relations and demanding adaptation. They had in common that they arose under the social conditions that exist in many countries. This happened when the situation was ambivalent for the man and woman concerned and when social attitudes are antagonistc or non-supportive.

Cullen characterized the moods according to stages of reproduction as confusing in the early stages of pregnancy, euphoria in the middle stages, fear during labour, and depression post-partum. The stressful state could be reduced by a clear and united sense of purpose of the couple, explanation and preparation in the antenatal period by health personnel, and closeness of a female relative or friend in the post-partum period.

PHYSIOLOGICAL MECHANISMS

For a full discussion of the hypothesis that increased catecholamine and corticosteroid secretion, through hypophysical stimulation by psychological stimuli arising from social situations might be a common pathogenic mechanism, the reader is referred to Volume 1 in this series.

Frankenhaeuser's demonstration of the tendency for women to respond less to stress, than men in terms of catecholamine excretion, was referred to above.

Persky noted that anxiety produced an increase in urinary corticosteroids and that administration of corticosteroids increased anxiety. He and Rahe referred to studies in which subjects who reacted to critical situations with the least anxiety and the most coping had the lowest corticosteroid changes.

Michael referred to experiments in which it was shown that ovariectomized subhuman primates were more likely to respond aggressively to male aggression. He briefly mentioned that women during the luteal phase were at high risk of death from all causes; poor examination performance; delinquent actions; and petty offences such as shop lifting.

Persky said that testosterone level was related to some extent to aggressivity, but Money had found a poor correlation between testosterone and corticosteroid levels.

PRECURSORS AND DISEASE

In Chapter 1 'precursors' were defined as 'malfunctions in mental or physical systems which have not resulted in disability but if continued are likely to do so', and 'disease' as 'disability caused by mental or somatic malfunction'. Disability was defined as 'failure in the performance of a task'. It was necessary to differentiate between essential and optimal performance. This definition could be applied to the individual, the family, or the community but what is disease for the individual is not necessarily disease for the family or community and vice versa. In discussion the participants found it useful to include social malfunctions and social disability.

Unwanted pregnancy
This common condition was thought to be clearly due to male/female relations. (For discussion on the risk of disease in the child resulting from an unwanted pregnancy the reader is referred to Volume 2 of this series.) An unwanted pregnancy did not always result in an unwanted child. The evidence that an unwanted pregnancy resulted in disease in the child was contradictory but on the whole in favour of high risk for mental and social disability. It was not clear to what extent unwanted pregnancy resulted in disability in the mother or father. That the mother, and to some extent the father, was often distressed in the short term, was a common experience in many countries. The extent to which this occurred and the risk of chronic disease developing was essentially a function of social conditions. The evidence from Scandinavian countries was that enlightened social measures and lack of social stigma was reducing the trauma of unwanted pregnancy. There was some discussion on the possibility that premarital conception was a cause of subsequent divorce. Hertoft was of the opinion, from his survey, that the association between premarital conception and divorce was due to the fact that they were both related to early age at marriage and that the latter was more likely to be causal of divorce than premarital conception. He hoped so, because premarital conception accounted for more than half the first births in his community.

Venereal disease
Tottie gave figures showing the increase in gonorrhoea in most countries, with the notable exception of China. He indicated a change in character — to a symptomless form in most women and 20 per cent of men, — its resistance to penicillin, and the presence of a rash.

The increase in cases of gonorrhoea that Tottie had noted in maladjusted adolescents was supported by

Hertoft's survey in which the majority of cases was found amongst young people who had been school drop-outs and had low-status jobs. Rahe's study of sailors showed that high-risk factors were leaving school early, trouble with supervisors at work or with the law, and low-status jobs. Social class was not a risk factor. He thought the common characteristic was an 'anti-authority attitude'.

There was general agreement that venereal disease was, in most countries, a behavioural problem. Some took the view that adolescents so affected were 'attempting to expiate the sin of sex'. Mead thought that these young people were attempting to call attention to themselves and were asking for help and much in need of it.

The change from pair-bonded sex relations to group sex noted in some countries was a basis for spread of venereal disease. But Tottie thought that the small groups in Sweden were in themselves not enough to account for increase in gonorrhoea and Mead pointed out that 'travel and anonymity' were the accelerating factors. She agreed that casual sex was primarily a function of density of population and anonymity, and said that in most primitive societies anonymity was absolutely impossible. There were festival occasions, when taboos were forgotten, and everybody copulated with everybody else; but everybody else was twenty people. They were very, very small groups that met no outsiders or travellers. In societies in which travelling salesmen, or sailors, moved from place to place, rapid transmission of venereal disease began. Mead cited the very interesting case in New Guinea now, where a road was built through the Highlands about 25 years ago, before which the people of New Guinea had no contact with modern society. It was said that this road promoted venereal disease.

'What it is actually doing is promoting travel, and anonymity, and people getting outside their own circles, and therefore not being subjects to the rules and regulations that existed before.'

In addition to change in the nature of the disease, Rahe thought that difficulties in prevention and treatment were due to the fact that often sex was so casual that the names of contacts were not known. Linnér referred to the adverse influence of making conditions for treatment e.g. in Massachusetts it was necessary for a 16-year-old girl's parents to be informed before a doctor could treat her. Money pointed out the importance of having treatment facilities available right on the spot. Tottie said there was reason to suppose that an intensified campaign to encourage the use of condoms would improve the situation a little. Meanwhile everyone hoped that a vaccine would be produced.

Impotence, frigidity, infertility, and spontaneous abortion

These conditions were all mentioned as *possible* effects of psychosocial factors. A subgroup chairman summarized:

Infertility is related to difficulties in heterosexual coitus, resulting from, say, impotence, vaginismus, premature ejaculation, etc. We considered the possibility that certain positions may be less conducive to conception than others, and we thought that infertility may, rarely perhaps, but nevertheless sometimes, be a result of preference for some special position or technique. We considered that stress could influence the production of antibodies, which in turn might affect fertility. We recorded the observation that anxiety and fear may adversely affect fertility because of the known effect it has on the closure of the oviducts.

Sexual arousal is thought to influence the composition and viscosity of cervical mucus, and also vaginal pH, and possibly the time of ovulation. The prostaglandins in the ejaculate cause uterine muscular contraction and hence influence fertility. Sexual desire may affect fertility in this same indirect way. There was some mention that too-frequent coitus is associated with a small volume of ejaculation on each occasion, and a small sperm-count, and this has been suggested as a cause for infertility. Sexual inadequacy, which we took to include impotence, frigidity, and allied conditions, is very often psychogenic. Masters has pointed out that it is always psychogenic in males under 60. Money strongly disagreed and thought that there was little doubt that certain organic situations made individuals more vulnerable to such psychosomatic trouble. Anxiety, fear, sense of obligation, and so forth, can all cause sexual dysfunction, as can mismatch in interpersonal relationships. We noted that whilst the pill has freed thousands from the fear of pregnancy which caused sexual dysfunction, this same emancipation from pregnancy has caused trouble for those few who feel that sexual activity is only justified by the possibility of conception. On the other hand there are people who, because they are not sure whether their partner has taken the pill or not, feel impotent. Impotence and anorgasmia can also be caused by irrational attitude towards menstruation and pregnancy. Lastly we pointed out that the stress of childcare plus concern over children interrupting coitus can cause sexual dysfunction.

'We could not say there was a clear indication that stimuli arising from male/female relationship or sex role can cause spontaneous abortion through psychological mechanisms.'

Menstrual disorders
The subgroup chairman summarized:

Psychogenic alteration or suppression of menstruation is well known. Brief fear and depression can have this affect; consequently any psychological trauma arising from male/female relationships, e.g. rejection or divorce, can perhaps influence menstruation. A 1967 survey in Minnesota was referred to which indicated that women who dislike the role of housewife suffered more menstrual pain than women who had jobs outside of the home; and it has been shown that hysterical females have more menstrual pain than normal females. Dysmenorrhoea has been reduced by the use of the pill. Many believe that rejection of the female role is the basic reason for the amenorrhoea of anorexia nervosa, although this is highly contentious.

Menopausal vaginal atrophy

'There is a persistent suggestion that regular sexual arousal and coitus retards or even prevents vaginal atrophy, and this, perhaps, operates through psychological rather than the purely organic mechanism.'

The paraphilias

Money summarized a good deal of the discussion on paraphilias:

The common characteristic that allows one to put these many manifestations together would seem to be that the paraphiliac is a person who is capable of being sexually aroused or 'turned on' by a signal 'that is different from the one ordinarily expected'. The usual terms for the stimulus in the past were deviant or perverse, but I think it is much better to be less judgmental and say an unconventional or atypical stimulus. The most important thing about this stimulus for the paraphiliac person, however, is that he or she — very rarely she — is dependent on that stimulus for the completeness of his arousal and achievement of orgasm. The classic example is the fetishist who is unable to get the experience of orgasm without contact with the fetish object. We talked about the fact that there is a compulsive feature characteristic to the paraphilias. Here again I bring up the comparison with a handwashing compulsion; these experiences which end in orgasm really turn out to be as little related to genuine eroticism and love as compulsive handwashing is related to genuine hygiene and cleanliness. I think of the example of a transvestite who, after he had made a big change in his life, and got relieved of his transvestism, said he used to need to have an orgasm four to five times a day to relieve the ugly inner tension that he experienced building up in him. When he had those orgasms with his wife, he was in fact — and this he said retrospectively when he could make the comparison — simply masturbating in her vagina. He told quite a different story about how he and his wife related together now in what sounds to me like a truly erotic relationship with sensitivity and affection, as compared with that former time. Another point here with regard to this compulsive character to the orgasms of the paraphiliac is that, when the men are treated with anti-androgen, which is often successful, they often don't report that they become impotent or lost their libido. The first thing they report is that they don't feel so nervous, and they are quite willing to fore-go the experience of libido and ejaculation for a while in the interests of calming this other compulsive nagging trip hammering that gets at them and expresses itself through sex.

Why are the paraphilias more frequent in males than in females? In fact the more bizarre paraphilias, for example coprophilia or necrophilia, simply have not yet been reported in females. Perhaps the explanation here is the same as with regard to differentiation of the foetus in which the principle always is that, shall I say it metaphorically, God made Eve first, and then put an injection needle of androgen into her and got Adam. It is more difficult in the sense that it takes one stage more to make a male, and that may in fact be involved in the phenomenon here of the paraphilias occurring more in males than in females. My personal conjecture here is, that it is part of nature's plan of things to have the male more responsive to the visual image, and thereby to become aroused and initiate sex. That could be interpreted in an anthropomorphic sort of way dealing with nature by saying that the woman is always reproductively available to the man, but the man is useless to the woman unless he gets an erection. So nature did need to provide some method of insuring that the male would be able to get an erection when he and the woman were interested in each other. It is not the only way in which it could have been done, but it is quite an effective way to have the man out scanning, so to speak, or girl-watching all the time, especially when he is a young adolescent. So the importance of the visual image — if one links it to the male in that way, whilst not saying that the visual image is not important to the female, but rather that it is a matter of a threshold difference — does give us a basis for at least getting some glimmer of understanding of why this extraordinary behaviour in sex that one finds in the paraphilias is so widespread amongst the males, but not among the females.

The paraphilias are never a response to sexual stress and strain in a partnership, but they always antidate it and they actually bring stress and strain into a sexual partnership. I believe one can understand the paraphilias only if one can capture the biographical history back to childhood, which is when they all had their beginning.... Then they manifest themselves in explicit form after they are 'fuelled up' by the sex hormones at puberty, if I may use that figure of speech.

However, there is another fascinating point here, which is that the number of the paraphilias, long as the list is, is still limited. I don't think, for example, one has ever recorded a paraphilia for carrot, in fact, for almost any foodstuffs, and I have never heard of a paraphilia for a piano or a television set. I think one finds the explanation of this limitation by looking again into phylogeny, the phyletic mechanism, and finding if there is some sort of explanation of why a certain category of paraphilia might enter into the human system. One nice example, a very obvious one I think, is that a great many paraphilias are associated with fabrics and things that you touch, so one can relate this to the great need among primates in infancy to have haptic stimulation, to be nuzzling up against fur or skin and to be able to cling.

I do want to emphasize, however, that the phyletic mechanism itself does not determine the paraphilia but only gives the foundation for it. It is the biographical experience that actually makes it occur. One might speculate in this connection with another example. There is a relatively high incidence of sadomasochistic paraphilias in British and German cultures. They are cultures which, especially in the earlier generations, put a premium on physical punishment of young children and on sexual taboos. Any sufficiently intense emotional experience can spill over to create an erection, a non-erotic erection, especially in little boys. This overflow, when under the tension of punishment in childhood, may set the contingency of the relationship between punishment and erection, which then later appears at adolescence as a compulsion. Interestingly enough, and we discussed a few cases of this type, one can see the beginnings of the paraphilia in an early childhood experience, if it was intense enough. But usually when you talk to the adolescent or the adult they are not able to bring this information out of memory, and in fact they often very exquisitely have it inhibited and repressed because it was a sufficiently painful experience. That means then that only the prospective studies will give us the full amount of information we need. I would emphasize in this respect the importance of the strength of the emotional experience.

We did discuss this with regard to homosexuality and the question was, could homosexual experience in childhood pre-ordain a boy or a girl to homosexuality later. I believe the evidence is that it does not have to, but one can find examples of a very intense experience. I gave one example of a boy of six who was being babysat by a teenager who was a frotteur, and the boy woke up to find the teenager had been lying beside him and ejaculated. The parents kept their heads pretty well, but they were too anxious to be able to ask the little boy exactly how he felt about it. When I talked to him he said he could not understand what on earth the big boy was doing and he thought he was probably going to murder him. And 10 years later, the little boy, who is now 16, came back to discuss a problem. He was having a serious problem in his girl-friend life, always picking exactly the wrong kind of girlfriend for him, the castrating type and I mean that literally almost, not just in the casual way that one uses that word sometimes. He was obsessed with the idea that he would have to try a homosexual experience to reconstruct exactly what had happened to him when he was six, and he was very distressed with the obsessive recurrence of this idea in his fantasies, in dreams and in his masturbation fantasies.

However, I think ordinary sexual play at childhood that involves casual kind of genital inspection would not leave a residue of the type that I have just mentioned. That other experience was so intense, also so mystifying. I can't help but quote yet another example with regard to the phyletic origins or possibilities of paraphilia, the matter of coprophilia, the origins of which had puzzled me beyond my endurance. But I was at White Sands, New Mexico, in the chimpanzee colony down there some years ago. I saw two little baby chimpanzees in the incubator, and they had been soiling themselves, and so I had at last the chance to ask what is the method of sanitation for chimpanzees when the mother takes care of the baby, and the answer was, she licks it clean. And so in the brain, I could presume in the limbic system, there really is a mechanism for eating faeces in the primate, and so one sees here the basis of how it can be misconnected to the erotic stimulus instead of the sanitation one. The basic mechanisms I think are not sex-specific, but again it is a threshold difference.

Money said that the subgroup also discussed the rather uncanny way in which a person afflicted with a paraphilia was able to attract a mate who somehow fitted in and complemented that disability. One example was of a woman who had an intense love affair with a transvestite, without knowing of his transvestitism. But the woman had previously acted as a nursemaid for her psychiatrically disabled brother, who was a chronic paranoid schizophrenic. So she was almost out looking for a psychiatric case to continue taking care of, and was able to adjust herself to the problem up to a point.

Mead added that the fact that both sexes were reared by the mother was far more important than we had allowed for. The male established heterosexual behaviour while he is relating to his mother, e.g. while breast-feeding. The connection with thumbsucking, which was much commoner in boys than in girls, could be traced back to breast-feeding when little boys played with their own haircurl or their mother's haircurl.

Mead thought that there was therefore more opportunity for a boy to experience either deficiencies or overemphases in his long period of relating to his mother, than for a girl, who was not establishing a heterosexual relationship at that point. She added that the opposite might be true if both sexes were reared by men. She agreed that there was a phylogenetic reason for both sexes to be reared by women but thought that if fathers could take as much care of children as mothers, we might open the way either to the disappearance of those paraphilias due to an over-emphasis of a mother/male child position, or to the appearance of paraphilias in females, where the paternal role was defective.

Money said that the Aborigines in Western Australia had no paraphilias.

Exactly. You also do not find the transitional object that is characteristic of our society, where we make a child sleep away from the parents. The child with a little piece of dirty blanket that he carries around all the time is a characteristic of modern society and of the extreme tactual alienation that is imposed on an infant that is made to sleep alone, very often almost from birth. I have never seen a transitional object in any primitive society, where babies sleep where they belong, which is near human skin. As a precursor of various forms of fetishism, I think that the transitional object, which is very often a blanket or a teddybear, is ideal. It has a soft fabric quality, and this is substituted for human skin quality.... Paraphilias can be seen partly as an outgrowth of our kind of civilization, where we expect a baby to lie on its back in an uninviting crib and commune with the ceiling.

Depression, suicide, and murder

Cullen referred to the importance of psychosocial factors in causation of *post-partum depression*. A positive attitude of the mother to child-bearing and child-rearing would be likely to reduce its frequency and severity. Ambivalence towards the motherhood role was likely to increase it. Mead thought that the isolation of women was a principal factor producing post-partum depressions. Statistically adequate studies had shown that post-partum depression was positively correlated with the absence of other female friends and relatives. She regretted that we had not discussed the implications of modern town-planning and the consequent isolation of women, which was not confined to our society. It was extreme in India for instance. People who had lived all their lives in a very close, warmly-knit community moved to the city to work. The men loved it; for the first time in their lives they had a little private life. Women on the other hand left totally isolated without female relatives or help, and this was a frightfully traumatic situation. Mead thought we had talked too much about the nuclear family, and too little about the provision of the kinds of communities in which we could diffuse the intensity of maternal and paternal roles, and sex relationship roles. In this type of community one would not demand of one's sex partner that they be good at everything — in bed, at cooking, skiing, accounting and so on — but a variety of other relationships would be possible. Mead said she would like to see much more emphasis on new kinds of communities, which support the possibility of women doing some things, and men doing other things, and there being plenty of people to look after the children. Many problems would vanish in such a community.

Depression and age. On this question of depression and its association with age, and the suggestion that older post-menopausal women and younger, more vigorous men are regarded as trustworthy by a society, Mead thought it was necessary to mention the work of Margaret Field, an anthropologist and a trained physician and psychiatrist, who had compared the depression of menopausal women in England and in Africa, and found an extraordinary association, with similar sets of fantasies. Although they were culturally very differently expressed in the women that Field had studied in England both sets of women experienced severe self-accusation, a feeling almost of having destroyed psychologically members of one's family. In Africa this was expressed as witchcraft, and women accused themselves of having killed their children, in a most overt and definite form. In both these fantasies occurred at the point of menopause, when reproduction was no longer possible, and when the menopausal symptoms were announcing to the woman that there would be no more children. Mead said that, added to this, in many societies there was the notion of a fixed number of ova and that these were used up, so that at the point of menopause a fixed number of potential children had been used up. In one society women accused themselves of having mistreated the children that were there, and in the other of having killed them. Mead thought this was all exceedingly suggestive in terms of menopausal female depression, and had to be taken very seriously into account.

Suicide. Mead thought that suicide was certainly linked with trauma connected with male/female pair-bond-type relationships. Suicide attempts were commoner among young females, elderly persons, and young persons who had lost a spouse. Marital problems were thought to be a common motive for suicide, in fact, anything that broke or spoilt the male/female emotional relationship predisposed towards depression and suicide. Depression resulting from troubled relationships or dissatisfaction with sex was very common.

Murder. Mead asked:

Why have we not discussed murder? I mean, murder is a consequence of misplaced sex roles, almost as often as suicide is. And the commonest murders, 75 per cent of the murders that occur in the United States, are in the family. One of the many things that married people experience is that there is no way out except murder or suicide, and that they are so attached to the partner they can't leave them.

Persky, referring to the fashionable tendency to attribute murder to excessive aggressivity to males with XYY chromosomes, stated that he had not found or seen any data which showed excessive testosterone in such people.

Cancer

The association between risk to cervical uterine cancer and promiscuity, probably more directly with chronic infections, was cited by Henry as a possible indicator of a relationship between psychosocial factors arising from male/female relationships and cancer. Both cancer of the body of the uterus and cancer of the breast was more common in childless women and in nuns. Very speculatively, Henry attributed the relatively high rates of cancer of the prostate in Caucasians in Hawaii compared with the low rates for Japanese and Chinese to a culturally expected higher sexual drive in the former (compared with elderly Japanese and Chinese males), which in some cases could not be met by sexual intercourse.

Disease in general

Rahe showed data associating high risk, in terms of frequency and severity to a large variety of diseases, and life-stress score. The correlations, though significant were low. He postulated that 'life stress' of various kinds might increase risk to a wide variety of disease but would be expressed in different people in different ways according to their particular weakness and other associated factors.

Male/female preponderance in disease

Henry said: 'Medalies' data from a prospective study in Israel supports the notion that male/female family relations will predispose to coronary heart disease. The latter developed twice as frequently in males who claimed that their wives were not loving or supportive when compared with the incidence in men who claimed the reverse.

Kagan, commenting on the high rate of sexual dissatisfaction shown in a survey by Gebhard between married couples (about 30 per cent) speculated that if other causes of marital friction were added there was probably a very high level of chronic 'family' stress in some communities. the recent widespread rise in the ratio of age-specific male to female mortality was mentioned in this connection. This rise in the male/female ratio was greatest in those countries where male/female mutual family care was likely to have diminished most in recent years. This gave additional support to the speculation that lack of male/female mutual care was having a greater effect on male than female health.

SEX EDUCATION

Although there was general agreement that sex education was needed for children (as well as adults) there was some doubt and much disagreement on the content and mode of administration. Hertoft said:

In Denmark we are now in a situation of transition. In the past the school has been reproached with neglecting sexual guidance, and it is praiseworthy that it is now beginning to make up for those times. But there are new dangers attached to this. First that the school may overrate its own importance in this field, and set itself on a pedestal. Second, by approaching the subject in too rational a fashion it might succeed, instead of helping the children and the young, in intimidating them, by not giving due respect to their individual ideas and fantasies.

I think people tend to forget what qualifications children have for accepting and understanding what is explained to them. Many are inclined to think that they are just a kind of miniature adult. A Danish psychologist, Iversen, seeks 'a more comprehensive attitude to the irrational and the emotional factors in small and older children, which represent their faithfulness to early childhood.' There is no doubt that too many well meaning educators in the sexual field have offended this faithfulness to early childhood, with clumsy attempts at guidance.

Sex guidance acts on only one personality level. Sexual adjustment and behaviour are related to all parts of the mind, some difficult to reach and difficult to influence. Therefore I think it best neither to overrate nor to underestimate sex guidance, but to recognize that it has an intrinsic value and that it serves no useful purpose to attribute to it an importance which it can hardly claim in an otherwise well-informed community.

The aim is, first and foremost, to provide each individual person with a certain fund of knowledge, which he may use to the extent which he himself finds correct and can manage. (Just as we find it quite natural that every person should have the opportunity of learning to read and write.) But such a fulfilment will not necessarily bring about a solution to difficulties which may be the result of man's sexual drive and actions.

The role of myth

A child should be told the whole truth but there is room for myth and folklore to make the story understandable to very young children. Hassler wondered whether the myth served the child or the adult. Mead thought there was a reciprocal relationship. Hertoft regarded myths as ways of explaining deep experiences. Money felt that a fairly tale type of presentation was useful but much thought needed to be given to the content. He said that, confronted with the need to communicate with children, he had made up his own legend concerning the origin of babies. This legend had been repeated back to him by the parents of the same child, showing that the parents and the child can communicate, using this story. The most important part of the story for the parents was the description of impregnation, a concept parents found difficult to approach, as a swimming race of the sperm. When they had surmounted that hurdle the parents could then usually find enough courage to be able to say that the penis had to fit into the vagina and pump the sperm out, so that they all have a fair chance in the swimming race. To make it easy for the children to remember, Money dramatized that of all those 300 million sperms there was only one winner; the children could then guess what the prize was. Money also added that children rather liked the idea that the baby had to come out head first, because otherwise it might get stuck — another way to help them remember the story.

Sex education for children in Sweden

Linnér said there had been a sex education programme for children since the 1940s which had been compulsory, and integrated into the school system, since 1956. The basis of equality in current sex education, which was given to boys and girls together, had been laid down in the proposal of a commission in 1976.

The moral implications of the sexual behaviour of men and women should be judged equally. The argument that women are not equal to men should be totally dismissed. And when you, Preben [Hertoft], talked about the difficulties in our sex education programme, I think we have shifted over a little. Earlier, we talked about reproductive organs, and then went on to foetus development, and we did not take up intercourse and how it happens. Now we are much more open with that, and, basically, I think we have taken into the programme the dual role of intercourse — for reproduction and for mututal joy and for personal joy. This has to be commenced early in the children's life and not in the teenager.

The use of diagrams and symbols

Linnér went on to illustrate a lesson on family planning for people between 16 and 18 years of age using the overhead charts and diagrams currently in use. Engström felt that such lessons should be 'pre-tested' to see how much understanding and misunderstanding they conveyed. Both Engström and Mead were concerned about the possible traumatic effect of some of the symbolism Linnér had shown, e.g. the pill being represented by an owl and endocrine secretion by blue and red spiders. Mead felt that it was a disadvantage to have to learn from diagrams and in this respect women, till now, had been at a disadvantage compared to men. Females had never had any access to a visual knowledge of their own interior reproductive organs, whereas males from the age of six months could inspect themselves, and, as soon as they could walk about, all other little males. There had been speculation that this delayed females' erotic responses, and the development of maternal response and that this would not happen without this inhibition on female exploration. One of the developments of the Women's Liberation movement in the United States was putting at the disposal of each woman a speculum with a mirror. For the first time in human history, women had had a chance to know what they looked like inside. In most societies women not only knew nothing about their own insides, but they knew nothing about any other woman's inside. Mead had worked in societies where a woman did not even loosen her grass-skirt at the time of delivery of a child. General experience with children's sexplay was that it tended to be heterosexual or between males, and that there was very little exploration by young females of each others' anatomy. Mead thought that giving children knowledge of the female interior anatomy could represent one of the most extraordinary shifts in sex education that could occur. If a male child was shown a diagram of his reproductive organs he could view it in the light of his own visual experience. But if he was presented with a diagram of a female, this could not be demonstrated by his female teacher's experience. This could be changed to the extent that all women could have some knowledge of their internal reproductive apparatus.

273

There would then be, to some extent, empirical under-writing of education. It was very easy to present diagrams, and statistics on venereal disease, and logical remarks about masturbation not driving you insane, but to be able to convey to children something of the affective, the emotional content of sex, was where we fell down most completely. There was a tremendous emphasis in most sex education courses on anatomy without affect, and without any experience either, so the teaching tended to be kinesthetic rather than visual.

Linnér pointed out that restrictions were often imposed by local value systems and referred to the necessity of illustrating sexual intercourse to school children in bizarre ways because of this e.g. in Japan (1971) recourse had been made to copulating hippo-potami.

Evaluation of the effect of sex education in childhood

Lazarus voiced the concern of many when he asked if there were any studies 'on what happens to children as they grow up into adults, as a consequence of one or another type of approach' in sex education. Gebhard mentioned that his Institute was currently analysing data from a controlled study on the short-term effects of sex education in high-school children. The analysis had only just commenced but it looked as if one of the early results was that children thought more about the subject, and were more adult in their attitudes to sex afterwards. Bancroft referred to

a rather limited study in England, evaluating the short-term or immediate effects of sex films in primary schools. The study was carried out by sociologists of the London School of Economics. They assessed the attitudes of the parents, and the knowledge of the children before and after these films, and although this is, of course, a relatively superficial assess-ment, there were certainly no obvious immediate harmful or disturbing consequences of this, which, perhaps, was at least reassuring.

Goodman said the National Institute of Mental Health was just considering embarking on a long-term study.

ACTION NOW

Reproduction and family planning

Gebhard and Linnér made the following recommenda-tions, with which there was little disagreement.

1. No female should be forced to bear an unwanted child. Contraception should be made available to every male and female, regardless of their marital and economic status. In addition, abortion on demand of the female should be made available in clinics and hospitals.

2. There should be social rewards for keeping families small, or even childless. These rewards should be in terms of special tax exemptions, financial bonuses, and social prestige. The small or childless families should not be stigmatised, as they are now, and our mass media and educational system must counteract the notion that people have an obligation to repro-duce.

3. There should be government-supported health centres,

medical services in industrial plants, youth centres, and so forth, which would provide family planning services. And lastly, in connection with this, we feel that there should be maternity and paternity leave of absence from industrial plants or employment without loss of earnings.

Child care

Gebhard and Linnér recommended:

1. That employment arrangements should be made so that parents can share in caring for the children.

2. Childcare centres should be supported by federal and local agencies, and larger industries, e.g. the larger industries to have their own childcare centres for their own employees; the federal or local agencies to have childcare centres for other segments of the population.

3. Educational systems and mass media must promote the idea that males should share in childcare. It is not going to do much good if we talk about sharing unless we can arrange matters so that males would be willing to do this.

4. There should be more professional and paraprofessional help available to parents to assist them in raising their children, because not all parents are equipped to do this effectively.

There was some opposition to the spirit of these recommendations based on the absence of knowledge of the effect on children of day care and paternal care and Kagan considered that large-scale application of these notions should await evaluation of their safety and efficiency on a small scale.

Mutual support in male/female pair relationships

Gebhard and Linnér's recommendations here were that

there should be sharing of domestic and other household duties. This seems very rational, but of course, it is a bone of con-tention. The only way this can be affected is for the educational system and mass media to emphasize that sharing is a good thing. Then roles can be interchanged without loss of self-esteem or loss of social prestige.

Efforts should be made to improve the economic and occupa-tional status of women, so as to provide equal opportunities for social and emotional growth and well-being. Such efforts would necessitate changing laws concerning employment, property rights, and legal privileges.

Although there was a feeling that generally women were underprivileged there was no universal feeling that an artificial attempt to bring about complete equality would be either desirable or free from danger.

Goodman and Gebhard felt that gender differences should be minimized at school and afterwards. Linnér and Odhnoff felt that men and women should at least be equally represented on administration and decision-making committees. Mead, summarizing for her sub-group, said

the enormous richness and range and variety of primate and human behaviour makes it desirable to avoid in our current stage of knowledge, the imposition of narrow educational objectives and male and female role relationships. It was felt very strongly that the attempt to eradicate previous inequalities in our own society over time, by imposing new fixed positions, was undesirable.

Emotional relations between men and women
Gebhard and Linnér's recommendations were:

1. Concerning the improvement of emotional relationships between men and women we feel that the educational system and mass media must provide the basic knowledge, anatomy, physiology, and sexuality, as necessary for a healthful and fulfilling relationship between the sexes; and that if education facilities are not available for all, some compensatory arrangements should be made to achieve the same goal, e.g. the free distribution of printed material or graphic material.

2. Individuals should be taught not only how to live in a marriage and family situation, or in other pair relationships, but they should also be taught how to cope with relationship problems following separation, divorce, or the death of a partner. We hear a great deal about education for married and family life, but we don't hear anything about education for divorce or widowhood, or education for simply the splitting up of a pair that has been married.

3. Attempts should be made to improve the affectional relationship between men and women, in order to enhance emotional growth, maturity, and health. And here again, we have to fall back on the educational system and mass media, which in some cases, I think, is rather a feeble crutch upon which to lean, but it is all we have at the moment. Special counselling facilities really ought to be available, as Dr. Money pointed out, for teaching people or helping people learning to love and express affection.

4. Lastly we simply have one category of recommendations concerning interpersonal crisis counselling, and there we have but one recommendation. That is that marriage and divorce counselling should be made far more available than they presently are. Such counselling could certainly be a part of a general health service, or part of a larger reproductive service, such as Dr. Hassler was mentioning. In addition to dealing with existing crises, such counselling might serve to avert or at least minimize subsequent crises. And such counselling would not only benefit the adult individuals involved, but obviously the children as well.

Counselling
The need for adolescent, premarriage, marital, and divorce counselling was referred to in some detail by Cullberg, Hertoft, Hynie, and others. Cullberg and Engström referred to the need of advice when perinatal death or death of a spouse was experienced. Unfortunately there seemed to be a conspiracy between nursing and medical staff and relatives to prevent the bereaved from expressing grief.

Mead reminded the meeting that the unit needing advice was in most cases not a man or woman but a pair, and Michael indicated from subhuman primates the wide variation in 'match' between mating pairs. Hassler took this further and felt that sometimes the unit for counselling should include mother, father, and child or some other relative.

Engström, speaking for a subgroup, felt that family issues 'should be viewed comprehensively as opposed to the current fragmented approaches. For example, fertility and genetic counselling, abortion, pregnancy supervision, contraception, etc. should all be pieces of the same scheme.'

'Love and life centres'. Money proposed multipurpose centres which would bring together all the disciplines for advising on the many aspects of male/female roles and relationships already mentioned. They would be the ultimate referral places for people with sexual problems and love problems, that needed to be specially treated, and people would go there in the same way that people travelled long distances to a major referral centre when they have other really tough medical problems. These places should be primarily behaviour-oriented rather than endocrinologically or genetically oriented, although the latter aspects would not be excluded.

Triage. In many areas facilities for advice are scattered and people just do not know where to go for advice. Cullen, Kagan, and Money felt that in every small community there ought to be some person who would be able to decide which problems could be dealt with on the spot, which problems could not, and in the latter case to whom the person should be referred.

Dial for help. Cullen and Money thought that the triage service might be supplemented by a telephone 'dial for help service', or alternatively the latter might be reserved for people who had a query that they would like to put completely anonymously.

Education of doctors and auxiliary medical personnel
Several participants felt that medical personnel should be educated to handle problems of the bereaved and at the very least not to avoid those distressed in this way.

Cullen thought that education about psychological factors and psychobiological factors 'basic to your orientation, whether you are advising about sex or genetics, should more often take place very early in the students' education and be continued throughout.'

Bancroft and Linnér gave examples of how the medical profession was often antagonistic to social changes, particularly when this meant delegating the doctors' function. Cullen thought that sometimes it was not just a matter of knowledge but a question of attitudes and basic philosophy.

Education for coping
Several participants felt that although a crisis counselling service was necessary for those in distress much could be done to reduce the number of people who need such a service. It would be best of all if people could cope with most of their own problems, and education could help in this. Cullberg thought that one way would be to present children and students with imaginary problems which they could attempt to solve, under supervision, and learn from in the same way as arithmetic exercises were used. As Money said, 'What teenagers need is to know how people find a resolution to their problems, and that is where we should concentrate our efforts.'

Sex educational films

A subgroup summary stated that films planned for educational purposes should be made. Films, with an accompanying handbook, could educate better than teachers, who took a long time to train and who might never be good at talking about sex. The subgroup thought there already were some films, as there were some novels, that could be used, and simply put on a list; but in either case there should be some kind of an explanatory handbook to at least lead the discussion. There could be three types of films; one on simple reproduction, which was the type of film which was rather well done today, and not too difficult to obtain, e.g. showing animation of sperm transport and fertilization of the egg, and so on. Then there would be films showing love, affection, and the human relationship in making love and copulating, which, although available today, were still quite difficult to obtain, and were too scarce, especially those catering for particular age levels. Finally, films were needed about problems of love — the crises, whether acute or insidious in onset, that threaten the long-term allegiance of a relationship, marital or otherwise. There were none of these films yet in existence.

Information gap

Linnér sid it was one thing to have information and another for people to be able to find it when they needed it. One approach to this was the local triage service (above). Another, Gebhard thought, was to make information available to those agencies that would use it. Mead pointed out that children in developed countries spent a great deal of time looking at television.

Gebhard and Mead said that central and local political objection to sex education had to be overcome. It took only about three people objecting to sale of literature on sex to have it removed from a nationwide chain store in the United States.

Information registers

Money proposed that registers should be made, published, and kept up-to-date of all agencies that were interested in dealing with sex and love problems, and that an annotated bibliography of books and films which have 'genuine, valid, and helpful information' should be published.

The role of WHO

Cronholm thought that for WHO to propose action there had to be unanimity concerning means and objectives in its member governments. Mead agreed that WHO should be responsible for promoting the implementation of areas where there is unanimity and should also have the task of clarifying issues where there was no unanimity 'without bigotry and without trying to force a position'. Hassler and Kagan thought that WHO was planning both these functions in its family planning programme.

RESEARCH PRIORITIES

Several participants throughout the discussions drew attention to the urgent need for knowledge and understanding before ideas that seemed reasonable but were so far untested were applied on a large scale.

Trost thought the difficulties were due to trying to use the same methods in the social sciences as are used in the natural sciences. Frankenhaeuser thought the end-product was less tangible in the social sciences and that administrators were therefore less interested in the developmental side of research and development in the latter than in natural sciences. She thought there was a great deal of knowledge that had been accumulated and which could be developed for practical purposes. Engström thought the complexity of social science which put people off research, should be regarded as an acceptable challenge.

Kagan proposed a strategy for ethical community research which had as its objectives the simultaneous evaluation of the use of a proposed health or social action (e.g. sex education) in terms of safety, efficiency and cost; testing one or more key hypotheses; and gathering additional low cost data which might be of some use at some later date (e.g. in system analysis) but which would be too expensive and too speculative to obtain for its own sake alone. Illustrations of the application of scientific principles through this strategy to social problems such as prevention of gonorrhoea, unwanted pregnancy or marital conflict were given (Chapter 31).

Priority topics for action research

Bancroft, Cullberg, Cullen, Kagan, Mead, Money, Trost, and others indicated priority areas for such evaluation, e.g.

(a) the essential features of child-rearing, with special reference to how optimal action could be obtained in different cultures e.g. the advantages or disadvantages of the father taking a larger share;

(b) the advantages and disadvantages of different forms of sex education and education for coping;

(c) the prevention of venereal disease and unwanted pregnancy in young people through peer-group teaching or by making preventive and therapeutic measures available in ways specially adapted to the adolescent 'culture';

(d) ways of reducing family conflict and the effect of this on health and well-being of members of the family;

(e) ways of improving mutual care in the male/female dyad and the effect of this on health and well-being;

(f) effects of different ways of administration of family planning on use, effectiveness, health, and wellbeing of the woman, husband, family, and community.

Although *abortion* was common and becoming more common the *psychological effects* were as yet insufficiently understood. Similarly there was need to understand more fully the psychological effects of *contraception* by the pill, intrauterine device, and vasectomy. Michael said that endocrine contraception was beginning to be used by young girls who had hardly experienced a normal menstrual cycle. Before this practice was extended it would be wise to understand its effects.

Cullen said that technological developments in endocrine assay made it possible to establish the effect of *psychological stimuli on ovulation and fertility*.

Mead thought it was important for rational education, social legislation, and planning to know whether *not having a child* was a physical or psychological deprivation for a woman.

Michael drew attention to gaps in our knowledge of the *needs of older people* for sexual activity and relations and of the psychobiological effects of the *male menopause*.

Money listed a number of research topics to which he would like to give priority (see Chapter 38).

Animal studies
Although results of experiments in animals could not be extrapolated directly to humans they did give ideas which, if of sufficient importance, could sometimes be tested relatively simply in humans. Henry said that the instinctive drive mechanisms and sympatho/adrenal/medullary and pituitary/adrenal/cortical mechanisms of all mammals had a great deal in common. Cullen added that the types of study organized by Michael in sub-human primates would permit the study of pair-bond relationships, which already had some relevance to studies in human beings. Henry's system of studying mice provided a flexible arrangement which allowed a study of cause and effect of social change on stress diseases. Answers to questions, which in humans either couldn't be put or would take many years to answer, could be obtained in such colonies in a relatively short time and with relatively small expense.

'Love and life centres'
Money described the possibilities for research in these. He thought a love and life centre would be first of all a service research centre. But antecedent to that he thought the centre should deal with parental love, the parent/child relationship, and the beginning of life; and then fraternal love, the term he used for the bonding between youngsters of the same age; in the next stage of life with partner love particularly sexual component; and finally with grandparental love. The centre would therefore be dealing with behaviour of human beings in all their interactions together with particular emphasis upon the stresses, strains, and crises of those interactions in order to find out how to solve them. Also, since it would be a research institute, the centre would make as much effort to understand successful relationships between people in their various

manifestation of love and sometimes, of course, the lack of it.

The emphasis should be on behavioural aspects, Money continued, because that was where there was the greatest lack in research around the world at the time — on the affairs of men and women, boy and girl. He did not expect the research would be exclusively behavioural, but rather that that would be the focus. The interest would be in correlating behavioural development and changes with some other variables. He did not envisage the centres as being exclusively biochemical institutes dealing with the sex hormones. He thought that biochemical research should be adjunctive, and closely parallel.

I have subdivided the main types of studies that I think should be undertaken. They would include observational studies, which could include written data from the subjects, such as using a checklist questionnaire, as, unhappy as I am with that form of data it is useful sometimes. Then there would be developmental studies, and I would rather like to put extreme emphasis on that because of my personal experience in realizing how much one can learn from following children for 20 years, as compared with how much data gets lost, when you take a 5 year cross-sectional study … then quit. I would also like to see cultural and social comparative studies, especially cross-cultural ones. There is still so much to be learned and so much that will soon be lost because of the rapidity of change around the planet. I expect also that there would be some 'social epidiomological' studies. I think of these as being statistical incidence studies with regard to various different variables that one may become interested in, especially those that relate to social and behavioural phenomena. I think also that in this kind of a centre we should be very much involved in animal fieldwork studies of the type that we hear of from Dr. Henry, and even from as far away as Tanzania, the type that Dr. Jane Goodall does and others working in their primary field studies.

Money added that one pay-off that could be obtained from these studies would be that one could have a public relations project in the form of one of the best types of naturalistic and small zoo, which could be attached to the centre. This would also serve the purpose of making it a very lively and attractive place for children to come to.

Dr. Mead suggested that one might have a glass incubator where children can watch the chickens pecking their way out of the egg, as she has seen in Connecticut, and as I have seen at the Natural History Museum in Chicago, as no doubt many of you have. I guess a few mice being born might be a good idea too, Dr. Henry? A very good beginning of sex education or rather, shall we say, reproduction education.

There is something of a question mark as to whether there should be animal laboratory studies, especially those that get closer to death than to life, because of the sacrifice of the animals at the end of the study. And perhaps the location of labs of this sort should be separated from a centre for human beings. But there certainly should be a very close relationship with this type of experiment, because it has so much relevance, especially in the primates, to human beings.

And I have left till last in this list of the types of studies that could be undertaken, the clinical studies, because I have a little extra to say in the way of subheading here. They would indeed be one of the very important branches of the work that would be undertaken in an institute or centre of this type, because they would offer medical, psychological, and psychiatric help to people in trouble, and use these same clinical populations as sources of accumulation of information to better understand the process of disorder or disease, or maladjustment, that is going on, and to learn how to correct it, half a generation, or a generation ahead. I would think here, particularly that the approach would be one of making correlations initially rather than any prediction, between developmental behaviour and various other variables. There would be first of all a correlation of present manifestation with antecedent experiences ... for instance whether the youngster was breast-fed or not, whether the father did a lot of baby tending or not, and so on. There would be correlation studies with genetics; with hormonal functionings and different patterns of hormonal functionings during different parts of the life cycle; correlations with anatomy and anatomical defects; correlations with various lesions and disease processes in various organs of the body affecting both the sexual system and the relationship system; correlational studies with pharmacologic products and treatment with them, or in the case of addiction drugs just simply addiction to them; and correlation studies with fertility or its lack, and the whole reproductive process and its alternations and dysfunctions.

Money felt it was necessary strongly to emphasize that for these types of clinical study related to behaviour it was necessary to train an entire new generation in how to keep records and use them. In the fields of psychiatry and the behavioural sciences record-keeping was 'quite shocking'. The case records were useless for the retrieval of information. He thought that the Maudsley Hospital in London was the only one to keep reliable records. Large groups of patients, homogenous for diagnosis, had been used for good follow-up studies. Many more places should use at least a simple punch-card type system, to be able to record data and obtain new insights.

Mead thought that we were trying to 're-connect' concepts and disciplines that had become separated. We were trying to put together the medically trained, who had not been trained in research, and those trained in research who had not been medically trained, and each of these with the paraprofessions. She thought Money's suggestion of having a Ph.D. in paramedicine a good one. The paraprofessional would thus be elevated and would perhaps then be treated with dignity.

'... We are trying to put together people of very different levels of training on a basis of human equality, where they can work together.' Mead also said that very few people knew where the word 'discipline' came from. We had invented it so that a nurse could sit down with a doctor at the same table, and discuss a case: it was a way of including those applied activities that were looked down on by these high-level, noble hard sciences. Mead said the word 'discipline' was invented for interdisciplinary work at a time when we were trying to put the organ back in the patient, and the patient back in the family, and we had not yet put the family back in the community. She thought therefore

one aim of a love and life centre would be to 'put together the fragmented professions that are at present in every degree of, or lack of degree of, cooperation.

The second thing that we are trying to put together is services in the communities that are now very widely scattered, with possibly special emphasis on those services that are related to reproductivity and parenthood and marriage and ageing, the whole set of services that are related to the life cycle. Dr. Money left one thing out, and that was filial love. You have parental love, fraternal love, partner love, grandparent love, and you left out filial love, so let's put that in too. Now, at present, you very often have prenatal services separated from abortion centres; genetic counselling in another place; and what we were considering, and what is being done in a few places, and I think it is being done to some extent in Sweden, is to put all these things together. Which means that the young parents before the baby is born, and then the baby itself, and as it grows up, will be included in the services of a centre of this sort. We would recommend the building-in of the collection of research data, as Dr. Hassler and Dr. Cullen talked about, into the records at the start, so that whenever service was given, where it involved a kind of clinical test for instance, that record would automatically be part then of a potential follow-up. There would be no services that did not have a research pay-off. And there would be no research that was separated from the services, but there would be an intimate relationship between the two. We would be recognizing the present demand that no one should ever be simply a guinea-pig, and that their participation in research should be voluntary, and that they should have real knowledge of what is happening.

A very important aspect of such an ongoing institution, of course, is the long-term records. Now, of course, whether you can get long-term records is very dependent on the stability of the population, and there will be a fairly high degree of wastage. Here I think it is important to mention something else, which Dr. Money and I have not talked about, and he may disapprove of. But that is a universal health care, so that people who leave such a centre, take with them a record of the shots that the child has had, the examinations it has had, and the medication it has had. Because at present we have people roaming around the world, being medicated by half a dozen agencies who pay no attention to anything else, with no records. In New Guinea, where people don't even have names that are stable, there is no telling how often a child may get the same shots of something of this sort. One of the things that such a centre would do, would be to give each person a health identity, which made it part of where ever they went to be treated in relation to their past, and this may, of course, in time be tied up with computer retrieval. But we would cease to give a child a shot and let it go again with no relation to anything else at all. So you would have an ongoing research outfit that was related to the population that was there, and to those that went away or who came to be reintegrated into it, when they came. We would be able to look at families over a long time. We would be able to look at the same family in which one child failed and another child succeeded. We would be able to ask the questions, for instance, about the relation between physical maturity in children and failure in school, or delinquency, and things of this sort, that have been postulated from studies that were only concerned with one of these issues, and could not be put into a much wider matrix.

I think Dr. Money has been mainly drawing a picture of a centre such as you might have in a large city or covering a whole region, but one would envisage more centres of the same

278

sort, which would deal with more everyday cares and which would hopefully separate childbirth from surgery.... Childbirth would be returned to being a natural event, not a disease. We would begin to relate these events of sickness and health to each other in the whole setting.

We emphasized the fact that young fathers are very heavily stressed but with our present set-up there is no access to the father. He is just put out in the hall, and they hope he will stay there, and there is no way in which anyone can relate to him. We have also stressed the fact that at present there is no medical profession that deals with the health of men, but only the health of children, females right through life, and males coming back in again very often when they are too ill to do very much about it. Such a centre would hopefully, put men, women, and children together in a relationship that could be followed.

INDEX

282

pre-coital, 106
technique, disagreement over, 106
Pharmacological effects on erotic sensation, 255
Phenylethanolamine N-methyltransferase 187
Philosophy,
Judeo-Christian, 72
religious, 72
Phobia,
heterosexual, 161
of cancer, 113
Phosphatase, acid, secretion, 159
Photographic material, restrictions concerning, 229
Phyletic mechanisms, 270
Phylogenesis, 6
Phylographic determinants, 19
Physical,
abnormalities, 149
attributes, 101
trouble over, 104
factors in sexual dysfunction, 63
state, innate, 24
stressors, 168
violence, 108
vulnerability, 171
Physicosocial stimuli, 147
Physiological,
arousal and behavioural efficiency, 136
determinants of sexual differentiation, 42
mechanisms, 268
nature of sexual arousal, 159
needs, 6, 143
reactions and distress, 171
response to psychosocial stimulation, 185
Physique, 18
and gender identity, 63
Pictorial representation, 155
Pill, the, 116, 152
as a 'scapegoat', 119, 127
endocrine aspects of, 126
interpersonal aspects of, 127
intrapsychic aspects of, 128
mental effects of, 126
physiological effects of, 126
psychological,
aspects of, 126
meaning of, 126
side-effects of, 126
sociological aspects of, 127
use of, 235
Pill-forgetters, psychological factors in, 118
Pituitary gland, 197
Placebo effects, 117
Planned parenthood, 73, 151
Planning family, 72, 123
Play,
boys', 243
doll, 11
girls', 243
neutral, 243
Playing areas, 222
Pleasure, sexual, 120
Plethysmographic techniques, 158
Plurality of sexual relationships, 19
Polarization, sexual, 98
Policy,
-makers, female, lack of, 215
making and sex roles, 247
social, 212, 217, 267
and research, 24
Political,
activity, lack of time for, 91
language, lack of insight into, 220
Population cages, 42, 44

Pornography, 154, 156
de-dramatization of, 229
Post-,
mature delivery, 252
menopausal,
females, 78
sexual behaviour, 16
natal,
differentiation, 262
events, influence of, 12
partum,
depression, 271
psychosis, 252
Potency, threat to, 119
Poverty of speech, 220
Power, equal, xiv
Powerlessness, sense of, 96
Prayer, 191
Pre-action phase, 154
Pre-coital petting, 106
Pre-copulatory phase, prolonged, 5
Precursors of disease, 6, 268
definition of, 4
Predisposing interacting variables, 147
Pre-ejaculatory emission, 158
Preferences, erotic, 16
Pregnancy, 22, 144
and emotional lability, 252
and health, 252
and irritability, 252
and mental health, 254
desire for, 119
effects on sex life, 16
failure to achieve, 152
fear of, 108, 120
freedom from, 117
frequent, 5
hormonal changes in, 16
motivation for, 252
number of, 186
premarital, 70
psychoendocrine relationships in, 254
psychological aspects of, 251
stressful events in, 254
unwanted, 6, 143, 268, 276
information on, 234
prevention of, 208
Premarital,
sex, 67, 130
sexual relations, 72, 119
traditions, 68
Premature,
delivery and extramarital pregnancy, 252
ejaculation, 62, 111, 150, 194
definition of, 194
Premenstrual,
distress, 198
tension, 118, 136
Premises, underlying, 3
Prenatal,
androgen, 10
androgenization, 255
deandrogenization, 255
Preparedness, coital, 120
Preponderance in disease, male/female, 272
Pre-school children, percentage of families
with, 88
Prevention,
evaluation of, 205
of damages, xv
of gonorrhea, 208
of psychosocial dysfunction, 212
of sexual inadequacy, 234
of stress, 203
of unwanted pregnancy, 208
Primary group function, 86

Primate models, 30
Principle, additive, 10
Priority topics for research, 276
Privacy, 18
of sexual acts, 253
Private homes, 94
Privatization of family, 93
Problems, 3
economic, 111
marital, 132
psychosomatic, 126
Procreation and sex, 128
Productive and reproductive roles,
coincidence of, 88
Professional advancement, reduction of
possibilities for, 92
Progestagens, mental actions of, 126
Progesterone, 33, 43, 46, 197
and sexual function, 34
Progestin-induced hermaphroditism, 10
Programme, psychobiological, definition of,
4
Projection, 115
Prolonged bleeding, 120
Promiscuity, 118, 120, 143
Property, provisions concerning, 84
Prophylactic measures, xv
Prostaglandins, 201
Prostate,
cancer of, 190
hyperplasia of, 145
Prostatic hypertrophy, 122
Prosthetic devices, 255
Prostitution, 164
Protection, 42
Protective intervening variables, 147
Provider-role, 73, 89
Proximity, 30
Pseudocyetic fantasies, 113
Pseudo-hermaphroditism, 149
Psyche and hormones, 199
Psychiatric,
disorders, and sexual functions, 251
facilities, sex ratios in utilization of, 97
Psychoactive drugs, sex differences in
reaction to, 138
Psychoanalytical approach to sex differences, 173
Psychobiological programme, 209
adequate, 147
definition of, 4
Psychoendocrine relationships in pregnancy, 254
Psychoendocrinology, 199
of aggression in marriage, 201
Psychological,
adjustment, adrenalin facilitating, 135
aspects of,
contraception, 116
parenthood, 251
pregnancy, 251
assistance, need for, 253
complications and sterilization, 252
stimuli, 6, 209
and fertility, 277
and ovulation, 277
stress and alcohol intoxication, 138
studies, 169
Psychoneurosis, 170
Psychopathic personality, 16
Psychopathology, sexual, 9, 14
Psychopharmacological effects of the pill,
116
Psychophysiological,
reactions, 168
reactivity male/female differences in, 167